HEALTH IN THE LATER YEARS

Third Edition

HEALTH IN THE LATER YEARS

Armeda Ferrini, PhD
California State University, Chico

Rebecca Ferrini, MD, MPH
*San Diego Hospice and
University of California, San Diego, School of Medicine*

Boston   Burr Ridge, IL   Dubuque, IA   Madison, WI   New York   San Francisco   St. Louis
Bangkok   Bogotá   Caracas   Lisbon   London   Madrid
Mexico City   Milan   New Delhi   Seoul   Singapore   Sydney   Taipei   Toronto

McGraw-Hill Higher Education

A Division of The McGraw-Hill Companies

HEALTH IN THE LATER YEARS, THIRD EDITION

3 4 5 6 7 8 9 0 QPF/QPF   0 9 8 7 6 5 4 3 2

ISBN 0–697–26263–4

Vice president and editorial director: *Kevin T. Kane*
Publisher: *Edward E. Bartell*
Editorial coordinator: *Kristine K. Fisher*
Senior marketing manager: *Pamela S. Cooper*
Project manager: *Mary Lee Harms*
Production supervisor: *Sandy Ludovissy*
Coordinator of freelance design: *Michelle D. Whitaker*
Senior photo research coordinator: *Lori Hancock*
Senior supplement coordinator: *David A. Welsh*
Compositor: *Precision Graphics*
Typeface: *10/12 Times Roman*
Printer: *Quebecor Printing Book Group/Fairfield, PA*

Freelance cover designer: *Kristyn A. Kalnes*
Cover images: (top) ©*Kevin Horan/Tony Stone Images;* (bottom) ©*SuperStock*

Library of Congress Cataloging-in-Publication Data

Ferrini, Armeda F.
    Health in the later years / Armeda F. Ferrini, Rebecca L. Ferrini.
  — 3rd ed.
        p.   cm.
    ISBN 0–697–26263–4
    1. Aged—Health and hygiene. 2. Health.   I. Ferrini, Rebecca L.
  II. Title.
  RA777.6.F46   2000
  613' .0438—dc21   99-31317
                                                       CIP

www.mhhe.com

CONTENTS

PREFACE

The population of older people in the United States is growing at a rate that is unprecedented in American history. Newspaper columnists, politicians, economists, talk show hosts, elder advocates, and health and social service professionals discuss the many and varied effects of the increasing aging population, both real and imagined, on our society. No matter what our age or career path, the continued growth in the number and proportion of older people in the United States impacts us all.

It is important to know about the process of aging, elders' health needs and problems, and the current and potential health and human services systems available to respond to their needs. Knowledge about illness, medications, physical activity, nutrition, sexuality, health care delivery, and death and dying is useful to facilitate our own healthy aging and that of our kin. For those planning careers in health and human services, this information is key to providing effective care to their future patients and clients.

Health status is an important variable in determining the length and quality of our later years. Older people commonly assert that, "when you have your health, you have everything." Most people begin to consider themselves as old when their health begins to fail. Although reading about ways to maintain health and reduce the effects of illness does not guarantee that we will change our behaviors to increase our chances of a long and healthy

life, it is a beginning. Further, such knowledge will enable those who work with elders to maximize the quality of life of those under their care.

This text is designed for use in college-level courses in health and aging. Students enrolled in these courses usually come from diverse fields, such as biology, medicine, dietetics, social work, psychology, nursing, sociology, recreation, public health, and allied health professions. Some students are preparing to work with older people, while others may just wish to know how to help themselves and their loved ones age successfully. Students often share this text with their older family members because it is written in a style that the layperson can understand. The material in this book can meet the needs of various audiences, including graduate students and professionals, who want to continue their education in health and aging.

Included in this edition are chapters addressing all major influences on health of the elderly. To meet the needs of students with little background in health, basic principles of physiology are included. However the authors do not oversimplify complex issues or shy away from discussing controversial subjects. The text is amply referenced to enable advanced students to study health issues in more depth. In this edition, more attention is paid to helping readers better understand the nature of research, hopefully enhancing their ability to read and interpret current research, both in professional journals and in the news.

For the third edition, the majority of the text has been rewritten and updated to reflect the rapid expansion of knowledge about health and aging. Among other changes, this edition includes more information on mental health and transitions in later life, pros and cons of managed care, and prescription medications. A new chapter on prevention and health promotion discusses ways to help elders make positive health behavioral changes. The burgeoning attention paid to complementary medicine is addressed with sections on types of alternative therapies and herbal remedies. We have added many new pedagogical tools geared to personalize student learning, such as "What Is Your Opinion?" inserts to stimulate the readers to develop their own views regarding many complex issues. New case studies, most from personal experience, illustrate the complexity of care involved in working with elders. The photographs, thanks to Marianne Gontarz, photographer and social worker, capture a vibrant, sensitive, and realistic portrait of older people.

We appreciate the valuable feedback by students at California State University—Chico, who were assigned earlier versions of this text in the course, "Health in the Later Years." These students often asserted that the text should be required for all college students, and most said they planned to keep the book for future reference after completing the course.

We thank Rick Narad, D. P. A., and Jeff Klein, Ph. D., for their invaluable computer savvy, saving us from several computer glitches and lost files as we collaborated on this book from across the state. We express gratitude to Jennifer Phelps, whose drawings illustrate normal anatomy. Finally, we would like to acknowledge Rebecca's children, Allison, Joshua, and especially the new baby, Davis (who was born and raised in Rebecca's lap during the last months of manuscript preparation) for their patience with their mother's and grandmother's endeavor.

We also wish to acknowledge the assistance of the following women at WCB/McGraw-Hill: Mary Lee Harms, Project Manager; Kristine Fisher, Editorial Coordinator; and Michelle Whitaker, Designer. Many thanks to: Professor Lawrence K. Kosecki, University of Hawaii at Manoa; Margaret V. Pepe, Kent State University; and Sue V. Saxon, University of South Florida, for reviewing the second edition of the text.

THE STUDY OF HEALTH AND AGING

Old and young, we are all on our last cruise.

Robert Louis Stevenson

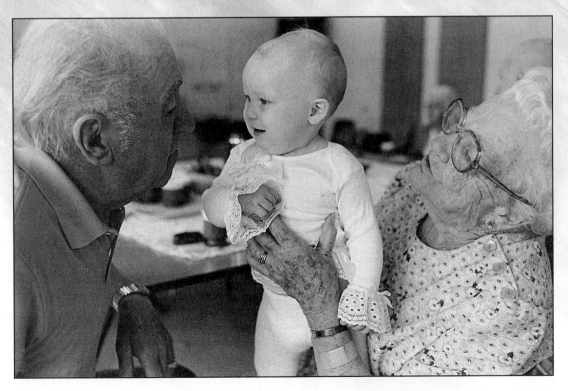

How Old is Old?

Although death and taxes are said to be inevitable, living to be old is not. It is only in the last century that a significant number of people have lived long enough to be classified as "old."

The definition of "old" varies over time, culture, and situation. Today, we consider age sixty-five or so to be old, whereas two hundred years ago, age fifty might have been considered old. One national study attempted to find out when Americans believe old age begins. According to a national study, the typical modern day response is it begins at age sixty-three for men and sixty-two for women. Younger people see old age beginning when the individual stops work or stops contributing to society, or for women, when the family is raised. But the older respondents are more likely to respond that old age depends on attitudes, good health, or activity level (Speas and Obenshain, 1995).

The age at which one is considered *old* may depend on the age of the person defining the word. A child may consider someone over twenty to be old, a teenager may think forty is over the hill, and a sixty-year-old may consider seventy as elderly. In essence, old is generally thought of as an age beyond one's own. Most elders do not consider themselves old until they become sick or dependent upon others.

Aging is a complex, continuous process that begins at maturity and continues until death. Although we commonly think of stages of life (childhood, young adulthood, middle age, elderly), it is difficult to pinpoint exactly when one stage begins and another ends.

The simplest way to classify age stages is by *chronological age.* In the United States, age sixty-five defines the beginning of old age because this is the age of full retirement benefits from Social Security. Researchers often use age sixty-five as a cutoff point to define old age, many businesses use this age to define "senior citizen discounts," and even elders themselves look at this age as the beginning of their later years.

Some gerontologists make distinctions between the young-old (sixty-five to seventy-four) and the old-old (seventy-five and above) because there are significant differences between these groups.

Terms Used to Describe Those 65 and Older

Many terms have been used to describe older people: senior citizens, golden agers, retired persons, mature adults, elderly, aged, and old people. There is no clear preference among older people for any of these terms. For instance, some people grimace at being called a senior citizen, while others like the term. Many gerontologists have chosen to adopt the term "elder" to describe those age sixty-five and older. This term is an attempt to redefine aging in a more positive way that connotes wisdom, respect, leadership, and accumulated knowledge. This text will use "elder" to reflect that attitude. The term "older people" will also be used to describe those sixty-five and older. This term makes it clear that aging is a continuum, with older people at one end and younger people at the other.

The Live Oak Project describes an elder as the following:

> An elder is a person who is still growing, still a learner, still with potential and whose life continues to have within it promise for, and connection to the future. An elder is still in pursuit of happiness, joy and pleasure, and her or his birthright to these remains intact. Moreover, an elder is a person who deserves respect and honor and whose work it is to synthesize wisdom from long life experience and formulate this into a legacy for future generations.

Generally, the young-old are more vigorous, have higher incomes, are more likely to be married, and have fewer health problems than the old-old. But even these divisions are not absolute.

Use of chronological age to determine old age is limiting in obvious ways. First, it is apparent that no abrupt change occurs on the eve of one's sixty-fifth birthday that automatically transforms a person from "middle-aged" to "elderly." Secondly, there are profound differences between individuals of the same age that make generalizations problematic. Some elders are in extremely good health well into old age, while some individuals in midlife exhibit many disabilities and illnesses. For this reason, many gerontologists distinguish chronological or numerical age, from *functional age,* the physiological capacity of the body. Thus, a marathon runner may have a chronological age of eighty, but physiologically function as well as a forty-year-old. Furthermore, we all know individuals who psychologically and socially grow old before their time. For example, individuals who use their age as an excuse for inactivity, dependence, and disengagement from society. In a sense, these individuals have died before their bodies. Without a doubt, *sociological* or *psychological age* is also an important part of aging.

Despite these caveats, the definition of "old" used in this text is the chronological age of sixty-five and older because most data are available in this form. When available, information on age subgroups will be included.

THE STUDY OF AGING

"Gerontology" is the term used to describe the study of aging. The word "gerontology" comes from the Greek terms *geron* and *-ontus,* which means "old man." Gerontology is a multidisciplinary field with a major focus on the biological, behavioral, and social sciences. However, gerontology may be applied to such diverse areas as anthropology, history, literature, and economics.

The term "geriatrics" refers to the medical care of older people. In contrast to gerontology, geriatrics is primarily concerned with changes that occur with age as a result of disease. Geriatricians and geriatric nurses are the more common medical professionals who specialize in meeting the medical needs of elders.

As the number of elders grow, the study of gerontology and geriatrics will become increasingly important. These experts provide guidance regarding social and public policy changes, medical care innovations, and future direction of medical services to respond to this increasing consumer pool.

Research Tools to Study Elders' Health

When scientists seek answers to research questions, a variety of research methods can be utilized that depend upon the question. Studies may try to assess the health status of a particular group (e.g., Why do white older men have a high rate of suicide? Why do African American women have a high death rate of breast cancer?), or may try to figure out what causes a disease (e.g., What influence does the environment have on prostate cancer?). Studies may try to determine what is the best treatment for a certain condition (e.g., Is mastectomy or lumpectomy better for breast cancer?) or identify and assess risk factors for disease (e.g., Do people with a sedentary lifestyle have a higher risk of developing heart disease than those who are active?).

Regardless of the research question, all studies utilize statistics to determine the relevance (or significance) of their results. Statistics is a scientific field that directs the collection, classification, description, interpretation, and presentation of data. Some statistics are used to summarize or describe a population, called *descriptive statistics.* If you wanted to report the average weight of elders in the population or the number of elders who were overweight, you would use descriptive statistics. *Inferential,* or *analytic statistics* uses more complicated statistical procedures to make generalizations about a population based on results of one study. For example, if a study found that people who smoke develop more lung cancer, analytic statistics would be used to determine how strong that association was and what the chance was that the results reported are "real."

All statistics are reported in terms of probability. If there is a 95 percent chance that the association or difference reported is not due to chance, this is commonly referred to as "statistically significant." Because something is statistically significant does not mean it is important or that it is even biologically significant. Likewise, if the conclusions of a study are not statistically significant, this does not mean they are *not* important. In general, larger studies are more likely to have statistically significant results. It is important to realize that statistical procedures are only tools to better understand health and its influences. Statistics usually do not allow a person to assert the statement, "Smoking causes cancer," but rather, "Smoking is highly associated with the development of lung cancer, especially in people who smoke more than one pack per day."

Observational and Interventional Studies

The design, or plan, of a study is classified into two broad categories: observational studies and interventional (experimental) studies. Neither type of study is intrinsically better than the other. Without exception, all studies have benefits, limitations, and situations where they are more or less useful. When reviewing the results of a study, it is important to be able to classify the study by type to better interpret the results. The following section will discuss the differences between observational and interventional studies, describe their subclassifications, and discuss their benefits and limitations.

Observational studies, as the name implies, look at and document what is occurring in a population to better understand it. In these studies, the investigator does not control or manipulate anything, just observes and records. For example, a researcher trying to understand the association between fiber intake and colon cancer may observe that people with colon cancer usually eat less fiber than people without colon cancer. Observational studies cannot predict "causality" or assert that one thing caused another. Even if a study shows clearly that people with colon cancer report a lower intake of fiber than those without colon cancer, this does not prove that fiber protects against the development of colon cancer. Some other, yet unidentified, factor may be more important than fiber (e.g., intake of fruits and vegetables, which contain fiber but also contain other nutrients).

Observational studies may use a variety of designs, but most commonly employ case-control or cohort designs. A *case-control study* compares a group of people who have developed a certain condition (e.g., colon cancer) with a group of people who do not have the condition, but are alike in other ways. Both groups may be asked to complete a questionnaire about their personal behavior (for example, about their diet and how much fiber they used to eat), then the researchers, using appropriate statistical techniques, compare the two groups. Using statistics, the researchers can "control for" (reduce the effect of) other differences between the groups so they can focus on what they are interested in. These studies are done to find out risk factors or characteristics that predispose a person to a disease. For example, they may control for age, other dietary habits, smoking history, and physical activity level. After statistically controlling for these factors, a conclusion can be drawn regarding the importance of fiber in the development of colon cancer. It is impossible, however, to control statistically for all the possible or potential factors that may interfere with the association you are trying to demonstrate.

In another type of observational study, called a *cohort study,* a researcher follows a group of people over a time period to find out what happens to them. These people may have risk factors, but generally have not developed disease. For example, a researcher may follow a group of smokers and a group of nonsmokers over ten years, then assess how many in each group developed lung cancer. The researchers do not have any influence upon who smokes or who doesn't, or who develops cancer. These studies are often large, expensive, and time-consuming because researchers must wait for years. It is still difficult to determine that smoking causes lung cancer by this type of study, because of confounding variables. *Confounding variables* are other factors that interfere with the association the researcher is studying. For example, it may be shown that alcoholics have a high risk of heart disease. Alcohol does not increase risk of heart disease, but smoking does, and people who drink a lot of alcohol are often those who smoke.

Another example of an observational study is a *field study*. In this study, researchers seek to uncover the relationship (or correlation) between variables in the natural setting by observing, questioning, and interviewing subjects. For instance, a researcher may interview a sample of elders who attend a senior center and a sample of elders who do not, to find out what characteristics or needs differ between the two groups. Questions on variables such as income, health and mobility status, personality characteristics, and degree of social support might be included in the interview. The answers to these questions from both groups are then compared statistically to determine if any of these variables relate to senior center use. Field studies are helpful because they use natural settings. However, they are limited by the types of research questions asked.

An *experimental study* tests the effect of an intervention on health status. In these studies, the investigator is more active in changing the environment. One type of experimental study is a laboratory study. In a laboratory experiment, the researcher can isolate what is to be studied by limiting the effect of extraneous variables. For instance, if a researcher wants to isolate the effects of low light on reading ability, other factors that might affect reading ability (e.g., background noise, size of print) can be controlled except the level of light intensity. However, since these studies are conducted in an artificial environment, the results may not be applicable to real life. The laboratory setting can cause alterations in the subjects' behavior, especially among elders. For instance, an older person may perform more poorly on an intelligence test in the laboratory than at home because of the anxiety induced by the artificial environment.

Laboratory experiments may also be conducted on animals. These experiments allow the investigator to perform experiments that may be unethical or impractical with human subjects. Because laboratory animals have short life spans, researchers can gather results more easily. For instance, researchers can manipulate weight, lifetime diet, or body temperature to see the effect on aging in one to two years, rather than seventy or so. Animals can be injected with drugs, be deprived of sleep, have organ transplants, or be sacrificed to examine organs—techniques that are impossible to conduct on humans. The biggest drawback to animal studies is that the results may not be generalizable to humans.

Field experiments are similar to laboratory experiments except that they are conducted in a natural environment. The field experiment manipulates a selected variable, while keeping others constant, to determine the effect of one particular variable. For instance, researchers might offer weekly lectures on accident prevention at a senior center to a select group of participants, and offer no such service to another group (the control). After a certain number of weeks of educational seminars, the researchers may determine how many accidents occurred in both groups and conclude that the educational presentations were or were not effective in reducing accidents. Field experiments may be more effective than laboratory studies because they are conducted in more natural situations; however, many variables cannot be controlled in the field. For instance, in the study described above, the researchers could not be sure that the accident risk decreased because of the information presented in the seminars, or because the participants' interest in accident prevention stimulated them to read more material on accident prevention and discuss the topic with friends and family.

The gold standard of interventional studies is the *clinical trial*. In a clinical trial, a researcher separates all the volunteers into two groups on a random basis. Some receive a particular treatment or intervention, and some do not. At the end of a time period, the researcher analyzes whether there are any differences between the two groups. Sometimes the group that doesn't get a treatment gets a placebo, or a "sham treatment." For example, one group may get a blue pill designed to reduce blood pressure, while the other group gets a blue pill made from sugar; at the end of the study, blood pressure is measured. Another example is that a group of women over age sixty are invited to be in a study. When they arrive, half are offered an educational pamphlet on breast cancer, and the other half receive a mammogram. Each year, the women are asked to return. After several years, the researchers see how many women died of breast cancer in each of the two groups. If fewer women died in the mammography group, the researchers may suggest that mammography reduces breast cancer deaths among women over age sixty.

Sometimes neither the patient nor the researcher measuring the outcome (called a double-blind study) knows who is in which group. Placebos and blinding strengthen the study by eliminating bias. For example, if the investigator knows who is getting the treatment and he really believes in the treatment, he may not be objective in evaluating how well the treatment is working, or may bias the patient in some way. Clinical trials are often very complex, time-consuming, and expensive. However, results from these studies are elevated in importance and have less bias.

There are various ways to collect information to answer a research question. *Survey research* commonly uses personal interviews, written questionnaires, or phone interviews to collect data on the incidence, distribution, and interrelationships of psychological and social variables. Survey research uses large or small population groups by selecting random samples that ideally represent the population as a whole. A good example of survey research is the National Health Interview Survey in which a large sample of elders are asked to report on several of their health habits. This type of study is advantageous because a great number of people can be assessed. However, like all methods that use interviewing, the respondents may not remember their health habits or may adapt answers to please the interviewer. Another disadvantage is that the sample of survey respondents may not represent all older people, but just a subgroup, such as those who are motivated or literate. For instance, those who respond to studies on elder sexuality may be more open, sexually active, or willing to discuss sexuality than the rest of the elder population.

Another type of survey research involves the reanalysis of data collected by someone else. In these types of studies, researchers utilize data from public documents and previously collected statistics, such as those collected by the U.S. Census Bureau, to answer particular research questions.

Cross-Sectional and Longitudinal Approaches

One of the most salient issues in the study of aging is ascertaining which changes are due to age and which are due to other factors. For instance, gerontologists who want to determine the effect of age upon function of a particular body system need to distinguish the effects of aging itself from other variables (e.g., poor nutrition, physical inactivity, chronic illness, cigarette smoking). All research attempting to distinguish the effect of age on particular variables utilizes either cross-sectional or longitudinal methodology.

In a *cross-sectional* approach, the researcher draws a sample of individuals from different age groups and collects data on the presence of a certain trait. For example, a cross-sectional study might measure attitudes about death by examining three age groups: twenty to thirty-nine year-olds, forty to fifty-nine year-olds, and those aged sixty to eighty. After the data are collected, the various age groups can be compared to ascertain their differences and similarities. In another example, to determine whether height is lost with advanced age, researchers may collect height data on various age groups and compare the averages to determine if inches in stature are lost in old age.

Cross-sectional analyses have many advantages and disadvantages. They can be accomplished over relatively short time periods and are less expensive than longitudinal analyses. The limitations of cross-sectional research can be illustrated using the two examples outlined above. In the first, an alternative conclusion from the data would be that elders are more apt to talk about death because they have more recent experience with the deaths of those close to them than younger persons. Thus, it may not be the age that causes a preoccupation with death, but rather recent experiences with the death of loved ones.

Cohort effects may also impact results in cross-sectional analyses. Each "generation" of people are born and live in a different time than those coming before or after. Thus, elders may report less sexual activity than younger groups, not because frequency of sexual intercourse decreases with age, but because elders were less likely to have sex when they were younger as well, or perhaps just less likely to talk to researchers about it! In the example above, the conclusion that older people lose stature with age may be erroneous because the researchers did not take into account the fact that average heights have increased with every decade in the United States. Thus, older people may not have significantly shrunk in stature with advancing age, but may have been shorter to begin with. Furthermore, cross-sectional studies do not take into account that older people may react differently to tests or laboratory situations than younger people, affecting test results.

Another systematic method to distinguish changes that occur among individuals with age is the *longitudinal study.* A series of measurements are taken on the same group of individuals over an extended period, generally for at least seven years. For instance, cognitive function may be tested in a group of fifty-year-olds, then these same individuals may be similarly retested at age sixty, seventy, and eighty. Because the same individuals are tested over an extended period of time, it is more likely that any changes uncovered are due to age, rather than generational differences. However, even longitudinal studies are not foolproof because physical condition, motivation, attitude, and other variables may affect the results and, unless accounted for, may be mistaken for age changes. Further, longitudinal studies by definition require a long-term commitment by the individuals in the study. It is difficult to keep track and maintain sufficient participants to gather sufficient information. Such studies are often quite costly. Finally, individuals may become familiar with the testing situation or interviewer with time, possibly influencing the study results.

A problem inherent in any research methodology is sampling. It is obvious that all older people cannot participate in every study, so researchers attempt to choose a sample that is representative of the entire population (in terms of income, education, living situation, and other variables) so they can generalize the results of the sample to the entire popula-tion. Many experiments use a random sample of individuals; however, since studies often rely on voluntary participation, the results may be biased. Those who volunteer for experiments may be more healthy, outgoing, intelligent, and independent than those who do not. On the other hand, many studies obtain their volunteers from clinic outpatients or those who are institutionalized. Obviously these populations do not represent the healthy elder population, and the presence of drug effects, chronic illness, and inactivity may affect the results.

WHY STUDY HEALTH AND AGING?

One of the most powerful incentives to study health as it relates to aging is a personal one. Information about the many variables affecting health status in the later years can help people make better-informed health choices to increase the quality of their later life.

Whether old age is to be endured in an unhealthy, debilitated state, or with energy and vigor is largely up to individual responsibility and the value placed on healthy behavior. One common response of an individual who is practicing an unhealthy behavior (e.g., smoking cigarettes, overeating) is, "I'm going to die anyway, might as well be from this." However, this reasoning is flawed. The chance of growing old with disabilities due to poor health behaviors is much greater than the chance of dying quickly from them. It is ironic that many of the diseases and disabilities formerly believed to be inevitable are now known to be caused by our own thoughtless behaviors. Thus, the short-term enjoyment of unhealthful activities exacts a long-term cost on health. Whereas health may not seem of great concern when young, when one becomes old, health becomes a crucial concern. Perhaps the most important reason to discuss health in later years is to get a perspective on the direction our own health behaviors may be leading us.

Aside from the impact on our personal lives, the study of health and aging will assist us to better manage the aging process of those close to us—our friends and families. It is more likely now than it was fifty years ago that our parents, grandparents,

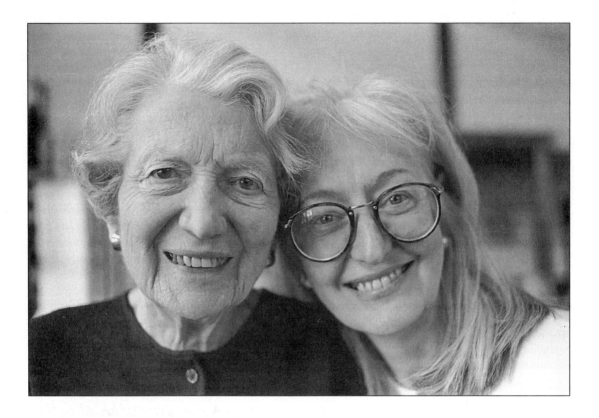

and other kin will live to old age. Also, it is more likely that family members will spend some of their lives dealing with impaired spouses or relatives. Accurate knowledge about health and disease, appropriate measures to minimize health problems, and available medical social services and means to finance them will be valuable in meeting that challenge.

The study of aging and health may enhance our professional careers. With the demographic shifts in the next few decades, the number of careers for those who choose to work directly with elders will increase dramatically. Researchers, teachers, social workers, physicians, nurses, nutritionists, counselors, psychologists, pharmacists, physical therapists, and many others with special knowledge of the needs of elders will be in demand. Those entering other careers, such as advertising, fashion designing, tourism, and mass media will do well to understand the needs and desires of elders as older consumers become an increased proportion of our total population.

Finally, as enlightened citizens and voters, it is our duty to be knowledgeable of the variety of issues regarding health and aging. Health care provision for all the nation's people is a critical economic, political, and moral issue. Health care expenditures currently account for 14 percent of the gross national product and cost the nation over a trillion dollars a year. The medical expenses of elders account for about a third of that expenditure, yet elders are paying more from their own pockets than they did before Medicare was enacted. With the expected population shifts, important issues will have to be faced: Who should pay for health care, and what should it include? How can health care policy be modified to better meet the needs of elders? Barring early death, sooner or later we will all join the ranks of elders, and will be either helped or harmed by these policy decisions. Answers to questions such as these are crucial for our nation and our future.

OUR NATION'S ELDERS: MYTHS AND FACTS

Wisdom would suggest that the most foolish and least affordable prejudice is that directed against a group which we must all join.

Alex Comfort

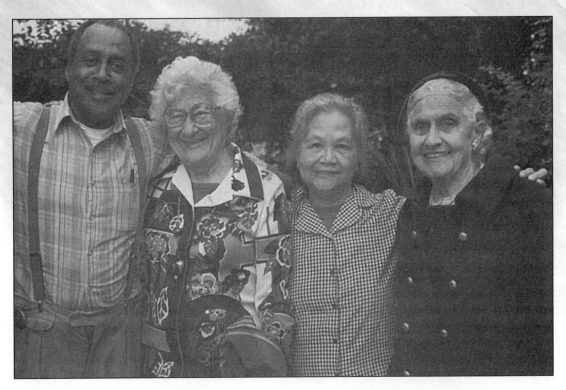

One of the first tasks in the study of aging and health is to be able to counteract some of the stereotypes that lead many to be prejudiced against elders. Several common myths will be discussed, and it is likely that the reader may think of many more. One way to counteract misconceptions about the older population is to replace them with accurate information gathered, analyzed, and published in professional journals and governmental documents by researchers in university and government agencies. In this chapter, we will address the status of the current population of elders by looking at data from several sources. Elders' life expectancy, marital status, living arrangements, income and poverty levels, educational level, and racial and ethnic composition all have an enormous impact upon health status and medical care needs.

If we are lucky enough to be alive in 2010, we will experience the beginning of the largest growth spurt of the older population in history when the baby boomer generation turns sixty-five. What impact might that demographic bubble make? It is estimated that racial and ethnic populations will expand faster than the white population, and minorities are expected to comprise one out of four elders by 2030. An overview of the four largest minority elder groups in the United States is presented to help you to better understand their health status and medical needs. If you are going into the health field, cultural sensitivity is an important prerequisite in serving one or more of these population groups: African Americans, Hispanic Americans, Asian and Pacific Islanders, and Native Americans.

AGEISM: THE MYTHS

Robert Butler, a prominent gerontologist, coined the term "ageism" to describe prejudice and discrimination against the old because of ignorance, misconceptions, and half-truths. Ageism is the assumption that personal traits of older individuals and their situations are due to age, not other factors. These generalizations, whether negative or positive, are usually based on limited experience with older people. Although some myths of aging

may be true for *some* older people, ageism is the practice of applying these stereotypes to *all* elders.

Ageism arises from those who view elders as separate or different, and as people who no longer experience the same thoughts and feelings as the rest of the population. Alex Comfort, another prominent gerontologist, asserts that like racism, ageism needs to be met by information, contradiction, and when necessary, confrontation. We need to reject ageism for ourselves, says Comfort, and refuse to impose it upon others. He puts it bluntly when he says, "By ignoring an oppressed minority, which we are inevitably going to join, we do not realize that we are slashing our own tires."[1]

Myths and stereotypes about elders affect how others feel about older people, reflecting their personal fears of being old. A study commissioned by the American Association of Retired Persons[2] revealed that American adults of all ages tend to believe that elders had more problems than elders actually reported. On the average, Americans estimated that elders had six of thirteen problems listed, but elders themselves reported an average of one of the thirteen potential problems. Interestingly, those between ages eighteen and sixty-four reported more personal problems (finances, job opportunities, availability of medical care, housing, and education) than did the elders.

Myths and stereotypes about elders also affect how elders view themselves. In the same study, older people had exaggerated views about the problems facing the elder population as a whole, even though they did not personally experience them. In essence, many elders also exhibit ageism, but see themselves as the exception.

The following are only a few of the many ageist attitudes perpetuated in American society. Much of the information presented here will be discussed more fully in the following chapters.

"After age sixty-five, life goes steadily downhill."

Sixty-five is not a magic age that defines the boundary between healthy middle age and total decrepitude. Aging is a dynamic process that begins the moment we are born. As a group, the health status of elders is poorer than that of

Stereotypes of the Ideal Aged American

Let us look at the stereotype of the ideal aged American as past folklore presents it. He or she is a white-haired, inactive, unemployed person, making no demands on anyone, least of all the family, docile in putting up with loneliness, rip-offs of every kind and boredom, and able to live on a pittance. He or she, although not demented, which would be a nuisance to other people, is slightly deficient in intellect and tiresome to talk to, because folklore says that old people are weak in the head, asexual, because old people are incapable of sexual activity, and it is unseemly if they are not. He or she is unemployable, because old age is second childhood and everyone knows that the old make a mess of simple work. Some credit points can be gained by visiting or by being nice to a few of these subhuman individuals, but most of them prefer their own company and the company of other aged unfortunates. Their main occupations are religion, grumbling, reminiscing, and attending the funerals of friends. If sick, they need not, and should not, be actively treated, and are best stored in unsupervised institutions run by racketeers who fleece them and hasten their demise. A few, who are amusing or active, are kept by society as pets. The rest are displaying unpardonable bad manners by continuing to live, and even on occasion by complaining of their treatment, when society has declared them unpeople and their patriotic duty is to lie down and die.

If this picture of aging offends you, visit a few of the places where old people are kept. If you dislike what you see, recognize that you have a few years to change it before the stereotype hits you. If it has hit you already, you will know it better than anyone and you will want any help available to fight back.[3]

younger groups. However, age changes vary among older people and are influenced by both psychological and environmental factors. In general, decrements associated with age are minor, and most individuals adapt well with little alteration in daily routine. Although some physical decrements and chronic diseases are associated with advanced age, the later years have many benefits. They can be a time to continue old roles and interests or develop new ones. Aging may bring more free time, independence from raising children, and lack of job-related stress.

"Old people are all alike."

There is more variability among elders than any other segment of the population. Individuals become more unique with age as their collection of experiences and attitudes exert a tremendous influence on adult development. Elders experience drastically differing rates of physiological and psychological aging and decline of health. The characteristics of an immobilized elder in a nursing home are very different from an elder marathon runner or statesperson of the same age. Furthermore, the age of an elderly person varies from sixty-five to over 100, a span of thirty-five years. Using that same age range in another group, we can see the variability; what does a fifteen-year-old have in common with a fifty-year-old? Although a text on aging has to focus on generalizations, there are many differences among elder subgroups.

"Old people are lonely and ignored by their families."

The common belief that elders are more likely to be lonely than other age groups is not substantiated by research. In fact, one study reported that elders are less lonely and more satisfied with social relationships than all other age groups. Those elders who are lonely are most likely to have recently lost a spouse or loved one.

The majority of elders are not ignored by their families. They remain in close contact, either in person or by phone. When given a choice between living alone or with their children, elders overwhelmingly prefer to live alone if they can afford it. And, contrary to popular belief, the great majority of frail elders are not relegated to institutions, but are cared for by family members. For every frail elder who is institutionalized, four equally frail elders are cared for at home by family members.

"Old age used to be better."

There is a widespread myth in our society that there was a "golden past" when multigenerational families lived in harmony on large farms, the elderly were venerated, and they were cared for with dignity. In fact this is untrue. In the first place, few people lived to be old; in the 1900s, the life expectancy for both men and women was under fifty years. When people died, it was often suddenly from acute conditions—people didn't linger on with multiple chronic illnesses as they do today. In the second place, elders then, as now, preferred to live alone and often did. Elders were often not revered; in fact, many historians show that some elders threatened to disinherit their children just to assure they would be cared for, or even be allowed to sit at the family table. In contrast, it is the norm nowadays for children to provide physical and emotional care to aging parents, and provide care for a longer period of time. Although providing such care is demanding, most would have it no other way.

"Old people are senile."

The term "senility" has often been used loosely to describe any memory loss and confusion in older people. However, memory loss and confusion are not normal accompaniments of aging and, when they are present, should prompt a work-up for a medical cause such as adverse effects of medication, dementia, or depression. Although it is true that the incidence of cognitive impairment increases with age, especially among those in their eighties and nineties, most elders are not cognitively impaired. This stereotype prompts a lot of worry among older people who are concerned that they are becoming senile. It is interesting that the young, or those around them, do not worry when they forget, but when an older person forgets, it is seen as significant.

"Old people have the good life."

Along with the many negative myths about old age, many people believe that elders have it easy and that life after retirement is paradise, with time to travel and rest. Although elders on the whole enjoy their later years, it is fallacious to think that old age is easy for all. In fact, old age is a time of loss for many elders—the loss of loved ones, the loss of health, the loss of physical appearance, and reduced financial resources. Many minority elders never live to retirement age, or they must continue to work because they have insufficient money to survive otherwise. Although aging is not a negative experience for most elders, there are negative aspects of growing old that must be addressed. These include coping with negative stereotypes, chronic illness of self or spouse, limitations in mobility, death of loved ones, increasing dependency, and reduced income.

"Most old people are sickly."

Most elders experience at least one chronic condition, and some have several. However, the majority of elders' health problems do not limit their ability to enjoy life and to manage their own households. Although concerns about those with severe health problems and the institutionalized should be addressed, many older people have no health problems at all. According to the most recent U.S. Census, about 10 percent of elders in the community need help in carrying out daily activities. Although many see elders as a "sickly" group, the majority of elders rank themselves in better health than others their age. About 70 percent of elders reported their health to be good or excellent in comparison with others their own age, and only 9 percent reported themselves to be in poor health.[4]

"Old people no longer have any sexual interest or ability."

Although there is a slight alteration in sexual response with age, older people in reasonably good health have satisfying sex lives. Interest in sex persists into old age, and many elders remain sexually active into their nineties. Those who do not are often those who were inactive as younger adults, those who lack a partner, or those who are very disabled.

"Most old people end up in nursing homes."

Only 4 percent of those sixty-five and older are in a nursing home at any one time. Contrary to popular opinion, nursing homes are not only used for living out one's final days; many people who enter nursing homes stay only a few weeks or months after hospitalization to recuperate. However, the likelihood of being placed in a nursing home increases sharply with advancing age. Only 1 percent of those sixty-five to seventy-four reside in a nursing home, but 15 percent of those eighty-five and older live there.[5]

OUR NATION'S ELDERS: THE FACTS

Physiological state is an important component in determining overall health status. However, a number of other social and economic considerations, such as marital status, living arrangements, education, income, degree of social support, and cultural background, exert a strong influence upon health status and behavior. The following cases exemplify the complex interactions among physiological, socioeconomic, and other environmental factors upon health.

> Case 1: The seventy-five-year-old Asian American woman is partially blind and walks with a cane because of osteoporosis. She is unable to drive but relies on public transportation to go to church and visit members of the historical society of which she is the chairperson. She is mentally alert, reads well with glasses, and has a positive attitude about life. She has some college education and lives alone.
>
> Case 2: The sixty-five-year-old African American man with a history of congestive heart failure lives in a three-story walk-up because he does not have enough money to move. His children live nearby and help him with housecleaning and meal preparation. However, he has refused their offer to stay with them. He has been prescribed medication for his heart trouble but takes it only when he experiences pain because he believes medicine should only be taken when one is sick.

> Case 3: The eighty-three-year-old white woman has recently returned from the hospital after hip surgery and is temporarily disabled. She needs physical therapy but cannot get there because she fears she will be attacked in the city neighborhood. Her neighbors help her fix meals, but she is very hesitant to ask for any other type of help because she is unable to pay for it.
>
> Case 4: The sixty-five-year-old woman is a retired dancer and continues to dance daily in a local studio. She is fully mobile and drives well. She is highly educated about the importance of diet and exercise in maintaining health. She lives with her husband in a house behind her adult daughter's family and helps with babysitting and light housework.

This section provides an overview of the demographic factors that directly or indirectly affect the health of older people. Demography is the study of the size, geographical distribution, and vital statistics of a particular group. Most demographic data available considers elders as those sixty-five and older. Furthermore, the information is generally presented in terms of average values and does not address the tremendous variation among individual elders. Thus, it is important not to use these general data to make predictions about the situation of a particular older person.

Unless noted otherwise, the facts and figures cited were gathered from *A Profile of Older Americans, 1998,* compiled from data from the Bureau of the Census, National Center on Health Statistics, and the Bureau of Labor Statistics. A yearly update can be found on the Administration on Aging web site: http://www.aoa.dhhs.gov/aoa/stats/profile/.

Number and Growth of the Older Population

The number and proportion of those over sixty-five continues to grow rapidly, and will accelerate over the next three decades (figure 1.1). At the beginning of the 20th century, less than one in twenty-five people in the United States was sixty-five or

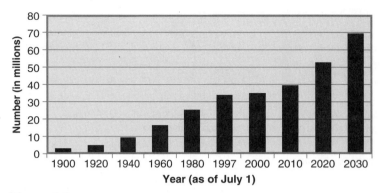

Figure 1.1

Number of Persons Sixty-five and Older: 1900 to 2030.

Note: Increments in years are uneven.

Based on data from the U.S. Bureau of the Census.

over (4.1 percent). By 1997, the percentage more than tripled: one person in eight (12.7 percent) was 65 and over—a total of over 34.1 million people. By 2030, elders will comprise more than 20 percent of the nation's total population.

The proportion of the population aged seventy-five-and-older is increasing the fastest. In 1997, the sixty-five through seventy-four age group was eight times larger than in 1900, but the seventy-five through eighty-four age group was sixteen times larger, and the eighty-five-and-older group was thirty-one times larger. Close to half of all elders are seventy-five and older.

The rapid growth of the older population is due to the fact that more people are surviving to old age. The increase was smaller in the 1990s because fewer babies were born during the Great Depression of the 1930s. The unprecedented increase in proportion of individuals reaching sixty-five is expected between 2010 and 2030 when the baby boomers "come of age."

The proportion of elderly ethnic minorities continues to increase. In 1997, about 15 percent of all elders were minorities; 8 percent were African American, about 5 percent were Hispanic American, 2 percent were Asian or Pacific Islanders, and less than 1 percent were Native American. By 2030, these minority populations are projected to represent 25 percent of the elderly population.

Historically, ethnic minorities have been underrepresented in the elder population because of their shorter life expectancy. As the life expectancy and birth rates of ethnic populations increase, however, they will comprise a greater proportion of the elder population. Many ethnic and racial elders have moved to the United States in later life because their children have sent for them. The two elder groups that will expand the most are Asian and Pacific Islanders and Hispanic Americans, who are all estimated to grow more than threefold.

The increased numbers and proportion of elders in the United States will have profound consequences on our society, especially upon the demand for medical care. Higher numbers of elders, especially those over seventy-five, increase the need for medical services, long-term care facilities, and home health services. Furthermore, publicly funded insurance programs that serve elders, such as Medicare and Medicaid, will have to carry a heavier burden.

It is expected that the future elderly population will be demographically different than the current one. Elders will be more highly educated, assertive, politically savvy, and financially secure. Remember, those who will be elderly in the future are those who were at one time called "hippies," "yuppies," and "DINKS" (double income, no kids). Might they become a powerful voting block to advocate for more health and social services?

Life Expectancy

Life expectancy for both men and women in the United States continues to increase. Those born today can expect to live more than twenty-five years longer than those born in 1900. In 1997, the average was 76.5 years. If a person survives to age sixty-five, life expectancy is recalculated, and generally many years of life expectancy are added. For instance, females reaching age sixty-five can expect to live another nineteen years, and men fifteen years. This is because once you have arrived at a certain age, you are a "survivor" who has "beaten the odds," and these characteristics translate to a longer life expectancy.

Gender has the largest influence on life expectancy, although the difference is narrowing somewhat. Women continue to live longer than men. As a result, there are more older women than older men. In 1997, there were 20 million elder women and 14 million elder men, making a sex ratio of 143 women for every 100 men. This sex ratio increases with age; after age 85, there are 248 women for every 100 men. No matter what ethnicity or race, the life expectancy of males continues to lag behind females. For instance, the life expectancy for white women born in 1997 was 79.3 years; for white men, 74.3; for African American women, 74.7 years; and for African American men, 67.3 years.

Ethnicity also has a strong influence upon life expectancy. In the United States, whites live longer than African Americans, and both live longer than Hispanic Americans. However, some Asian American groups live longer than whites. In 1997, the death rate for Asian Americans was 40 percent less than for whites, and African Americans had a death rate of 50 percent more than whites. Native Americans have the shortest life expectancies of all minority groups. The life expectancy of Native Americans is estimated to be as much as eight years less than the average for the general population. The reduced life expectancy among ethnic and racial groups is thought to be due primarily to poverty and reduced access to health care.

Regardless of gender, ethnicity, or race, life expectancy has increased rapidly in the last century largely because of reduced deaths of infants and children, primarily through control of infectious diseases. A greater proportion of the population is now living to be old, even very old. There are currently 40,000 centenarians in the United States, or approximately one centenarian for 10,000 people. In fact, it is estimated that there are more people over the age of 100 alive today than all those who ever lived to be 100 prior to the twentieth century.[6]

Although life expectancy is still increasing, it is now beginning to level off. Some researchers assert that advances in disability-free life expectancy have not kept pace with advances in life expectancy. Thus, instead of living longer, healthier lives, Americans may be spending more years in a disabled state. However, these conclusions have been challenged by those who believe that the onset of disability is now occurring at more advanced age and that even disabled elders are still functional.[7] Recent national figures indicate a decline in the proportion of people over age 65 who are disabled from previous years.[8]

Housing and Geographic Distribution

More than three-fourths of older people live in their own homes with a median value of $81,956 (1995), and most have paid off their mortgage. Half of their homes were built prior to 1960. Many live in the same homes in which they raised a family, and those houses may be older, in need of repair, or too large for one or two people. Almost one-quarter of elders are tenants. Some of these tenants live in public or subsidized housing. As expected, the median income of those who rent their homes is lower ($10,151) than the median income of those who own their homes ($21,627). The percentage of total income spent on housing (including maintenance and repair) in 1995 was higher for elders than younger adults (35 percent versus 27 percent).

Elders are less likely to change residences than younger groups. In 1997, only 5 percent had moved in the past year compared to 18 percent of the population under age sixty-five. Even when older people do move, 80 percent stay in the same state.

Over three-fourths of older people in the United States live in metropolitan areas, either in the city or in the suburbs. More than one-third of these elders live in the inner city. White elders are more concentrated in the suburbs, while ethnic elders are more predominant in the central cities. About one in five elders lives in rural areas, primarily small towns. In 1997, the states with the highest number of older people were California (3.6 million), Florida (2.7 million), and New York (2.4 million). Those states with the highest proportion of older people were Florida (18 percent), Pennsylvania (16 percent), Rhode Island (16 percent), West Virginia (15 percent) and Iowa (15 percent).

Marital Status and Living Arrangements

Marriage is generally very beneficial for both partners in later life. It can provide companionship, help with daily living activities and personal care when a partner needs assistance, and a higher household income compared to those who are sin-

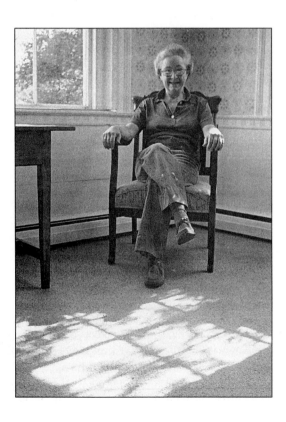

gle. Those who are married are less likely to need home health services and institutional care.

Most elders are married during the early part of their later years. However, with advancing age, failing health and death of companions, more become widowed. Because women live longer than men and have a tendency to marry men older than themselves, women are more likely to become widowed. Older men are nearly twice as likely to be married than older women. In 1997, 74 percent of older men and 42 percent of older women reported being married. In 1997, almost half of older American women were widows, almost four times more than the number of widowers. Two-thirds of women age seventy-five and older were widowed, while two-thirds of men this age were married.[9]

Although divorced older persons who have not remarried represented only 7 percent of all older persons in 1997 (2.2 million), the proportion of those who have been divorced has increased five times as fast as the older population as a whole since 1990. It is estimated that the proportion of elders who have been divorced may climb to 50 percent by 2020.

Two-thirds of the nation's older people who are not institutionalized live in a family setting. Living arrangements generally reflect marital status—those who are married are more likely to live with families. However, the number of elders living with family members decreases with advancing age. And older women are less likely to live with their families than older men, mostly because most older men are married and most older women are widowed. In 1997, 80 percent of elderly men lived with their families compared to 57 percent of women that age. After age 85, only 47 percent of elders lived in a family setting. About 13 percent (8 percent of men and 17 percent of women) were not living with a spouse, but instead lived with children, siblings, or other relatives, while another 2 percent lived with nonrelatives.

The proportion of elders living alone is increasing. In 1997, almost one-third of older people lived alone (41 percent of older women and 17 percent of older men). The likelihood of living alone increases with advancing age. Among women 85 and older, about three out of five live alone. Most elders choose to live alone and prefer that lifestyle to living with adult children. However, living alone can be a liability because these elders are more likely to have lower incomes and are at greater risk of institutionalization than those who live with families.

Marital status, living arrangements, and the availability of children play a major role in determining whether an older person needs formal care. Although most older people have some relatives, a few have no living children. In 1990, for example, one-fourth of white women over 85 and one-third of African American women over 85 had no living children. However, when the parents of the baby boomers are very old, it is likely that the percent of those who are childless will decrease. Looking even farther into the future, the baby boomers themselves have a relatively high percentage of childlessness, and may need to depend on formal services.[10]

Only about 4 percent of the total population of elders resides in nursing homes at any one time.[4] When a spouse or child is not present, elders are more likely to be institutionalized. Current trends, such as the increasing divorce rate, tendency to have fewer children, and more women in the work force, will likely affect the living arrangements of future elders.

Education

As a group, older people have completed less schooling than younger adults. However, this gap continues to narrow: from 1970 to 1997, the percentage of elders completing high school more than doubled, from 28 percent to 66 percent. In 1997, about 15 percent of those sixty-five years and older had a bachelor's degree or higher. However, the percentages vary by race and ethnic origin: 68 percent of whites, 44 percent of African Americans, and 30 percent of Hispanic Americans completed high school. Since the

baby boomers are the most educated cohorts in history, it is expected that this percentage will continue to climb. Nonetheless, it is likely there will still be significant disparities in educational level among elder subgroups, particularly minority immigrants.

Although elders may have fewer years of formal education than other adults, they do not stop enrolling in educational programs. Some elders choose to enroll in community classes, and others are enrolled in courses at community colleges and universities that offer reduced-tuition programs to attract older people. As the educational level of the elder population increases, it is expected that many retirees will return to education to enhance their quality of life, develop their interests, and acquire new skills.

Income and Employment

There have been dramatic changes in the level of income of elders over the past few decades. With the onset of Medicare and Social Security, elders are no longer the most financially vulnerable age group. With increased protection from high medical bills and a guaranteed income, elders have more financial security than ever before. However, there are still significant disparities among elder groups. Elder women, particularly those over age eighty-five, the infirm, the institutionalized, and elder minorities still suffer from insufficient incomes, and many are barely able to subsist.

As a group, elders in the United States have a lower annual income than other adults groups (children have the highest poverty level). For all older persons reporting income in 1997, more than one-third reported less than $10,000 (figure 1.2). Only 21 percent reported $25,000 or more. In 1997, the median annual income was $17,768 for elderly men, and $10,062 for elderly women. In families headed by elders, the annual household income averaged $30,660 ($31,167 for whites; $23,420 for African Americans; $22,677 for Hispanic Americans), approximately 60 percent of the median income of the twenty-five to sixty-four age group. In 1997, about 14 percent of families

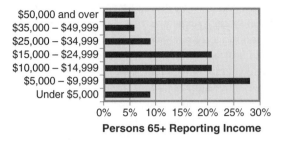

Figure 1.2
Percent Distribution by Income: 1997.

$13,049 median for 31.4 million persons 65+ reporting income.

Based on data from the U.S. Bureau of the Census.

headed by elders had incomes below $15,000, but 42 percent had incomes of $35,000 or more.

In 1999, the federal poverty level for those sixty-five and over was $8,112 per year for individuals and $14,412 for those living in a family. About 10 percent of elders lived in poverty in 1997, which is slightly less than the poverty rate for other adults. Another 6.4 percent of elderly were classified as "near poor" with incomes up to 25 percent above the poverty level. The current poverty rate among elders is not as high as in 1970, when 25 percent of elders had incomes below the poverty level, or in 1959 when 33 percent of elders were poor. Even though a lower percentage of elders are subsisting below the poverty line, a disproportionately high number are still living on marginal incomes. When the percentage of poor is added to the percentage of near-poor elders, 17 percent are considered either poor or near poor.

There is a great disparity in income level with race and ethnicity. One of eleven white elders is poor or near poor, but one in four African Americans and Hispanic Americans is poor or near poor. In addition, being a woman increases the risk of poverty. Older women have a higher poverty rate than older men (13 percent versus 7 percent). Also, older people living alone were more likely to be poor than those living with relatives (21 percent versus 6 percent). Being female, ethnic, and living alone increase the risk of poverty. For example, 40 percent of older African American women living

alone were poor in 1997. And those who are over 85 generally have the lowest income of all.

In 1996, elders received income from a number of sources including Social Security (91 percent), assets (63 percent), public and private pensions (41 percent), earnings (21 percent) and public assistance (6 percent). Older households are significantly less likely than younger households to receive public assistance, including food stamps and Medicaid.

Almost two of three elders receive a portion of their income from assets. Assets include annuities, income properties, and savings. The median net worth (assets minus liabilities) of older households ($86,300 for sixty-five and older and $77,700 for those seventy-five and older) was well above the U.S. median of $37,600 in 1993. However, there is wide variation among elders in number of assets. Net worth of their assets was below $10,000 for 16 percent of older households and above $250,000 for 17 percent. Although national figures show that elders have accumulated significantly more assets than younger adults, their major asset is a home, which cannot be easily liquidated. Further, minority groups have far fewer assets than whites.

Earnings are an important source of income for younger elders; those aged sixty-five to sixty-seven received 35 percent of their income from earnings, but only 4 percent of the income of those eighty and older was from earnings. Only 12 percent of older people are in the labor force. Twice as many men as women work after sixty-five, and of those who work, half are employed part-time. Those elders who work are more likely to be self-employed than other age groups. The elder population comprises almost 3 percent of the labor force.

Health Status and Health Care

In 1995, almost 30 percent of older persons classified their health as fair or poor (compared to about 10 percent of all persons). Men and women differed little on their evaluation of their health, although African Americans reported poorer health. On the positive side, 70 percent reported their health as good or excellent.

Morbidity (or illness) rates provide information about the incidence of disease and disability. Elders have the highest morbidity rates of all age groups because of their high prevalence of chronic illness. Most elders have at least one chronic condition. In 1994, the most common conditions reported by those sixty-five and older were arthritis (50 percent), hypertension (36 percent), heart disease (32 percent), and hearing impairments (29 percent). As expected, the number of illnesses and their severity increases with advancing age. Elders are less likely to report that they suffer from psychological disorders than younger groups, but rates of cognitive impairment (such as dementia) increase with age. Alzheimer's disease is the leading cause of cognitive impairment.

Limitations in activity due to chronic conditions increase with age. In 1995, more than one-third of older persons reported a limitation of activity (preparing meals, managing money, using the telephone, doing housework and taking medications) due to a chronic health problem. Ten percent of the elder population reported they were unable to perform a major daily activity (including bathing, dressing, eating, and getting around the house). Both these figures are significantly greater than the activity limitations reported by people under sixty-five.

Because elders have a higher prevalence of chronic illness than the rest of the population, they have longer hospital stays, visit physicians more often, and are prescribed more drugs than younger groups. Also, older people are the prime users of long-term care institutions.

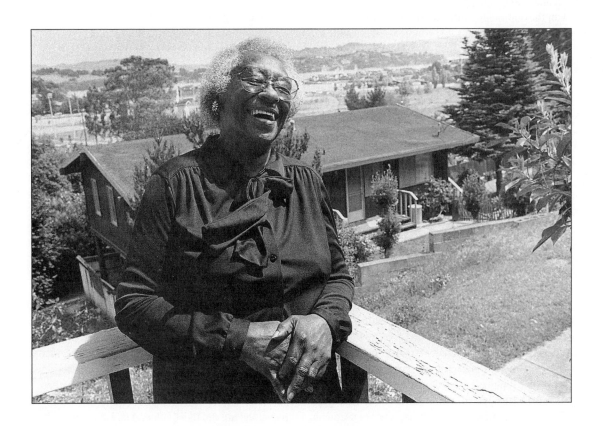

In 1995, four out of five elders received health and medial services through Medicare (the federal insurance program for all aged sixty-five and older), with an average payment for each individual of $15,000. Further, one in three elders received services under Medicaid (the federal and state medical program for the poor, blind, and disabled of all ages), with an average annual bill of $9,000.

RACIAL AND ETHNIC DIVERSITY AMONG ELDERS

Today's elderly are a highly diverse group and an important aspect of this diversity is race and ethnicity. The status and resources of several racial and ethnic elder groups are reflective of the continued social and economic discrimination experienced throughout their lives. Many also face cultural and language barriers. In general, minority elders are more likely to have less education, substandard housing, more poverty, and poorer health than the dominant white culture. In this section, the health of four groups of minority elders will be considered as they are the four predominant groups both in numbers and their history of being disadvantaged in the United States: African Americans, Hispanic Americans, Native Americans, and Asian Pacific Islanders.

The four minority groups comprise only 15 percent of the total elder population, but their numbers are increasing due to higher fertility rates and gains in life expectancy over the past few years. Currently, the growth of the minority elderly population is outpacing the growth of the white population: by the year 2030, the Bureau of the Census estimates that one in four elders (25 percent) will be nonwhite. The fastest rate of growth of minority elders will be among the oldest old (those 85 years and older). As mentioned earlier, the fastest growing groups are Asian Pacific Islanders and Hispanic Americans, projected to increase more than threefold by 2030.

Although the minority groups are incredibly diverse, they have two characteristics in common—high poverty level and racial discrimination. Differences in language, education, appearance, and customs have kept many minorities out of well-paying jobs, positions of authority, and consequent

financial security, which all began during their working years, leaving most with no resources for their later years. Despite the negative impact of discrimination throughout their lives, these elders possess some unique resources. Identification with an ethnic group and cultural traditions are a source of support in the later years. In addition, ethnic groups tend to maintain stronger extended social networks, both within the family and the local community. However, acculturation is changing this to a greater or lesser degree among some groups.

Even within each group, there is much variation in education level, financial status, cultural background, length of time in the United States, family structure, geographical distribution, and degree of adherence to cultural practices. The Native American and Asian Pacific Islander groups in particular include many subpopulations, each with its own cultural heritage and language. Statistics necessarily focus on generalities, but the reader should be aware of the diversity within these ethnic and racial groups as it strongly influences their health and medical care needs and their response to the medical care system.

African Americans

The African American population (also called Black Americans, or blacks) is the largest group of minority elders in the United States, comprising about 8 percent of the total elder population. Just as in other elder populations, there are more elder African American women than African American men; most elder men are married, and most elder women are widowed. Even though the life expectancy of African Americans is increasing, it still lags behind that of whites. The life expectancy of African American women is 4.5 years shorter than that of white women, and the life expectancy of African American men is seven years shorter than that of white men.

A high proportion of elderly African Americans are living in poverty. Older African Americans are almost three times as likely to be poor as aged whites (African Americans, 26 percent; whites 9 percent), and aged African American women who live alone are the most vulnerable. Like other ethnic minorities, elder African Americans are generally less educated, have had lower-paying jobs, and have less financial security than their white cohorts. Because of their job record, they have not contributed as much to Social Security. Thus, in their later years, they continue to be poor. Because they are also less likely to have pensions and assets than their white counterparts, they are more likely to depend on Social Security for the mainstay of their income. However, all elder African Americans are not poor. Those with a college education and professional careers in their working years have similar income levels as white elders.

As a group, African American elders are more apt to suffer from chronic health problems than their white counterparts; about half have chronic conditions as compared with just over a third of whites. Although heart disease, cancer, and stroke are the three major causes of death in both African Americans and whites, these diseases are more prevalent in the African American population. Since most African Americans have endured a lifetime of prejudice, some experts assert that the high incidence of hypertension in the population is reflective of the stress that results from societal pressure and low social status. African American elders also have a higher prevalence of glaucoma, diabetes, and prostate cancer. When compared with whites their age, African American elders have more restricted activity, disability, and lost work days per year.

African Americans visit physicians less often and stay longer in the hospital, and often postpone seeking medical attention until health problems become severe. They are also less likely to use home health services and nursing homes than white elders. It is hypothesized that health professionals' prejudicial attitudes toward African Americans may, in some cases, deny needed access to health and social services, or not offer services of adequate quality.[11]

Hispanic Americans

Today there are about a million older Hispanic Americans (also called Latinos) living in the United States. Their numbers are growing at a faster rate than the elder white population. Individuals within the group are highly diverse: the largest group origi-nates from Mexico, a significant number comes from Cuba and Puerto Rico, and fewer originate in other Central and South American countries. The largest concentrations live in California, Texas, New York, and Florida. The Hispanic American population is considerably younger than the white population. This age difference is due to higher fertility rates, shorter life expectancies, and historical patterns of immigration and emigration. For instance, many middle-aged and elder Hispanic Americans voluntarily return to their homeland. However, some elders arrive in the United States in their later years as their children send for them.

Demographic data on the Hispanic American population are often inadequate. Hispanic Americans are often classified as white, many are unable to read or speak English. Because many are here illegally, they are suspicious of census takers. Of all minority elderly, those of Hispanic background are the least educated. Forty percent of elderly Hispanic Americans do not speak English, and they are only half as likely to finish high school as the white elderly population. Lack of education and inability to speak English have forced them into jobs with low pay and no pension or health insurance benefits. They are less likely to be drawing on Social Security because of erratic employment in farm and service industries or because their wages were paid "under the table." They are more likely to depend on Supplemental Security Income, the federal assistance program for the poor. Half the Hispanic American elderly are immigrants, and some of those have arrived illegally.

Elderly Hispanic Americans are almost three times as likely to be poor as the white population, 24 percent live below the poverty level compared to 9 percent of white elders. As in all elder populations, poverty rates among Hispanic Americans are higher among older women than among older men.

As a group, elder Hispanic Americans suffer poorer health than their white counterparts. They are more likely to suffer from diabetes and heart disease and less likely to comply with medication therapy or change their behavior to enhance their health status. Elder Hispanic Americans average significantly more annual physician visits than white elders, and they are more likely to be hospitalized. However, they are less likely to be covered by Medicare or to have private insurance. Elder Hispanic Americans are more likely to have disabilities that interfere with daily activities; researchers estimate that 40 percent of them have at least one functional limitation and that they are two to three times more likely to have long-term-care needs than elders who are not.[12]

Hispanic American elders rely more heavily on their families than do white elders. As a group they are least likely to live alone than other elder groups. Three factors are involved: they may not have enough money to have a separate household, they have more disabilities and cannot function independently, and they have strong family ties. Traditionally, Hispanic American elders are highly respected by their children and are the core of the extended family network. They act as repositories of cultural traditions, values, and history. More than the younger Hispanic Americans, they have retained their native language and culture. In comparison to whites, Hispanic Americans often have more kin in town, interact more frequently with relatives, and are more likely to help family members out financially. However, as adult children are quickly being integrated into American culture, the extended family network of the Spanish-speaking population is disintegrating, threatening the emotional and financial support of Hispanic American elders.

In general, elder Hispanic Americans are cynical and suspicious of governmental institutions and workers. With the exception of going to the doctor, they are less likely to utilize social and educational programs, mainly because many cannot speak or read English. However, their underutilization of services does not mean that the services are not needed.

Native Americans

Native American elders (American Indians, Eskimos, and Aleutians) comprise less than 1 percent of the U.S. elder population. About one-quarter of Native American elderly live on American Indian reservations or Alaskan Native villages. Over half are located in the southwestern states. The Native American group is comprised of over 500 tribes and 150 tribal languages.

Native Americans do not live as long as whites. From 1985 through 1987, the Indian Health Service figures reported average life expectancy at birth for Native Americans to be only 70.5 years, more than four years less than that of the general population at that time. Some Indian Health Service areas had figures approximately eight years less than the U.S. figure.[13] Less than 6 percent of the Native American population lives to be sixty-five or older.

Besides having the shortest life expectancy, Native Americans are the poorest minority group in the United States. Because of the high unemployment rate among Native Americans (50 percent), most elders are ineligible for Social Security benefits and must depend on government support as their sole source of income. Some experts believe they should be eligible for Social Security benefits earlier than the rest of the population since many Native Americans do not live long enough to collect their benefits.

Although the majority of younger Native Americans have moved from reservations to urban areas, for the most part, their elders still live on reservations or in rural areas. On the average, the quality of their housing is very poor. A report on housing conditions among Native American elders noted that their homes are five times more likely to lack plumbing and fourteen times less likely to have sewage disposal than other homes in the country. Furthermore, many of their homes are overcrowded, 50 percent have areas that lack flooring, almost 50 percent use only wood-burning stoves for heat, 13 percent have no refrigerator, and 75 percent lack telephones.[14]

As a group, elder Native Americans are less educated than other elders in the United States. Nearly 12 percent of all Native American elders have had no formal education. Furthermore, less than one in four of their elders have graduated from high school.

Many Native Americans have an extended family network with a strong commitment to their elders. Furthermore, because of the high rate of unemployment among the younger population, the family often stays together because the elder in the family may be the only one with a steady income. Due to the high unemployment rate, elders may provide a significant proportion of the family income through government subsidies. This provision of support may indirectly preserve the status of elders within the family. However, traditional family support is ineffective in families with no resources, and many Native American elders are left impoverished on the reservation when their children leave to seek a better life.

Native Americans have the unenviable reputation of having the poorest health status in the United States. This population has a shorter life expectancy, higher rates of alcoholism, and higher accident rates than any other minority group. Death rates for tuberculosis and diabetes among the Native American population are significantly greater than the general population. Other major health problems of Native American elders include pneumonia, high blood pressure, and malnutrition. Almost three-fourths of Native American elders have health impairments severe enough to affect their ability to complete tasks of daily living. It is believed that their higher proportion of illness and disability is due to insufficient funds to purchase nutritious food and reduced access to medical care.

Despite the high prevalence of illness among elder Native Americans, most rarely see a physician. On the reservations, the Indian Health Service is responsible for their health care. Those who do not live on the reservation or belong to a registered tribe must seek care outside the Indian Health Service. Furthermore, older Native Americans are more likely to have a different view of disease and healing, and are more likely to rely on ritual folk healing than visit a physician.

Even though health care expenditures have increased consistently for the rest of the population, per capita health care expenditures for Native Americans have not. Because the U.S. Congress and the Bureau of Indian Affairs, not the individual states, are responsible for developing and implementing programs to meet the health and social service needs of Native Americans, older Native Americans may not have access to government-assistance programs available to the rest of

the population. As a result, they are at higher risk for substandard housing, poverty, malnutrition, and poor health.

In sum, the poor state of health of elder Native Americans is exacerbated by their low income and educational level, shorter life expectancy, serious health problems, poor housing, and lack of access to and stringent governmental controls on health and social service programs for Native Americans.

Asian and Pacific Islander Americans

Asian Americans represent the fastest growing racial group aged sixty-five and older in the United States. This population includes sixty ethnic groups from twenty different countries. The largest four subgroups are Chinese (24 percent), Japanese (24 percent), Filipino (8 percent), and Korean (5 percent). The population also includes people immigrating from East India, Cambodia, Guam, Hawaii, Samoa, Vietnam, Thailand, Laos, Malaysia, and more. Some arrived at the turn of the century and have lived here for generations; others may have arrived in the 1970s. Asian/Pacific Islander American elders comprise less than 2 percent of the total U.S. population. Information on Asian American (this term includes Pacific Islanders as well) elders is very sparse and is mostly limited to the two largest Asian groups, the Japanese and Chinese.

The majority of Asian Americans in the United States live in urban areas in three states: California, New York, and Hawaii. Although a subgroup of younger Asian Americans have a higher median income and a lower unemployment and poverty rate than the national average, elder Asian Americans still suffer the same poverty, discrimination, and language difficulties as other ethnic minorities. Many receive no Social Security benefits because they were employed as seasonal farm workers or self-employed.

As in all elder populations in the United States, the majority of elder Asian/Pacific Islander American men are married, while the majority of women are widowed. However, unlike other white ethnic populations, there are more elder Asian American men than women, partly due to larger numbers of men immigrating here.

In aggregate, the health status of Asian/Pacific Islander Americans is similar to white elders. However, generalizations about these populations ignore the tremendous diversity among populations: some have better health than whites and others have poorer health. Asian elders are less likely to smoke or drink, and report better health, longer life expectancy and fewer functional limitations than their white counterparts.[15] As a group, they have the lowest mortality rate in the United States, more than 40 percent lower than the white population.[16]

Health status relates somewhat to acculturation. With acculturation comes some positive effects (increased reliance on preventive care, better communication with medical providers) as well as some negative effects (change from traditional low-fat Asian diets to high-fat American diets). Asian American elders have a higher incidence of some types of cancers, hypertension, and infectious diseases such as hepatitis and tuberculosis. As a group, elder Asian Americans have a higher incidence of suicide—three times that of their white counterparts.

Like other minorities, elder Asian Americans are less likely to utilize medical care services than white elders, probably because of language barriers and unfamiliarity with Western medicine. They may be recent immigrants and may not have access to Medicare or Medicaid services. Many do not have private health insurance.[17] However, they are likely to seek emergency room care, preferring Western medical services for emergencies or severe symptoms.[18]

Traditional Asian culture dictates that children should care for their elder parents who are venerated for their wisdom and experience. For Asian Americans, however, filial piety has begun to take a back seat to such traditional American values as independence and self-reliance. Still, aged Chinese and Japanese Americans tend to retain the old ways, living in small, close-knit groups with others who share their language and culture. However, such strong social support tends to isolate these populations from the rest of society.

WORKING WITH MINORITY ELDERS: OBSTACLES AND OPPORTUNITIES

Health care professionals are in a good position to appreciate the challenges posed by differing cultures. As one social scientist stated, "Western medicine values sterility, order, quiet and isolation of the patient from others in order to achieve healing. This is very detrimental to patients who come from a culture where increased attention and intense social interaction with family—both near and distant kin—is necessary for healing."[19] These following cases illustrate factors to be considered in working with ethnic minority elders in health care settings.

Mr. W., an elderly Asian American man with liver cancer, would sit placidly in his hospital bed during various tests and visits from specialists. Because he did not speak English, little communication was directed towards him, although he was always smiling and allowed any examination. Chemotherapy was administered, based on the expectation that this is what he would want. His granddaughter, who was working full-time, would take calls at work and act as a translator. She mentioned that he felt nauseated and had pain, but she was not able to follow-up on whether those symptoms were treated. She did not tell him that his illness was terminal. When Mr. W. began to get weaker, a large number of family members would come and sit at his bedside, spilling over into other areas of the hospital and bringing pungent foods to tempt his appetite. They crowded into his room, which he shared with two other patients, and someone was present at all times. Visits by medical personnel and updates about the patient's medical status were communicated through the granddaughter, who was expected to relay it to her relatives. When the patient died, the granddaughter called and asked for his body to remain in the bed for hours, which is a Buddhist tradition. The hospital denied her request, informing her that they required the bed immediately.

Mrs. G., a 67-year-old Hispanic American woman with diabetes, high blood pressure, and

Obstacles to Effective Health Care Delivery to Minority Elders

Economic and Educational
- They may not be eligible for Medicare.
- They are more likely to have a low income level.
- They are less likely to be able to pay for services.
- They are more likely to have a low educational level.
- They are not likely to understand medical and bureaucratic jargon.

Cultural
- They are less likely to be able to speak and understand English.
- They are less likely to know about available services, eligibility standards, and application procedures.
- They are more likely to have many health care needs.
- They are more likely to distrust the health system.
- They may have had prior negative experiences.
- They may not be legal U.S. residents.
- Their loved ones may not be in this country.
- They may have strong values about healing and may be using other types of healing therapies at the same time (herbs, traditional healer).
- They may have particular beliefs about shots, pills, taking blood, and X-rays.
- They may not communicate, and their silence may be misinterpreted.
- They may be there because of family pressure, not because they want to be.
- They are more likely to use a kin network for emotional support.
- Their values and world view affect their health and illness beliefs and practices.
- They are more likely to have traditional views of health beliefs and illness behavior.

Geographical
- Fewer services are available in remote areas, so the elder must travel long distances.
- Public or private transportation may not be available.
- In urban areas, crime may deter elders from leaving home to seek services.
- Family and friends may not be nearby to accompany them.

Institutional
- The service provider may be biased that minority groups take care of their own elders.
- Services may be fragmented with different qualifications for care.
- The care facility may require excessive paperwork, making it confusing for the illiterate.
- The facility may not have personnel who can speak their language.
- There may be a shortage of outreach personnel.
- Educational materials targeting common health problems of specific populations are not common.
- Community support for long-term care for minority groups is inadequate.
- Unavailability or reduced availability of services is a problem.
- Discrimination by provider resulting in no care or poor care is common.
- There may be a cultural insensitivity towards the minority consumer.
- Minorities have little, if any, input on program planning.

Facilitating Minority Elder Access to Needed Services
- Learn about the needs of the population.
- Advocate on their behalf for needed services.
- Train health and human service workers to be culturally sensitive.
- Recruit more minority service personnel.
- Help clients to understand available services and how to go about receiving them.
- Develop and distribute written materials in their language.
- Tailor programs and services to specific populations, considering their language, culture, and history.
- Integrate family and native healers into the care-giving team.
- Enforce civil rights laws and strengthen policies that prohibit discrimination against poor and minorities.
- Secure effective transportation to facilitate use of service.
- Encourage hiring of bilingual staff.
- Use available translation services rather than relying on family members or untrained staff.

obesity, required amputation surgery of her lower foot because of poor circulation and an ulcer that would not heal. She was visited at home by a home health nurse. The nurse found the house quite crowded, with the woman living with a daughter, grandchildren, and a niece in a two-bedroom apartment. Her daughters all worked and were unable to change the dressings on the wound. Mrs. G. took her medications sporadically, based on her own assessment of how she felt and whether she needed them. Her family would go across the border to Mexico and bring back medications—some of them homeopathic, and some of them versions of U.S. prescription drugs—that she would also take as she needed. She expected her daughters to care for her and was upset to discover that the doctor had talked to them about placing her in a nursing home.

Although working with ethnic elders can present some challenges, most health and social service professionals find these populations particularly gratifying. For example, minority elders may be more grateful and appreciative of services provided. Because of lower educational attainment, they may benefit tremendously from relatively simple educational efforts (for example, recommendations and explanations of mammograms). In many cases, their larger extended families often mean that more loved ones are available to provide help in the home, reducing the need for institutionalization. Cultural sensitivity, willingness to learn and change, and motivation to find better ways to meet the needs of minority elders are prerequisites for effective services to this group.

SUMMARY

When studying about elders and their health status, it is important to debunk widely held myths of aging. These myths arise from *ageism,* negatively stereotyping and discriminating against older people because of half-truths, ignorance, or misconceptions. Familiarity with demographic data is crucial to understanding elders and the multiple factors that affect their health status. Information concerning the living situation, financial status, health care utilization, morbidity, and geographical distribution of older people allows a realistic appraisal of their characteristics and needs. Statistical data may lead one to the erroneous conclusion that elders are a homogeneous population, rather than a widely varied group. Nevertheless, statistical information is invaluable in dispelling stereotypes about elders and planning to meet the future demands of that group. Finally, since the elder group is one we eventually will all join, the information can assist us to be more realistic about our later life.

ACTIVITIES

1. Visit the document section of your library and look up the demographic characteristics of elders in your community. Find the proportion of older people, proportion of ethnic group elders, income, and other pertinent material. Compare with national figures.

2. Using the material you gathered for question 1, what health needs can you predict for your community? Interview a public health official, social worker, or planner of the local Area Agency of Aging to get other perspectives on the status and needs of elders in your community.

3. Collect materials that reflect myths and stereotypes about elders. Pay particular attention to advertisements, birthday cards.

4. Analyze current television programming, newscasts, and television commercials to determine whether the media's view of older people is consistent with the demographic picture presented here.

5. List stereotypical views you have held or that you have heard your friends say about older people. What information do you now have to counteract those myths?

6. Do the statistics outlined in this chapter accurately define the elders you know? How do your friends or

relatives differ? Discuss some of these facts and figures about elders with your friends and family. Which ones were surprising? Which of these statistics reinforced or dispelled your stereotypes of elders?

7. The median income in 1997 for an older woman was $10,062. Use this figure to develop a monthly budget. What expenses could not be covered in your budget? List the ways her income might interfere with the quality of her life.

8. Interview an elder and write a brief case history. How do demographic characteristics (e.g., marital status, income, family support) contribute to his or her health status? How does this elder report personal health in comparison with others his or her age?

9. Given the expected increase in the proportion of elders in 2030, project how society will have to change to better meet the future health care needs.

BIBLIOGRAPHY

1. Comfort, A. 1976. *A good age.* New York: Simon and Schuster.

2. Speas, K., and Obenshain, B. 1995. *Images of aging in America. Final Report.* 1995 FGI Research for American Association of Retired Persons, Washington, D.C.

3. Comfort, A. 1976. *A good age.* New York: Simon and Schuster.

4. U.S. Bureau of the Census. 1990. Persons needing assistance with everyday activities. *Statistical Brief* SB 12–90. U.S. Department of Commerce.

5. Dey, A.N. 1997. *Characteristics of elderly nursing home residents: data from the 1995 National Nursing Home Survey. Advance data from vital and health statistics,* no. 289. Hyattsville, MD: National Center for Health Statistics.

6. Beard, B.B. 1990. Centenarians: the new generation. In Wilson, N.K. and Wilson, A.J.E., (eds.). *Centenarians.* New York: Greenwood Press.

7. Rogers, A., Rogers, R.G., and Belanger, A. 1990. Longer life but worse health? *The Gerontologist* 30(5):640–49.

8. Manton, K.G., Corder, L., and Stallard, E. 1997. Chronic disability trends in the US elderly populations: 1982–1995. *Proc Nat Acad Sci USA.* 94:2593–98. Proceedings of the National Academy of Science, USA.

9. Shoen, R, and Weineck, R. W. 1993. The slowing metabolism of marriage: figures from the 1988 Marital Status Life Tables. *Demography* 30:740–41.

10. Himes, C.L. 1992. Future caregivers: projected family structures of older people. *Journal of Gerontology* 47:S23–26.

11. Mui, A.C., Burnette, D. 1994. Long-term care service use by frail elders: is ethnicity a factor? *The Gerontologist* 34:190–98.

12. Adams, J., 1989. *Poverty and poor health among elderly Hispanic Americans.* Baltimore. A Report of the Commonwealth Fund Commission on Elderly People Living Alone.

13. Indian Health Service. 1990. *Regional differences in Indian health.* Washington, D.C.: Public Health Service.

14. Rhoades, E.R., Reyes, L.L., and Buzzard, G.D. 1987. The organization of health services for Indian people. *Public Health Reports* 102:352–56.

15. Tanjasiri, S.P., Wallace, S.P., and Shibata, K. 1995. Picture imperfect: hidden problems among Asian Pacific Islander elderly. *The Gerontologist* 35:753–60.

16. Ventura, S.J., Anderson, R.N., and Martin, J.A. 1998. *Births and deaths: preliminary data for 1997. National vital statistics reports,* vol. 47 no. 4. Hyattsville, MD: National Center for Health Statistics.

17. Tanjasiri, S.P., Wallace, S.P., and Shibata, K. 1995. Picture imperfect: hidden problems among Asian Pacific Islander elderly. *The Gerontologist* 35:753–60.

18. Boult, L., and Boult, C. 1995. Underuse of physician services by older Asian-Americans. *Journal of the American Geriatric Society* 43:408–11.

19. Barker, J.C. 1994. Recognizing cultural differences: health care providers and elderly patients. *Gerontology and Geriatrics Education* 15:9–21.

2

BIOLOGIC AGING THEORIES AND LONGEVITY

Young man,
Seize every minute
Of your time.
The days fly by;
Ere long you too
Will grow old.

Tsu Yeh

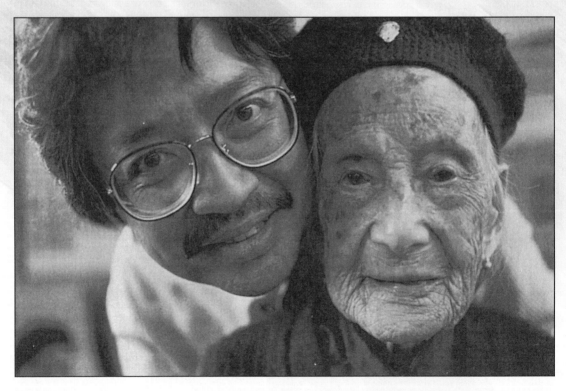

Why do we age and die? What factors influence the rate of aging and determine how long we live? What can we do to increase our chances of a long life? And would we *want* to live forever? These are the types of questions spurring researchers all over the world as they search for dietary, cultural, psychological, physiological, and biochemical factors associated with longevity.

Interest in why we age and how the aging process may be thwarted must have existed from the time our species started to live long enough to see the aging process. Currently, interest is focused on the cellular and genetic basis of aging. Despite extensive scientific inquiry, the how and why we age remains a mystery. In fact, each new discovery raises more questions than answers.

This chapter will begin by describing the many factors that affect how long we will live. Some of these are under our control, while others are not. The next section discusses what is known about why our bodies age, mainly looking deep into the genes that make-up each body cell. Finally, we will explore efforts that scientists have made to counteract the effects of aging.

FACTORS INFLUENCING LONGEVITY

Gerontologists generally consider 110 to 120 years to be the maximum limit of human life, yet most people live less than two-thirds of that. Why do so few reach this upper limit? In an attempt to answer this question, scientists have identified a number of genetic and environmental factors that are associated with longevity. Some believe heredity to be the primary determinant, while others assert that psychosocial and lifestyle factors are more significant. Regardless of which determinants are most important, most agree that several factors influence our length of life: some are beyond our control (e.g., genetics, gender), and others are modifiable lifestyle choices (e.g., smoking, weight control, and physical activity). Since none of us can change our genetic make-up, we can choose a healthy lifestyle, making the best of what we have. As Robert Louis Stevenson said:

"Life is not a matter of getting good cards, but of playing a poor hand well."

When we study the factors that influence longevity, we must realize the tremendous variability among individuals. Although there are a few individuals with poor health habits who live long lives, and conversely, some with good health habits who die prematurely, on the average, choosing a healthy lifestyle increases our chance of living long and well. Although certain factors are associated with longevity, there is no simple formula or collection of traits that guarantees any one of us a long life.

Heredity and Parental Influences

A running joke among gerontologists when asked how best to live long is the response, "The best way to live long is to choose long-lived parents." Clearly, longevity has a genetic component. For example, both life span and cause of death are more similar in identical twins than in fraternal twins. Parental longevity is significantly correlated with longevity of the offspring—an observation that is likely related to both genes and parenting style. Parents probably influence the longevity of their children in the way they raise them—by their diet, activity level, their ways of managing stress, and whether or not they have harmful habits (such as being a couch potato or a smokestack). Further support for the theory that genes are the basis of longevity is the wealth of research conducted to better understand the relationship of genes and disease. The Human Genome Project, an awe-inspiring attempt to understand the entire human genetic code, is making many exciting discoveries. Genes that play a role in diseases such as diabetes, cancers, and heart disease are being identified. The genes that determine Werner's syndrome, a disease causing rapidly accelerating aging and premature death, have been located and identified.

Gender

There is a strong relationship between gender and longevity. In almost every country, among all racial groups, females live longer than males. This differential holds in all age groups, even in the prenatal period. In those few countries where men live longer than women, researchers have attributed this differential to a high rate of maternal death during childbirth, and in some cases, to the neglect or infanticide of girls. In the United States, men have a higher death rate for the top fifteen causes of death, except for Alzheimer's disease. In 1997, the average life expectancy for males was 73.6 years; for females, it was 79.2. Both genetic and behavioral explanations have been proposed to explain this sex differential in longevity.[1]

An obvious reason why females live longer than males is because, at least in our culture, males are at higher risk for accidents, homicide, and suicide, and are more likely to smoke and drink excessively than females. Also, men are less likely to visit doctors and practice positive health behaviors than women. However, they do engage in more physical activity than women. Experts believe that

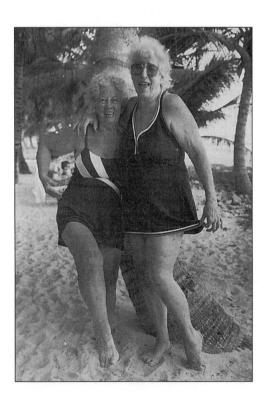

much of the sex differential in mortality is due to males' aggressive and competitive personality, which causes them to participate in more risky behaviors. Although these factors certainly account for some of the difference in life expectancy, they do not account for all of them.

Since females of almost all animal species have a longer life expectancy, scientists hypothesize that females have a genetic advantage that enables them to live longer than males. The physiological basis for this advantage is the subject of ongoing research.[2] The X chromosome (females have two, males have one) carries important genes for immune system functioning and possibly those that repair damage within the cell. This might make females more resistant to infectious diseases and cell damage. Females may also produce more antioxidant chemicals that inactivate harmful chemicals and prevent damage to genetic material. The X chromosome also directs production of sex hormones, namely estrogens. Estrogens influence blood levels of cholesterol, producing more high-density lipoproteins (HDL, or "good" cholesterol) and less low-density lipoproteins (LDL, or "bad" cholesterol). Estrogens also protect women against heart disease, atherosclerosis, and osteoporosis. Females become more susceptible to these conditions after menopause, when estrogen production is reduced. However, even then, their rate of heart disease is lower than their male counterparts. Women also have lower metabolic rates than men, which may partly explain their increased longevity.

In the past, it was believed that testosterone, produced in greater quantity by men than women, was responsible for the differences in life expectancies. Testosterone is produced in the male testes and in the adrenal glands in both sexes. Before laws to protect people who participated in research were in effect, one study of mentally retarded adults found that castration (removal of the testes) increased life expectancy; castrated men lived an average of 13.5 years longer than their virile counterparts and 6.7 years longer than women.[3] However, current research suggests that the picture is much more complicated. Men with lower levels of testosterone and other androgens (male hormones) actually have higher mortality than those with higher levels, and the range of "normal" is very broad. Testosterone replacement therapy can improve cholesterol levels, mood, muscle mass, and sexual function in men who have abnormally low levels of testosterone. It is clear that too little is known about hormones to fully explain the gender differences in longevity.

Ethnicity

Life expectancy varies significantly among ethnic groups in the United States. For instance, African Americans, Hispanic Americans, and Native Americans have a shorter life expectancy than whites. Higher mortality rates for most nonwhite groups are not due to genetic factors, but primarily to the consequences of poverty and discrimination. African Americans, Native Americans, and Hispanic Americans have significantly lower incomes than their white counterparts, resulting in poorer diet and limited access to adequate medical care. Psychological stress, related to social position, low income, and discrimination, may also play a role.

Cigarette Smoking

Experts agree that the single-most important action an individual can take to increase life expectancy is to not smoke cigarettes. The link between tobacco use, serious health problems, and decreased life expectancy is well documented. People who smoke cigarettes die significantly earlier than those who do not, mainly because of an increased incidence of lung cancer and heart disease. The risk of illness and death is directly related to the degree of cigarette smoke exposure: number of cigarettes smoked per day, total years of smoking, and degree of inhalation. The Surgeon General's Reports estimate that 30 percent of both cancer and cardiovascular disease deaths are caused by cigarette smoking[4,5] But the good news is that quitting decreases the rate of disease and premature death. Healthy people who quit smoking between age thirty and seventy-four will gain approximately three years of life, with higher gains for those who

stop when younger.[6] Insurance companies are well aware of the higher mortality rates of smokers and offer reduced premiums for nonsmokers.

Genetic and Acquired Disease

Genetic and acquired diseases significantly determine life expectancy. Many inherited genetic diseases (e.g., hemophilia, sickle cell anemia, Down's syndrome, and juvenile diabetes) and acquired health problems (heart disease, cancer, and Alzheimer's disease) decrease life expectancy.

Obesity

A number of epidemiological studies report a correlation between obesity and decreased life expectancy in humans. Obesity has been correlated with an increased risk of sudden death and increased likelihood of those diseases that increase mortality rate: diabetes, coronary heart disease, and hypertension. However, there is a controversy about whether obesity itself creates a decreased life expectancy or whether obesity accompanies other more important risk factors, such as sedentary lifestyle or high-fat diet, which cause premature death.

Physical Activity

Most experts agree that a high level of physical activity retards many age-associated changes, reduces the incidence of some diseases, and increases longevity. The physiological benefits of physical activity that influence longevity are well-documented: exercise strengthens the heart, decreases the likelihood of obesity, increases the good cholesterol in the blood, and reduces blood clot formation. These benefits will be more fully discussed in the chapter on physical activity.

Many studies have documented that a higher level of physical activity is associated with a lower death rate, not only from heart disease but from all causes of mortality. The higher the degree of fitness, the lower the risk of death. Even individuals who increase their activity level in midlife can realize a significant reduction in death rate. Although fewer studies have documented the relationship of high physical activity and longevity among women and older people, results thus far indicate similar benefits. Studies are being conducted now to determine the level of physical activity needed to increase length of life.

Alcohol Use

Light consumption of alcohol is associated with health benefits. Light drinkers reduce their risk of death from cardiovascular disease by one-third, and reduce their overall death rate by about 10 percent, compared to those who abstain.[7] Light to moderate use is defined as one to two drinks a day. Suggested biological mechanisms for the benefits of alcohol are that alcohol increases the production of certain beneficial types of blood cholesterol (HDLs), and alcohol may decrease the clotting tendencies of the blood.

It is still not clear whether the association of alcohol consumption with longer life is due primarily to the alcohol consumption itself. For example, it may be that moderate drinkers as a group have other lifestyle characteristics in common that predispose them to living longer. As a group, teetotalers have a lower socioeconomic status than moderate drinkers. They may also have more rigid personalities that make them more susceptible to stress. On the other hand, it may be that those who do not drink have health problems that prohibit them from drinking, including alcoholism.

Heavy drinking (drinking three or more alcoholic drinks a day) is associated with reduced life expectancy and a higher risk for a number of physical and mental health disorders, such as liver damage, nutritional deficiencies, cardiovascular problems, nervous system conditions, suicide, accidents, and certain cancers. Heavy drinkers also are at significantly higher risk of early death.

Marital Status

Data gathered on deaths and death rates for the United States in 1996 clearly show that people who were married at the time of their death lived longer than those who were widowed or divorced. And people who never married had the highest death rates. The never married group had over twice the rate of death (117 percent) of those who were married. The death rates for the widowed and divorced were 86 percent and 78 percent higher than those who were currently married at the time of their death.[8]

Exactly how might marriage promote longevity? Studies consistently show that individuals with few social relationships have more illnesses and die earlier from a variety of causes than those who have a good social support network.[9] The advantage of being married, it seems, is not just a matter of togetherness. Marriage also promotes healthful habits. Excessive rates of smoking and drinking are more common among the single, divorced, and widowed than among married men.[10] Another reason may be that a proportion of those who remain single or get divorced may have

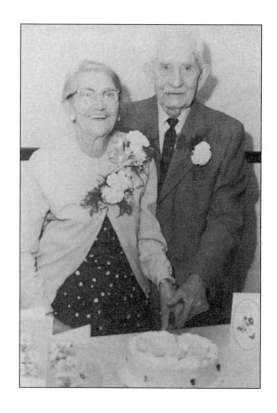

mental or physical illnesses or disabilities that predispose them to an earlier death.

Since societal mores still regard married life as the ideal, being single may induce stress. The stress of losing a spouse of many decades during old age may also contribute to the shortened life expectancy observed among those not currently married when death occurs. The increasing trend of couples to live together, gaining the benefits of marriage without the formalities, may alter these statistics in the future.

Psychological Factors

Mounting evidence supports the hypothesis that some people are resilient to the effects of stress and disease while others are vulnerable and disease-prone. It is hypothesized that negativity in daily interactions, or a repressed/depressed personality style wherein bad feelings are "bottled up," may be associated with a high risk of illness and premature death, comparable to having high blood pressure or high cholesterol.[11] Personality traits, such as bitterness, hostility, and a suspicious, frustrated nature, are associated with increased cardiovascular disease and premature death. Conversely, individuals able to handle stress constructively may live longer. Such personality traits may influence longevity by affecting hormones, immune function, cholesterol level, or other biochemical processes within the body. Further, negative personality characteristics may predispose some individuals to select life-shortening behavioral patterns (such as smoking cigarettes and drinking alcohol).

Social Class: Education, Income, and Occupation

Because income level, education, occupation, and social class are so closely interrelated, it is difficult to isolate which are the most important determinants of longevity. High education level and occupational level are correlated with a higher income and standard of living. And people in the middle and upper classes live considerably longer than those in the lower classes. It is clear that higher educational attainments and social class, more prestigious occupations, and above-average income levels contribute to greater longevity.

Cultural Factors

It is well-documented that life expectancy varies widely from one country to the next. In general, people from developed countries have a longer life expectancy than those from less-developed countries. However, much of the influence on life expectancy in less-developed countries is explained by their increased rates of infant and maternal mortality; many individuals die very young, but others can live to be very old. Multiple factors affect rates of longevity, such as sanitation and prevalence of infectious diseases, dietary factors, and access to health care.

Physical Environment

A number of factors in the external environment may affect longevity. Radiation, air pollution, radon, water quality, and the geochemical environment have been associated with variations in life expectancy.

Humans are exposed to low levels of radiation every day. This low-level radiation can impair cell function by causing mutations in the genetic code. Higher levels of radiation can shorten life by accelerating the aging process. Radiation is thought to damage the immune system, making the body less resistant to infection. Leukemia and tumor development are more prevalent after irradiation. Researchers estimate that a single radiation dose of one roentgen ages humans the equivalent of five to ten days.[12]

Death rates in areas with dense air pollution are higher than those in pollution-free communities. As the threats of ground-water pollution, acid rain, and increased pollution of air and water increase with technological advancements, it is likely that the effects of pollution on human health and longevity will be greater.

BIOLOGIC THEORIES OF AGING

There is probably no area of scientific inquiry that abounds with as many untested or untestable theories as does the biology of aging.

Leonard Hayflick

With aging, two phenomena are present: a physiological decline in many body systems and an increased prevalence of disease. Each process influences the other; it is difficult to separate how much of the decline is due to disease and how much is a result of aging. Although we have some control over the onset of disease, aging itself is inevitable. But how does it happen? Many scientists have made it their life's work to search for the answer to this question.

Within the past thirty years, many theories of aging have been put forth, with the idea that there was one single process of aging. The theories vary and are dependent on the specialty of the researcher. They were divided into two main camps. Some believed aging results from a series of random, accidental events (i.e., the process of aging could be attributed to an accumulation of errors in important molecules, the results of waste products in the cell, or results of wear and tear). The other camp believed that aging is programmed into the genes, and the master plan is already laid out. There might be death genes, or hormones secreted at a certain time, or another mechanism that directs the cell to die.

Within the last few years, most experts generally concur that one theory will not explain the aging process. Mounting evidence points to many parallel, and often linked, causes, some of which are genetically controlled, that work together to produce the frailty we know as old age.[13] Instead of looking at each theory separately, we will discuss some areas of research that have proved the most promising in understanding the complex and inevitable process of aging.

To begin to understand the aging process, we must first look at individual cells. Human cells cannot grow and divide forever; instead they have a finite life span. For instance, human embryo cells may divide no more than forty to sixty times before death. Leonard Hayflick, a pre-eminent researcher in longevity and aging, reported cells have the capacity to remember their maximum life span: the older the cell donor, the fewer times it divides before it dies.[14] Even if a cell has divided twenty times, is frozen, and then thawed, it continues to reproduce about thirty more times before death. Interestingly, most people die long before they reach the limit of their cells. Hayflick hypothesizes that as the cells gradually grow older, a number of biochemical decrements occur that decrease cell function and reproductive capacity.[15]

Many theories of aging focus on accumulation of cell damage as a key component in cellular aging and death. This damage can be caused by free radicals, waste products or accumulation of errors or cross-linkages in the DNA (the chemical make-up of the genes) within the cell.

Perhaps the most widely accepted theory of cell damage involves free radicals. Free radicals are parts of molecules that have either an extra or missing electron that makes them highly reactive and likely to combine with and destroy essential cell components, especially DNA. Free radicals are the normal by-products of necessary chemical reactions in cells. For instance, free radicals are produced when the cells metabolize oxygen to make energy to maintain itself. Free radicals also occur when the cell is exposed to environmental chemicals (such as tobacco smoke or radiation) or nitrites (used as preservatives).

Fortunately, the body produces enzymes to inactivate free radicals before they cause damage by hooking on and inactivating an important chemical. Also, cells produce enzymes that can repair free radical damage. Melatonin produced in the pineal gland has also been found to be a strong antioxidant. Further, some vitamins and minerals, such as vitamin E, vitamin C, vitamin A, and selenium, help to inactivate free radicals, leading some individuals to supplement their diet to assist in the process.

Although enzymes made by the cells "mop up" much of the damage caused by free radicals, their efficiency wanes with age. The destruction accumulates over time, likely contributing to cell

Overview of Cell Reproduction and Repair

Because many theories of aging focus on the genetics of cells, a basic understanding of cell reproduction and repair is necessary. The body is composed of millions of cells, each specialized for a particular function. Some cells (neurons) conduct electrical messages from one part of the body to another, some cells (blood cells) serve to carry oxygen to body tissues, and some cells (somatic) combine with other cells to form tissues and body organs.

Most cells in the body can reproduce by dividing in two, a process called *mitosis*. After growth and development are completed, mitosis is the usual process for the body to replace damaged cells. Mitosis results in two cells that look identical to the parent cell. If one cell dies, another can divide and make a new one just like it. Cells that can divide are called *mitotic cells*. However, some cells in the body cannot divide after the individual reaches maturity (called *postmitotic cells*). This is true of neurons and muscle cells. Once these cells die, they are never replaced. However, postmitotic cells have complicated mechanisms to repair cellular damage.

The pieces of information that direct cell function, called *genes*, are located on *chromosomes* inside each cell nucleus. Humans have twenty-three chromosome pairs, one of each pair contributed by each parent. Chromosomes are often referred to as DNA because they are composed of deoxyribonucleic acid. Chromosomes carry genetic messages, which direct the cell's assembly of amino acid building blocks into proteins that are ultimately used in the cell for growth, maintenance, and repair. The directions are in a chemical code composed of four types of *nucleotides* (A, C, T, G), each of which stands for a different chemical. These letter nucleotides are arranged on the chromosome in precise three-letter word combinations called *codons* that are interpreted by a compound called ribonucleic acid or RNA. The RNA molecule reads a group, or sentence, of these codons within the cell nucleus. It then moves to the cytoplasm where it directs the synthesis of a specific protein, following the directions specified in the genetic code.

Almost every cell in the body has an identical and complete set of genetic information. Thus a nerve cell in the brain and a cell in the kidney are identical genetically, even thought they have very different functions. Although every cell contains all the information for development and maintenance of the body, only that section of the information that is applicable to a particular cell is used, and the rest of the genetic information is ignored.

A *mutation* is any alteration in the genetic code that can be caused by a number of factors including radiation and chemical exposure. Mutations may be insignificant if they affect a part of the genetic code that is not used by that particular cell or if the cell can easily repair the damage. However, mutations can be lethal to a cell if they affect a gene that is crucial to cell function.

malfunction and eventual cell death. Individuals with high serum levels of antioxidant chemicals and postmenopausal women taking estrogen manifest lower rates of DNA damage.[16]

Free radicals can damage genetic material, especially DNA, preventing it from making important enzymes needed for cell metabolism or from dividing correctly. They can also cause damage to other cell components, such as the mitochondria (site of oxygen metabolism), other cell membranes, or connective tissue. For example, free radical damage to the inner wall of blood vessels can cause abnormal blood clotting and the formation of atherosclerotic plaques, increasing the risk of heart disease and stroke. Damage to connective tissue can cause increased stiffening of the blood vessels and lungs and skin wrinkling.

The effect of free radical damage on the cell's DNA combined with the decreased efficiency of the cell to repair such mistakes, can lead to an accumulation of errors in the genetic material, altering its ability to function properly. This can lead to abnormal cell growth or cancerous tumors. Damage may also reduce cell efficiency if the cell is unable to make key chemicals because of damaged DNA instructions.

Free radical damage is thought to have the greatest impact on the nerve and muscle cells. Because these cells do not commonly divide after maturity, they are likely to be less able to repair damage to their genetic material as they age, ultimately affecting the entire neuromuscular and endocrine system.[17]

It has been suggested that cell growth, maturity, and decline are programmed as part of the DNA within the genes for each cell. Some researchers believe that the ability to self-destruct serves an important function of cells. They assert that in some cases, it is advantageous for a cell to kill itself. For instance, if a cell is infected with a virus or contains tumor potential, it is in the best interest of the organism for the cell to self-destruct. Likewise in the process of maturation and cell division, some cells need to die to make room for new ones. Researchers are seeking special sets of genes that make enzymes that kill the cell.

The immune system is often thought to play a key role in the aging process of cells and eventual cell death. The immune system defends the body against foreign invaders—such as bacteria or viruses, or even incompatible blood products. Components of the immune system are highly skilled at differentiating "self" (natural body components) from "invaders" and destroying all that is foreign, including infected body cells and abnormal or cancerous cells. With age, as errors accumulate, the body is more likely to produce immune cells that make mistakes, inadvertently attacking normal cells or tissues, or failing to attack aberrant ones. Alteration in hormonal levels with advancing age may play an important role in the decline of immune function.

Some questions have been answered about the process of cell deterioration and death, but there remains much more to be learned about this physiological, yet very mystical, process of growing old. We now know that human aging is influenced by many factors: some mechanisms occur inside the cell, and others influence cell function by producing chemicals in another part of the body (the nervous, endocrine, and immune systems). It is evident that free radical damage to cell genetic material and other components is an important contributor to senescence and eventual death.

Both the accidental and programmed theories of how we age have merit. However, it is very difficult at this point to understand the role each plays. Even though we know that a number of changes within the cell are associated with aging, one of the greatest difficulties researchers encounter is determining which changes are the underlying causes of aging and which are only manifestations of a process that originated elsewhere. Most likely, a combination of these events, and some yet undiscovered, contributes to the complex and intriguing process of aging.

Learning more about the biological process of aging will not only satisfy our curiosity regarding how we age, but will also serve to prolong youth and forestall deterioration. Such knowledge will be of most use in combating common degenerative diseases that accompany aging.

ATTEMPTS TO EXTEND LENGTH OF LIFE

Although immortality continues to be beyond our grasp, scientists throughout the world still seek ways to deter aging and extend life. Researchers have not yet discovered the fountain of youth, but their attempts continue to provide a better understanding of why and how we age.

Before we continue, it is important to distinguish the difference between life expectancy and life span. *Life expectancy* is the number of years an individual can expect to live and varies with time period and culture. For instance, the average life expectancy of a female infant born in the United States in 1997 was 79.2 years. As infectious diseases are controlled and health and sanitary conditions improve, life expectancy increases. In contrast, *life span* is the maximum length of time

At Age 121, Oldest Person Takes Up Rap

ARLES, France (AP)–She's old. She's bad. And for her age she's rad.

Jeanne Calment marked her 121st birthday Wednesday by celebrating her appearance on the rap music scene—an art form a century younger than she is.

At Arles' City Hall in southern France, Mrs. Calment celebrated a birthday that calls for 10 dozen candles, plus one. She is blind, nearly deaf and uses a wheelchair, but her mind and her wit are quite intact.

"I'm afraid of nothing, and I don't complain," she said. "I have only one wrinkle, and I'm sitting on it."

The *Guinness Book of World Records* lists Calment as the oldest living person whose birth date can be authenticated by reliable records.

There's a contender for the title—a former slave in Brazil who says she's 124. But because of doubts about Mari do Carmo Geronimo's birth certificate, record-keepers recognize only Mrs. Calment.

All the fuss didn't bother her at her 121st birthday bash. Elegant in a white blouse and black suit, her normally snowy hair purple-rinsed for the occasion, Mrs. Calment sat through a brief ceremony in City Hall's ornate ballroom.

She didn't make a speech, but halfway through the local mayor's long-winded tribute, she asked loudly: "Has he finished yet?"

Mrs. Calment has become Arles' greatest attraction since the artist Vincent Van Gogh, who spent a year here in 1888. She met him that year when he came to her uncle's shop to buy paints, and remembers him as "dirty, badly dressed and disagreeable."

Today, a Paris production company will release "Time's Mistress." On the four-track CD, Mrs. Calment recounts her memories over a musical background of rap, techno and farandole, a regional dance tune dating to the Middle Ages.

From *Chico Enterprise-Record* Feb 22, 1996 © Associated Press.

---

an individual can live under ideal conditions. Thus, even though life expectancy has increased, life span has remained relatively constant at 110 to 120 years for the past 2,000 years of human evolution. The purported age of Methuselah in the Bible and, more recently, reports of extreme longevity among inhabitants of remote mountain villages have not been substantiated. A French woman, Jeanne Calment, holds the world record for longevity. She was 122 years old when she died in 1997.

This section will discuss selected research attempts to increase length of life. The following attempts are more likely to increase life expectancy, rather than life span. Because most experiments have been conducted on animal subjects, the effect of these treatments on human longevity cannot be directly measured and is largely hypothetical.

Caloric Restriction

Studies to determine the relationship between calorie restriction and life extension have been ongoing for more than half a century, and the relationship is now well-documented in small laboratory animals. The pioneering studies of Cornell University researcher, Clive McCay, found that underfeeding rats right after weaning significantly extended their life.[18] One group was fed a normal, well-balanced diet while the other ingested the same vitamins and minerals, but only one-third the calories. The rats on the restricted diet had slower growth and development and were smaller in size than the control group, but they lived 60 percent longer than those on a normal diet. Subsequent research decades later confirmed and expanded McCay's original findings. Not only was there an increase in longevity, but there were also delays in almost all age-associated diseases: tumors, heart disease, kidney disease, and autoimmune disease.[19]

Although some of the same physiological results might be expected in humans, conducting such studies would be impossible. But, the closest species to humans are primates. Currently, an extensive long-term study is underway to determine the calorie-restricting effects on long-lived animals, specifically with rhesus monkeys. Half are receiving as much food as they like, and the

Historical Attempts to Postpone Aging

Throughout history, individuals of nearly every culture have sought to prolong youth and postpone the inevitable aging process. Perhaps the best-known seeker of immortality was Ponce de Leon, who set sail to find the fountain of youth, thought to exist on the isle of Bimini, but who arrived in Florida instead.

Myths abound regarding the relationship of sexuality and longevity. Some people have attempted to prolong youth by increasing sexual activity, restraining from ejaculation, or encouraging abstinence. The Shakers, a nearly extinct religious sect in the United States, believed that sexual abstinence prolonged the length of life. Conversely, to ensure long life one ancient sect in central India participated in ritual sexual activity with special sacred prostitutes.

Others believed semen to have special life-enhancing powers. Ko Hung, a fourth-century Chinese philosopher, believed the loss of semen from a man's body would shorten life, but prolonged sexual activity would lengthen it. He advised, "the art of commerce with a woman consists in refraining from ejaculation. I must admit," he also lamented, "that I have not yet personally gotten all the directions involved in the art."[20] In the late nineteenth century, a renowned French professor injected himself with an extract of crushed dog testicles and reported that it restored the strength and vitality of his youth. Around the same period, vain attempts were made in America to graft ape and goat testicles onto aging men to increase virility and vitality.[21]

The Roman Hermippus attributed his long life (115 years) to inhaling the breath of young maidens (or young boys, depending on the translator). Much later other immortalists believed aging to be caused by deleterious toxins in the intestines that had to be diluted by buttermilk and yogurt or purged with daily enemas or strong laxatives.[21]

These attempts to postpone aging seem foolhardy, but most modern attempts are as ineffective. Our magazines advertise that royal queen bee jelly, youth tonics, negative ion generators, or oriental herb remedies will produce miraculous results for only $29.95 plus tax. The wistful search for eternal youth continues as it has since the dawn of civilization—only the methods change with time and culture.

---

other half are receiving 30 percent fewer calories. It will be decades before the study is completed, but thus far, those monkeys who receive less food have lower blood pressure, better cholesterol readings, lower diabetes risk, slower metabolism, and a slightly lower body temperature. The study will also look at the effects on cognition and behavior.[22]

How caloric restriction extends life and reduces disease is not clear. Some experts assert that a slower metabolism reduces the amount of oxygen consumed, and fewer free radicals are produced from oxygenation to damage cells, especially DNA and the energy-producing mechanism of the cell, the mitochondria.[23] Underfeeding may also increase the cell's ability to repair damage from free radicals. Finally, it may reduce the chance that the genes that might cause cancer will be expressed. Underfeeding may result in reduced cell turnover, decreased metabolic rate, and delayed maturity. On the other hand, Hayflick hypothesizes that those animals that receive all the food they want were overfed, so those animals were likely exhibiting a shortened life expectancy when compared to their natural state of underfeeding in the wild.[24]

Even if caloric restriction is shown to be beneficial, it is unlikely that many Americans will significantly alter their diets to take advantage of its benefits. Experience has shown how difficult it is to get people to make health behavioral changes known to extend life (such as reducing dietary fat intake or stopping smoking). The dietary regimens imposed on laboratory animals are far too severe for human subjects who might be less willing to trade stunted growth, delayed maturity, or hunger pains for the possibility of a longer life.

Melatonin

Another interesting offshoot of the studies on caloric restriction is the observation that mice on calorie-restricted diets have higher levels of melatonin in their blood than their counterparts on regular diets. Melatonin is a hormone that is released from the pineal gland in the brain, mostly at night, and its levels decrease with age. It is already known to be important in inducing sleep and coordinating cyclic processes in the body. This hormone seems very important in "phase shifting," the re-setting of the biological clock for travelers (jet lag), the blind, and those who must work at night.

Melatonin has been hyped in the popular press as an antiaging substance. It is a very powerful antioxidant, it may boost the immune system, and, since it decreases with age, supplementation might improve many age-associated declines. Although the compound is relatively nontoxic, incorrect or poorly timed dosages can interfere with the body's natural biological clock. Further, the dosages in the health food stores are more than needed to fall asleep or to improve sleep quality. Thus far, no studies report an anti-aging effect of melatonin in humans. The National Institute on Aging is planning to study melatonin's safety and long-term effects.

DHEA

Dihydroepiandrostenedione (DHEA) is probably the most popular anti-aging drug in our country at this time. The promoters of this drug assert it to be a panacea for aging, reducing a wide variety of illnesses. DHEA is made from cholesterol by the adrenal glands and can be easily converted to estrogen and testosterone in the body. It is also one of the most common hormones in the body. The level of DHEA increases at puberty, peaks in the 20s and 30s, then rapidly declines and, by the age of 70, is only about 20 percent of that present in young adulthood. It has been documented that people with high naturally occurring levels of DHEA have better health and a longer life than those with lower levels. However, no studies have been conducted to show that low DHEA levels are responsible.

Many researchers suspect that DHEA deficiency in older persons is an important contributor to immune system declines, problems with insulin metabolism, and increasing rates of cancer with age.[25] Preliminary animal and human studies find DHEA supplementation may protect against heart disease (men only), enhance immunity, improve cholesterol readings, increase insulin sensitivity, and generate an enhanced well being. But not one of these benefits has yet been shown in a large randomized placebo-controlled clinical trial. The National Institute on Aging supports animal research of DHEA to study its anti-aging effects, but more research needs to be conducted on humans to document the benefits of treatment and the risks of side effects.

DHEA is fraught with problems. Because it is a hormone that is converted to testosterone and estrogen in the body, it has potential side effects, especially among women: breast cancer, reduced levels of good cholesterol, growth of facial hair, and possibly increased rate of heart disease. It may increase prostate cancer. Studies of DHEA often use laboratory animals, lack control groups, or study people with abnormally low DHEA levels; little is known about who would benefit from treatment. Preparations available in health food stores often contain extremely small dosages that are insufficient to cause a biological effect in humans (doses of 25 to 50 mg/day are required). Also, taking the hormone for long periods of time might suppress the body's ability to manufacture its own DHEA and possibly other hormones, with a variety of consequences.[26] Finally, the long-term effects of this powerful hormone are still unknown.

Despite the preliminary nature of the results, health stores, newspapers and magazines, and even the Internet are promoting the "fountain of youth" drug to the unsuspecting public. Even though some preliminary studies show promise, most scientists believe it is premature to recommend the hormone DHEA to anyone as there is insufficient evidence of its dosage, purity, and long-term effects.[27]

Antioxidant Therapy

High blood levels of antioxidants are associated with longevity and a reduced risk of heart disease and cancer. New research suggests that antioxidants may also delay the development of Alzheimer's disease.[28] People who consume diets high in antioxidants, including fresh fruits and vegetables and whole grains, also have a greater life expectancy. Although evidence is inconclusive at this point, some scientists believe that dietary supplements of antioxidants may reduce the cell damage caused by free radicals. Antioxidants include the vitamins A, beta-carotene, C, E, and bioflavenoids and the minerals selenium, manganese, copper, zinc, and molybdenum.

Large-scale studies are ongoing to test whether antioxidant supplements are effective in reducing illness and extending life. In light of such findings, many gerontologists and laypeople supplement their diets with antioxidant vitamins "just in case." However, overdoses of some vitamins and minerals (especially vitamin E and selenium), although rare, may be harmful. Further, antioxidant formulations in pill form often do not contain the wide variety of antioxidant chemicals found in whole foods, particularly fresh produce and grains. See the nutrition chapter for further discussion of antioxidant supplements.

Prescription Drugs

The public forks over millions of dollars each year on quick-fix treatments to live longer (or just look more youthful). Hoping for longevity, many people take megadoses of vitamins or amino acid concentrates. Others order life-enhancing compounds by mail or travel to other countries to receive "live-cell" injections or drugs not approved in the United States.

Researchers continue to develop drugs that may allow people to live longer, healthier lives. One widely used medication, estrogen, taken by women after menopause when their own production of this hormone slows dramatically, may be very effective at life extension by decreasing the rate of cardiovascular disease, the number-one killer of American women.

Other drugs already in use may someday be used to slow the aging process. Deprenyl, a drug approved for Parkinson's disease and depression, shows promise in slowing some aging processes.[29] Advocates believe that deprenyl protects brain cells that make dopamine, a brain chemical controlling body movements. Controlled experiments with rats given deprenyl show an increase in longevity, sexual functioning, and learning performance. However, the use of deprenyl for increasing life expectancy and improving function in normal elders is still experimental.

In 1990, a flurry of excitement occurred when researchers reported their results of experiments with human growth hormone injections on a small group of elderly men. They asserted that as people age, the secretion of the growth hormone by the pituitary gland declines quickly, causing many physiological deficits. They provided evidence that the hormone reversed some of the age-related decline in muscle and fat accumulation, and their subjects looked younger and leaner.[30] Similar results were reported among elderly women. Growth hormone is available only by prescription. It is administered by self-injection, and the cost for a year's treatment is more than $12,000.

Several years later, another group of researchers experimented again with a group of older men, this time to find out if the hormone would increase their muscle strength. Although they did confirm that lean body mass increased and fat mass dropped, the men had no change in muscle strength or endurance. They concluded that the drug made no improvement in elders' functioning.[31] Further, excess growth hormone may cause hypertension, diabetes, and nausea, to name a few. Currently, the National Institute on Aging is funding clinical studies at several centers throughout the United States to see if the hormone can reduce frailty among older people.

Scientists in Europe prescribe more anti-aging drugs for their patients than do American physicians. Many drugs are only available for use in Europe since they have not been approved for use in the United States. Some may turn out to be extremely useful, while others are likely to be nostrums. Piracetam and L059—drugs purported to enhance memory, attention span, and learning—are prescribed in Europe for healthy elders. Another drug, centrophenoxine, thought to have both antioxidant and memory-improving properties, increases the longevity of laboratory animals. It is used in Europe for reversal of normal aging as well as for elders with dementia. Phosphatidylserine, a component of cell membranes, may help stabilize membranes or affect neurotransmitters in the brain. In double-blind studies in the United States and abroad on Alzheimer's patients, the drug improved memory, and benefits persisted after the drug was discontinued. Again, this drug has not been approved by the FDA.

A perusal of even the most reputable methods of extending productive life reveals that, although some hold promise, very few have large-scale placebo-controlled trials on human subjects that support their effectiveness. Clearly, much of their success is likely due to a "placebo effect," namely a *belief* that the treatment is working. Treatments that either promote longer life or postpone the diseases and symptoms of old age will continue to make headlines. As consumers, it is important to make rational decisions about new longevity treatments that do nothing more than give false hope and take our money.

What is Your Opinion? The Consequences of Life Extension

Scientists' projections of a future in which all people live to be very old are largely speculative and dependent upon many variables. Will science find a means to extend life expectancy to the current maximum of 110 to 120 years? Will the life span be extended to 200 years or more? Will humans be able to retain youthful physiques until death, or will they just age more slowly?

Not everyone believes life extension is desirable. More people living longer would strain our environmental and economic resources. More old people would mean a limited space for the young and more pressure on our food supply and energy demand. Further, a higher proportion of older people will be retired and will need to be supported by a smaller proportion of working adults. Even if life expectancy increased by only ten years, drastic policy adjustments would be needed for retirement, Social Security, and Medicare.

The possible consequences of life extension on our political, economic, social, and value systems are approached more often by science fiction writers than gerontologists. If there were more old people and fewer young, would this decrease the influx of creative new ideas or would even more knowledge accumulate on the basis of elders' wisdom? Would the government have to interfere with the freedom to bear children to curb overpopulation? If the old no longer experienced the physical symptoms of aging, what effect might this have on our culture? Would people devote more energy to avoid overpopulation, pollution, and nuclear war if they lived longer to personally experience the consequences?

The goal of research on life extension is to expand the number of productive years with the highest level of physical health and mental abilities. To live longer without vitality is a foolish, even cruel, endeavor. Some may consider the time and money spent on such research as futile. On the other hand, when a method to prolong our good years is discovered, which of us would turn down the opportunity?

Some gerontologists believe that the quest to extend life in the laboratory is misplaced. They assert that the goal should not be to extend the length of life, but to enhance the quality of life in the later years by modifying the factors that we already know to affect the rate of aging and onset of disease (e.g., cigarette smoking). In this way, the individual remains healthy and vital until the very last days of life, then dies quickly. Good health habits, a rewarding social situation, and a positive mental attitude are more likely to extend life than the treatments discussed above.

Man's subconscious quest for a measure of immortality continues unabated; yet paradoxically, he jeopardizes his small share in the immortality of his species by his actions.

Leonard Schuman

SUMMARY

One of life's enduring questions is, "Why do we age, and how might it be prevented, or at least postponed?" We now know there are many and varied factors that influence the length of life. A number of genetic determinants, such as gender, ethnicity and race, familial history, and predisposition to genetic diseases play a role. However, there are a number of factors that are associated with a longer life that are under our control: eating healthfully, abstaining from cigarette smoking, participating in regular physical activity, and learning how to cope with stress. Changing our destructive habits may not guarantee a longer life, but it will at least increase our chance for a healthier old age.

A number of gerontologists are conducting experiments to support hypotheses on why and how we age at the cellular level. To better understand why the body deteriorates, even in the absence of disease, researchers are trying to understand the genetic basis of aging and how the endocrine and immune systems fit into the aging puzzle. They have already documented the importance of the finite life span of our body cells and the accumulation of damage to cells, predominantly from free radicals.

Based on epidemiological associations and biological theories of aging, researchers are studying many ways to prolong life. Perhaps the best is dietary restriction, whereby laboratory animals maintain better health and longer lives if fed a well-balanced diet that is low in calories. Other methods show promise, but they have not been subject to rigorous scientific scrutiny in humans. Some methods may affect life expectancy, the amount of time an individual can expect to live, but few affect life span, the maximum time a human can live, which is 110 to 120 years. Thus far, no "magic bullet" has been discovered that ensures a longer life. Although more difficult than mindlessly swallowing a pill, the tried-and-true way to improve the quality of remaining life, and perhaps its length, is to begin a program to change negative health behaviors (such as stopping smoking, increasing physical activity, losing weight, or altering diet). In the long haul, it will show more results than the "quick fix" of unproven longevity drugs.

ACTIVITIES

1. What is the single-most important thing you could do to prolong your life? What is the most difficult? How long do you want to live? Ask these questions to people of different ages—your parents, grandparents, children. How do their answers differ? Why?

2. Collect and analyze five advertisements from magazines or newspapers that boast their product's ability to increase or reduce the rate of aging. How could you determine if they are fraudulent?

3. Devise an experiment or set of experiments where you attempt to isolate one of the factors that

influence longevity. Would your experiment show a causal relationship or merely a correlation between the factor and longevity? Can you see the difficulty in isolating one factor?

4. If everyone lived to be 120 years old, what would be the effect on our society—politically, socially, economically, medically, and psychologically? What might some of the consequences be, and how might we surmount them?

5. How long do you want to live? Why? Would you want to live longer if you could be guaranteed good health? Do you think it would be a good idea to extend the life span? Why or why not?

6. Debate: Life extension studies should be supported by the United States government.

7. Imagine that you are given an opportunity to take an anti-aging drug guaranteed to double your life span. Would you take it? Why or why not?

8. Interview a long-lived individual. What personal characteristics enabled he or she to live long? Can you see additional positive characteristics ? Write up the material in the form of a biography.

BIBLIOGRAPHY

1. Ventura, S. J., Anderson, R.N., Martin, J.A., et al. 1998. *Births and deaths: Preliminary data for 1997. National vital statistics reports,* vol. 47, no. 4 Hyattsville, MD: National Center for Health Statistics.

2. Magnani, M., and Accorsi, A. 1993. The female longevity phenomenon. *Mechanisms of Aging and Development* 72:89–95.

3. Hamilton, J.B. 1948. The role of testicular secretions as indicated by the effects of castration in men and by studies of pathological condition and the short life span associated with maleness. *Recent Progress in Hormone Research* 3:357–322.

4. U.S. Department of Health and Human Services, report of the Surgeon General. 1982. *The health consequences of smoking: Cancer.* Washington, D.C.: Public Health Service.

5. U.S. Department of Health and Human Services, report of the Surgeon General. 1983. *The health consequences of smoking: Cardiovascular disease.* Washington, D.C.: Public Health Service.

6. Grover, S.A., Gray-Donald, K., Joseph, L., Abrahamowicz, M., and Coupal, L. 1994. Life expectancy following dietary modification or smoking cessation. *Archives of Internal Medicine* 154:1697–704.

7. Klatsky, A.L., and Friedman, G.D. 1995. Annotation: alcohol and longevity. *American Journal of Public Health* 85:16–18.

8. Peters, K.D., Kochanek, K.D., and Murphy, S.L. 1988. *Deaths: final data for 1996. National vital statistics reports,* vol. 47 no. 9. Hyattsville, MD: National Center for Health Statistics.

9. House, J.S., Landis, K.R., and Umberson, D. 1988. Social relationships and health. *Science* 241:540–44.

10. Rosengren, A., Wedel, H., and Wilhemsen, L. 1989. Marital status and mortality in middle-aged Swedish men. *Journal of Epidemiology* 129:54–64.

11. Friedman, H.S., Hawley, P.H., and Tucker, J.S. 1994. Personality, health and longevity. *Current Directions of Psychological Science* 3:37–41.

12. Hershey, D. 1974. *Lifespan and factors affecting it.*

13. Rusting, R.L. 1992. Why do we age? *Scientific American* December: 130–41.

14. Hayflick, L. 1961. The limited *in vitro* lifetime of human diploid cell strains. *Experimental Cell Research* 37:614–36.

15. Hayflick, L. 1975. Current theories of biological aging. *Federation Proceedings* 34:9–13.

16. Wei, Q., Matanoski, G.M., Farmer, E.R., et al. 1993. DNA repair and aging in basal cell carcinoma: a molecular epidemiology study. *Proceedings of the National Academy of Science, USA* 90:1614–18.

17. Strehler, B.L. 1980. A critique of theories of biological aging. In *Aging—its chemistry,* A.A. Dietz, ed. Washington, D.C.: American Association for Clinical Chemistry.

18. McCay, C.M., and Maynard, L.A. 1939. Retarded growth, life span, ultimate body size and age changes in the albino rat after feeding diets restricted in calories. *Journal of Nutrition* 18:1–13.

19. Walford, R.L. 1990. The clinical promise of diet restriction. *Geriatrics* 45:81–87.

20. Long, K. 1989. Historical notes: *Longevity* June:88.

21. Walford, R.L. 1983. *Maximum life span.* New York: Norton & Co.

22. Mlot, C. 1997. Running on one-third empty. *Science News* 151:162–63.

23. Weindruch, R. 1996. Caloric restriction and aging. *Scientific American* January 46–52.

24. Hayflick, L. 1996. *How and why we age.* New York: Ballentine Books.

25. Casson, P.R., and Buster, J.E. 1995. DHEA administration to humans: Panacea or palaver? *Seminars in Reproductive Endocrinology* 13:247–56.

26. Rosch, P.J. 1995. DHEA, electrical stimulation, and the fountain of youth (editorial). *Stress Medicine* 11:211–14.

27. Skolnick, A.A. 1996. Scientific verdict still out on DHEA. *Journal of the American Medical Association* 276:1365–1367.

28. Harman, D. 1993. Free radical theory of aging. A hypothesis on pathogenesis of senile dementia of the Alzheimer's type. *Age* 16:23–30.

29. Parkinson's Study Group. 1989. Effect of deprenyl on the progression of disability in early Parkinson's disease. *New England Journal of Medicine* 331:1364–371.

30. Rudman, D., Feller, A.G., Nagraj, H.S., et al. 1990. Effects of human growth hormone in men over 60 years old. *New England Journal of Medicine* 323:1–6.

31. Papadakis, M.A., Grady, D., Black, D., et al. 1996. Growth hormone replacement in healthy older men improves body composition but not functional ability. *Annals of Internal Medicine* 124:708–16.

THE BODY AND ITS
AGE CHANGES

How old would you be if you didn't know how old you was?

Satchel Paige

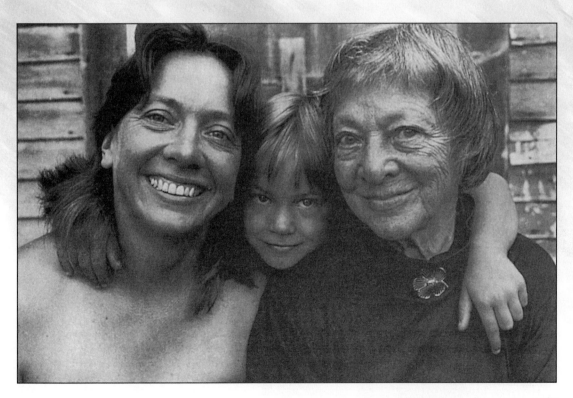

If you were asked to list the ways the human body changes as it ages, you would probably start with wrinkled skin and graying hair. As obvious as these changes are to the casual observer, they have no effect on a person's physical health. Other changes associated with the aging process, although not as visible, are more likely to result in reduced efficiency of some body systems and organs. These include inherited traits and environmental factors, such as chronic diseases, exercise and dietary history, and cigarette smoking. It is very difficult to separate these factors from the aging process itself.

This chapter will describe the role and function of each body system and its major age-associated changes. The term "age-associated" will be used throughout the text to describe changes that commonly occur with age. Even though many of these changes are inevitable, it must be stressed that the rate of decline is highly variable, with many older adults maintaining functional abilities that rival those many years younger. We have all seen extra-ordinarily "young" eighty-year-olds and inordinately "old" forty-year-olds.

STUDYING THE PHYSIOLOGICAL PROCESS OF AGING

It is important to take a scientific approach to the study of physiological aging to distinguish normal aging processes from those resulting from disease or lifestyle. How can this best be accomplished? The easiest way to determine if a physiological change is due to age is to conduct a cross-sectional study. Gather a sample of healthy older adults, measure a physiological variable (e.g., the extent of muscle mass in the upper arm), and compare these results with the same measurements in a sample of young adults.

However, cross-sectional research has several limitations. First, there is a "cohort effect." Every generation is somewhat different than the next. For example, elders over 70 years may be less likely to engage in regular physical activity, both now and

---

Measuring Age Changes

If there is a single indisputable fact about normal aging, it is the magnitude of individual variability. Take gray hair, for instance. We all know people who began to gray in their twenties and others who do not gray until they reach sixty or later. If we choose at random men in their twenties, forties, and sixties to study graying of hair, we might conclude that gray hair begins in the twenties, disappears in the forties (because by chance we chose middle-aged men who were not gray), and reappears in the sixties. Or that gray hair never occurs (because we happened to choose only men who were not gray or who were completely bald). This is called a cross-sectional study and, as the examples indicate, it is often a flawed method for studying age changes. The changes seen in such a study can be associated with aging only by inference—a dangerous business.

The best way to study age changes is by doing a longitudinal study. To study the graying of men's hair longitudinally, one would choose the largest number of young men possible, then study each one periodically until he ages or dies. In this way you would find the truth—that as men grow older the likelihood that their hair will turn gray increases, although the graying may start at a different time in each participant. You can also determine the rate of graying (for example, the number of gray hairs per year), which cannot be done in a cross-sectional study.

A story presently circulating in gerontological circles illustrates the dangers of interpreting cross-sectional studies in aging. It seems that a group of naive gerontologists decided to do a cross-sectional study on aging in Miami. When the study was complete, they found that most people there are born Hispanic and die Jewish![1]

when they were younger, because such activities were never encouraged. So, in this example, even though older adults would have less muscle mass, it could be erroneously attributed to an "age change" but is probably a reflection of past and present level of physical activity. Secondly, because it is often difficult to distinguish changes due to age from those due to chronic diseases, it is important that subjects are thoroughly examined and found to be healthy. Even when healthy people are chosen, there is usually great variability from one person to another in any age change measured. Finally, there may be a "survivor effect." For example, if obese individuals are more likely to die young than those who are of average or below-average weight, then when older subjects are compared with younger subjects, it appears that weight is lost in the later years. In fact, those who survive into old age have not lost weight.

A longitudinal research design circumvents the limitations of the cross-sectional approach to the study of age changes. The longitudinal approach selects a group of healthy people to study over a long period of time (sometimes decades), regularly taking physiological measurements. Thus, elders are not compared to younger subjects, but to their own past measurements. These studies show how certain physiological measures change over time.

Even longitudinal studies have their drawbacks. They are very costly because individuals need to be measured regularly over a period of several years. And, the people in the sample must commit to be available over the years of the study. Further, those people who volunteer to participate in a long-term study tend to be white, healthier, better educated, and have a higher income than the general elder population. Finally, the outcomes of longitudinal studies might not be available for many years.

DEFINING AGE CHANGES

It is often difficult to distinguish between physiological changes that often accompany old age from those that are due to aging itself. For a decrement to be considered the result of aging, five requirements must be fulfilled.[2] The decline must be *universal,* that is, it occurs in all members of the species to a certain degree. The decline must be *intrinsic* (e.g., caused by age or genetics) and not due to environmental influences. The onset of the decline must be *progressive*—a gradual process rather than a specific event. Changes due to age have to be *irreversible,* although it may be possible to slow the process. Finally, the change must be *deleterious,* that is, must lead to a loss of function.

Although these requirements seem clear-cut, in almost all cases, it remains very difficult to distinguish which physical decrements are due to aging and which are due to other factors. Cross-cultural studies of physiological changes accompanying age are sparse, so the requirement of universality remains unfulfilled in most cases. Additionally, it is virtually impossible for researchers to determine whether a decrement is the result of the aging process, or due to disease, poor diet, physical inactivity, environmental contaminants, mental state, or even decrements in another body system. Furthermore, when the "average" decline is reported, it includes some individuals who maintain or even improve in function and others who are totally debilitated.

Growing old is inevitable, but the rate of aging is highly individual. Chronological age is not a good indicator of biologic age after midlife. Without a doubt, genetic, environmental, and lifestyle differences play an important role in the rate of aging. Furthermore, the degree at which each organ declines varies within each of us. For instance, a seventy-year-old woman may have excellent vision and hearing, but have poor lung capacity. The ability to adapt to such changes also varies among individuals. Some elders adapt easily to heavy losses and are minimally affected in their daily routine, while others have minimal losses but adapt so poorly that they require major lifestyle changes. Whether an elder is debilitated or challenged by a loss of body function depends on the person's physiology, emotional state, and presence of social support.

The study of the physiological age changes of each body system is important in order to differentiate disease states from normal aging processes. Because elders often have chronic illnesses in addition to normal age changes, it is often difficult for health professionals and elders themselves to determine if a complaint is a symptom of disease or "old age." If physicians erroneously attribute symptoms to old age, they may miss treatable conditions. When elders themselves attribute their symptoms to age, they may not seek treatment. For example, an elderly man with severe joint pain that limits his mobility may not bring his problem to the attention of his physician because he believes aches and pains are just part of growing old. In reality, his pain may be due to any of several treatable conditions.

Knowledge of the physiological aging process gives us a realistic view of aging. The body does not suddenly become frail at age sixty-five. Even though there may be some decrements attributed to aging, these do not significantly affect a person's everyday functioning. Alex Comfort believes that most age changes are primarily due to sociological pressures: our youth-oriented society and ageist attitudes affect our feelings of self-worth and do more to age us than the natural physiological process.[3] Further, there is a difference between "usual" aging (what is average for the population) and "successful" aging (achieving the maximal functional capability in the later years).[4]

As Cicero stated, "It is not old age that is at fault, but rather our attitude towards it." Although this chapter focuses on age-related decline, it is important to realize that none of these decrements are serious. The deterioration caused by disease has a much more significant effect on health and lifestyle. Those who understand the physiological changes of aging should not use this knowledge to restrict elder's job access, intellectual pursuits, leisure activities, or to unnecessarily label them as feeble. The intent is not to categorize older people as different, but to emphasize that everyone experiences gradual changes with advancing age. Many changes are occurring in your body even as you read this page—some cells are no longer functioning as effectively, and others are gradually dying. Eventually those changes will be interpreted as signs of aging as they become more visible to us and to those around us.

THE INTEGUMENTARY SYSTEM

The skin and its accessory organs comprise the integument, the largest and most visible body system. The skin has many functions. It protects underlying tissues from harmful environmental influences and minimizes water loss. The large surface of the skin and its capacity to sweat and shiver is important in the regulation of body temperature. Through sweating, the skin also serves to eliminate salts and other waste products. A variety of sensory receptors in the skin permit us to respond to environmental changes such as heat, cold, pain, or light touch. Upon exposure to ultraviolet light, the skin synthesizes vitamin D from a hormone in the skin. Vitamin D plays a vital role in building bone. The subcutaneous fat cushions the body from injury and forms a large part of energy reserves. The skin is also able to absorb certain drugs, and dermal patches are becoming a common method to administer medication.

The skin has two layers: the epidermis (outer layer) and the dermis (inner layer). The epidermis is covered by a layer of dead cells on the skin surface that is constantly worn away as newer cells form beneath. Skin cells thicken and harden as they are pushed toward the surface. The pigment, melanin, is produced in the epidermis and protects the body from sunlight by absorbing light energy. Skin color is dependent upon the amount of melanin in the epidermal cells. Individuals with dark complexions have more melanin than those with fair complexions.

The dermis consists of nerve endings, blood capillaries, hair follicles, sweat and sebaceous oil glands, and connective tissue. The capillaries supply nutrients to all skin cells and are very important in regulating body temperature. When we are too hot, the capillaries dilate and the skin feels warm as heat leaves the body. When we are cold, the capillaries constrict, directing blood away from the skin, towards the body core. Specialized nerve endings, receptive to heat, cold, touch, pressure, and pain, are found in the dermis. The layer below the skin connects the skin to the organs beneath it. It has more blood vessels, nerves, connective tissue, and fat. The fat serves as a shock absorber to protect internal organs, and the blood vessels control body heat.

Age-Associated Changes in the Integumentary System

No one dies of old skin.

Leonard Hayflick

The speed and extent of skin changes vary among individuals and are strongly influenced by heredity, hormone balance, cigarette smoke, and sun exposure. Experts agree that the vast majority of the skin changes we associate with aging are due to too much sun. Only a few facial furrows, such as laugh lines around the eyes and between the nose and upper lip, and others created by habitual facial expressions are believed to be a consequence of aging. The elastin fibers that keep the skin taught loosen over time, allowing the skin to sag.

In general, older skin tends to be more wrinkled, folded, mottled, and dry than younger skin, especially among whites. The skin becomes more fragile and translucent with age due to the thinning of the dermis and epidermis. The connections between the epidermis and the dermis flatten out, making the two layers more easily separable, resulting in an increased propensity for the skin to tear. The skin may also feel rough because the outermost layer of the epidermis cannot replace its cells as readily. Fewer sebaceous glands are available to lubricate the skin. The collagen and elastin connective tissues become less uniform and are replaced with inelastic fibrous tissue, reducing the resilience of the skin. The effect is greatest on skin exposed to sun, and least on unexposed areas.

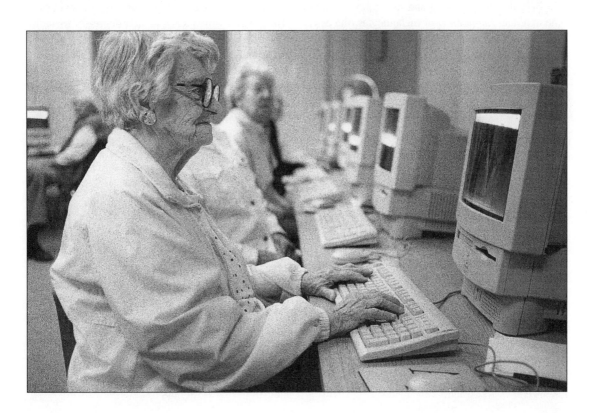

The amount of active sweat ducts in the skin diminishes with age. Although the decline reduces the potential for body odor, it decreases the ability to perspire and to regulate body temperature.

Blood circulation in the skin is reduced with age. This explains why elders feel cold more than do younger people. The capillaries become fragile and more susceptible to rupture with even a slight injury. That is why older people bruise more easily and their wounds heal more slowly. Sunlight accelerates the loss of elasticity in the walls of the capillaries that feed the skin, resulting in a permanent dilation. They are commonly called spider veins. The sun is also thought to damage the walls of the vessels, which also increases the likelihood of bruising.

With advancing age, the skin's ability to produce vitamin D from sunlight is reduced significantly when compared to its production during youth. Obtaining vitamin D from supplemented foods is much more important in the later years.

Both the aging process and sun exposure combine to reduce the number of melanocytes (the cells that produce the pigment melanin) and in turn, melanin production itself. Further, the reduced melanin increases susceptibility to sun damage. The melanin that remains may clump, causing pigmented blotches on the skin or larger dark areas, commonly called liver spots. These can be removed by cryosurgery (freezing with liquid nitrogen), electrocautery (burning with low-dose electricity), or laser surgery (vaporizing with a focused light beam). Retin-A has been documented to fade age spots.

Because the face is more likely to be exposed to sun and wind than the rest of the body, it is the most likely to show damage, especially wrinkles and pigment changes. The skin is stretched when facial muscles move in characteristic expressions. With age, the skin is less likely to return to its original shape so that, by age forty, most have creases that reflect habitual facial expressions. Additionally, solar (actinic) keratosis, or roughened whitish patches, commonly appear on the face and other sun-exposed areas in old age. These may develop into skin cancers and should be monitored by a physician.

Subcutaneous fat smoothes the contours of the body. With advancing age, subcutaneous fat is generally reduced in the face, hands, shins, and feet and increases in the midsection of men and women and the thighs of women. Less subcutaneous fat, combined with diminished skin elasticity and gravity, causes the skin to sag and fold. These changes make underlying bones, tendons, and blood vessels more prominent. A reduction in muscle mass further contributes to the loosening of the skin.

Although most people consider wrinkled, loose, leathery skin a necessary accompaniment to old age, much of the mottling, roughening, and wrinkling is due to sun damage. Sunlight damages elastic fibers in the skin, causing wrinkling and sagging. Sunlight also stimulates the development of age spots and premalignant and malignant (cancerous) skin lesions. A certain degree of irreversible skin damage occurs with each prolonged exposure and accumulates to cause what we call aged skin. Thus, the degree of skin degeneration is directly related to the amount of sun exposure. Black skin, which has a greater degree of melanin, resists sun damage, ages more slowly, and deteriorates much later in life than white skin. Those with freckled or fair complexions, red or blond hair, and blue eyes are most susceptible to sunlight damage to their skin.

Cigarette smoking can profoundly alter the texture of the skin, creating tiny vertical wrinkles around the lips and increased wrinkling in the area around the eyes. This explains why cigarette smokers look about five years older than those who do not smoke.

With advanced age, nails grow more slowly and appear thinner and duller. The crescent at the bottom of the nail may disappear, and the nail may develop longitudinal ridges. Also, the nail may become thickened and hard to cut. Some elders, especially those with deteriorating vision, poor coordination, obesity, or arthritis, may be unable to cut their own toenails. They may need to see a podiatrist to prevent foot discomfort, infections, and mobility problems.

Graying hair in the middle years, widely recognized as an age change, is caused by a reduction

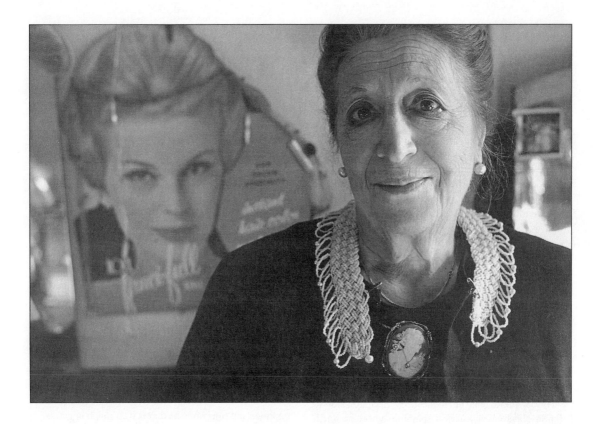

of hair pigment. Almost everyone experiences a change in the texture and thickness of their hair as they grow older. The number of hairs on the scalp, pubic area, and underarms are reduced. In males, some hairs become coarser, particularly on the ear ridges and eyebrows, and in the ears and nostrils. In women, hairs may coarsen on the upper lip and chin because of changes in the balance of sex hormones.

Perhaps the most dramatic alteration in hair distribution is baldness among men. About half of the male population can expect some degree of baldness, which may begin as early as the late teens or not until the late forties. Although both males and females may carry the gene for baldness, the gene must be activated by the male hormone testosterone, so only males are affected. Typically, hair loss begins when hair follicles shrink and produce finer and shorter hair, eventually resulting in a ring of hair above the ears and around the back of the head. Females with the genetic trait do not exhibit baldness, although their hair may thin.

Because baldness is a sign of old age, much money is spent on potions to postpone or reduce hair loss. Minoxidil (Rogaine), a drug for high blood pressure, reduces hair loss in men and women who rub the medication into their scalp daily over a period of several months. This medication is now available over the counter. However, the drug is ineffective in many cases. The individual must have had recent hair loss and it must be in the crown of the head, not the hairline. Even when these stipulations are fulfilled, the drug works only half the time, and even then, the hair that grows back is very fine. Perhaps the biggest drawback is that the drug must be used daily and, when it is stopped, hair loss follows. Further, the cost per month is prohibitive for many, especially due to its spotty success. Research continues on other drugs

What is Your Opinion? Reversing Wrinkles

Everyone wants to live a long life, but no one wants to look old.

Albert Kligman

Although wrinkling and age spots have little effect on longevity, they may profoundly affect feelings of self-worth, especially for people who strive to look youthful. Society places more pressure on women than men to maintain a youthful appearance. Thus, women are a receptive market for a lucrative cosmetic industry that offers formulas to delay wrinkling, age spots, and loosening of skin. Cosmetics do little more than lubricate the superficial layers of the skin, causing it to appear less roughened and dry. Currently, the best way to reduce wrinkles is prevention: reduce sun exposure and don't smoke.

But wrinkles come to all of us to a greater or lesser degree. Many techniques are available to counteract the imprint of the sun upon the skin. To a great extent, the choices depend on the pocketbook. Tiny wrinkles can be reduced by dermabrasion—mild abrasion that uses a spinning wheel or brush that removes the outer skin layer—or a chemical peel that does the same but with acid. When the skin regenerates, it is smoother. A newer technique to remove the sun-damaged outer skin layer is called laser resurfacing. This technique destroys the outer skin layer by using a focused light beam to vaporize the water in the skin cells. No matter how the top layer of skin is removed, the technique depends upon the regeneration of smoother skin during the healing process

Most people rely on creams, many of which do no more than temporarily hydrate the skin. Perhaps the most effective cream documented to reduce the degree of skin wrinkles and some precancerous skin conditions is tretinoin or Retin-A, a vitamin A–derived cream. This drug seems to work by increasing the depth of the epidermis, skin circulation, cell turnover, and connective tissue synthesis. However, the drug can be irritating to some individuals and increases sensitivity to the sun. Currently, it is sold only by prescription in the United States.

Another method of reducing wrinkles is injecting collagen (taken from elsewhere in the body or from cows) into the wrinkle, reducing the shadows caused by wrinkles and skin folds. Collagen injections are temporary, and last up to two years. Silicone implants and injections have received much negative publicity and are no longer recommended. Cosmetic surgery is the most expensive way to look younger and is more effective than the nonsurgical approaches. Common procedures are face lifts, eyelid lifts, and neck tightening.

---

to retard hair loss. Other methods to combat baldness and thinning hair are surgical hair transplants and hairpieces.

THE MUSCULOSKELETAL SYSTEM

Muscles and bones work together to protect and support the organs of the body; preserve body structure, posture, and stability; and enable body movement. The skeleton consists of over 200 bones; cartilage and ligaments bind bones together at the joints. Bone is a specialized type of connective tissue composed of calcium, salts, and some other minerals. Although bones look very inactive, live bone tissue is constantly being reformed as salts in the bone and calcium in the blood are continuously interchanged. The bone stores calcium and other minerals and releases them into the bloodstream when calcium is needed in other parts of the body. The bone also produces red and white blood cells in the bone marrow.

In general, the strength and thickness of bone depends on physical activity. When skeletal muscles contract, they pull on the ligaments attached to the bones, causing the bones to thicken and strengthen. Physical exercise increases bone mass by causing stress on the bones. Without physical activity, bones become weaker and thinner. People who have physically taxing jobs or are athletes have thicker and heavier bones than those who are sedentary. Bones lose calcium with inactivity, thus reducing bone mass and bone strength. In general, men have more bone mass than women in all age groups.

Muscles support the skeleton and account for almost one-half the body weight. Active muscles release a large amount of heat that is conducted to other body tissues by the blood to maintain body temperature. Muscles can be divided into three categories based on their structure: skeletal (or striated), smooth, and cardiac. Skeletal muscles are primarily attached to the skeleton and act upon the bones to produce voluntary actions such as those needed for posture, facial expressions, and locomotion. In contrast, smooth muscles are mainly involuntary and line the walls of the digestive tract, windpipe, bladder, and blood vessels. The movement of smooth muscles is slow and sustained, often wavelike. Cardiac muscle is composed of a network of fibers that contract as a unit. These muscles initiate their own contractions and are responsible for the continual pumping action of the heart.

Just as bones are strengthened with physical activity, skeletal muscles become strengthened by use. A muscle that is not used decreases significantly in size and strength (sarcopenia). Muscles can atrophy rapidly, as one can tell by observing how much thinner an arm or leg looks when immobilized by a cast. It occurs more slowly over a long period of time among those who are sedentary.

Age-Associated Changes in the Musculoskeletal System

There is disagreement among researchers regarding how much muscle is lost with age and at what age sarcopenia begins. It was believed that muscle mass began to decline only in the later years; however, current research suggests that slow muscle wasting begins in the thirties, even among those who are physically active.[5] Progressive loss of

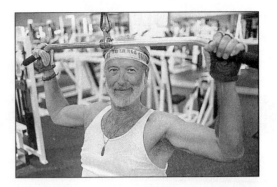

muscular strength is related to a loss of muscle mass with age. In elders, individual muscle fibers may be atrophied, or the number of fibers may be reduced. The old-old are more likely to have more rapid loss of muscle mass and strength. However, it is questionable whether it is due to disease, disuse, or the aging process. Among women, muscle mass decreases more quickly at menopause, especially in the first three postmenopausal years.[6]

Rapid loss of muscular strength and mass with age is not inevitable, as physical activity can reduce muscle atrophy at any age. Longitudinal studies report that elders who maintain higher levels of activity have less deterioration of muscle mass and strength than those with lower activity levels. In contrast, those who are immobile show very high rates of muscular atrophy. Even when an exercise regimen is initiated late in life, studies commonly report that deterioration can be significantly slowed or reversed. For more information on increasing muscle mass among elders with exercise, see chapter 4.

One consequence of the loss of muscle mass with age is an alteration in the basal metabolic rate, the number of calories the body burns at rest. Because muscle tissue needs more oxygen than other tissues, when muscle mass declines, fewer calories are needed to fuel the body. The basal metabolic rate begins to decline in young adulthood. To avoid gaining weight, a person must consume fewer calories. It is estimated that the body needs about twelve fewer calories a day for each year of age after age thirty. For example, a

60-year-old person would need 360 fewer calories per day than a 30-year-old.

A loss of muscle means a greater relative proportion of body fat. Even though the total body fat remains relatively constant in adulthood, the proportion of fat increases because the proportion of muscle declines. The average 25-year-old woman is composed of about 25 percent fat, whereas the average elder woman is more than 40 percent fat. Also, fat distribution changes in middle age. For men, fat becomes more prominent in the middle torso and for women, the middle torso, hips, buttocks, and thighs. Total body weight generally increases until age fifty-five, then it begins to fall, mostly due to loss of muscle, bone, and water.[1]

Joints become less flexible with age, creating minor stiffness and limited movement. Although joint degeneration is associated with old age, the aging of the joints begins even before skeletal maturity. Thus, joint problems may occur in adults of any age and increase in frequency as aging progresses. Calcification, fraying, or cracking in the cartilage and ligaments contribute to joint movement difficulties. Cartilage may become eroded in heavily used joints (especially the knee and hands) causing bone pain, stiffness, and loss of flexibility. In joint pain of the knee, obesity plays a significant role. Limitations in limb and neck joints may cause moderate alterations in posture, gait, and balance. Although extremely common, joint problems are not inevitable in old age. Like muscles, joint problems can be reduced with regular exercise, and in some cases, weight loss.

Reduction in bone strength and mass is associated with advancing age. The bones lose mineral content and become more porous and susceptible to fractures. Experts believe this occurs because the rate of bone rebuilding does not keep pace with the rate of bone breakdown. Although bone loss is inevitable with age, the degree and rate are highly variable. A strong determinant of bone mass in the later years is the amount of bone mass built up before the mid-twenties. Gender also plays a significant role in bone loss. Women commonly lose up to 30 percent of their bone mass over their lifetime, whereas men lose about half that amount.

For women, the most rapid bone loss occurs within five to ten years after menopause. Since women start with a lower bone mass than men, such loss can be significant. Because of this difference, it is important that women build up bone mass before maturity.

Since bone density increases when bones are stressed and become brittle with disuse, it is clear that physical inactivity plays a significant role in bone thinning. Other variables such as a diet deficient in calcium, fluoride, or low levels of vitamin D and estrogen also play a role. The good news is that bone loss can be slowed with exercise, hormonal therapy (for women), calcium supplementation, and prescription drugs. While some bone thinning is thought to accompany old age, osteoporosis is a chronic disease characterized by excessive bone loss and increased susceptibility to fracture (see chapter 8).

Reduced bone mass affects elders by increasing minor aches and pains and fractures. Furthermore, when older bones break, they take longer to heal. Ironically, the immobility necessary to heal can further exacerbate bone loss. Finally, brittle bones may further reduce physical activity because elders become overly cautious, inadvertently promoting further decline.

It is rare to see an older person with the erect posture of a young person. This is because the changes in muscles and bones produce alterations in posture with advanced age. Further, bad posture in youth is accentuated with advancing age. Some elders may assume a stooped posture: head and neck held forward, bent or stooped shoulders, forward thrust of the hips, and slightly bent knees. These changes may be caused by compression of the vertebral disks in the spinal column, a decrease in elasticity of joints and ligaments, a loss of strength and shortening of tendons or muscles, or degenerative changes in the central nervous system. Gravitational compression of the vertebral disks in the spinal column also lead to a gradual reduction of height. It is estimated that women lose two inches over their life span and men lose 1.25 inches.[1] However, osteoporosis, spinal deformity or injury, foot problems, and obesity, have a greater effect on posture than the normal aging process.

Poor posture affects a number of bodily functions. It interferes with stability and balance, increases back problems, and may also impede movement. Curvatures of the back may reduce lung capacity or compress internal organs. Lastly, poor posture detracts from general appearance, contributing to a decreased sense of self-worth. It is important to note that good posture can be maintained with exercise and is not inevitable in old age.

THE CARDIOVASCULAR SYSTEM

The cardiovascular system transports nutrients and wastes through the body. The system includes the heart, blood vessels (arteries, capillaries, and veins), and the blood. The heart is a muscular pump that rhythmically moves blood and dissolved substances through the body vessels to every cell in the body. Oxygen from the lungs,

nutrients from the digestive system, hormones from the endocrine glands, and antibodies from the immune system are transported to body cells, and waste products are moved from the cells to the lungs and kidneys for removal through the blood. Blood also maintains body temperature by transferring the heat generated by the skeletal muscles to the rest of the body.

The heart muscle consists of four chambers, two upper (atria) and two lower (ventricles) (figure 3.1). The atria and the ventricles are separated by valves that control the timing and amount of blood flow in each of the chambers and between the large arteries and the ventricles. The right side of the heart receives deoxygenated blood from the veins and pumps it to the lungs to be oxygenated. Oxygen-laden blood returns to the left side of the heart to be pumped to the rest of the body via the arterial system. Special arteries, called coronary arteries, supply the heart muscle with blood. The heart beats about seventy-two beats a minute and pumps about 170 gallons of blood in an hour.

Unlike other types of muscle, the muscle fibers in the heart wall initiate contractions that spread through specialized fibers to all parts of the heart. Some heart fibers, called pacemaker cells, initiate a rhythm of contraction that signals the other heart muscle fibers to contract. Heart rate can be altered by hormones or by nerve signals from the brain.

The heart pumps blood into high-pressure arteries that transport it to vital body organs. Blood then flows into the capillaries, which have highly permeable walls, allowing substances in the blood (nutrients, hormones, oxygen) to exchange with carbon dioxide and waste products in the fluid around body cells. Deoxygenated blood then flows into low-pressure, storage vessels: the veins. Blood must flow uphill to return to the heart, which is slower than the flow in the arteries. Some veins contain one-way valves to assist blood in returning to the heart and prevent back flow. Skeletal muscle movements and the muscle contractions in respiration are important in helping blood to return to the heart. When

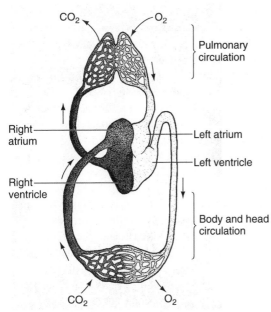

Figure 3.1
The circulatory system

blood is drawn at the physician's office, it is most likely venous blood.

Age-Associated Changes in the Cardiovascular System

With advancing age, elders experience some reduction in cardiovascular efficiency and maximal cardiac function. Although few changes occur in the heart at rest, maximal exercise tolerance is known to decrease with advancing age. Both longitudinal and cross-sectional studies have documented a decrease in maximum heart rate (level achieved with exercise) with advancing age. The decline in heart rate occurs at a constant rate from birth and can be estimated by subtracting one's age from 220. However, this number is highly variable and is not related to health problems. Because elders cannot increase their heart rate with exercise as much as younger adults, they are able to maintain the amount of blood leaving the heart (cardiac output) by increasing the amount of blood pumped with each beat.[7]

Most age-related alterations in cardiac efficiency affect only peak levels of performance and do not affect the ability to carry out daily activities. Additionally, cardiovascular performance in elders is highly correlated with level of physical fitness. Elders who exercise regularly maintain a higher level of cardiovascular function when compared to their inactive cohorts.

Certain structural changes in the aging heart may contribute to decreased maximal efficiency and increased risk of cardiovascular disease. The walls thicken and the heart increases in weight with age. This weight gain increases the pumping force of the heart and may compensate for the slightly increased blood pressure that usually occurs with age. The heart valves become stiffer and more likely to calcify. The coronary arteries supplying the heart muscle with blood become twisted while the aorta, the major vessel carrying blood out of the heart, becomes larger.[8]

Changes in the arteries throughout the body may contribute to the reduced cardiovascular efficiency in elders. Arterial walls become thicker and progressively less elastic with age due to calcification, resulting in a smaller artery diameter and a hardening of connective tissue. This decrement is called arteriosclerosis, or hardening of the arteries. *Arteriosclerosis* occurs whether or not vascular disease is present: it is an age-related condition, and is not associated with lifestyle. Over time, these changes contribute to a gradual increase in systolic blood pressure (the top number in blood pressure readings referring to the pressure of the blood on the walls of the arteries when the heart is beating) but the diastolic blood pressure (the bottom number denoting the pressure of the blood on the walls of the arteries at rest) does not change. In contrast, *atherosclerosis,* the build-up of cholesterol within the walls of the arteries, is a disease that is caused by a combination of genetic and behavioral influences. Atherosclerosis progresses with age, and, in the United States, it even appears among children.

Effects of age upon the venous system have not been studied as extensively as the arterial system. Researchers do know that the veins become thicker and more twisted, and some of the larger veins increase in capacity due to decreased elasticity of the walls. Deterioration of the venous valves creates increased venous pressure and pooling of blood in some areas, causing varicose veins in some middle-aged and older people.

The amount of blood flow to the internal organs diminishes with age. Since many body organs lose mass with age, this decreased blood flow may be in response to a reduced need for oxygen and nutrients by each organ.

THE LYMPHATIC SYSTEM

The lymphatic system has two major functions. The first is to collect excess fluid from around cells and return it to the bloodstream. The second function is protective. Lymph nodes, located throughout the body, contain immune cells that inactivate bacteria and viruses and filter foreign matter from bodily fluids. These lymph nodes enlarge when a person has an infection or is invaded by cancerous cells. They are located in the neck, under the arms, inside the chest and abdomen, in the groin, and around joints such as the elbow. Two other organs of the lymphatic system are related to the lymph nodes: the thymus and the spleen.

The thymus, located in the center of the upper chest cavity, plays an important role in the immune system. It contains a large number of lymphocytes, a type of blood cell that produces substances that destroy foreign cells and stimulate other parts of the immune system to act. Most of the lymphocytes are inactive, but some of them leave the thymus. The thymus secretes a hormone, thymosin, that stimulates the immune action of those lymphocytes that have migrated to other tissues. The thymus starts to degenerate after puberty, and mature adults have only a small percent of the original mass. Levels of thymosin decline in early adulthood and disappear by the later years. Many research questions still need to be answered about the function of the thymus.

The spleen, the largest lymphatic organ, is located in the upper left part of the abdomen. Its function is to store blood. When the body needs more blood because of exercise or hemorrhage, the blood stored in the spleen is expelled into circulation. Also, the spleen filters blood as do the lymph nodes. In addition, some of its cells (phagocytes) destroy damaged red blood cells, and others (lymphocytes) help to defend the body against infection.

The role of the immune system is to protect the body from invasion and colonization of bacteria, viruses, and fungi, and to destroy its own defective body cells. It does this by detecting, inactivating, and removing foreign invaders. The immune system also protects the body from cancerous cells and from "foreign bodies" such as transplants. Immune cells (lymphocytes) are made continually throughout life in the bone marrow and fluctuate in response to stress or infection.

Our bodies are at constant war with foreign invaders, and many physiological mechanisms serve to overcome its adversaries. For example, the skin provides a strong barrier against invasion by microorganisms, stomach acid deactivates organisms that we may swallow, and enzymes in the mucous membranes (mouth, nose, vagina) inactivate invaders. Additionally, the body has many internal lines of defense. The liver, spleen, and lymph nodes filter the blood and contain many antibodies and immune cells to attack invaders. When there is an infection, these organs become more important and may enlarge. Perhaps the most important mechanism of the immune system is the white blood cells, specialized cells that seek out and destroy foreign bodies. White blood cells may do their work while circulating in the blood or body fluids, or in the spleen or lymph nodes.

The following is a sketchy description of the very complex immunity process that is still not completely understood. The primary players are two types of white blood cells: lymphocytes and macrophages. Picture these cells as an intelligence and communications network that cooperates to form an immune response. The lymphocytes can be divided into two major groups: B cells, which produce antibodies, and T cells, which are able to switch the immune response on and off.

In the presence of infection, the B cells make specialized proteins, called antibodies, that bind to small parts on the surfaces of bacteria or viruses and target them for destruction. The body makes several different kinds of antibodies to combat a single microorganism. These antibodies also protect us against future infection from the same type of bacteria or virus. For instance, if you have had measles, you will carry antibodies that are specifically directed against measles for the rest of your life. T cell lymphocytes can have multiple functions, depending on their type: T-helper cells aid B cell function, T-killer cells attack bacteria or foreign cells, and T-suppressor cells protect the body's own cells from attack by the immune system. Macrophages also serve an important immune function by engulfing and digesting invaders.

Age-Associated Changes in the Lymphatic System

Although scientists generally believe that immune function declines with age, the changes are highly variable, and many studies find little differences in immune processes between the young and the old on many measures. However, studies demonstrate reduced numbers of lymphocytes with advancing age. The general consensus is that there is a slight decrease in T-helper cells, and possibly increased activity of T-suppressor cells. Older people's antibody production does not respond as vigorously to foreign antigens as that of younger adults. There is evidence that elders have a diminished capacity to kill cancer cells, starting in middle age. Neutrophils, another type of white blood cell, become less efficient with advanced age. However, the ability of the bone marrow to manufacture B cells that make antibodies continues at youthful levels through old age. There is also evidence that the levels of some immune-activating substances produced by the T cells, called lymphokines, actually increase with age.

With advancing age and peaking around age seventy, the body seems to make an increased number of antibodies in response to slightly changed proteins in its own tissues. Researchers thought that such an increase in autoantibodies might cause autoimmune disorders, a host of diseases (e.g., rheumatoid arthritis) that occur in people of all ages. However, even though these antibodies increase with age, there is no evidence that autoimmune diseases are more common in the later years. In fact, they are more likely to occur in the middle years.

THE RESPIRATORY SYSTEM

All body cells require oxygen to survive. Since cells and tissues are unable to store oxygen, a new supply must be delivered continuously by the bloodstream or the cells will die. The waste product of oxygen metabolism, carbon dioxide, is excreted from the body cells into the circulatory system. The major function of the respiratory system is to transfer oxygen from the air into the bloodstream and to remove carbon dioxide from the bloodstream into the environment. Figure 3.2 illustrates the structure of the respiratory system.

Air enters the nostrils and is filtered, warmed, and moistened in the nasal cavity. Air then passes through the pharynx, a flexible tube that also carries food to the esophagus, then through the larynx (voice box) to the trachea (windpipe). The trachea divides into two tubes, called bronchi, and these continue to divide and subdivide into smaller and smaller cartilage-ringed branches that reach deep into both lungs. The bronchial tubes are lined with cells that secrete mucus. Protruding cells with hairlike projections (cilia) trap foreign particles that are inhaled and moved upward to the pharynx. Once in the pharynx, mucus and foreign material pass through the esophagus and into the stomach.

Each of the smallest tubes, bronchioles, ends in a tiny air sac called an alveolus. Nearly a billion microscopic balloonlike alveoli are housed in the lungs, giving the lungs a spongy appearance. The walls of the alveoli are one cell thick and covered with capillaries. They are the site for oxygen and carbon dioxide exchange. Oxygen passes through alveolar walls and binds to hemoglobin molecules inside red blood cells in the bloodstream. Carbon dioxide, the waste product of oxygenation, dissolves in the blood, then moves through the alveoli walls to be exhaled.

The mechanism of breathing is very complex. With each inspiration, the diaphragm (a sheet of muscles separating the chest from the abdomen) contracts, which causes the diaphragm to lower. This creates a decreased pressure inside the lungs that causes air to enter the respiratory passages. Upon exhalation, the diaphragm muscle relaxes, bowing upwards again. This constricts the lungs and forces the air out. Movement of the intercostal muscles (between the ribs) increases the depth of inhalation or expiration by lifting the chest. When extra respiratory effort is needed (such as during intensive exercise or in cases of chronic lung disease), muscles in the neck, shoulders, and abdomen become involved.

The rate and depth of breathing are regulated by a respiratory control center in the brain. Either high levels of carbon dioxide or low levels of oxygen in the blood can trigger an increase in breathing rate or depth by altering the muscle contractions.

Age-Associated Changes in the Respiratory System

The respiratory system is constantly exposed to environmental pollutants. Because of this exposure, it is extremely difficult to differentiate the extent of respiratory deterioration due to age from that

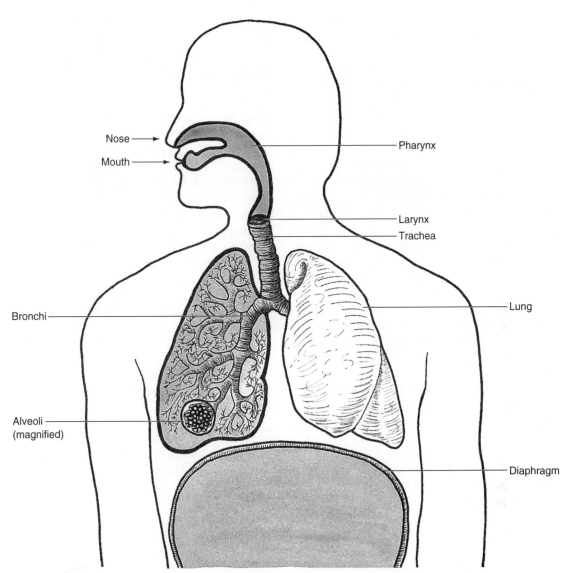

Figure 3.2
The respiratory system

caused by accumulated pollutant damage. Although there are noticeable respiratory decrements associated with age, the degree and rate of loss also depend upon the state of the other body systems, overall health status, and extent of physical activity.

The main effect of age on the respiratory system is the reduced amount of oxygen taken up by the blood. With age, air tends to distribute less evenly within the lung, which lowers the efficiency of gas exchange. Lung tissue becomes less elastic with age, decreasing the amount of time the airways in the lungs are kept open. This decrease in elasticity affects the amount of air that can fill the alveoli, especially in the lower portion of the lung. Respiration becomes less efficient because blood still flows through the areas that are poorly ventilated.

Gas exchange is also limited by other age-related factors. The alveolar walls break down and flatten, reducing the area for gas exchange. The chest wall muscles and skeleton become more rigid, which increase the effort of breathing and reduce the ability of the lungs to expand during inspiration and compress during exhalation. Because of this, maximum breathing rate decreases with age.

The most consistent change in breathing capacity with age is a decrease in *vital capacity,* which is the amount of air that is moved in and out of the lungs when a person is inhaling and exhaling as hard as possible. An increase in *residual lung volume* is commonly noted with age. Residual volume is the amount of air left in the lungs after a maximal exhalation. The air that stays in the lungs is not replaced with each breath and therefore is not available for oxygen–carbon dioxide exchange.

Decreased pulmonary efficiency has little effect on daily functioning. However, *maximum exertion levels* or the length of time older people can sustain heavy physical activity may be affected. Elders may need more rest periods during heavy physical exertion because they tire more easily and take longer to recover. Decreased pulmonary efficiency can lower the metabolic rate and decrease the oxygen supply to body tissues, especially during heavy physical exertion. In general, elders are less able to cope with environmental pollutants and are more susceptible to pulmonary distress or death during periods of high pollution. As in other age changes, a tremendous variation exists among elders regarding these measures of pulmonary efficiency. A systematic aerobic exercise program can help many elders to minimize most of these decrements. On the other hand, cigarette smoking exacerbates them.

THE DIGESTIVE SYSTEM

The digestive system is a modified, muscular tube that extends from the mouth to the anus (figure 3.3). Portions of this tube are specialized for dif-ferent functions. Each plays a role in the breakdown of food into usable nutrients, absorbing them into the blood and temporarily storing the waste products until elimination. Accessory structures, such as the pancreas and gallbladder, release chemicals into the canal to facilitate digestion and absorption. Other body systems also affect the workings of the digestive system. The nervous system regulates the contractions of the muscles in the wall of the alimentary canal and the blood flow to these organs. Digestion also involves the secretion of enzymes and hormones by the endocrine system. The cardiovascular system transports food molecules from the digestive system to body cells.

Digestion begins in the mouth where teeth mechanically break down the food particles. Saliva, secreted by three major pairs of salivary glands, moistens the food and secretes an enzyme that breaks down complex carbohydrates into simple sugar molecules. Salivary secretions also help taste bud functioning and keep the oral cavity clean. The tongue mixes food with saliva and also moves food from the mouth into the passageway of the esophagus.

When food is swallowed, rhythmic muscular contractions of the esophagus push food towards the stomach. When the esophagus contracts, a valve opens at the entrance to the stomach. As the sphincter closes, the muscular stomach wall churns, as it works on the food. Although the stomach's major function is storage, some digestion occurs there. An enzyme (pepsin) and hydrochloric acid initiate the digestion of proteins. Gastric juice also contains other enzymes, one of which aids in the absorption of vitamin B_{12}. This mixture of partially digested food and secretions then passes from the stomach into the first part of the small intestine, the duodenum.

The small intestine, almost 10 feet in length, is the main site for the absorption of nutrients, water, and salts. The pancreas opens into the small intestine, secreting bicarbonate to neutralize the strong stomach acid, and enzymes to break down carbohydrates, fats, and proteins. Bile, produced by the liver and stored in the gallbladder, helps the

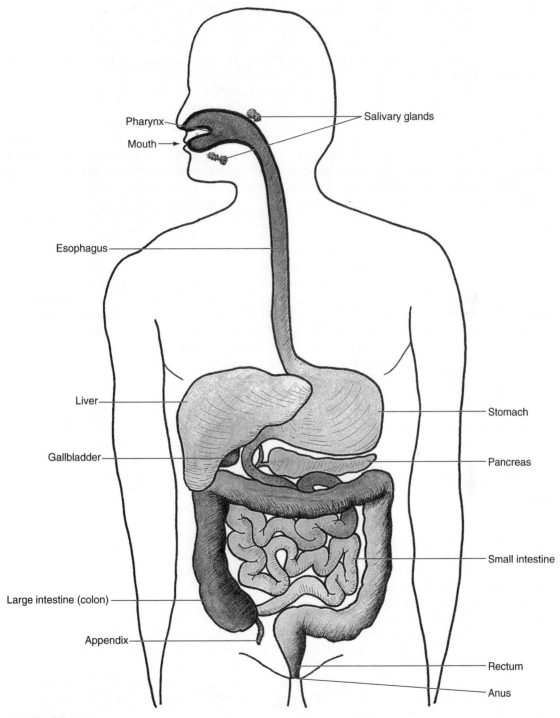

Figure 3.3
The digestive system

body absorb fats and cholesterol. Bile also contains waste products from the liver, such as bilirubin, that are excreted in feces. Bile passes through the bile duct to the duodenum. The lining of the duodenum also secretes a number of different enzymes that further break down proteins, complex starches, sugars, and fats.

As the food moves through the small intestine, fingerlike outgrowths (villi) of the internal wall with hairlike projections (microvilli) absorb the water, salts, and small molecules of the meal into the bloodstream. After four to six hours in the small intestine, the unabsorbed contents empty into the large intestine through another valve, then into the large intestine.

The large intestine consists of the colon, the rectum, and the anal canal. The appendix is a tubular appendage that extends from the entrance of the large intestine. It has no digestive function; however, it contains lymphatic tissue that may resist infection. Although the large intestine has little significance in absorbing nutrients, it absorbs water and salts, and forms and stores solid feces. When the muscular terminal portion of the colon (the rectum) is filled, feces are eliminated through the anal sphincter. Feces usually contain 50 to 75 percent water, indigestible plant matter, dead cells, and bacteria.

Age-Associated Changes in the Digestive System

The digestive system has a high turnover of cells and a substantial reserve capacity, enabling it to withstand considerable decrements before any effect is noted on digestive functioning. Perhaps the most obvious change in the digestive system associated with advancing age is tooth loss. However, tooth loss is not a normal part of aging. About 85 percent of those over age sixty have at least some of their natural teeth. However, the oldest-old, those with the least education, African Americans, and people living in the northeastern United States are more likely to be missing teeth or have no teeth at all.[9] Factors influencing tooth loss are poor oral hygiene, malnutrition, diabetes,

gum disease, or drugs that dry out the mouth. Teeth do wear down with age, but with normal diets, the rate of wear is insignificant. There is also some evidence that gums recede from the teeth with advancing age, but researchers do not know whether this is a true age change or the result of poor dental hygiene.

Experts predict that, in the future, more people will retain their original teeth. Younger generations have grown up with a bevy of oral care products, fluoridated water, improved dental hygiene, and more frequent checkups.

Although pepsin production in the stomach is reduced in middle age, healthy older people show no additional decline. Structurally, there is a reduced blood flow through the intestinal mucosa in older people. There is some evidence that reduced absorption of calcium, iron, and vitamins B_1 and B_{12} is common in late life. However, if an older person is healthy and eats well, this is not a problem. No significant functional changes in the gallbladder, liver, or pancreatic secretions into the intestine have been reported.

THE URINARY SYSTEM

As each body cell breaks down food into molecules necessary for cell growth and energy, waste products are formed and are transported away from the tissues by the lymph and blood. The respiratory system eliminates one waste product, carbon dioxide, from the body. The urinary system rids the body of other waste products and toxic substances. Aside from its excretory function, the urinary system also regulates the amount and composition of body fluids.

The urinary system is composed of a pair of kidneys, each attached to a muscular tube, the ureter, that transports urine from the kidneys to the bladder. The bladder stores the urine until the urethra, a narrow tube connected to the bladder, carries the urine outside the body (figure 3.4).

The kidneys are located behind the digestive organs in the abdomen and are each about four inches long. They are composed of millions of tubules called nephrons that serve as the filtering

The bladder, an expandable muscular sac, stores the urine. When the bladder is about half-full, sensors in its wall signal the brain, resulting in the urge to urinate. When the time is appropriate, an individual relaxes the sphincter at the opening of the bladder and squeezes down on the bladder, emptying the urine into the urethra. In males, the urethra is about eight inches long; in females, about two inches. The male urethra also carries semen.

Age-Associated Changes in the Urinary System

During middle age, the kidney becomes gradually less efficient at filtering the blood. With age, both kidney weight and blood flow to the kidney decrease. Whether the decreased blood flow is due to reduced cardiovascular efficiency or to a decreased need for blood by the kidney because of its reduced mass is not known. In addition, some nephrons look different: researchers believe that many become nonfunctional with advancing age.

Although age-related decrements in kidney efficiency have been reported many times in cross-sectional studies, kidney function may not decline as dramatically as originally thought. The Baltimore Longitudinal Study of Aging reported that many subjects maintained stable kidney function.[10] Perhaps the elders in other studies had diseases (cardiovascular or diabetes) that affected their kidney function. Thus, most experts now conclude that some decline in kidney function is expected, but the severity and rate of decline are highly variable.

A reduced filtering capacity has little noticeable effect on daily living because the organ has a great reserve capacity. However, reduced kidney efficiency may be noticeable during stress or dehydration. For instance, the kidneys of elders may not be able to make urine as concentrated as younger people. Thus, when dehydrated, the body may lose more water through urination. And, the decreased filtration rate affects the excretion of some drugs. If the main route of drug excretion is through the urine, these drugs may remain active longer in older

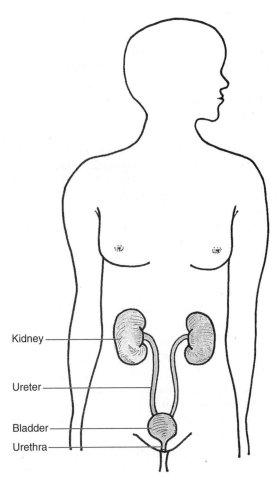

Figure 3.4
The urinary system

Kidney

Ureter

Bladder

Urethra

system of the kidney. They selectively remove a small amount of waste from the blood, returning almost all the fluid and nutrients back to the body. The waste products and water become urine, which pass through the kidney into the ureters and then to the bladder. The kidney regulates the concentration of urine. When we are dehydrated, our kidneys make more concentrated urine to conserve water; when we drink a lot of water, the kidney makes the urine more dilute. The urinary filtration system is very efficient: the entire volume of blood in the body is filtered almost fifty times a day.

people. To accommodate for reduced kidney efficiency in elders, physicians should adjust the dosage of drugs that are excreted by the kidney.

Early studies report that, with advanced age, the bladder can hold less fluid and more urine remains in the bladder after voiding. As a result, older people may need to urinate more often, even waking up at night to urinate. Incomplete emptying may predispose elders to bladder infections. Also, younger adults generally receive a neural message that their bladder is becoming full; the message in elders may be delayed. The reduced time differential between awareness and involuntary urination may result in "accidents" and anxiety. As in many other age changes, there is great variability in loss of bladder efficiency among elders.

THE NERVOUS SYSTEM

All body functions are monitored and controlled by a complex communication network composed of the nervous and endocrine systems. In general, these systems function well into advanced age. However age-associated changes in the neurosensory system, particularly those affecting hearing and vision, are inevitable in the later years.

The nervous system has two main components: the central and the peripheral. The central nervous organs (brain and spinal cord) gather input from the sensory organs, integrate it, and send output messages to the peripheral nervous system. The peripheral nervous system controls the work of body organs, glands, and muscles. Both the central and peripheral nervous systems are composed of nerve cells, or neurons, which store and conduct information. Neurons transmit information to each other using both chemical and electrical means. Some neurons, called sensory neurons, are specialized to receive information from the outside world. Others, motor neurons, are specialized to conduct messages to the muscles. Glial cells in the brain and spinal cord protect and nourish the neurons.

The brain consists of approximately 100 billion neurons that transmit information, both within the brain and to nerves in other parts of the body. The brain is extraordinarily complex, and many of its functions are not well-understood. Each area of the brain has a different purpose. The largest portion, the cerebrum, is responsible for intellectual activities: speech, thought, learning, memory, and reasoning. The cerebrum also interprets messages from the sense organs and controls voluntary muscle action. The cerebellum coordinates voluntary muscle movements and maintains muscle tone, posture, and equilibrium. The brain stem connects the spinal cord and brain and is the main relay center for messages traveling to and from the brain. It controls involuntary processes: heartbeat, blood pressure, respiration, temperature, and the release of some hormones.

The spinal cord is a bundle of nerves encased within the vertebral bones of the spine. Spinal cord neurons receive messages from various body parts and transmit directions to the brain or to other parts of the body. Neurons that branch out from the spinal column and brain constitute the peripheral nervous system. Some of these peripheral nerves regulate voluntary actions (such as movement of the skeletal muscles in the arms and legs). Others regulate involuntary actions such as breathing, digestion, and hormonal release. Sensory messages are received in the skin and other organs and are transmitted to the spinal cord.

Age-Associated Changes in the Nervous System

Because the nervous system controls and coordinates other body activities, decrements in the nervous system affect the whole body. Some age-associated changes in the structure of the nervous system are well-documented. However, the effect of these changes on nervous system function is still speculative. Although some elders may exhibit decrements in nervous system functioning, the differences are highly variable and are more likely to be caused by other factors besides age.

Starting in the twenties, brain weight starts to decline, and in very advanced age, it has lost about

Exercising Your Memory

Mnemonics, the art of improving short-term recall and ferreting out stored facts, depends on strong visual images and meaningful associations: it's a system for cross-indexing stored information in arresting ways. These methods take only a little time to master. They work because they seize the attention and demand concentration. The more outrageous the connections, the better.

Use "loci" (latin for "places"). Take a string of facts to be remembered: (for instance, points you want to cover in a talk). Match each one to a specific site you can visualize easily—your living room, perhaps, or your street. If you're giving a talk on substance abuse, make a tour of the living room, stationing your introductory remarks on drug cartels on the table left of the fireplace. On the mantel, store what you're planning to say about government policy. To the right of the fireplace, in the bookcase, situate drug education—and so forth, around the room. When you give your talk, make another mental tour of the room and "pick up" your notes. You can adapt the same loci to something more innocuous, like a grocery list: pasta on the table, tomato sauce on the mantel, salad greens in the bookcase.

Make up rhymes. Nobody ever forgets the useful "I before E, except after C." But to remember home chores, make up your own rhymes: "Skitty, skat, let in the cat," for instance. The cornier the better.

Compose mental pictures, particularly when you're trying to remember a name: Helen Decker, say, might conjure up a vision of Helen of Troy on shipboard.

Repeat or rehearse new facts. "How do you do, Helen," you say when introduced at a party. A few minutes later you say to yourself, "That's Helen Decker." And a minute or so after that, "Can I get you anything to drink, Helen?" You probably won't forget Helen's name.

Make up acronyms or sentences. "Maple" could help an out-of-towner in New York City remember the order of Madison, Park, and Lexington Avenues. "The postman at Sutter's Mill was bushed from pining for California" could help a visitor remember the order of five San Francisco streets, Post, Sutter, Bush, Pine, and California.

Chunk or regroup clusters of data to give them a pattern. Telephone numbers are already partially grouped, but you can give them further meaning. Helen's three-number exchange, 744, is easy to remember, but you won't forget the rest of the number either, 4591, when you reflect that she looks to be about 45, almost halfway to 91.

Write things down. Writing notes and making lists will often fix things in your mind. You may not even have to refer to your notes or lists.

Structure your life. Even the hook for the house keys by the back door is a mnemonic device: you'll always look there first. Similarly, keep your checkbook in the drawer of your desk, or park your reading glasses on the night table.

Ease your mind. If you feel you are forgetting too much, consider the following:

- Give yourself time. The sky won't fall in if you forget a name or a number, and if you employ a few delaying tactics (don't rush right up to the friend whose name you've forgotten), the missing data may surface. If they don't, don't make a big fuss over it. Just admit you've forgotten.
- Don't expect too much. If you're nervous about forgetting, you usually do.
- Play games. Crossword puzzles, Scrabble, and card games are all good exercises for improving memory.
- Improve your mind. Going to lectures, taking classes, and joining groups will introduce new stimuli and keep your neurons transmitting.

Excerpted with permission from the University of California, Berkeley Wellness Letter © Health Letter Associates, 1991. For information, call 800-829-9170.

10 percent of its mass, mostly in the frontal and temporal lobes. Declines in brain weight may be due to reduction in size rather than number of neurons.[11] <u>With a decreased brain size, there is a corresponding reduction in blood supply to the brain.</u>

Structural changes occur in some neurons and glial cells, although there is no evidence that it affects function. Glial cells increase in number in some parts of the brain and decrease in others with advancing age. Furthermore, <u>neurons accumulate lipofuscin</u>, an age-associated pigment. It used to be thought that small amounts of plaque and tangles in the brain were a normal accompaniment of aging, but it now appears that this may not be the case because elders without cognitive impairment often have none of these features.[12] We now know that these changes are a confirmation of Alzheimer's disease.

Cognitive function includes measures of memory, intelligence, and speed of processing new information. Alterations in cognitive function with age are variable and difficult to separate from the consequences of disease or lack of intellectual activity that may accompany aging. It is easy to see how vision and hearing loss, chronic illness, educational level and motivation may affect elders' performance on cognitive tests. For example, one study compared the memory performance of older adults with two groups of young adults— those attending college and those who did not. The young college students performed better than their noncollege peers and the older adult group. However, the older adult group performed as well as the younger group who did not go to college.[13]

Older people perform more poorly on timed tests of cognitive or motor function than their younger peers, but perform about the same on tests that do not have a time limit. Of note, 15 to 20 percent of older people exhibit no change in mental function with age. Among elders whose performance does appear to be declining with age, cognitive changes are reversible with minimal training.[14]

It is commonly believed, by young and old alike, that memory declines with age; hence the comment, "I must be getting old," when a name is forgotten or car keys are misplaced. In general,

elders manifest a gradual and modest decline in short-term memory (e.g., remembering what one had for breakfast).

However, memory is a very complex cognitive skill and can be affected by a number of other factors, especially mental state. Memory loss is also a consequence of dehydration, drug reactions, low blood sugar, anemia, hypothyroidism, or a stroke. Memory decrements are highly variable in older people and are less common in educated elders. Memory has been shown to improve with practice.

Generally, an older person's perception of memory loss is far worse than the reality. One researcher asked a group of older men and woman to estimate the extent of their memory loss. Then the elders were objectively tested to determine their actual impairment. Although each usually had some impairment, the extent was not nearly as great as the person had estimated. Even more interesting, very few reported that memory failure is even a minor handicap in their everyday functioning.[15]

With age, elders also exhibit a reduction in the speed at which new information is processed. It has been suggested that the reduction in speed may be due to the need to sort through a larger store of memories for the correct answer. Studies suggest that verbal intelligence is stable at least into the eighties.

A number of studies have demonstrated that reaction time lengthens with age. Visual and auditory reflexes and time to complete a physical or mental task decline 20 percent or more from youth to old age. This decline may be due to physiological alterations in the neural pathway, alterations in vision or hearing, difficulty with testing situations, or increased cautiousness with age. Chronic illness and physical inactivity may also play a role. Even though there is a statistically significant lengthening of reaction time with age, in real life, this translates into an increase of only hundredths of a second, and does not interfere with most everyday activities.

A positive finding about the brains of older people is that some of their brain cells send out new branches, or connections, to other neurons.

Researchers speculate that the branching facilitates communication within the brain.

THE SENSORY SYSTEM

The nervous system depends on its specialized sensory receptors to gather information about the internal and external environment. The receptors include those needed for vision, hearing, smell, taste, touch, equilibrium, temperature, and pain sensation. Although each sensory receptor responds to only one type of input, all convert the input into electrochemical impulses that travel along peripheral nerves to the central nervous system for processing.

Sensory decrements are the most crucial physiological changes associated with the aging process because they affect an individual's perceptions and response to the world. Since visual and hearing changes are gradual, elders may not seek medical attention because they adapt to the deficits.

Vision

Eyelashes, eyelids, tear glands, and tear ducts protect the eye from dirt, injury, or dryness. The sclera is the white, outer layer of the eyeball (figure 3.5). The cornea is a transparent membrane that covers the front of the eyeball. The iris is the circular, colored part of the eye that lies behind the

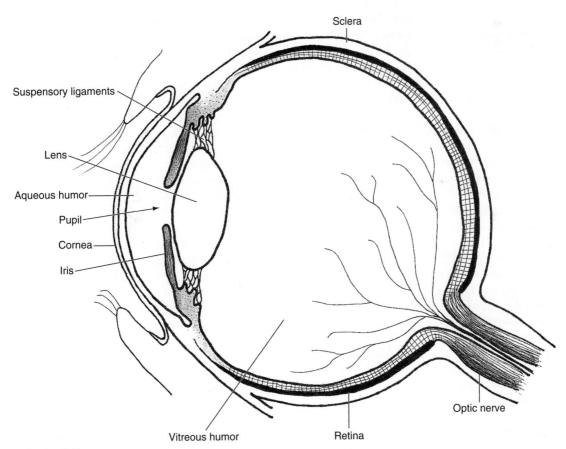

Figure 3.5
The structure of the eye

cornea and in front of the lens. The opening at the center of the iris is the pupil. When the light is dim, the pupil opening expands to allow more light to stimulate the receptors. When the light is bright, the pupil contracts to protect the receptors from damage from intense light.

The lens is located behind the pupil and is suspended by ligaments. The function of the lens is to focus light rays entering the pupil so they merge to a point on the retina located in the back of the eye. The lens focuses the image by changing its shape with the help of supporting muscles. This capacity allows for sharp vision at any distance. In some people, the shape of the eyeball or lens focuses light rays at a point beyond the retinal surface, which causes farsightedness or hyperopia (an inability to focus on near objects). In others, light rays come to a focus at a point in front of the retina instead of directly on it, causing nearsightedness or myopia (an inability to focus on distant objects). Both disorders can usually be corrected with eyeglasses or contact lenses.

Vision receptors are located in the retina and consist of rods to distinguish general outlines, and cones for color vision and sharp outlines. The rods and cones connect with neurons to form the optic nerve. A blind spot, where the optic nerve connects to the retina, has no visual receptors. Viscous fluids (the aqueous humor in front of the lens and the vitreous humor behind it) maintain proper eye pressure and fluid balance to allow the eye to function properly.

Age-Associated Changes in Vision

Reduced visual acuity is one of the most significant changes that occur in the aging process, especially the gradual changes that occur in the lens. With advancing age, the lens thickens, yellows, clouds, and becomes less elastic. The thickening of the lens reduces the amount of light that can pass through the lens. Visual clarity is further reduced by a clouding of the lens, called a cataract. The term is derived from the Latin word *cataracta* which means "waterfall," because the visual effect can be likened to looking through a sheet of water. A normal lens allows light to pass

to the back of the eye but a cataract disperses and reduces the incoming light. In the early stages, elders experience a dulling of colors, difficulty with glare, and problems with night driving. Any clouding of the lens is considered to be a cataract; however, depending on the cataract's size, location, and density, it may or may not impair vision.

Most cataracts are associated with advanced age, but diabetes, cigarette smoking, chemicals, alcohol, some medications, and sun exposure can cause or accelerate cataract formation. There is mounting evidence that antioxidant vitamins, especially vitamins C and carotenoids, reduce cataract formation.[16] Cataracts can occur when UV-B rays in sunlight alter the proteins in the lens of the eye. Even inexpensive sunglasses absorb UV-B rays.

Cataracts are considered to be the leading cause of reversible blindness in the United States. In our country, more than three-fourths of all adults over sixty have some degree of cataract formation. Some individuals do not even know they have a cataract; others cannot see well enough to do the things they need or want to do. The older one is, the more likely he or she will have cataracts. Further, women are more likely than men to have a cataract, and African Americans are more likely than whites to have one. However, not all people with cataracts have a significant vision loss. It is estimated that less than one in ten is legally blind from them, and few will need surgery. Whether a person needs surgery or not depends on the effect of the cataract on vision and overall function, visual needs (everyday activities, hobbies, and occupation), and the potential surgery risks. Since cataracts almost always develop slowly, surgery may be postponed or never become necessary for many. Some experts believe that cataracts are inevitable, if one lives long enough.

When cataracts cause impaired vision, surgery is usually recommended. Cataract surgery is the most common operation performed on Medicare patients: about 1.35 million cataract extractions are conducted in the United States each year. Cataract surgery has become quite sophisticated, and procedures vary. Most surgeries are performed on an outpatient basis.

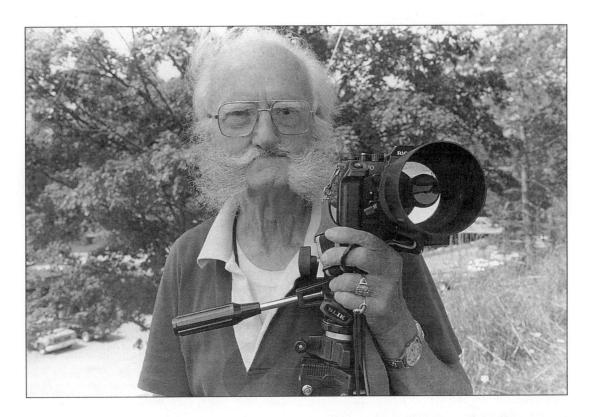

How Do I Decide Whether to Have Cataract Surgery

- I need to drive, but there is too much glare from the sun or headlights.
- I do not see well enough to do my best at work.
- I do not see well enough to do the things I need to do at home.
- I do not see well enough to do things I like to do (read, watch TV, sew, play cards).
- I am afraid I will bump into something or fall.
- Because of my cataract, I am not as independent as I would like to be.
- My glasses do not help me see well enough.
- My eyesight bothers me a lot.[17]

Cataract surgery involves removing the lens from the lens capsule and implanting an artificial lens, a plastic disk, in its place. A newer technique allows a smaller incision of the lens capsule, softening of the lens by ultrasound, and removing it through a needle (called phacoemulsification). There is no evidence that one procedure should be chosen over another.

Cataract surgery has a high success rate, although patients may need to wear glasses or contacts afterwards for optimal vision. In a few cases, blurred vision occurs months after the surgery due to the clouding of the lens capsule. This condition can be treated with the use of a laser beam to make a tiny hole in the capsule to let light pass (called YAG capsulotomy). Not only is vision improved with cataract surgery, but also most elders report an increased health-related quality of life.[18] Unfortunately, nursing home residents have undetected cataracts because they do not have regular eye exams. Many who are legally blind from them could be successfully treated, increasing their quality of life.[19]

The likelihood of undergoing cataract surgery may be affected by factors other than poor vision; race, sex, geographic location, and type of medical reimbursement plan play a role. For instance, women are more likely than men to undergo the surgery, and whites are more likely than African Americans to have cataract surgery. Since African Americans are four times more likely to become blind from cataracts, this is of special concern. Further, the likelihood of surgery is significantly greater in regions with the highest concentration of optometrists and those with the greatest allowable surgery charges by Medicare. There is also a geographical North-South gradient: those in the South are more likely to have cataract surgery that those living in the North. This might be because higher sun exposure is associated with a higher cataract risk.[20] One large study of Medicare beneficiaries in southern California reported a significant difference in cataract surgery rates between those in fee-for-service settings and managed care plans: those in the fee-for-service plan were twice as likely to undergo surgery as those in the managed care plan. Whether this is due to an overuse of surgery in pre-paid plans or an underuse in managed care plans is not yet known.[21]

Almost everyone begins to have problems with near vision in middle age, called presbyopia. The lens becomes less elastic, decreasing its ability to bend to focus on close objects. A common symptom of presbyopia is the need to hold reading material farther and farther away. Presbyopia usually starts around age forty, and by age sixty, the lens is incapable of focusing at close distance. Presbyopia responds very well to corrective lenses or a magnifying glass for reading and close work. Some people may need bifocals, which are glasses that incorporate one prescription for close focus and another for distant focus. Because many people associate bifocals with old age, they may delay getting the vision correction they need. However, opticians can grind bifocals to look like ordinary glasses. Bifocal contact lenses are a newer alterna-

tive that may work for some. Another alternative is contact lenses, fitting one eye for close vision and the other eye for distant vision.

Another universal change in the eye is that the lens becomes yellowed with advanced age. Because more light is necessary to stimulate the light receptors in the retina, night vision is impaired.

The amount of light entering the eye is also reduced because of age-related reductions in pupil size and thickening of the cornea. The reduction in pupil size is caused by atrophy of the muscle that dilates the pupil. As the pupil becomes less responsive, the eye loses its ability to adapt to abrupt changes from light to darkness. Finally, with age, the fluids in the eye become cloudy, further reducing light sensitivity.

The cornea becomes thickened and less transparent with age. The thickened cornea causes light to scatter inside the retina, making glare more of a problem. To further increase visual acuity in elders, the amount of glare in the environment should be minimized. Generally, individuals who are sixty years old need three times the light to read than when they were twenty. Thus, great improvements in vision are possible by installing higher wattage light bulbs in elders' living space. The yellowing of the lens reduces light to the retina, and it also impairs the ability to differentiate blue, green, and violet. This is an important consideration in designing written material for elders.

Because most of the visual decrements accompanying aging occur gradually, elders adapt and their lifestyle is relatively unaffected. Elders can also adjust to many vision problems by purchasing corrective lenses. Those with presbyopia may be able to use inexpensive nonprescription magnifying eyeglasses. These will not, however, correct for other vision problems and should only be worn for reading and close work.

Elders should have eye examinations every two to five years to detect glaucoma, cataracts, and other visual problems. Unfortunately, as of this writing, neither vision examinations nor corrective lenses are covered by Medicare, although treatment of eye diseases is reimbursed. However, for those who qualify, Medicaid (MediCal in California) may pay all or part of the expense of eye examinations and corrective lenses. In some communities, the Lion's Club assists individuals with expenses related to vision problems. A toll-free number sponsored by the American Academy of Ophthalmology—1-800-222-3937 (EYES)—helps identify doctors who will examine elders for free.

Three types of health professionals deal with eye care. An *ophthalmologist,* a physician with special training in eye diseases, can diagnose eye disease, perform eye surgery, and prescribe correction for inadequate vision. An *optometrist,* though not a physician, is trained to examine for visual defects and prescribe proper correction. If a disease is suspected or surgery is required, the client is referred to an ophthalmologist. An *optician,* following the directions of the ophthalmologist or optometrist, grinds and fits the lenses.

Hearing

The ear is composed of three distinct sections. Sound waves enter the outer ear, are conducted into the middle ear, and are translated into nerve impulses in the inner ear (figure 3.6). Specialized receptor cells in the inner ear transmit sound messages to the brain for processing. The inner ear is also important in maintaining body equilibrium as special fluid-filled canals signal the brain whenever they sense motion.

The most visible structure of hearing is the cartilaginous outer ear (pinna). Inside is an auditory canal lined with hair and wax-secreting glands. Ear wax (cerumen) cleans and protects the ear from dirt, repels water, wards off infection, and prevents dryness. The funnel-shaped canal collects sound waves and guides them to the eardrum (tympanic membrane), which separates the outer from the middle ear.

In the middle ear, three small bones—the hammer (malleus), anvil (incus), and stirrup (stapes)—work together to transmit sound vibrations from the eardrum through the middle ear. The eustachian tube connects the throat and middle ear. This connection maintains equal pressure outside and inside the head, permitting the eardrum to vibrate normally. This explains why swallowing can relieve pressure in the ears during an airplane flight since this equalizes the pressure on both sides of the eardrum. Extreme pressure differences may cause the eardrum to rupture.

Sound waves are transformed into nerve impulses in the inner ear. The inner ear is completely filled with fluid and houses the cochlea, a snail-shaped tunnel also filled with fluid. The cochlea contains rows of cells that convert sound into electrical impulses and transmit them to the brain. These cells respond selectively to sounds of different frequencies, depending on their location on the membrane within the cochlea.

Age-Associated Changes in Hearing

Hearing loss is very common among older adults; however, many researchers believe these deficits are attributable more to an accumulation of noise damage than actual age changes. Elders in less technologically advanced cultures do not exhibit hearing loss to the extent of those in our society. In the United States, hearing sensitivity declines gradually with age, beginning in adolescence and continuing to old age. Overall, about 10 percent of the total population in the United States have a hearing deficit, with elders disproportionately represented. About one in three elders over age sixty-five has a hearing loss, and this increases with advancing age. Men are almost twice as likely to have hearing loss than women, and the loss is evident earlier in life. This gender difference may be due to physiological differences or different noise exposure history.

There is evidence that over the past thirty years, a higher proportion of those fifty and older are hard of hearing. It is hypothesized that the increase is due to more workplace noise and drug use that affects hearing acuity.[22] Many hearing authorities predict there will be even more widespread hearing difficulties because of the increasing noise in our country (e.g., city noises, rock concerts, and Walkmen). Very loud noises, such as explosions, immediately destroy the sensory cells of the inner ear, but lower-level chronic noise inflames the hearing mechanism, slowly destroying the sensory

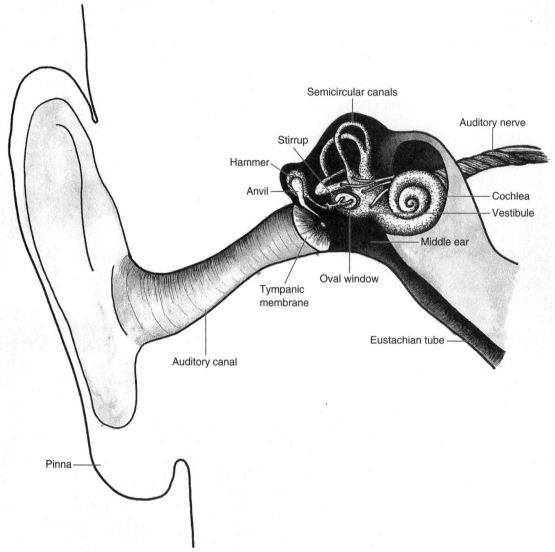

Figure 3.6
The structure of the ear

cells. There is marked variation among individuals regarding noise susceptibility and hearing loss, but generally the danger level begins at eighty to eighty-five decibels (e.g., garbage disposal rumbling) and increases at higher levels (e.g., rock concerts, video arcades, firearms). The louder the sound, the less time it takes a person to suffer hearing damage. For example, one can listen to a lawn mower for eight hours without damage, but only tolerate fifteen minutes of a loud rock concert or car horn. Temporary hearing loss or ringing in the ears after exposure to loud noise are warning signs in some individuals. Noise damage can be reduced with protective devices such as ear plugs. Hearing loss is not only caused by excessive noise, it can also result from disease (measles, meningitis, repeated ear infections) and some medications (e.g., antibiotics and diuretics).

Presbycusis is the term used to describe the hearing loss associated with the aging process. The word "presbycusis" originates in the Greek roots *presby* meaning "old" and *cusis* meaning "hearing." It is estimated that presbycusis is a common condition afflicting older adults, affecting about one-third of those over age seventy-five. This type of hearing loss affects both ears and affects the part of the ear that senses and transmits auditory information, the cochlea. With presbycusis, elders typically do not complain of hearing difficulty, but rather of an inability to understand ordinary speech (particularly high-frequency consonant sounds such as f, g, s, z, t, sh, and ch). This problem is confounded by their difficulty in screening out interfering noises and a slowed processing of auditory information. Communication with an elder with presbycusis is optimized when one speaks slowly in a quiet room.

Both family members and professionals who work with elders can easily assess hearing acuity by observing the following behaviors that may indicate a hearing problem.

1. Preferring radio or television at a higher volume than others in the room.
2. Complaining that others are not speaking clearly or loudly enough.
3. Consistently turning one side of head toward the speaker or cupping ear with hand.
4. Commonly asking others to repeat phrases or words or frequently saying "What?" or "Huh?"
5. Having difficulty hearing at large gatherings with background noise, such as lectures, church sermons, and social events.
6. Having difficulty in locating the origin of sounds.
7. Confusing words or making silly mistakes.
8. Understanding men's voices better than women's.

In addition to presbycusis, elders may suffer hearing loss due to other age-associated changes in the ear. The wall of the outer cartilaginous portion of the auditory canal collapses inward with advancing age, narrowing the passage and making the canal less efficient in receiving and channeling sound waves to the middle ear. Furthermore, earwax tends to thicken and accumulate with age, which may occlude the auditory canal, contributing to hearing loss. A significant proportion of hearing loss in elders may be due to build-up of earwax. Swabs to clean the ear canal should not be used because they can compress the earwax deeper into the ear canal. Over-the-counter wax-softening agents or irrigation of the canal by a medical professional can alleviate this problem.

Reduced ability to hear commonly has significant psychological effects. Decreased hearing sensitivity may limit enjoyment of social activities and the stimulation that other people and television provide. Paranoid ideas and behavior, withdrawal from other people, depression, suspiciousness, and lack of contact with reality may occur in those with gradual hearing loss. Family members and friends may also withdraw from the hearing-impaired person because they are frustrated by efforts to communicate. Conversation then dwindles to the necessities. Furthermore, people who are hard of hearing are commonly misjudged as senile because they appear inattentive or withdrawn.

For most people, these effects can be minimized by wearing a hearing aid. In one study, elder men with hearing loss improved in cognitive and communication skills, social interactions, and emotional well-being after being fitted for a hearing aid whereas a comparable group without hearing aids showed no improvement.[23] Although hearing aids amplify sound, they cannot distinguish between speech and background noise, despite claims to the contrary. However, hearing aids are becoming more and more sophisticated. Some have a built-in hearing aid as part of their eyeglass frame. Some are worn behind the ear with a clear plastic tube that transmits sound into the ear canal. Others fit in the outer ear, and a few are custom-fit in the ear canal and are not visible to observers. Some have several channels that allow reception tailored to the environment; others are programmable, responding to hearing loss changes.

Tips in Communicating with the Hearing-Impaired Individual

1. Speak clearly, distinctly, and slowly; do not shout or exaggerate your mouth movements.
2. Face the individual when talking and look him or her in the eyes. If the person to whom you are speaking is in a wheelchair, lower yourself to eye level.
3. Be sure there is enough light for the person to see you speaking but there is no glare.
4. Try to avoid noisy areas.
5. Give visual cues, such as hand movements and facial expressions in addition to your verbal message.
6. If you are asked to repeat what you said, find other words to say the same thing.
7. In a group situation, sit in a circle so everyone can see one another's lip movement and expressions. Clue them into the conversation by summarizing occasionally.
8. Be patient. Don't create the feeling that you are in a hurry.
9. Learn to read the individual's reaction to be certain she or he heard and understood what was said.
10. Keep hands, scarves, and tobacco away from your mouth. Don't chew gum, eat, or smoke while talking.
11. Get the person's attention before you start to speak.
12. Don't talk from too far away.
13. Make an attempt to discuss topics other than what is absolutely necessary, even though these are harder to communicate. Don't resort to curt, necessary exchanges.

Although a variety of hearing aids are available, all use the same mechanism. A tiny microphone in the aid converts sound to electrical impulses. An amplifier boosts the signal to a speaker, which changes it into sounds. The newer digital technology uses a microchip to convert sound waves into digital signals, and a computer chip is programmed to suppress background noise. However, it may cost up to $1,000 more, and the difference in effectiveness is small. Cochlear implants (electronic devices surgically placed in the inner ear), are possible for those with serious hearing deficits.

Despite the available technology, only one in four elderly persons who may benefit from a hearing aid wears one. This may be due to the fact that most hearing aids do not restore hearing to a normal level; instead, they amplify all sounds, which can be annoying. Additionally, hearing aids are often fitted incorrectly and are uncomfortable to wear. Some older people may refuse to wear a hearing aid for cosmetic reasons or because they believe it to be a sign of growing old. Furthermore, many elders cannot afford to purchase a hearing aid since neither the examination nor the appliance is covered by Medicare. Hearing aid costs range from $500 to $4,000, depending on their size and complexity. However, as in eyeglasses, Medicaid may pay for all or part of the cost if the individual qualifies.

Even when elders do wear hearing aids, the aids may not be in good repair. One study of British nursing home residents reported that half the hearing aids were not working, generally due to dead batteries.[24] Those residents with malfunctioning aids appeared isolated, confused, and had other social behavior changes.

A number of health professionals are available to assist elders with hearing problems. Physicians, either an *otologist* (ear specialist) or an *otolaryngologist* (ear, nose, and throat specialist), can diagnose the problem and determine if surgical or medical treatment is necessary, or if a hearing aid is indicated. *Audiologists* are highly trained, nonmedical specialists who can evaluate hearing problems and counsel a patient on hearing aids and rehabilitation. A *hearing aid dispenser* measures hearing loss, helps to select the proper aid, custom-fits the apparatus, and explains proper use and care techniques. Hearing aid dispensers must be licensed by the state to perform these tasks, but they are not qualified to diagnose hearing problems or to prescribe medication. Selecting a hearing aid is a difficult, expensive and time-consuming process and there is some variability among hearing aid dispensers in the quality of their work.

To participate in a simple screening by phone in your area, call 1-800-222-EARS. To find an audiologist in your area, or for advice on hearing aids or protection, call the American Speech-Language Hearing Association Consumer Helpline (1-800-638-8255). For information on protecting yourself from hearing loss, call the National Hearing Conservation Association at 515-266-2189.

Elders may also be interested in hearing ear dogs, pets trained to respond to the phone or doorbell. For more information, contact Dogs for the Deaf at 13260 Highway 238, Jacksonville, OR 97530.

Taste and Smell

The sensory organs of taste, called taste buds, are located predominantly on the tongue, although a few may be found in other places in the mouth. Taste buds are activated by chemicals from food when they are dissolved in saliva. When the receptor is triggered, it sends a taste message to the brain. There are certain types of cells that sense different tastes. Although it used to be thought that humans could detect four main tastes (sweet, salty, bitter, and sour), experimental data have shown that the full range of taste quality is broader (e.g., chalky, metallic, fat).[25] Each taste bud is thought to contain multiple types of taste cells and serves to synthesize taste sensations. The more taste buds, the better the sense of taste. Taste buds constantly regenerate, with a lifespan of about 10 days. The sense of smell further influences taste.

Most mammals have a highly developed sense of smell because this sense is crucial in their ability to find food, select a mate, and detect danger. However, humans depend on other senses to a greater extent, and their sense of smell is less developed. Dogs, for instance, have forty times more olfactory surface area than humans. Little research has been conducted to determine the type of smell receptors or the variety of odors humans can differentiate, perhaps because it is difficult to quantify odors.

Humans sense smells through a group of receptor cells (about 1/4 inch in diameter) located high in the nose. Smell receptors have a high turnover, about thirty days. These cells are very easily fatigued; a receptor will get used to a smell and stop sending messages to the brain after only a minute of exposure. The sense of smell influences the ability to taste and enjoy food, to be aware of dangers (such as gas fumes, burning electrical wires, smoke, or spoiled or burning food), and to detect body odors or pleasant smells.

Age-Associated Changes in Taste and Smell

Many adults have a reduced ability to taste and smell as they age; however, there is no clear evidence that aging itself is responsible. There are, however, fewer taste receptors and slower nerve transmissions with age, although the losses are highly variable.[26] Those elders who experience a noticeable loss of taste acuity generally have other medical conditions. Some medical problems cause noticeable loss in taste and smell, especially disorders involving nasal congestion. Alzheimer's disease also reduces ability to taste and smell, likely due to cognitive deficits. Other common causes are dentures, poor oral hygiene, and particularly, cigarette smoking. Medication side effects also play a role, especially those that cause dry mouth. Nutritional deficiencies, especially low zinc intake, reduce taste acuity.

The loss of taste and smell can have a significant effect upon an elder's health. A reduced ability to taste and smell makes it difficult for elders to adjust their food intake as they can no longer rely on their cues for salty, fatty, or sugary foods. For instance, loss of salt perception may make it harder for those with high blood pressure to restrict salt. Further, elders are less likely to detect the bad taste of spoiled food, putting them at a high risk for food poisoning. Those with a reduced sense of smell are less likely to respond to smoke, gas leaks, and other toxic fumes.

Reduced ability to taste or smell also makes eating less enjoyable, reducing the motivation to eat. Undernutrition is a major cause of involuntary weight loss, increased disease susceptibility, and reduced immune function among elders. A way to reduce the impact of poor taste and smell ability is to augment the natural taste of foods.

Balance and Equilibrium

There are three components of balance or equilibrium: the vestibular system, the visual system, and peripheral balance receptors. The major sense organ of balance is the vestibular system, located in the semicircular canals of the inner ear (figure 3.6). Three jelly-filled canals lie in each side of the head. Inside each canal are numerous receptor cells with hairlike projections imbedded in the jelly. When the head moves, the fluid moves and presses against these projections. These cells then send a message to the brain that the head is changing position. The brain reacts by sending motor impulses that either contract or relax particular involuntary muscles to maintain balance.

As long as two of the three components continue to function well, there should be little decrement in balance. However, if two systems are inadequate (e.g., an elder has vestibular problems and is in a dark room), the risk of an accident or fall is increased.

Age-Associated Changes in Balance and Equilibrium

Elders more commonly experience vertigo (a sense that the surroundings are spinning) and dizziness (light-headedness and unsteadiness). However, these symptoms are common side effects of many medications. Elders are also somewhat more likely to suffer from postural hypotension, a condition in which the cardiovascular system responds to a position change slower than usual, causing dizziness or

lightheadedness when one moves quickly from lying or sitting to standing.

Somatic Receptors

Somatic receptors respond to touch, pressure, heat, cold, pain, or body position in space and are located both in and outside the body. Upon stimulation, the receptors send impulses through nerve pathways to the spinal cord and brain for processing.

Touch and pressure receptors are located in the skin. The hairless portions of the skin (lips, fingertips, palms, genitals, and soles of the feet) are particularly sensitive to touch because they have a higher concentration of touch receptors. Once exposed to a particular touch for a time, the receptors adapt. This explains why we do not "feel" our clothing all day. Receptors that respond to heavy pressure are found deeper in the skin.

Thermoreceptors respond to either cold or heat. They sense changes in temperature, but once exposed to a certain temperature for a period of time, they adapt or cease to respond until there is another alteration in temperature.

Pain receptors are widely distributed throughout the skin and internal organs. Unlike the cold and heat receptors, the pain receptors do not rapidly adapt to a stimulus but continue to send messages to the brain as long as the pain continues.

Receptors that respond to changes in body position are located mainly around the joints. These sense changes in joint movement and relay the message to the brain.

Age-Associated Changes in the Somatic Receptors

Measuring age-related changes in the somatic senses is difficult since studies must rely on subjective responses to pain or temperature change rather than objective criteria. However, experts think that somatic receptors become less sensitive with age. Elders may need a greater stimulus before the nerve endings fire and send a message to the brain.

Elders may experience a decreased sensitivity to pain with advancing age. However, evidence supporting a physiological mechanism for this reduced sensitivity is lacking. Pain perception varies by situation, gender, culture, and personality. Elders may be less likely to report pain, have a higher threshold for pain, or feel less pain because of age changes in the receptors. A decreased ability to feel pain may carry both positive and negative consequences. Elders may be better able to cope with common, painful chronic diseases (e.g., arthritis). On the other hand, since pain signals danger, an elder with decreased pain sensitivity may be unaware of disease symptoms or minor injuries.

Although not necessarily an age change, many elders exhibit a decreased perception of heat and cold. Experts believe that reduced sensitivity to heat may contribute to the high incidence of burns among older people. Extremes in temperature are more likely to affect elders, and they recover more slowly after exposure to temperature stress.

THE ENDOCRINE SYSTEM

Body functions are regulated and coordinated through the interdependent workings of the nervous and endocrine systems. As previously described, the nervous system rapidly transmits electrochemical impulses across nerve fibers that send messages to and from the brain and spinal cord. The endocrine system transmits its chemical messages (hormones) much more slowly through the bloodstream, and its effects last longer.

Endocrine glands, located in the brain and other parts of the body, manufacture and release chemical messengers or hormones. A variety of metabolic activities are mediated by the endocrine system. Figure 3.7 illustrates the locations of the major endocrine glands. Each hormone has a different molecular structure and function, although all generally slow or speed a particular metabolic process. Hormones travel through the bloodstream until they attach themselves to the receptors located on the cells they are designed to reach (called target cells). Those hormones that do not combine with a receptor are usually inactivated by the kidneys or liver and released as waste.

Age-Associated Changes in the Endocrine System

Comparatively little is known about the endocrine system, and even less is understood about the effect

---

I Have Noticed

Everything is farther away than it used to be. It is even twice as far to the corner as they have added a hill.

I have given up running for the bus; it leaves earlier than it used to.

It seems to me they are making the stairs steeper than in the old days. And have you noticed the smaller print they use in newspapers?

There is no sense in asking anyone to read aloud anymore, as everyone speaks in such a low voice I can hardly hear them.

The material in dresses is so skimpy now, especially around the hips and waist, that it is almost impossible to reach one's shoelaces.

And the sizes don't run the way they used to. The 12s and 14s are much smaller.

Even people are changing. They are so much younger than they used to be when I was their age. On the other hand, people my own age are so much older than I am.

I ran into an old classmate the other day and she has aged so much she didn't recognize me.

I got to thinking about the poor dear while I was combing my hair this morning and in so doing I glanced at my own reflection. Really now, they don't even make good mirrors like they used to.

—Anonymous

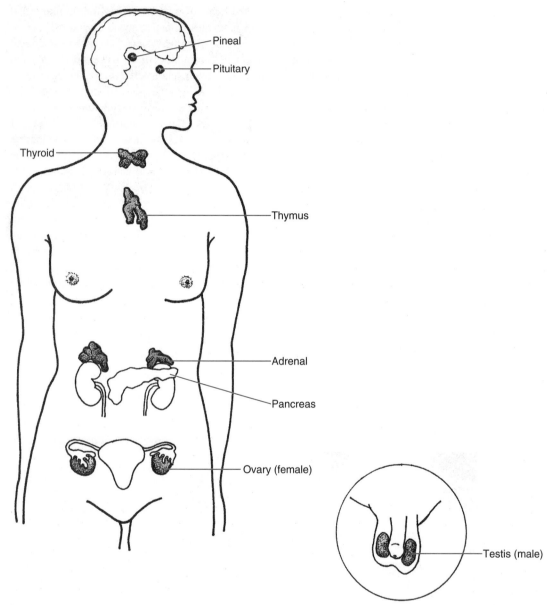

Figure 3.7
Major glands of the endocrine system

of aging on the function of each gland. The compli-cated interrelationship between the endocrine glands and the circulatory and nervous systems makes the distinction even more difficult. However, many hormones have been reported to decrease with increased age: estrogens, androgens, insulin, and thyroid and growth hormones. Further, hor-mone receptors frequently decline in numbers or efficiency with age. It can be difficult to determine whether the concentration of hormones decreasing or the receptors on the target cells do not respond as readily.

The most-studied endocrine gland is the pancreas and its associated hormone, insulin. After eating, food is broken down and absorbed, and its chemical components travel throughout the bloodstream. The liver converts some of the components into glucose, which the body cells use for energy. However, to extract the glucose from the bloodstream, the cells require insulin.

Those with Type I diabetes (also known as juvenile diabetes) do not produce insulin; thus, the cells cannot take up the glucose from the bloodstream. This may result in a very high glucose level in the blood (hyperglycemia) while the body cells are "starving in the midst of plenty" because there is no insulin to facilitate the entry of glucose into the cells. In contrast, those with Type II diabetes (also called adult-onset diabetes) have a defect that makes their cells resistant to insulin. Thus, the body must release very high levels of insulin to allow glucose to be taken up by cells. Insulin resistance is associated with high levels of glucose, high levels of insulin, and an accelerated rate of atherosclerosis.

With age, there is a decline in the ability of the blood to maintain normal glucose and blood sugar levels. There is also a decline of sensitivity of the cells to insulin. However, this is only partly attributed to advancing age and more likely a combination of aging, obesity, alteration in body fat distribution, and physical inactivity.

Levels of adrenal and thyroid hormones tend to decrease with age. Reduced thyroid hormone levels result in a decreased metabolic rate.[27] Cortisone levels also decline, likely due to decreased need for this stress hormone.[28] Although the thymus gland shrinks significantly after maturity, thymosin levels remain constant throughout adulthood. Changes in male and female sex hormones will be discussed in the next section.

THE REPRODUCTIVE SYSTEM

Proper functioning of the reproductive system depends on a complex interrelationship among the hormones of the pituitary, hypothalamus, and testes or ovaries. These hormones control the development of secondary sex characteristics, sexual arousal and activity, sperm production in men, and for women, egg production and the ability to bear and nurse children. Secondary sex characteristics include lower-pitched voice and facial and chest hair in men, and milk glands in breasts and body fat deposits on hips and buttocks in women. In the later years, the primary function of the system is sexual arousal and activity, and maintenance of secondary sex characteristics.

After menopause, women lose the capacity to reproduce. Elderly men, although still capable, are rarely interested in fathering children. This section will describe the male and female reproductive systems and their age-associated physiological changes. Psychological and social aspects of aging and sexuality, changes in sexual response with age, sexual dysfunction, and therapy will be discussed in chapter 6.

The Female

The hypothalamus, ovaries, and anterior pituitary glands secrete hormones that modulate the female's menstrual cycles, pregnancy, and the development and maintenance of secondary sexual characteristics. A pair of ovaries, located in the lower abdomen, produce estrogens (female hormones) and ova (figure 3.8).

The uterus is a muscular, pear-shaped organ held in place by four ligaments and located in front of the rectum. The vagina is a muscular tube that serves as the birth passageway and receives the erect penis during sexual intercourse. The external genital organs include the vulva, composed of the outer and inner lips (labia majora and labia minora) and the organ of sexual arousal, the clitoris. During excitation, the labia and the clitoris become engorged with blood and are sensitive to tactile stimulation. When sexually stimulated, the veins around the vagina become engorged with blood, resulting in a pressure that forces a liquid to pass from the veins through the surface cells of the vagina. The liquid provides a coating for the entire vagina. A pair of Bartholin's

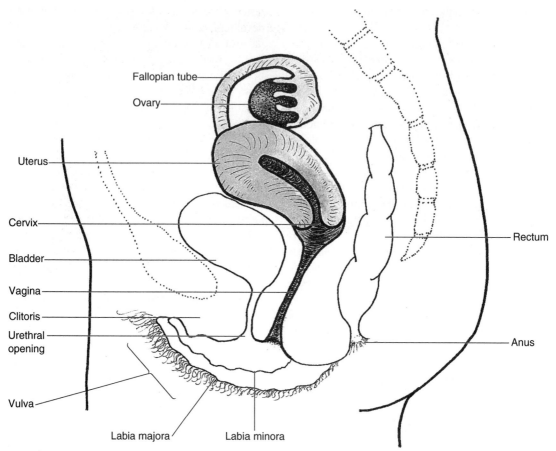

Figure 3.8
The female reprouctive system

glands, located on either side of the vaginal opening, secrete a small amount of mucus that facilitates genital sexual activity.

Age-Associated Changes in the Female Reprouctive System

Perhaps the most well-known age change for women is menopause, defined as the cessation of menstrual periods. However, menopause is not a discrete event, rather a gradual process. In their forties, women begin to experience hormonal changes that result in a gradual reduction in fertility and increasing variability in length and intensity of menstrual periods, until, at approximately age fifty,

menses and fertility cease. When a woman completes two years without a period, she has gone through menopause. The term "climacteric" refers to the duration of the period of hormonal fluctuations, which may last up to fifteen years.

During the climacteric, the menstrual cycle decreases in length and regularity due to the decreased ovarian production of estradiol, one of the most potent of the estrogen hormones. After menopause, estradiol production drops even further, and cyclical variation in hormone production ceases. However, this does not mean that the body no longer produces estrogens. In fact, androstenedione, a hormone secreted by the ovaries and the adrenal glands, is converted into estrone in fatty tissues. Estrone is a less potent form of estrogen that compensates somewhat for the decreased estradiol production.

Ovaries shrink when they cease to be stimulated to produce estrogens, likewise the uterus and fallopian tubes become smaller. The external genitalia lose subcutaneous fat, and pubic hair thins. Reduction in circulating estrogens causes the vaginal walls to be less elastic and thinner with decreased lubrication and decreased acidity. Reduced vaginal acidity increases the risk for yeast and bacterial infections. However, it is still questionable whether alterations in vaginal lubrication and elasticity are more related to disuse (e.g., reduced sexual activity) rather than age alone. Thinner walls make the vagina more prone to irritation or infection. Clitoral sensation remains throughout life so that older women retain the capacity for orgasm. Changes in sexual response will be discussed in chapter 6.

The hormonal changes accompanying menopause have dramatic consequences for women. A reduced estradiol production is associated with an increased rate of bone loss (osteoporosis), unfavorable alterations in cholesterol levels, and an increased risk of cardiovascular disease. After menopause, many women notice a change in the way their body fat is distributed, with a tendency for fat to accumulate on the abdomen. This alteration is related to an increased risk of diabetes and heart disease. Women may also experience other symptoms related to low estradiol levels, especially hot flashes and vaginal dryness.

Many women choose to undergo hormonal replacement therapy to reduce the short-term symptoms (vaginal dryness, hot flashes) and the long-term consequences of menopause (thinned bones and reduced heart disease risk). It is estimated that one-third the women in the United States have taken hormones to ameliorate the negative symptoms of menopause. There are many ways to take hormones, but generally women take two hormones cyclically, creating simulated monthly menses. Some women choose to take a lower continuous dose of the two hormones simultaneously, which does not result in cyclic bleeding.

A discussion of the risks and benefits of hormonal replacement therapy is found in chapter 10.

The Male

The male reproductive system consists of the penis, testes, scrotum, accessory ducts, and fluid-producing glands (figure 3.9). Two oval-shaped testes that produce sperm and secrete testosterone (the male sex hormone) are contained within the scrotum. Under the control of the pituitary gland, the testes produce viable sperm and male secondary sex characteristics. The testes release the sperm into the epididymis, where sperm cells mature and are stored. The epididymis empties into the vas deferens. Two glands, the seminal vesicles and the prostate, empty into the vas deferens. The seminal vesicles contribute fluid to aid the movement of the sperm. The prostate gland, a chestnut-shaped structure surrounding the first inch of the urethra, deposits fluid in the urethra, which activates the sperm.

Upon ejaculation, both the sperm and the fluid from the seminal vesicles enter the ejaculatory ducts. Semen is forcibly ejaculated from the urethra through the penis, a cylindrical-shaped organ equipped to carry both urine and semen. The penis is composed of erectile tissue enabling it to enlarge with sexual excitation.

Age-Associated Changes in the Male Reproductive System

Like many other changes with age, most functional changes in the male reproductive system are highly variable and depend on the man's psychological status, presence of disease, and drug use. Older men have more difficulty achieving and maintaining erections, and they have decreased ejaculatory force than younger adults. In addition, a longer time interval is required for a second erection. (Changes in sexuality with age will be more thoroughly discussed in chapter 6). Males experience a universal, age-related decline in the number of viable sperm. Even though the sperm count per ejaculation remains the same, the proportion of immature sperm increases with advanced age. Nevertheless, men generally retain the ability to father a child into very old age.

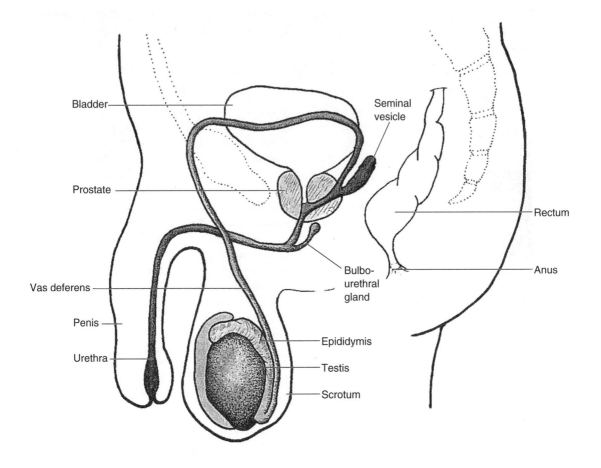

Figure 3.9
The male reproductive system

Perhaps the most well-documented structural alteration with age is the enlargement of the prostate. When it enlarges, it may constrict the urethra, causing difficulty in urinating. The gland begins to enlarge in the fourth decade, and by age eighty, almost all men have an enlarged prostate. This condition is known as benign prostatic hypertrophy. Although sexual performance is not altered, it can cause symptoms of urinary frequency, urgency, decreased force of stream, and

urinary retention. Benign prostatic hypertrophy will be discussed further in chapter 8.

Although not all studies document the same effect, it is thought that testosterone levels decline gradually with age. Levels of estradiol also diminish with age in men; this is likely because men produce estradiol from testosterone. Men who are ill or inactive have even more dramatic decreases in testosterone levels. The decline in testosterone is highly variable, however, with some healthy, physically fit older men maintaining levels that are higher than some younger men. Because testosterone is important in maintenance of muscle and bone mass and sexual desire, lower levels may predispose men to muscle wasting, osteoporosis, bone fractures, and decreased libido. There is even some research suggesting that declines in testosterone are related to declines in HDL (the good cholesterol) with age.

Among those men with abnormally low levels of testosterone, supplemental testosterone (called androgen replacement therapy) may improve muscle mass, bone density, energy and mood, libido, sexual functioning, and well-being. The therapy involves an injection every other week, or a patch on the scrotom or other area of the skin. However, the long-term effects of androgen replacement therapy, especially as it may relate to cardiovascular disease or prostate growth or cancer, is unknown, and its use is not recommended in men with normal testosterone levels. Most studies have not been conducted in men over sixty-five. Unlike older women with estrogen decline, not all older men experience a significant testosterone loss. Factors other than age are likely to be more important that age-associated changes in sex hormone level.

SUMMARY

Age-associated changes in body systems vary greatly. Although some structural alterations occur in almost every body system with age, functional effects are relatively minor and have little effect on daily life.

Skin becomes more wrinkled and less elastic, and hair may become thinned and gray. Elders lose muscular strength, joint flexibility, and bone strength and mass, but the losses are highly variable among individuals. The cardiovascular system becomes less efficient, especially at maximal exertion. Some aspects of immune function decline with age, although studies are not conclusive in this area. Lungs become less elastic with age, decreasing the efficiency of gas exchange. Because the digestive system has high reserve capacity, age has little effect on its function. With age, the kidneys become somewhat less efficient at filtering wastes from the blood, which may increase the length of time an active drug remains in the body. Because of this, physicians should adjust the dosages of elders' prescriptions and medications.

Changes in the communication networks of the body—the sensory, neural, and endocrine systems—can affect an individual's internal equilibrium as well as the ability to respond to the environment. The most significant age-associated changes occur in vision and hearing. Structural changes in the eye cause presbyopia and a decreased visual acuity in low light and color discrimination. Cataracts are so common that they are considered to be an age-associated change. Environmental noise and structural changes in the ear result in an almost universal hearing loss with age, especially in the high frequencies (presbycusis). However, eyeglasses and hearing aids significantly reduce the impact of changes in vision and hearing.

Some structural changes occur with age in the nervous system, however loss in function is minimal, if at all. Similarly, alterations in taste, smell, equilibrium, and somatic receptors are minimal. Perhaps the greatest endocrine system change for women is a decline of estrogen production in the ovaries. Age changes in the genital system are minimal: healthy men and women maintain the capacity for sexual activity and orgasm throughout life.

Changes occurring in body systems are highly variable among individuals. Some older individuals function physiologically better than some middle-aged persons. Most of the declines we associate with aging are due not to aging itself, but to disease processes, environmental factors, or modifiable behaviors such as cigarette smoking, physical inactivity, and poor nutrition. However, understanding the systems that are affected by age can help us interact more effectively with the elderly.

ACTIVITIES

1. List the health behaviors you currently practice that may hasten your aging process. Which systems do these habits affect? How might these behaviors affect your functioning ten years from now? Twenty years? What practices enhance your health?

2. Make a list of physiological changes you believe are inevitable with aging. Which of these changes have you seen in all the elders you know? How are the elders you know affected by these aging processes? How do they adjust?

3. Draw or describe your appearance and lifestyle at age eighty. What physiological changes did you illustrate? Which changes may be minimized by different health habits?

4. Individuals of all ages often say, "I must be getting old." Explain the circumstances surrounding why you or others say this. Are they valid features of aging, or are they due to disease or environmental factors?

5. Select a characteristic of older people that you believe is an age change. Using the criteria given and recent literature, design a study that would demonstrate whether your supposition is valid.

6. Design a commercial, printed advertisement, or a radio spot aimed at young people advocating sunscreen use. How did you convince the public to take care of their skin before they notice damage?

7. Many companies prosper from products designed to make the public feel or look younger. Collect advertisements that promote this theme and share them with your classmates. Are claims valid? If not, write a letter to one of the companies protesting its false advertising.

8. A number of activities enable students to simulate age-related sensory and mobility decrements. Try some of the following and discuss the possible effects on daily routine and self-concept. To simulate decreased touch sensitivity, put rubber cement on your fingertips. To simulate decreased visual acuity, put Vaseline on your eyeglasses. Place cotton or plugs in your ears to simulate hearing losses. Ace bandages wrapped around joints simulates stiffness. A scarf tied from the neck to the belt can simulate postural changes. A student may spend the whole day using a wheelchair or walker. If your college has a theater department, ask to be made-up and dressed as an elder and then go shopping. Record your feelings and the reaction of others. Can you think of other simulation activities?

9. Interview a person who has visual or hearing loss. How does the loss affect his or her lifestyle? How has she or he compensated for this loss?

10. Compile a list of resources for visual and hearing-impaired elders and their families in your community.

11. Collect fliers, booklets, and newsletters geared for elder use and analyze the suitability of paper color, typeface, content, and layout. Ask elders which are the easiest to read.

12. Design a flier educating elders about age-associated changes using a user-friendly style.

13. What loud sounds have you been exposed to that may have permanently affected your hearing? List sounds that are common in your home and community that may cause hearing loss. Would you be embarrassed to wear a hearing aid? Talk with your parents and grandparents about their attitude about hearing loss and hearing aids.

BIBLIOGRAPHY

1. Hayflick, L. 1996. *How and why we age.* New York: Ballantine Books.

2. Rowlatt, C., and Franks, L.M. 1978. Aging in tissues and cells. In *Geriatric medicine and gerontology,* J.C. Brocklehurst, ed. New York: Churchill and Livingstone.

3. Comfort, A. 1976. *A good age.* New York: Simon and Schuster.

4. Rowe, J.W., and Kahn, R.L. 1987. Human aging: Usual and successful. *Science* 237:143–49.

5. Raloff, J. 1996. Vanishing flesh. *Science News* 150(August 10):90–91.

6. Aloia, J.F., McGowan, D.M., Vaswani, A.N., et al. 1991. Relationship of menopause to skeletal and muscle mass. *American Journal of Clinical Nutrition* 53:1378–83.

7. Rodenheffer, R.J., Gerstenblith, G., and Becker, L.C., et al. 1984. Exercise cardiac output is maintained with advancing age in healthy human subjects: Cardiac dilatation and increased stroke volume compensate for diminished heart rate. *Circulation* 60:203–13.

8. Kitzman, D.W., and Edwards, W.D. 1990. Minireview: Age-related changes in the anatomy of the normal human heart. *Journal of Gerontology* 45:M33–M39.

9. Marcus, S.E., Kaste, L.M., and Brown, L.J. 1994. Prevalence and demographic correlates of tooth loss among the elderly in the United States. *Special Care in Denstistry* 14:123–27.

10. Lindeman, R.D., Tobin, J., Shock, N.W. 1985. Longitudinal studies on the rate of decline of renal function with age. *Journal of the American Geriatrics Society* 33: 278–285.

11. Terry, R.D., DeTeresa, R., and Hansen, L.A. 1987. Neocortical cell counts in normal human adult aging. *Annals of Neurology* 21:530–39.

12. Morris, J.C., McKeel, D.W., and Storandt, M., et al. 1991. Very mild Alzheimer's disease: Informant-based clinical, psychometric, and pathological distinctions from normal aging. *Neurology* 41:469–78.

13. Ratner, H.H., Schell, D.A., and Crimmins, A., et al. 1987. Changes in adults' prose recall: Aging or cognitive demands? *Developmental Psychology* 23:521–25.

14. Schaie, K.W., and Willis, S. 1986. Can decline in adult intellectual functioning be reversed? *Developmental Psychology* 22:223–32.

15. Sunderland, A., Watts, K., Baddeley, A.D., and Harris, J.E. 1986. Subjective memory assessment and test performance in elderly adults. *Journal of Gerontology* 41:376–84.

16. Varma, S.D. 1991. Scientific basis for medical therapy of cataracts by antioxidants. *American Journal of Clinical Nutrition* 53(1 Supp):335S–345S.

17. Wolfe, S.M., ed. 1998. "Cataracts in adults: A patient's guide." *Health Letter* 14:2.

18. Mangione, C.M., Phillips, R.S., and Lawrence, M.G., et al. 1997. Improved visual function and attenuation of declines in health-related quality of life after cataract extraction. *Archives of Opthamology* 112:1419–25.

19. Tielsch, J.M., Javitt, J.C., and Coleman, A., et al. 1995. The prevalence of blindness and visual impairment among nursing home residents in Baltimore. *New England Journal of Medicine* 332:1205–9.

20. Javitt, J.C., Kendix, M., Tielsch, J.M., et al. 1995. Geographic variation in utilization of cataract surgery. *Medical Care* 33:90–105.

21. Goldzweig, C.L., Mittman, M.S., Carter, G.M., et al. 1997. Variations in cataract extraction rates in Medicare prepaid and fee-for-service settings. *Journal of the American Medical Association* 277:1765–68.

22. Wallhagen, M.I., Strawbridge, W.J., Cohen, R.D., and Kaplan, G.A. 1997. An increasing prevalence of hearing impairment and associated risk factors over three decades of the Alameda County Study. *American Journal of Public Health* 87:440–42.

23. Mulrow, D.D., Aguilar, C., and Endicott, J.E., et al. 1990. Quality of life changes and hearing impairment: A randomized trial. *Annals of Internal Medicine* 113:188–94.

24. Anand, J.K. 1989. Hearing loss leading to impaired ability to communicate in residents of homes for the elderly. *British Medical Journal* 298:1429–30.

25. Schiffman, S.S. 1997. Taste and smell losses in normal aging and disease. *Journal of the American Medical Association* 278:1357–62.

26. Morrison, E.E., and Costanzo, R.M. 1992. Morphology of olfactory epithelium in humans and other vertebrates. *Microscopy Research Techniques* 23:49–61.

27. Felicetta, J.V. 1990. The aging thyroid. *Consultant* (September):59–71.

28. Wolfsen, A.R. 1982. Aging and the adrenals. In *Endocrine aspects of aging,* S.G. Korenman, ed. New York: Elsevier Biomedical.

4

PHYSICAL
ACTIVITY

Those who think they have no time for bodily exercise will sooner or later have to find time for illness.

Earl of Derby

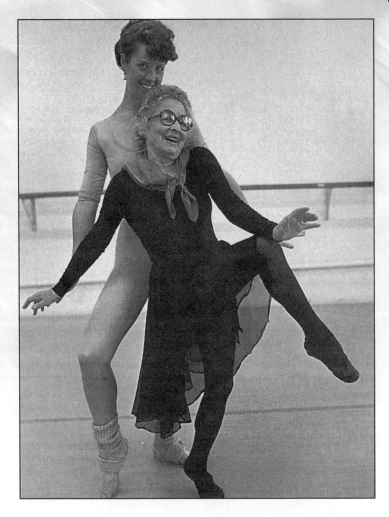

Before the Industrial Age, most people were not concerned about getting sufficient physical exercise because their active daily routine kept their muscles and hearts strong. As the workplace and home become more mechanized, fewer people get sufficient physical activity from their occupations and household chores. Most people must make an effort to become more active because it is easier to sit in front of the television or computer screen than to go for a walk or swim a few laps. Elderly people are even less likely to engage in physical activity than their younger counterparts, despite its proven value for all age groups. This chapter will discuss components of physical fitness, the benefits of keeping active, the pitfalls of inactivity, and the role activity plays in the prevention and treatment of several health problems. Patterns of physical activity in elders, their attitudes toward exercise, and ways to promote a more active lifestyle in that group will also be addressed.

COMPONENTS OF PHYSICAL FITNESS

It is important to learn the difference between physical activity, exercise, and physical fitness. *Physical activity* is defined as any bodily movement produced by skeletal muscles that results in the expenditure of energy. *Physical fitness* is a set of attributes that people have or achieve that relates to the ability to perform physical activity.[1] Not only does physical fitness enable us to have the energy needed to complete a given task, but it also allows us to generate the strength needed to perform that task. At any age, being physically fit enhances our quality of life, allowing us to meet ordinary and unexpected demands of daily life with ease. For elders, fitness may mean the ability to live independently, do household chores, shop for food, engage in active leisure pursuits, and withstand illness and injury. There are many components of physical fitness: cardiovascular endurance, muscle strength and endurance, joint flexibility, and coordination and balance. However, physical fitness is a state of conditioning that can rapidly be lost without continuous bouts of physical activity. *Exercise* is a type of physical activity that can be defined as "planned,

structured, and repetitive bodily movement done to improve or maintain one or more components of physical fitness."[1] Some exercises are better than others for the type of fitness desired. For instance, jogging increases endurance, while dancing increases balance and flexibility.

Exercises that increase **cardiovascular endurance** are called *aerobic,* meaning "with oxygen." These types of exercises maintain an elevated heart rate by repetitive or rhythmic motions of the two largest muscle groups, those that move the legs and arms. Aerobic exercises, such as jogging, walking, aerobic dance, martial arts, shoveling, sweeping, swimming, bicycling, cross-country skiing, and rowing strengthen the heart and lungs. Indeed, this component of physical fitness has been studied the most and has the most scientific evidence of benefit to overall health and disease prevention. Aerobic exercises increase ability to withstand illness, decrease morbidity from heart disease or diabetes, and are associated with weight loss and other favorable changes in body physiology. However, other aspects of physical fitness should not be neglected: muscular strength and endurance, joint flexibility, balance, and coordination.

The more intensely an individual exercises aerobically, the more oxygen must be inhaled and the harder the heart has to work. Thus, the most commonly accepted measurement of cardiovascular fitness is called *maximal oxygen consumption.* This is the amount of oxygen taken in and distributed to working muscles when a person is exercising at maximum rate. Highly fit individuals have a higher maximum oxygen consumption than their sedentary counterparts. In the laboratory, maximal oxygen consumption is used to estimate intensity of exercise.

Exercises that increase muscle strength and endurance, but not cardiovascular fitness, are called *anaerobic,* meaning "without oxygen." These exercises require so much muscle exertion that oxygen cannot be supplied to muscle tissues fast enough. Thus, the tissues begin to get their energy from a chemical pathway that does not require as much oxygen. Although these exercises may increase muscle strength and endurance, they do not strengthen the heart and lungs. Anaerobic exercises include sprinting, isometric or static exercises (e.g., grip squeezes), and weight lifting.

Endurance is the ability of a muscle to sustain work over a period of time, either to keep a muscle contracted or to continually contract and relax the muscle. Muscular endurance is required to hold a heavy object for a long time or to continually repeat a motion, such as hammering, kneading bread, or sawing. Both aerobic exercises and anaerobic exercises increase muscular endurance.

Strength is the ability to apply force by muscle contraction. Muscles develop strength when they contract against resistance. Strength is important in a wide variety of daily activities including opening a jar and carrying groceries. Strong muscles in the back and abdomen are important to preserve posture and prevent backache, while muscles of the shoulders and legs are important in mobility and daily activities. Aerobic exercises build up abdominal, leg, and upper body strength. The syndrome of painful knees and tired legs in older people is alleviated considerably by quadricep-strengthening exercises. Calisthenics, brisk walking, jogging, weight training, or biking may also increase strength.

Flexibility is the ability to move the joints through a maximum range of motion without undue strain. Flexibility improves posture, physical performance, and reduces the risk of joint injuries or strains. A person who is flexible can easily pick up an object from the floor, look behind, or reach a high cabinet. Flexibility in the neck and extremities help prevent muscle strain, while flexibility of the spine prevents low back pain and postural deformities. Inactivity, joint disease, and injuries to the joints and surrounding tissues can decrease flexibility. People can enhance their flexibility by exercising each joint separately with slow, regular, repeated stretching exercises. Ballet, modern dance, yoga, and aquatic exercises enhance flexibility.

Balance is an important component of physical fitness and is affected by many of the chronic diseases of old age. Problems with balance are a major reason for falls and other accidents among elders. Older people can improve their balance with practice. Dancing, yoga, martial arts, standing or hopping on one foot, and walking on a straight line improve balance.

Coordination is the ability to synchronize different actions of the body with each other and with vision. Agility is the ability to coordinate such movements and change directions quickly and safely. Racquet sports, martial arts, aerobics, and dancing may provide the highest degree of training for coordination and agility.

Whether young or old, the goal of developing a personal fitness plan is to seek a balance among different fitness components. Even those with physical limitations can find some form of activity that is enjoyable and beneficial.

BENEFITS OF PHYSICAL ACTIVITY

Regular physical activity is well-documented to slow, or even reverse, many of the so-called age-related physical decrements. It also delays the onset or progression of several diseases and is believed to improve psychological well-being. And, for elders, physical activity is related to maintaining independence. It has been estimated that as many as 250,000 deaths a year in the United States, or about 12 percent of total deaths, can be attributed to a lack of regular physical activity.[2] The only other health behavior that causes more deaths than a sedentary lifestyle is cigarette smoking.

In 1996, the Surgeon General released a report, *Physical Activity and Health,* that reviewed the role of physical activity in the prevention of disease. The report concluded that physical activity reduces the risk for developing or dying from coronary heart disease, adult-onset diabetes, hypertension, and colon cancer.[3] It also reduces symptoms of anxiety and depression, and contributes to the development and maintenance of healthier bones, muscles and joints, and helps control weight. Physical activity enables older adults to maintain the ability to live independently and reduces the incidence of falling and fractures. Further, the report stated that many of the health benefits from an active lifestyle can be

Chopstick-Wielding 'Wrong Old Lady' Nabs Purse-Thief

SAN FRANCISCO (AP)—Pity the poor purse snatcher who made the mistake of picking on 73-year-old Louise Burt.

"I didn't give him a chance. He picked on the wrong old lady," said Burt as she recounted how she chased the would-be thief through San Francisco's Mission District Tuesday.

"Kid, I ran after that son-of-a-b—. I chased him to hell-and-gone. Then the police caught him."

Burt was en route to a bingo game at a senior citizens' center with a couple of chums when someone grabbed her purse. Dressed in a black pantsuit and pumps with 2 1/2-inch heels, her waist-length silver-gold hair anchored with lacquered chopsticks, Burt gave chase.

"That guy took off like a deer and I was right behind him," said the intended victim, whose purse contained her keys, about $10, a transit pass, and her police whistle.

"I was so beside myself I wanted to kill him. I pulled out the chopsticks out of my hair to stab him if I could," she said. "My hair fell down and was hanging down to my fanny. I must have looked like a witch but I got superpower from somewhere and kept right after him." Swearing and shouting for help, she chased the thief down one street, through an alley and up another street into a public housing project where police officers Cherelyn Barnett and Melvin Thornton joined the pursuit.

"We were on (foot) patrol when we saw—and heard her—chasing the guy," said Thornton. "Did she run. We finally overtook her and went after him."

Thornton caught the man on a roof-top.

"He took one look at me, dropped the purse and jumped off the roof, two stories down to the ground," said the officer. "It must have been a 20-to-25-foot drop."

Thornton ran downstairs where he found William Jones, 22, cowering beneath a car with two broken ankles.

(Reprinted with permission of the Associated Press.)

---

achieved with a moderate level of activity—150 calories a day nearly every day, which is equivalent to a 30-minute brisk walk. Even though the exercise doesn't need to be vigorous, the degree of benefit is related to the length and intensity: the longer and more vigorous the exercise, the greater the benefits.

Although a lifetime of physical activity is best for health and a long life, even middle-aged and older individuals who were previously sedentary can achieve health benefits when they begin a program of physical activity. This section discusses some of the benefits associated with physical activity: decreased death rate, changes in fat and energy metabolism, increased cardiovascular endurance, decreased serum cholesterol and insulin levels, increased bone mass, muscle strength and joint mobility, and psychological benefits. Although most studies have been conducted on white, middle-aged men, a growing number of trials are including women and the elderly.

Although we know that exercise extends life and prevents disease, exactly how it works is the topic of multiple ongoing studies. Is exercise itself beneficial, or is it just that those who exercise are thinner? Are the benefits of exercise due to the increased metabolic rate, change in distribution of body fat, or the changes in the level of insulin or fats? Perhaps exercise itself is not important, but rather that those who exercise are likely to practice other healthy behaviors, such as eating right and not smoking. It is likely that a combination of these and other, still undiscovered, factors account for the benefits of exercise on health.

Decreased Death Rate

Data from a variety of studies have provided solid evidence of an inverse relationship between the level of cardiorespiratory fitness and all-cause mortality: the more fit an individual is, the lower the risk of both cardiovascular disease and death from any cause. In one study, the moderate fitness group had a 60 percent reduction in death rate when compared to the low-fitness group. When the high-fitness group was compared to the low-fitness group, there was a 68 percent reduction in death rate.[4]

Individuals who increase their activity level can also reduce their risk of death. One large longitudinal study compared the death rates of sedentary middle-aged men with their more active peers, and found a significant difference in mortality rate. Several years later, they measured the sedentary men again, this time comparing the death rates of those who were still sedentary with those who became more physically active. They reported a 65 percent reduction in death rate among those sedentary men who subsequently became more active when compared to the other members of their group who remained unfit.[5]

Fewer studies have been conducted on women and elders, but the results indicate similar benefits. A recent study of more than 40,000 post-menopausal women confirmed that regular vigorous exercise resulted in a reduced death rate. Also, those who exercised moderately two to four times weekly were 30 percent less likely to die prematurely, and increasing benefits were reported with more vigorous activity levels.[6] Another longitudinal study of over 700 retired men reported that those who walked less than a mile a day had nearly twice the mortality rate of those who walked more than two miles a day. In that study, the longer the distance walked, the lower the mortality rate.[7]

Although multiple studies find that people who engage in a lifetime of physical activity live longer than those who are inactive, there is no consensus on how much activity is enough to have an effect on mortality. An early study of Harvard alumni found that those who regularly engaged in walking, stair climbing, and sports had a lower mortality rate, especially from cardiovascular and respiratory conditions, than their more sedentary counterparts. The researchers asserted that the amount of additional life attributable to exercise was about two years.[8] Another large study of middle-aged men several years later reported that only those who engaged in vigorous physical activity had a reduced mortality rate: those with moderate exercise did not reduce their mortality rate at all.

Vigorous exercise was defined as burning 1,500 calories a week, or walking briskly four to five miles for at least forty-five minutes a day, five days a week, or jogging at least an hour three times a week. In that study, the reduced mortality of those who exercised vigorously was equivalent to the difference in mortality risk between a pack-a-day smoker and a nonsmoker.[9]

Increased Metabolic Rate and Decreased Body Fat

Exercise causes a temporary increase in the speed at which the body burns calories, or metabolic rate. Even if total calories ingested remain the same, an increase in metabolic rate through exercise leads to weight loss. It is common knowledge that more calories are burned during exercise, but it is now known that an increased metabolic rate persists even after exercise is completed. If exercise is vigorous and practiced regularly, the increased metabolic rate results in a weight loss above the caloric expenditure of the exercise itself. In contrast, dieting without exercise reduces metabolic rate, thus burning fewer calories.

Those who engage in vigorous physical activities generally have less body fat and more muscle mass than those who are sedentary. The body fat of the average older person is generally about 30 percent, while that of an older professional athlete may be half that percentage. Furthermore, body fat can be reduced with a regular aerobic exercise program. Studies show that older people participating in exercise programs can decrease body fat levels and increase metabolic rate, even at moderate exercise intensity. In addition, research shows that if regular strength training is part of a weight loss program, muscle mass is increased, even though total weight is decreased. In contrast, dieting without strength training results in muscle loss.[10]

Changes in Blood Fats and Insulin Resistance

There is much evidence that aerobic exercise reduces the incidence of cardiovascular disease by changing the relative balance of blood fats, subsequently slowing the progression of atherosclerosis. Many experts assert that a low level of high-density lipoprotein cholesterol (HDL) is the single most powerful predictor of heart disease. High levels of HDLs are associated with a *lower* risk of heart disease, while high levels of low-density lipoprotein cholesterol (LDL) and triglycerides are associated with a higher risk. Regular aerobic exercise acts to decrease both LDLs and triglycerides and increase HDLs in both men and women.

Although exercise alone can elevate HDL, some experts believe it is the weight loss resulting from the exercise that is responsible for the changes in lipid composition. The greater the intensity, frequency, and duration of exercise, the more likely blood levels of triglycerides and LDL will decrease. Because most studies on the effect of exercise on lipids have been conducted on men, there is less evidence of these favorable effects upon women.[11]

As people age, their body cells are less likely to respond to the insulin circulating in their blood (called lowered insulin sensitivity). Because the glucose (sugar) carried in the blood that has been broken down from food cannot get into the body cells to produce energy, the blood contains too much glucose. Even older people without diabetes require higher doses of insulin for their body to use circulating sugars. These higher insulin levels are associated with an increased risk of atherosclerosis, obesity, and cardiovascular disease. With exercise, the body cells become more sensitive to insulin, and glucose passes into the cells more easily. Consequently, the pancreas secretes less insulin, and blood sugar levels fall to more healthful ranges.

Increased Cardiovascular Endurance

In sedentary individuals, cardiovascular capacity declines from age thirty, and this decline may even accelerate after age sixty-five.[12] Although some of the decline may be related to aging, a significant portion is likely due to weight gain and heart muscle atrophy from inactivity. Vigorous aerobic exercise improves many variables affecting cardiovascular function: it strengthens the heart muscle, allowing a higher volume of blood to be expelled with each beat of the heart, thus increasing its efficiency and creating less strain on the heart. Exercise also lowers the resting heart rate and blood pressure, improves blood return to the heart, and reduces harmful blood cholesterol and blood clotting. It is now well-documented that the decline in cardiovascular function can be slowed, or even reversed, with regular, vigorous physical activity.

Elders who engage in aerobic exercise are able to reduce the age-associated decline in aerobic capacity. The improvements are even greater in elders who were formerly sedentary. A number of reports indicate that an aerobic exercise program initiated in later life can significantly improve cardiovascular endurance. Ideally, individuals should engage in moderate intensity exercise programs throughout life. However, most people exercise sporadically. New evidence finds that even with lapses in exercise that persist for more than two months, cardiovascular losses are small and upon resuming exercise, elders are able to rapidly recondition.[13]

How much physical activity should be accomplished to maintain a moderate or high level of cardiorespiratory fitness? In one study, over 13,000 subjects between twenty and eighty-seven were questioned on the type and duration of physical activities they accomplished each week. Their responses were compared to their fitness level as measured by a maximal exercise test. In this study, those who had a moderate to high level of cardiorespiratory fitness took the equivalent of a brisk walk of approximately thirty minutes on most days of the week. This level of activity generally held for both males, females, and all adult age groups.[14]

Increased Bone Mass

A reduction in bone mass is associated with advanced age and inactivity, consequently increasing minor aches and pains and, more seriously, debilitating fractures. Elders with brittle bones may become overly cautious about physical activity, inadvertently promoting further decline. When older bones are injured, they take longer to heal.

Sure, You'll Get Older. So What?

"I JUST CAN'T GO and find somebody to ask for help every time I want to lift a finger," said Marjorie Newlin, explaining why she took up body-building.

We were at a gym in Philadelphia where Newlin was training for the National Physique Committee's Philadelphia Bodybuilding Champi-onships. Newlin sat down at the leg-press machine, bracing her feet against a platform connected to 180 pounds of cast iron. She pushed it back and forth 12 times, then paused and did three more sets of 12. Not bad for a 78-year-old grandmother of four who started weight-lifting just six years ago.

Newlin, who has won 25 trophies so far, said it was never her intention to bare her sculpted muscles in pub-lic. She began lifting weights to become strong enough to handle everyday tasks, like keeping her cat supplied with kitty litter. A few years ago, her supermarket had a sale on 50-pound bags, but Newlin couldn't find anyone to lift them off the shelf. That's no longer a problem. Nor is the upkeep of her two-story home. "I always felt I could do whatever I want to," she said, "and now I know I can." Newlin shovels snow, cuts grass, and hauls a 50-pound fan up from the basement every spring. "I couldn't do all this before without being worn out."

Newlin always enjoyed exer-cising. After finishing her work-day as a registered nurse, she'd often stop into a health club for a stint on the treadmill or stationary bike. But after retiring in 1987 to care for her terminally ill husband, Newlin decided to take up weight training. She knew resistance training with free weights and machines builds strength, sta-mina, and endurance, and it prevents osteoporosis.

One day Newlin entered Rivers Gym, a mecca for serious body-builders, then owned by Bob Rivers. It wasn't long before Rivers spotted her commitment and potential. "Rain, shine, cold weather—I'd look up, and she'd be there," he recalled.

Rivers took charge of Newlin's training. At first he was concerned about pushing her too hard, but as Newlin's strength increased weekly, Rivers noticed she could perform feats that people many years younger couldn't. "It was amazing to watch a 72-year-old body in that condition," he noted. Rivers decided that it was time for Newlin to compete, but when

Deborah Holloway

he showed her the teeny-weeny bikini she'd be wearing to display her mus-cles, she said, "No way!" Then she reconsidered.

"I knew the contest meant a lot to him," said Newlin, "so I thought, 'I'll do this once—but I'm not going to do it again!" She won. "When the judge announced her age, the audience went haywire," Rivers recalled. Newlin had a different take: "I thought they were applauding because the old lady made it onto the stage," she joked.

The soft-spoken bodybuilder said she would like to see at least one belief about aging changed: "An older person can exercise with weights and build muscle," Newlin asserted. Her current trainer, the Rev. Richard Brown III, agreed. "She's opened my eyes to seniors," he said. Recently, Brown started Newlin on the "dead lift"—hoisting a 45-pound barbell up from the floor. Already she has increased the weight to 65 pounds.

How does she see herself next year, at age 79? "Well, I could add 50 pounds to the dead lift by next year," she replied. "And I should be able to bench-press 100." She hopes to grow steadily stronger or at least maintain her present strength.

"People say, 'When you get to this age, you can't do this and you can't do that,' but that's not the way it is," she added. "I never con-sidered my age when I went to the gym." In fact, Newlin never thought about her age at all until she attracted so much attention. "I see some people so terrified about getting older, but it's going to hap-pen if you're still alive," she said, laughing.

The immobility necessary for healing further exacerbates bone loss.

Exercise increases bone mineral content and consequent bone strength. Bones become stronger through the pull of muscle contraction and the forces of gravity upon them. Those engaging in a higher level of physical activity have a higher bone mineral content than sedentary individuals. A group of long distance runners ages fifty to seventy-two were compared with a matched group of inactive people. Both male and female runners had 40 percent more bone mineral than the control group.[15] Additionally, weight-bearing exercise programs increase bone mineral density in both men and women.

Improved Muscle Strength

A decrease in muscle strength is an important factor leading to physical limitations and disabilities in old age. The muscular strength of a sedentary

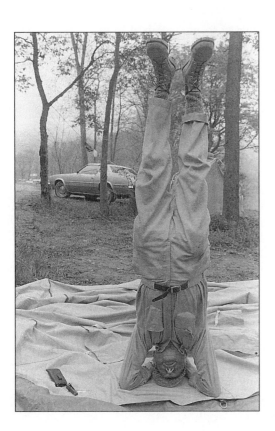

elder is estimated to be only 60 to 70 percent of the level in young adults.[16] Muscle strength increases with aerobic and anaerobic exercises, even if exercises are begun late in life. With prolonged exercise, the muscles get larger, develop an increased blood supply, and work more efficiently. There have been multiple studies on the effect of exercise that document significant increases in muscle strength in older adults, even among the very old.[17] Elders can significantly increase muscle strength with weight training almost as much as younger individuals.[18] Even frail elders in skilled nursing facilities can increase mobility with strength training. One study of institutionalized frail elders (average age, eighty-seven), underwent a weight-training regimen three times a week for ten weeks. As a result, muscle strength more than doubled, and the ability to climb stairs and walk increased significantly.[19] Regular exercise, particularly strength training, can combat sarcopenia, muscle loss associated with aging.

Positive Psychological Effects

Studies are beginning to support the widespread experience of those who regularly exercise: it reduces stress, improves the ability to sleep, and enhances feelings of well-being. Those who exercise regularly report a lower risk of depression and improved mood when compared with those who do not exercise. Exercise may exert its effect on mood by release of endorphins, natural pain-killing chemicals that promote feelings of well-being, or possibly through alteration of hormone levels. Exercise also has positive psychological effects (distraction from problems, feeling more attractive or capable, interaction with others) that may be responsible for the positive effects reported after exercise.

Although there is general support for the claim that exercise confers psychological benefits to its participants, many of the studies that have attempted to document such effects suffer methodological problems. Thus far, the effectiveness of exercise programs in treating depression, anxiety, and other negative mood states is not well-documented.[20] However, evidence continues to accumulate, and the studies are becoming more sophisticated. One study divided a group of mildly depressed elders living in the community into two groups: one group participated in a ten-week supervised weight-training program while the other group attended health education sessions without exercise. In addition to gaining strength, those in the weight-training group significantly reduced self-reported depression when compared to the matched group who underwent the health education program.[21] Another study compared institutionalized elders who participated in a reminiscence group with a group who participated in seated exercises twice a week. Aside from physiological gains, the exercise group reported less depression.[22]

Limited research on elders has shown that exercise can have a tranquilizing effect. In a classic study, the effect of a single "dose" of mild exercise was compared with a tranquilizer on reducing muscle tension in ten elderly subjects. The only treatment that significantly lowered electrical activity in muscles was exercise: a fifteen-minute walk at a moderate rate was sufficient to bring about the desired muscle relaxant effect, and it persisted for about one hour.[23]

Although there is much anecdotal evidence that physical exercise enhances the ability to fall asleep easily and to sleep well, a recent study was able to document that older adults with moderate sleep complaints increased both their ease of getting to sleep and sleep duration with regular exercise. The regimen included four training sessions a week of thirty to forty minutes of low-impact aerobics and brisk walking.[24] Since exercise has no side effects and is inexpensive, prescribing exercise instead of medication could eventually be the physician's first line of treatment for sleep problems.

Exercise, particularly aerobic exercise, may improve memory, reaction time, and cognitive function in elders, although study results in this area are mixed.[25] For example, elders participating in exercise programs improved their performance on tests of reaction time, memory, visual organization, and mental flexibility.[26] However, another study found no improvement in cognition after a year-long endurance training program.[27] One study of Alzheimer's patients revealed that those elders who engaged in a walking program three times a week improved communication skills compared to their counterparts who spent the same amount of time in conversation.[28] Just as with its psychological effects, it is difficult to determine whether exercise exerts its effects through altered physiology (e.g., increased circulation of blood to the brain) or through psychological factors (e.g., increased socialization).

HAZARDS OF INACTIVITY

> Look at a patient lying in bed.
> What a pathetic picture he makes.
> The blood clotting in his veins,
> the lime draining from his bones,
> the scybala stacking up in his colon,
> the flesh rotting from his sweat,
> the urine leaking from his distended bladder,
> and the spirit evaporating from his soul.[29]

In the nineteenth century, strict bed rest was believed to promote healing and was prescribed for many illnesses common in old age: tuberculosis, congestive heart failure, and heart attacks. However, studies of World War II veterans suggested that rehabilitation and increased activity improved recovery. With space travel and its studies on weightlessness, additional evidence was gathered on the negative consequence of inactivity and the benefits of movement.

Inactivity, especially if it is prolonged, is detrimental to individuals of any age. Many people mistakenly attribute many signs and symptoms of inactivity to the "normal aging process," when, in fact, they are related more to a sedentary lifestyle. Increased tiredness, decreased ability to tolerate physical exertion, reduced muscle strength, and joint stiffness are all factors associated with aging that can be dramatically improved with physical activity, no matter what the age or extent of initial ability. While it is true that there is some natural decline in ability to exercise, elders who are physically active are likely to stay well longer than those who are not. Further, they generally maintain more youthful physiques, better pulmonary function, cardiac function, and increased muscle mass and muscle strength than the inactive.[30]

Currently, there is substantial evidence that prolonged inactivity delays recovery, reduces ability to function, and promotes deterioration of almost every body system (table 4.1.) Also, immobility creates a cycle of further immobility, taking its toll on every body system, creating even more disability, and eventual death.

Those who are hospitalized or in a nursing home are at high risk for deconditioning from immobility. Illness or recovery from surgery, as well as institutional policies and norms, promote bed rest and limit activity. One study of hospitalized elders found that one in four were totally inactive

during their first week of hospitalization. Only half of those who did walk walked at least every other day. Those who were immobile had no documentation of range of motion or strengthening exercises, and physical therapy was rarely provided.[31]

To counteract the negative cycle of immobility, everyone should be encouraged to maximize activity to the extent possible while in the hospital and at home—even if it is no more than dangling their legs from the side of the bed or doing range-of-motion exercises. Muscle contraction exercises while in bed and appropriate positioning in bed can also prevent muscle weakness. Other strategies to minimize the harmful effects of bed rest include use of bedside commodes, standing the patient briefly when

---

TABLE 4.1	**Effects of Immobility on the Body**

- **Cardiovascular system**
  Orthostatic hypotension
  Heart works harder
  Increased resting heart rate
  Risk of blood clots in legs
  Anemia
  Decreased cardiac reserve
  Decreased volume blood pumped per heartbeat

- **Respiratory system**
  Decreased max O_2 consumption
  Decreased chest expansion
  Decreased clearance of secretions
  Reduced coughing
  Oxygen/carbon dioxide imbalance
  Decreased aerobic capacity

- **Gastrointestinal system**
  Lack of appetite
  Slowed food transit time
  Constipation

- **Skin**
  Decubitus ulcer risk

- **Musculoskeletal system**
  Increased fracture risk
  Accelerated bone breakdown
  Osteoporosis risk increased
  Decreased muscle strength and size
  Reduced range of motion in joints

- **Urinary system**
  Reduced bladder function
  Increased calcium breakdown
  Impaired bladder emptying
  Urinary infection

- **Metabolism**
  Increased triglycerides
  Increased LDL cholesterol
  Reduced metabolic rate
  Altered drug metabolism
  Tissue atrophy
  Protein deficiency
  Loss of body water, blood volume
  Reduced insulin resistance
  Mineral imbalances

- **Psychosocial effects**
  Sensory deprivation
  Anxiety and depression
  Decreased learning capacity
  Decreased problem-solving ability
  Decreased motivation
  Exaggerated or inappropriate emotions
  Increased dependence
  Disorientation

transferring from bed to chair, encouraging the wearing of street clothes, and providing mobility aids to patients to encourage walking (e.g., walkers and canes). Whenever possible, physical or occupational therapists should be utilized to improve the individual's physical tolerance for activity. A good axiom, taught to medical students over fifty years ago by Dr. Asher, still holds true today:

> Teach us that we may dread
> Unnecessary time in bed
> Get people up and we may save
> Our patient from an early grave.[29]

PHYSICAL ACTIVITY TO REDUCE CHRONIC ILLNESS

"If exercise could be packed into a pill, it would be the single most widely prescribed, and beneficial, medicine in the nation."

Robert Butler

Previously, we have discussed the multitude of physiological and psychological benefits of exercise. Regular exercise also delays the onset, progression, and possibly the effects of some diseases. And, most importantly, it may also allow a person with a chronic illness to maximize function and stay independent as long as possible.

Individuals with chronic illnesses may fall into a cycle of reduced physical activity that results in deconditioning and its associated symptoms, creating a vicious cycle of fatigue that further decreases the ability to engage in physical activity. In addition, many chronic illnesses hasten the cycle of debilitation. Even though physical activity has been shown to prevent or reduce the impact of many chronic illnesses, those affected often need individualized evaluation and counseling before embarking on an exercise regimen.

Motivating someone who is chronically ill to initiate an exercise program can be very difficult. They may believe their situation is hopeless, or the exercise itself may temporarily worsen their discomfort by causing fatigue, pain, and breathlessness. Initial attempts to exercise may not be successful because of unrealistic expectations. Further, continued monitoring is important to maintain an effective and systematic exercise regimen, not commonly done by physicians. The following section discusses the role that physical activity plays in several chronic diseases, both in prevention and rehabilitation.

Heart Disease

Heart disease is the primary cause of death and disability in the United States today. A sedentary lifestyle is the primary risk factor for heart disease.[32] The role of exercise in the prevention of atherosclerosis and coronary heart disease is well-documented: it provides strong protection by controlling weight, reducing blood pressure, increasing the level of protective HDL cholesterol, reducing blood clotting, and lowering blood insulin levels.

In addition to preventing coronary heart disease, regular and sustained physical activity is an important part of treating cardiovascular disease. People with cardiac diseases, including congestive heart failure, angina, and history of heart attacks, can generally exercise safely after evaluation. Exercise allows those with angina pain to do more work before feeling chest pain by reducing resting heart rate and oxygen needs of the heart. In one study, men with stable angina were randomized to receive routine care or routine care plus exercise. In general, those who exercised three to four hours a week halted the progression of the angina: those who exercised five to six hours a week made the disease regress. After one year, only 10 percent of the participants in the exercise group worsened as opposed to half those in the group who did not exercise.[33] Among those with cardiac diseases, exercise is also associated with improvements in exercise capacity and strength, improved sense of well-being, and improved cardiovascular risk factors such as lipid levels, blood pressure and weight.

Prescribed exercise is an important component of cardiac rehabilitation programs. Studies have been conducted to determine whether cardiac rehabilitation programs initiated after a heart attack protect against future attacks or death. It is clear that these programs increase many measures of cardiovascular physical fitness of those who participate (e.g., cholesterol levels, reduced body fat, improve exercise capacity).[34] However, there is no evidence that cardiac rehabilitation exercise training reduces the risk of a future nonfatal heart attack. Although no individual study is able to document that cardiac rehabilitation programs reduce death rate from cardiovascular disease, when several small studies are grouped and analyzed (a meta-analysis), significant reductions in cardiac deaths are noted among those undergoing cardiac rehabilitation, at least among middle-aged men.[35]

Cardiac rehabilitation programs offer other benefits such as education and stress reduction that improve the participants' quality of life. The success rate of cardiac rehabilitation programs is comparable to other far more invasive and expensive therapies. Nevertheless, although there are many candidates for such programs, only 11 to 20 percent of heart attack patients participate. Even though elders show comparable improvements in cardiovascular fitness to middle-aged men, they are less likely to be referred to, and to participate in, cardiac rehabilitation programs, especially elder women.[35]

Before exercise is recommended to cardiac patients, a full medical evaluation, including an exercise stress test, is generally necessary. The most beneficial exercise prescription is to train three times weekly for twenty to forty minutes at 70 to 85 percent of maximum heart rate.[35] If patients experience chest pain at a certain heart rate during an exercise treadmill test, they should keep their heart rate at least ten points below that level. Patients with cardiac disease are generally cautioned against heavy lifting and heavy static or isometric exercises (e.g., hand grip, power weight lifting). However, these patients do benefit from strength training—generally using eight to twelve repetitions of weights that are about 40 to 50 percent of their maximum strength.[36] Ideally, exercises should emphasize both the upper and lower extremities. Most cardiac medications do not interfere with the ability to exercise. Sometimes nitroglycerine is prescribed

prior to exercising to allow higher intensity exercise without angina pain.

Hypertension

Those who exercise regularly and vigorously have a lower incidence of hypertension than those who do not, and this is true even among those who are overweight. Regular aerobic exercise decreases blood pressure and reduces the increase in blood pressure that often accompanies aging. One longitudinal study found that men who exercised regularly had no change in blood pressure over more than twenty years while those who were sedentary increased their blood pressure.[37]

Older individuals with hypertension need to know that they can safely exercise to reduce their blood pressure, and even if they cannot reduce their blood pressure to the normal range, they can reduce their chance of dying from hypertension-related complications. Guidelines for exercise for those with hypertension are similar to guidelines for recommended physical activity: moderate intensity (walk, jog, bike) for thirty minutes most days.[38] High-intensity, anaerobic, or static exercises may be dangerous for those with hypertension and should be avoided as they cause a temporary increase in blood pressure.

Peripheral Vascular Disease

Peripheral vascular disease, also called intermittant claudication, causes severe cramping leg pain when walking. It is a significant cause of disability among older people. The standard medical treatment is drug treatment and surgery. Drug treatment is expensive and is seldom successful. Surgery is also expensive, and carries risks of cardiovascular complications. However, exercise is a low-risk, inexpensive, and noninvasive alternative to drugs and surgery. Walking is the exercise of choice for those with peripheral vascular disease. An analysis of several studies regarding exercise to improve the pain of intermittant claudication reports that walking at least thirty minutes three times a week is an effective treatment. The exercise prescription is to walk to the point of pain and limping, followed by a short rest, then continuing to walk, until a total of twenty to thirty minutes are completed. Exercising in this manner lengthens the time it takes before the symptoms appear.[39] It is believed that exercise may help develop collateral circulation in the extremities, both reducing the time it takes before pain ensues and decreasing the intensity of pain.

Adult-Onset Diabetes

Regular exercise plays a significant role both in the prevention and the treatment of adult-onset diabetes (type II diabetes). Adult-onset diabetes is less likely to develop in individuals who exercise than those who do not. The relationship between physical activity and reduced risk of adult-onset diabetes is consistent among studies, documenting the more exercise, the lower risk of diabetes, even among those who are obese. Exercise works through reducing weight and body fat, as diabetes is more likely to occur among the obese. Further, exercise has been shown to increase glucose tolerance and insulin sensitivity. One large study of over 21,000 male physicians reported that, even if vigorous exercise occurred only once a week, the risk of diabetes was reduced by over 20 percent.[40] These results were confirmed in a large study of Japanese American men.[41] In another large study of women, it was found that middle-aged women who engaged in regular physical activity reduced their risk of acquiring diabetes by 33 percent.[42] After nine months of vigorous endurance exercise training, elders exhibited a significant increase in glucose tolerance and reduced insulin levels, similar to the positive changes achieved in younger samples.[43]

In addition to preventing diabetes, exercise is one of the cornerstones of non-drug therapy for adult-onset diabetes. Diabetics who exercise regularly need fewer oral medications and insulin because their body cells are more sensitive to their own insulin production. The Council on Exercise recommends that diabetics participate in aerobic exercise at 50 to 70 percent of an individual's max-

imum oxygen intake for twenty to forty-five minutes at least three days a week.[44] More recently, Mayer-Davis and colleagues, after studying almost 11,500 men and women, report that exercise does not have to be vigorous to have an effect on insulin sensitivity. Moderate intensity physical activity on most days was successful in increasing insulin sensitivity. Further, the exercise should be appropriate to the person's general physical condition and lifestyle.[45]

Because diabetes is often associated with other illnesses, such as cardiovascular disease, hypertension, and peripheral vascular disease, diabetics should undergo exercise treadmill testing prior to beginning a moderately vigorous exercise program. In addition, as exercise can lower blood sugar and insulin needs, careful monitoring of blood sugar to prevent hypoglycemia (not enough sugar getting into the body cells), is warranted. For diabetics to continually reap the benefits of improved glucose tolerance and insulin sensitivity, exercise must be performed regularly as gains are lost several days after the last bout of exercise.

Obesity

Physical inactivity is a major contributor to the increasing number of overweight people in Western society. National studies show that about one-third of overweight men and 41 percent of overweight women are inactive, and the proportion of those who are inactive increases with age. By age seventy, 45 percent of men and 57 percent of women who are overweight are inactive.[46] Obesity is associated with a number of chronic health problems, including premature death, adult-onset diabetes, arthritis, hypertension, vascular disease, and respiratory problems. Physical activity can promote weight loss that positively affects the other variables associated with obesity.

Weight is a function of energy output and input. Those who increase food intake and do not increase activity levels will gain weight. Conversely, those who maintain the same caloric intake and increase activity will lose weight. Thus, exercise is a major factor in regulating body fat content.

Numerous studies report that aerobic exercise reduces body fat and increases lean body mass. One pound of body fat is lost for every 3,500 calories of energy expended. The primary goal of exercise for those who are overweight is to burn up 2,000 to 3,000 calories a week to lose weight. In elders, generally lower-intensity and longer-duration exercises are recommended to reduce injuries. As weight is lost, individuals may shift to higher-intensity workouts to improve cardiovascular endurance. Those who are only moderately obese can select from a wide variety of exercise activities, but generally fitness walking is recommended. Those who are more severely obese may suffer from other conditions that limit their ability to exercise (joint pains, reduced functional capacity, reduced range of motion) and may require even lower intensity exercise regimens (e.g., stationary bicycling or water

aerobics). Table 4.2 provides a list of various exercise activities and calories burned by each.

Exercise recommendations for those who are overweight should be accompanied by dietary counseling. It is important not to simultaneously begin a strict diet and an exercise program. People on calorie-restricted diets with or without exercise often lose muscle tissue as well as fat. However, when aerobic exercise is combined with a sensible diet, lean body mass is preserved and even increased, but body fat is decreased. Likewise, strength training (e.g., resistance weight training) can prevent loss of lean body mass and provides other benefits such as increased strength. Those who exercise frequently are also more likely to maintain the weight loss. Because of the high dropout rate in exercise intervention programs for weight control, exercise is

---

TABLE 4.2   Calories Burned by Various Exercises

Here's how many calories a 150-pound man or woman burns by doing any of these activities for a half hour. (If you weigh less, you burn fewer calories; if you weigh more, you burn more.)

Exercise	Calories Burned per Half Hour
LEISURE	
Dancing, folk or square	190
Dancing, general	150
Horseback riding	140
Stretching or yoga	140
Walking (4 mph)	140
Walking (3 mph)	120
Frisbee or bowling	100
Shuffleboard	100
Cooking	80
Walking, strolling	70
SPORTS	
Hockey or lacrosse	270
Skiing, cross-country	270
Swimming laps, slowly to moderately	270
Aerobics, high impact	240
Ice skating or roller skating	240
Jogging	240
Soccer	240
Tennis	240
Bicycling, light	200
Swimming, leisurely	200
Treadmill or stair exercise, moderate	200
Aerobics, low impact	170
Baseball or softball	170
Bicycling, stationary	170
Skiing, downhill, light	170
Calisthenics, light to moderate	150
Golf	150
Ping pong	140
Water aerobics or coaching sports	140
Weightlifting, light to moderate	100
AROUND THE HOUSE	
Mowing the lawn (hand mower)	200
Gardening	170
Walking up stairs	170
Household cleaning, heavy (washing the car, washing windows, etc.)	150
Lawn mowing (power mower)	150
Wall or house painting	150
Raking leaves	140
Food shopping, with a grocery cart	120
Walking the dog	120
Walking down stairs	100
Household cleaning, light (dusting, etc.)	80

Excerpted from Ainsworth, B.E., Haskell, W.L., Leon, A.S. et al. 1993. Compendium of physical activities: classification of energy costs of human physical activities. *Medicine and Science in Sports and Exercise* 25:71–80.

Exercise for Weight Loss

A t approximately twenty minutes into an aerobic exercise session your body shifts into what is called the "fat-burning phase." At this point, although you are still using all energy sources, your body begins to burn fat as the primary energy source. During this phase we are able to attack greater amounts of stored fat. Therefore, once we reach this phase, the longer we exercise, the more stored fat we will burn. An ideal program for weight loss is to exercise at an intensity of 70 percent to 85 percent of the maximum heart rate (MHR) for thirty to sixty minutes four to five times a week. People just starting a fitness program should begin exercising in a range of 60 percent to 70 percent of their MHR and slowly progress to 70 percent to 85 percent. Participating in a strength-training program on an every-other-day basis can also supplement this type of training by increasing muscle mass, which in turn burns greater amounts of fat.

Excerpted from National Exercise for Life Institute, 1994. P.O. Box 2000, Excelsior, MN.

more successful when performed in a group under close supervision.

Respiratory Diseases

Because individuals with pulmonary disease often lose additional lung capacity because of lack of physical activity, exercise is highly recommended to counteract that effect. Exercise cannot repair damaged lung tissue, but it can improve lung function and prevent further deterioration caused by inactivity. Exercise can increase oxygen consumption and utilization, improve breathing, reduce resting heart rate, and increase the tolerance for work.

Walking is the exercise of choice for patients with chronic obstructive pulmonary disease (COPD). Before beginning an exercise program, those with COPD should also undergo an exercise treadmill test, while oxygen intake is measured. If they have insufficient oxygen intake, supplementary oxygen may be required before or during exercise. Commonly, exercise causes shortness of breath and fatigue in individuals who have pulmonary disease, so a closely supervised program is recommended. These individuals are often more successful if they exercise after using bronchiodilator inhalants.

Osteoporosis

A sedentary lifestyle is a major contributor to the rate and extent of bone loss in osteoporosis. A number of studies show a high correlation between level of physical activity and bone mass in older women. Weight-bearing exercises are recommended to prevent, or, at least reduce the decline in, bone loss in both premenopausal and postmenopausal women and can significantly decrease the incidence of hip and leg fractures in both sexes. Results of randomized controlled trials confirm the positive effects of an exercise program on bone density, muscle mass, strength, and balance in older sedentary women ages fifty to seventy who participated in high-intensity strength-training exercises with resistance machines for forty-five minutes twice a week for one year.[47]

Exercise has been shown to reduce the risk of hip fracture. In one study of elder women, those who reported the highest activity level had the fewest hip and spinal fractures. The difference between the inactive and active women was about the same as the level of protection given by hormone replacement therapy. Even those who performed low-intensity activities for at least an hour a week had significant reductions in risk for hip fracture.[48] A regular exercise program, even if initiated late in life and among

Getting Stronger by Using Weights

Resistance training is exercise that builds strength by working your muscles against resistance. This can be done by lifting weights or by pushing against immovable objects with the arms or legs. Resistance training can provide many benefits. By increasing your strength and flexibility, daily activities such as getting out of bed, toileting, and getting up stairs become much easier. Resistance training may also prevent falls and help you walk faster.

You don't need to buy weights to resistance train at home. (Lifting weights is preferable to pushing against an immovable object.) You can make your own weights by filling bags or old socks with beans, pennies, or sand. Plastic water bottles partially filled with water or sand also make inexpensive alternatives.

Before starting a resistance training program, you should talk to your doctor. Together, you can assess your goals, needs, and current fitness level, and the doctor can suggest specific strengthening exercises. The following guidelines can help you start resistance training and make the exercise more enjoyable by reducing your risk of injury.

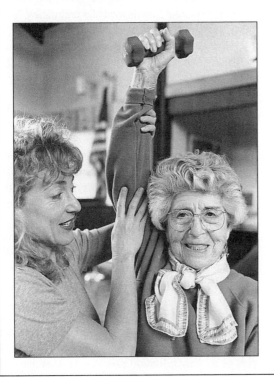

GETTING STRONGER SAFELY

1. Set aside a specific time of day to exercise. Choose a time when you usually are not tired.
2. Try to exercise every other day.
3. Wear socks and shoes that fit well. Ask your doctor what kind are best for you.
4. Before starting your resistance exercises, warm up the muscles you will be using by doing low-level calisthenics for ten to fifteen minutes.
5. Gently stretch your muscles (no bouncing) after warming up.
6. Start resistance training in your comfort range. The exercises should not cause pain or stiffness, or make you feel breathless or off balance. A weight that you can lift comfortably ten times is probably a good one to start with.
7. Lift the weight slowly, taking six seconds to lift it through the entire range of movement.
8. How you breathe when lifting the weight is important. You should inhale before lifting, exhale while lifting, and inhale again while lowering the weight. *Never hold your breath while lifting.*
9. Rest a few seconds between lifts.
10. Concentrate on a few muscle groups each session. Your doctor can choose those that cause the most problems.
11. Do each exercise about 10 times. As you get stronger, you may be able to do two or three sets of each exercise.
12. Don't use the same muscles each time you exercise. Give your muscles regular rest breaks. For instance, you might want to work your legs on Monday and your arms on Wednesday.
13. Try to lift a little more weight a few more times each week, but do not increase the weight or number of lifts more than once each week. If you have to hold your breath to lift, you are probably using too much weight.
14. If you have problems, do not increase the amount of weight or the number of lifts without talking to your doctor.
15. Slowly stretch your muscles for five to ten minutes after each exercise session.

Excerpted from Barry, H.C., Rich, BSE, and Carlson, R.T. 1993. How exercise can benefit older persons. *The Physician and Sports Medicine* 21:133-134.

the very frail, can slow or reverse the rate of bone demineralization.

Arthritis

Arthritis is the most commonly reported cause of activity limitation in elders, and limitations become more prevalent with advanced age. Patients with rheumatoid arthritis or osteoarthritis often suffer from physical deconditioning, leading to a vicious cycle of joint pain leading to further reductions in movement.

Effects of the disease itself, the consequences of therapy, and fear of recurring pain and disability are strong forces that encourage inactivity. Growing evidence points to the role of exercise in ameliorating the pain and disability associated with arthritis. Results of randomized controlled trials of those with arthritis reveal an overall improvement in ability and fitness from exercise programs, particularly aerobic exercise. In a review and analysis of several studies regarding exercise therapy for osteoarthritis and rheumatoid arthritis, it was concluded that exercise exerted a favorable effect. In studies of exercise and rheumatoid arthritis, stretching exercises improved range of joint motion, and aerobic exercise improved observed disability, oxygen uptake, muscle strength, and range of motion in joints. In studies of exercise and osteoarthritis, improvement in oxygen uptake, pain, and disability was reported by those who participated in aerobic exercise.[49]

Whether the person has rheumatoid arthritis or osteoarthritis, exercise must start gently and progress gradually. And, because those with rheumatoid arthritis commonly have morning stiffness, and those with osteoarthritis have more pain at the end of the day, exercise time needs to be adjusted.

The guidelines of the American College of Rheumatology for treatment of osteoarthritis of the knee assert that aerobic and resistance exercises reduce pain and disability.[50] One study by Dr. Ettinger and colleagues found that an aerobic or weight resistance program produced modest, but consistent improvements in pain and functional status in a group of elders over age sixty with osteo-

arthritis of the knee.[51] Another study documented decreased pain, decreased use of arthritis medication, and improved walking ability in elders age forty to eighty-nine who participated in an eight-week program of fitness walking.[52]

Despite the evidence that an individualized exercise program reduces the pain and disability associated with arthritis, one researcher reported that only one-fourth of those with osteoarthritis said that their primary physician recommended exercise. Of those who received advice, 64 percent began an exercise program. In comparison, of those who didn't receive advice from their doctor to exercise, only 23 percent did. This is a strong indicator of the power of physicians in getting their patients to exercise. Physicians need to play a more active role in encouraging and assessing exercise programs for that group. This includes showing them specific exercises as well as accompanying the demonstration with printed instructions.[53]

Generally an exercise program for those with arthritis begins with passive range-of-motion exercises and progresses to aerobic exercise and weight training to increase cardiovascular endurance, flexibility, and muscle strength.[54] Swimming or water exercises are particularly effective in elders because they place less stress on joints.

Lower Back Pain

Lower back pain is an extremely common complaint among adults; almost everyone has low back pain sometime in their lives. Most commonly, lower back pain occurs when muscles in the back and abdomen are too weak to keep the back in proper alignment. As a result, posture while lifting, sitting, standing, and walking is poor, increasing the risk of back injury. Physical inactivity is an important contributor to chronic back pain because a back with poor muscle tone is especially susceptible to fatigue, strain, injury, and tension.

Whether medication, manipulative treatment by a chiropractor or surgery are used to allay back pain, physical activity is recommended as a critical part of the rehabilitation process. An exercise pre-

Proper Lifting Techniques

- Use your legs, not your back.
- Bring objects close to your body before lifting.
- Avoid twisting or turning your body when lifting.
- Know your limits: don't try to lift more than you can easily handle.

scription improves physical conditioning to build activity tolerance and overcome individual limitations due to back symptoms. The goals are to strengthen muscles in the abdomen and back to improve posture, strengthen the leg muscles used in lifting, and improve flexibility and aerobic endurance. It is recommended that low-stress exercises be conducted to improve general stamina, then after two weeks, conditioning exercises be added to strengthen trunk muscles, and finally specific training to increase tolerance in carrying out daily activities. A moderate exercise program designed to strengthen the abdomen and back muscles should be performed regularly for lasting improvement.[57]

Cancer

Physical inactivity may play a role in the development of several types of cancer, with the strongest associations found in cancers of the colon and breast. A number of epidemiological studies have proposed an inverse relationship between physical activity level and colon cancer risk: the higher the level of exercise, the lower the risk for colon cancer. In a study of 47,000 middle-aged and elderly male physicians, it was reported that those who engaged in leisure-time physical activity at least three times a week were significantly less likely to develop colon cancer or polyps than those who were sedentary. This association was strong even when other factors were controlled, such as family history, dietary patterns, smoking,

and obesity. The most active men (who jogged four hours a week) had about half the risk for colon cancer as those who did not exercise.[56] It is believed that exercise works by increasing bowel activity, so that cancer-producing substances do not linger in the colon. Since obesity is also a strong risk factor for colon cancer, physical activity may also work indirectly to reduce colon cancer by weight loss.

There is evidence of a relationship between physical activity and a decreased risk of breast cancer among pre- and postmenopausal women. Since half the breast cancer cases occur in women over sixty-five, exercise might play a significant role in breast cancer prevention among postmenopausal women. In an epidemiological study of over 25,000 Norwegian women, a high level of physical activity was associated with a significant reduction in the risk of breast cancer among women who reported exercising regularly (four hours a week for three to five years). Even though the risk reduction was higher in women before menopause, the relationship was found in postmenopausal women as well.[57] In another study of almost 2,000 women over sixty-five, researchers reported the same relationship even among those with disabilities who engaged in only moderate levels of physical activity.[58]

There are many ways that physical activity might lower breast cancer risk. Evidence has accumulated that both obesity and elevated concentrations of estrogen hormones increase breast cancer risk. Physical activity may influence the production, metabolism and excretion of estrogen. Alternatively, exercise may decrease obesity or enhance immune function.

Falls

Deterioration of muscle strength, balance, and reaction time among elders is associated with an increased incidence of falls, disability, and a reduced mobility. Research is accumulating that exercise can reduce the frequency of falls, especially those exercises that improve muscle weakness, gait, and balance.

It's Never Too Late
Maria Fiaterone, M.D.

Aging in modern society is in many respects an "exercise deficiency syndrome" which contributes to an excess rate of heart disease, diabetes, obesity, hypertension, high cholesterol, arthritis, osteoporosis, falls, and other chronic problems. Cumulatively, these diseases, as well as fatigue, muscle weakness, low endurance, stiffness, impaired balance, and low self-efficacy may result in a syndrome we call frailty.

Frailty, if difficult to define, is not hard to recognize. Ask a child to show you what an old person looks like. They will stoop over, pretend to have a cane in one hand, shakily grab furniture for support with the other, and slowly walk across the room. This mobility impairment, fear of falling, and weakness they so readily identify and mimic is at the center of frailty and is increasingly prevalent in our ever-graying society.

Is there a medical treatment for frailty? Is there a way to prevent it? Needless to say, if we could pre-vent all of the diseases which contribute to it we would minimize its impact. But much of it has nothing to do with a discreet disease. Instead it is an expression of poor exercise tolerance simply due to disuse or underuse of the muscles and heart.

Consider 80-year-old Jack LaLane. Is he frail? He is old, he has wrinkles, he has gray hair, but no one would call him frail. This is because exercise, particularly resistance training, or weight-lifting exercise, which he has advocated since his youth, has a remarkable preventive and restorative effect on the body. Exercise in the aged, even those up to 100 years of age, has now been shown to increase strength, muscle mass, aerobic capacity, bone density, flexibility, balance, neurological speed of movement, functional abilities, and overall activity level. Along with these physical changes, improvements with respect to depression, morale, insomnia, and self-efficacy have been documented.

There is no pill that can perform even remotely as powerfully in this regard. Many older women who begin strength training are stronger than their daughters at the end of six months of weight lifting. Older men in their sixties and seventies who have lifted weights for many years have muscles that look and perform identically to those of 20 year-old men. Obviously, exercise cannot prevent all age-related changes in physical functioning, nor can it avert all diseases, but we have become much too complacent at accepting as inevitable changes that are now clearly documented to be preventable or reversible even in extreme old age. Less frailty will mean more independence, fewer injurious falls, lower nursing home admission rates, decreased health care costs, and improved quality and perhaps quantity of life. "Life is short. Play hard" is a popular slogan, geared towards the competitiveness of youth. We would say, rather, "Life is long. Play well." The consequences of not playing are real and frightening. The rewards of a lifetime of healthful exercise, or of taking it up for the first time in your nineties, are enormous. Start now, and be fit for your life.

Excerpted from *Perspectives in Health Promotion and Aging* 1996; vol. II (4): p. 7. American Association of Retired Persons.

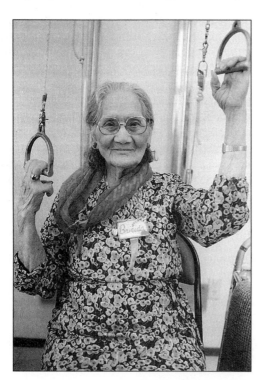

Although frail elders are not likely to participate in aerobic programs, flexibility and strength exercises can improve functions of daily living, such as getting up from a chair or toilet and out of a bath. Several exercise programs designed to improve balance and mobility among older people have been shown to reduce the risk of falling.[59,60]

ELDERS' ACTIVITY LEVEL AND ATTITUDES TOWARD EXERCISE

A large proportion of the nation's population is sedentary, and the older we get, the more inactive we become. A large national survey revealed that only about one in four adults participate in regular sustained physical activity (thirty minutes a day, five days a week).[61] Further, almost 30 percent of the adult population in the United States participates in no leisure-time physical activity, and the proportion of inactivity increases with age. By age seventy-five, almost half the respondents reported they engaged in no leisure-time physical activity.[62]

Given the many benefits of physical activity, why don't more elders exercise? In order to understand why elders are the most inactive age group, we need to look beyond age. What other variables affect their attitudes about exercise?

Elders may be poorly educated about the importance of exercise upon health and well-being because most schools had no physical education when they were growing up. Furthermore, much of the information about the benefits of exercise has only been recently understood. They may not have developed the habit of physical activity because they may have worked long hours and had other responsibilities that prevented them from developing the interest and skill in physical activity. Elders may have kept physically fit during their youth through daily activities, so exercise for its own sake was uncommon. It will be interesting to see whether the exercise patterns of the next generation of elders will differ.

National surveys report that women spend less time in physical activities and are more likely to be inactive than men. The traditional gender role for women is that physical exercise for its own sake is inappropriate, and women got all the activity they needed by their domestic activities. Such life-long customs and values are not easy to change.

Elders likely support the common belief that one should slow down in old age. Further, elders tend to exaggerate the risks involved in vigorous exercise after middle age so they do not exercise because they fear an accident or overexertion. And, they may overrate the health benefits of light, sporadic exercise and underrate their own physical capabilities.

Elders may not exercise because of a lack of encouragement from physicians. Many physicians are poorly informed about the beneficial effects of exercise or unaware of the exercise capabilities of even the most disabled patients. Physicians may actually discourage exercise by advising their elder patients to "take it easy" or avoid stairs or overexertion and may overestimate the hazards of exercise in elders with chronic diseases. They may focus their energy on treating their patients' acute problems rather than proposing long-term changes.

Many older people do not like to exercise. And, just as any other age group, they may not be motivated to increase their activity level. It is far easier to take a pill to reduce disease symptoms than perform daily, perhaps initially painful, exercises, especially when the benefits may not be immediate. Some people may even be dissatisfied when exercise is prescribed because they believe that doctors are trained and paid to provide modern drugs, not exercise that the patients must do themselves. Prescribing exercise forces patients to take control of their own symptoms, instead of relying on a cure by drug or surgical intervention.

In addition, older people do not have the same opportunities for exercise as younger people. Some elders have physical disabilities that reduce their ability to exercise vigorously. Others may live in unsafe neighborhoods. Also, many communities do not provide exercise programming for elders, and even when they do, seldom is transportation provided.

Despite the barriers to exercise among the elderly, their participation is on the rise. Health clubs are beginning to cater to their rising senior clientele, offering special classes or incentives for those over sixty-five to begin and continue exercising. The increased public focus on fitness activities, such as mall walking, has a special appeal to older people. Further, the aging of a more health-conscious generation will likely contribute to rising participation in exercise among elders.

EXERCISE PROMOTION

The physician is in an excellent position to educate and encourage their elder patients to exercise as most older people are very responsive to doctors' orders. However, multiple surveys find that many physicians do not routinely take an exercise history. Although many physicians discuss exercise with their patients, the discussion may be vague, for example, "You would benefit from losing some weight and exercising a little more." The majority of physicians are not trained in prescribing exercise. When they do, they seldom specify type, duration, frequency, and intensity, and they rarely monitor their patients. Further, they may not take time to talk with patients or have the staff to assist patients to begin and maintain an exercise program.[63]

Physicians may not prescribe exercise to their patients because they are often unaware of the techniques used to assess fitness level, prescribe an exercise regimen, or motivate patients. Unfortunately, information on exercise physiology is rarely a significant part of the medical school curriculum and continuing medical education. Physicians are even less certain about how to assess whether their patients are exercising, how to encourage patients to exercise, and how to monitor exercise appropriately. Appropriate discussion and prescription of exercise can be time-consuming, especially if it is not incorporated into a routine.

Physicians' attitudes and practices related to exercise and the development of exercise prescriptions are important. One survey of 168 physician respondents reported that almost half the physicians questioned said they required an exercise history as part of the initial exam, and almost all encouraged their patients to participate in regular exercise programs. However, 70 percent did not develop exercise prescriptions, and only one of four was familiar with the exercise prescription guidelines developed by the American College of Sports Medicine. Only 3 percent had ever taken a course related to exercise physiology and the development of exercise programs, even though more than 75 percent felt the content should be part of the medical school curriculum.[63]

In response to the need for physicians to become more active in counseling their patients in initiating and maintaining effective physical activity regimens, the Centers for Disease Control developed a manual for physicians, using the acronym PACE (Physical Activity Counseling and Evaluation). Three interactive counseling protocols were designed to help physicians to tailor the exercise message to the patient's readiness to change. One protocol helps the physician to motivate those who are currently uninterested in physical activity to consider it seriously, called "Getting out of Your Chair." Another protocol assists the physician to design a physical activity program for those interested in starting, called "Planning the First Step." And, there is a protocol for the physician to help those who want to maintain their active lifestyle, called "Keeping the PACE."[64] For more information and purchase of materials, write Project PACE, Student Health Services, San Diego State University, 5500 Campanile Drive, San Diego, CA 92182.

This section will discuss the role of the physician in exercise promotion. Factors affecting the motivation to start and continue an exercise program will also be addressed.

Medical Assessment

A medical assessment is an important tool for the health professional to encourage physical activity among elders. Information from the assessment can be used to prescribe an individualized exercise

Walk Your Way to Feeling Better

Walking provides many benefits and can be tailored to suit your needs or preferences—even if you need little exercise. Walking can make you feel better. It can ease stiffness, increase your ability to get around without assistance, improve your cardiovascular fitness, reduce your stress, and help control your weight. Before starting a walking program, you should think about your own goals and needs. Have your physician help you assess your current fitness level. The following guidelines can help you enjoy walking by reducing your risk of injury. Walking to music or with a friend can make the activity even more fun. If you have questions about your walking program, your doctor should be able to help answer them.

STEPS FOR SUCCESS

1. Set aside a specific time of day to walk. Choose a time when you are usually not tired.
2. Try to walk every other day.
3. Wear comfortable socks and supportive shoes that fit well. Ask your doctor for specific recommendations.
4. Before starting your walk, warm up the muscles you will be using by doing low-level calisthenics for ten to fifteen minutes.
5. Gently stretch your muscles (no bouncing) after warming up. Try to touch your toes while sitting in a chair with your knees bent.
6. Start walking within your comfort range. Walking should not cause pain or stiffness, nor should it make you feel breathless or off balance.
7. Try to walk a little farther and a little faster each week, but do not increase your distance or pace more than once a week.
8. If you have problems such as chest discomfort, shortness of breath, or leg pain, do not increase your distance or pace without first talking to your doctor.
9. After walking, stretch your muscles again for five to ten minutes.
10. Delay your postexercise shower until you reach your resting heart rate.

IF YOU HAVE VERY LIMITED CAPABILITIES

If you have difficulty getting up or need a walker, cane, or other mobility aid to go from place to place, you need to begin with very limited exercise. You may not be able to start walking right away. Before starting an exercise program, your doctor should help you determine your goals. He or she may suggest beginning with exercises to increase your flexibility and strength. A nurse or a physical therapist may need to help you with these exercises. Once your doctor says you can begin walking, you should start small. You may not want to try to walk any set distance at first. Using time as your goal may be helpful. For example, you may want to start by trying to walk for two or three minutes at a time. Try to increase your exercise time by two minutes each week.

IF YOU HAVE SLIGHTLY LIMITED CAPABILITIES

If you can move around, but it takes time and sometimes assistance, you can probably walk short distances, such as to the bathroom or kitchen, but not very often. Before you start a walking program, your doctor should help you determine your goals. At first, you may be able to walk five to ten minutes over short distances. You should try to increase your walking by five minutes or fifty yards each week.

IF YOU HAVE FEW LIMITATIONS

If you can walk in your home with few problems and can walk 200 yards with ease, you are relatively mobile. You should begin by walking ten to fifteen minutes every other day. Increase your exercise time by five to ten minutes each week. You should also try to increase your distance 100 yards per week. You may also consider other forms of activity such as swimming and low- to moderate-intensity water aerobics.

Excerpted from Barry, H.C., Rich, BSE, and Carlson, R.T. 1993. How exercise can benefit older persons. *The Physician and Sports Medicine* 21:133, 134. Reproduced with permission of McGraw-Hill, Inc.

program that is consistent with the patient's current health status and fitness level. This evaluation may also reveal diseases or disorders that may inhibit exercise or require special precautions.

Included in a medical assessment is a medical history, physical examination, laboratory work, and exercise testing. A medical history requests information concerning present and past levels of physical activity, physical symptoms suggesting conditions that would limit physical mobility, and current medications that impact on the ability and type of exercise to be prescribed. The physical examination includes the measurement of resting heart rate, blood pressure, body weight, and evidence of cardiovascular disease. Laboratory studies might include blood count, urine analysis, tests for fasting blood sugar and blood lipids, and a resting electrocardiogram. An exercise stress test, such as performance on a treadmill or bicycle, may be used as part of a medical assessment to determine a person's capacity for strenuous exercise.

There are conflicting views on who should have a medical assessment before starting an exercise program. The American College of Sports Medicine recommends that men over age forty and women over age fifty who plan to exercise at more than 60 percent of their maximum heart rate should consult their physician. However, these standards may have inadvertently contributed to the view that exercise is dangerous, preventing many healthy people from starting a fitness program. Many experts believe that healthy persons can begin a gradual, sensible exercise program on their own without seeing a doctor if they have (1) no history of heart trouble, hypertension, arthritis, or diabetes, (2) no family history of premature coronary artery disease, and (3) no exercise-related breathlessness, faintness, dizziness, or pain or pressure in the chest, neck, shoulder, or arm. For the very old and frail elderly, an exercise treadmill test may serve as a barrier to participation in exercise as many would not be able to complete the test. For these individuals, undertaking a low-intensity exercise program to improve balance, strength, and flexibility (e.g., chair exercises, walking) is safe and beneficial.

The Exercise Prescription

An exercise prescription is an exercise regimen tailored to an individual's physical condition by a physician or other skilled professional. The prescription is designed to change the patient's current physical activity level by developing a reasonable strategy that will not be a burden and will have a likelihood of continuance. The overall goal is to assist the patient to improve health and the quality of life, not to develop an athlete.

Exercise may be prescribed to maximize physical fitness, prevent illnesses and disorders due to inactivity, treat an existing illness or disorder, or rehabilitate after a crisis, such as a heart attack or stroke. Depending on the goal, specific types of exercises may be suggested to improve muscular strength and endurance, increase joint flexibility, reduce bone loss, or improve cardiovascular endurance. For instance, weight lifting may be prescribed to increase muscular strength and endurance, vigorous walking to enhance cardiovascular endurance and bone mass, and range-of-motion exercises to improve joint flexibility. Exercise may also be prescribed as part of a weight reduction plan.

A balanced exercise prescription includes aerobic activities for cardiovascular endurance, resistance exercises for strengthening the muscles, and exercises to improve joint flexibility. The prescribed exercises should be enjoyable and should fit into the person's daily routine. Socialization while exercising provides mental and intellectual stimulation and improves the sustainability of the program.

A gradual program of moderate exercise has a greater chance of success than an overly vigorous one, and will also confer many health benefits on its participants.

An exercise prescription should specify the following: exercise type, frequency, intensity, and duration. There should also be directions on how to progress to higher exercise levels.

How Much Exercise Is Enough?

I n 1990, The American College of Sports Medicine issued exercise recommendations for healthy adults: vigorous exercise (70 to 85 percent of maximum heart rate) for twenty to sixty minutes three to five times a week.[65] However, some believed that their recommendations were too stringent since it is unreasonable to expect that sedentary individuals will be able to begin and sustain such a vigorous exercise routine. In 1995, the group released supplementary guidelines to include more moderate, short-term exercise bouts to encourage sedentary people to begin exercising. The recommendations are that every U.S. adult should accumulate thirty minutes or more of moderate-intensity physical activity on most, preferably all, days of the week.[66]

Although any activity is better than none, short bouts of exercise are not as beneficial as higher-intensity training. The value of moderate physical activity has been documented to reduce the risk of many chronic illnesses, but if physical fitness is the goal, a higher level of exertion is required (about four times a week for thirty to forty-five minutes at 70 to 90 percent of maximum heart rate). Likewise, if weight loss is a goal, vigorously exercising five times a week for forty-five to sixty minutes at 45 to 60 percent of the maximum heart rate is recommended. Thus, a different protocol is used for reducing disease risk, increasing aerobic fitness, and attaining weight loss.

Type of Exercise

The first consideration is to select an activity that is enjoyable and can be accomplished reasonably. To promote cardiovascular fitness, activities that use large muscle groups should be emphasized. Active elders may enjoy aerobic dance, bicycling, swimming, and jogging. More sedentary elders may enjoy walking or water aerobics. For those who are exercising to lose weight, the more vigorous and sustained the exercise, the more calories burned.

A well-rounded exercise program includes activities that improve muscle strength and endurance, such as lifting weights. In general, the older and more frail the individual, the more important muscle-strengthening exercises and flexibility exercises become. Joint flexibility, balance, and coordination exercises should also be included, such as tai chi, yoga, dance, and calisthenics.

Frequency of Training

In 1990, the American College of Sports Medicine recommended that vigorous exercise should be

conducted three days a week to achieve a variety of benefits, especially in the cardiorespiratory system. In 1995, the organization recommended that moderate exercise almost every day of the week will also confer substantial health benefits. They further suggested that exercise may be accomplished once a day, or may be accumulated in several short bouts during the course of the day—intermittant activity also confers substantial benefits. The short bouts need to be at least as strenuous as brisk walking.[66] For elders with reduced endurance, several short sessions of low-intensity exercises within a day may be easier than once-a-day exercises. However, for those who must participate in low-intensity exercise, those with diabetes, and those who want to lose weight, daily exercise is preferable.

Intensity of Training

There are several ways to measure aerobic exercise intensity, but measuring heart rate, estimating perceived exertion, and performing a talk test are the easiest to perform while exercising. To measure heart rate, a pulse can be taken at the wrist or the side of the neck while exercising. Taking a pulse enables the person to know when the percentage of maximum heart rate is reached. Maximum heart rate is calculated loosely as 220 beats per minute minus the person's age. So, a seventy-year-old person has a maximum heart rate of 150 beats per minute. If the exercise prescription is 60 percent of maximum heart rate, exercise should be sustained at 90 beats per minute. Perceived exertion correlates well with physiological measures of intensity (table 4.3). Aerobic exercise should be performed between 11 and 13 on the exercise intensity scale shown in table 4.3. The greatest benefits in aerobic fitness are achieved when the perceived exertion is between 15 and 17 on the exercise intensity scale. In the talk test, those undergoing aerobic exercise should have enough breath to carry on a light conversation, sing, or whistle, but breathing should be fairly labored.

In the past, exercise guidelines recommended relatively intense aerobic exercise to be performed at 70 to 85 percent of maximum heart rate for at least twenty minutes three to four times a week. Although this is a reasonable goal for an active person, supplemental recommendations are that physical activity of moderate intensity (60 to 75 percent target heart rate) is also effective if the exercise is conducted for a longer duration. For physically inactive patients, the intensity should be tailored to health status and lifestyle. Strenuous activities should be deemphasized, and mild to moderate activity should be encouraged. For most elders, a good initiation into regular exercise is brisk walking several times a week for at least thirty minutes.

For weight training, current recommendations are to accomplish one set (eight to twenty repetitions) of eight to ten major muscle groups at least two days a week. To strengthen a muscle, it must be exercised to the point of fatigue. The standard recommendation is exercising eight to ten muscle groups two times a week, but weight training can

TABLE 4.3	Exercise Intensity Scale	
The Borg Category Rating Scale		
Least effort		
6		
7	Very, very light	
8		
9	Very light	
10		
11	Fairly light	**Endurance**
12		**Training**
13	Somewhat hard	**Zone**
14		
15	Hard	**Strength**
16		**Training**
17	Very hard	**Zone**
18		
19	Very, very hard	
20		
Maximum effort		

Borg, G. 1970. Perceived exertion as an indicator of somatic stress. *Scandanavian Journal of Rehabilitation Medicine*; 293: 92–98.

be accomplished daily if fewer muscle groups are exercised and the muscle group has not been exercised the previous day.

Duration of Training

In 1995, the American College of Sports Medicine recommended a duration of thirty minutes or more of moderate-intensity physical activity on most, preferably all, days of the week. Moderate activity is defined as the equivalent of two miles of brisk walking, or the expenditure of 200 calories per day.[66] The 1990 recommendations from the same organization were harder to achieve: twenty to sixty minutes of continuous aerobic activity three days a week. The newer guidelines suggest a more moderate pace, and hopefully a more realistic one, to encourage even the most sedentary to begin exercising. Elders, especially the very old, often benefit from shorter duration of exercise at more frequent intervals, such as moderate exercise in eight- to ten-minute intervals, to total thirty minutes a day.

Exercise Progression

Intensity, duration, and frequency of exercise should increase with time so the demands on the body keep ahead of the improvement made. Such overloading can develop muscle strength and improve cardiovascular endurance. The level of exercise should move from initial conditioning (four to ten weeks), through improvement to maintenance level (after about six months). During the improvement phases, exercise duration is increased every few weeks until thirty to sixty minutes is reached. After exercise can be continued for twenty minutes, the intensity can also be increased. During the maintenance phase, elders may vary their type of exercise to prevent boredom.

Progression is often quite individual and is based on the individuals' health status, physical capacity, personal goals, and motivation. Elders who have been sedentary should begin slowly, building up intensity and duration with time. Beginning an exercise program with vigorous exercise is associated with a high risk of injury and high dropout rate.

Expected Outcome

An exercise prescription is written to accomplish specific goals and expected outcomes so the elder is able to observe progress toward achievement of those goals. For example, the outcome of the prescription may include the ability to walk for a longer time before tiring, pain reduction, increased range of joint motion, increased muscle strength, weight loss, or ease of getting to sleep. Frequent monitoring of the exercise prescription, including sharing improved measurements with the client, will enhance continuation and success of the prescribed exercise. It will also provide an opportunity to modify the prescription if needed.

General Instructions

Elders beginning an exercise program need to be informed of the importance of warming up and cooling down, appropriate stretching exercises, and other ways to prevent injury. Most important, they should be aware of warning signs that exercise should be discontinued (chest pain, increased shortness of breath, bone or joint pains).

Because exercise programs have a high dropout rate, every effort should be made to make the prescription fit the individual's motivation, ability, and lifestyle. Above all, the exercise prescription should be realistic, since too much exercise may cause discomfort, fatigue, and feelings of failure and too little may not produce a fitness gain. Furthermore, the prescription should be developed mutually by the individual and the health professional so it can become an integrated part of the person's daily routine. Finally, the person needs to be held accountable for meeting his or her exercise goals. Success at achieving exercise goals can be evaluated by use of an exercise diary or charts so that progress can be reinforced. Elders also need to be educated of the benefits of performing the exercises and should be reinforced with each visit. If the health professional monitors the elder's progress and offers frequent feedback and reinforcement, there is a greater chance that the exercise goals will succeed (see chapter 11).

Risks and Complications of Exercise

Like a drug prescription, an exercise prescription has risks and complications that depend on health and fitness level. A few health conditions prohibit vigorous exercise: some types of angina, irregular heartbeat, congestive heart failure, or severe cases of hypertension, anemia, or obesity. A number of other health problems require medical supervision before and during a rigorous exercise program. These include some infections, poorly controlled diabetes, pulmonary disease, severe mental illness, angina, or a recent heart attack. Also, those on particular therapeutic drugs, such as beta blockers or digitalis, should be closely observed during an exercise program.

As part of the exercise prescription, the professional must make the elder aware of symptoms that may occur during a workout that may be hazardous. They are chest, arm, neck, or jaw pain, significant increase in shortness of breath, light-headedness or fainting, irregular heartbeat, nausea or vomiting during or after exercise, prolonged fatigue after exercise, weakness or uncoordinated movements, or unexplained weight or exercise-tolerance changes. These warning signs could indicate an underlying disease or a need to alter the exercise prescription. If any of the above symptoms occur, the elder should be directed to stop exercising and contact a physician.

The fear that exercise will induce a heart attack inhibits many elders from exercising. There is no evidence to suggest that even strenuous exercise is harmful to the normal heart. However, vigorous exercise can precipitate a heart attack in someone with cardiac disease or who is usually quite sedentary. For sedentary individuals, the risk of having a heart attack is 107 times higher while exercising strenuously.[67] If symptoms of a heart attack occur while exercising, such as shortness of breath and crushing chest pressure, an elder should immediately stop and seek medical attention. However, frequent exercise lowers the risk of having a heart attack. Thus, the small risk of having a heart attack while exercising should not preclude exercising.

Elders should be encouraged to drink fluids before, during, and after exercising to prevent dehydration, instead of waiting to "feel thirsty." They have a higher risk of hyperthermia (heat stress) and hypothermia (cold stress) and should be encouraged to dress appropriately for the weather. They may also fail to notice injuries such as blisters due to reduced sensation and should select shoes and socks carefully and regularly inspect their feet. Because elders may have poor vision, hearing, or balance, they may be at higher risk of falls, especially after dark.

The most common risk of exercise for all age groups is musculoskeletal problems due to too much physical activity: muscle soreness, shin splints, tension strains, stress fractures, bone bruises, joint pain, and low back pain. In elders, previous strains and fractures, inactivity, osteoporosis, illness, degenerative changes, nutritional deficiencies, hormone imbalances, or diabetes may affect the response to exercise. However, the benefits of a regular exercise program heavily outweigh the risks, and carefully prescribed, moderate, regular exercise is beneficial for almost everyone.

Implementing Effective Fitness Programs

As discussed earlier, the benefits of exercise are significant, even if started in the middle and later years. Although most people might agree that exercise is good for you, few are motivated to begin and continue a regular exercise program. Some experts feel that even the word "exercise" can serve as a barrier because this term has negative connotations for some. Instead, the use of the term "physical activity" may emphasize the life-long, daily nature of fitness goals. Encouraging elders to become more active, rather than to exercise, may be more palatable. Many positive changes can occur with simple changes in daily habits, such as walking more, taking the stairs instead of the elevator, or routinely parking farther away from the intended destination.

Although virtually everyone can realize the benefits of physical activity, the level of motivation to initiate and maintain an exercise program may differ. The most common reason for elders not participating in an exercise program is poor health and lack of interest. However, even those in poor health can receive many health benefits with an individualized exercise regimen. For elders, generally the most important motive for exercising is for health. But motivation to be healthy may not be enough to sustain a long-term fitness program.

Many individuals who begin a fitness program exercise sporadically and often tire of the activity within a few days or weeks. Less than half those who begin an exercise regimen are still participating after three or six months. Persistence in a physical conditioning program often depends

Why People Are Likely to Exercise[68]

The health professional should learn to motivate people to include regular exercise as part of their daily routine, because, for maximum benefit, exercise should be a lifelong habit. Those who develop and implement exercise programs should make an effort to learn the different backgrounds and needs of their participants to increase their chance of success. The following are the basic considerations relevant to any group that influence their beginning and continuing an exercise program. Individuals are more likely to exercise if they:

- perceive a net benefit
- choose an enjoyable activity
- feel competent doing an activity
- feel safe doing the activity
- can easily access the activity on a regular basis
- can fit the activity into the daily schedule
- feel that the activity does not generate excessive financial or social costs
- experience a minimum of negative consequences (including injury, loss of time, negative peer pressure)
- are able to successfully address issues of competing time demands
- recognize the need to balance "labor-saving devices" and sedentary activities with activities that involve a higher level of physical exertion

on whether the program and its effects meet initial expectations. Studies show that exercisers are more likely to persist in their program if the goals they set and achieve are their own goals, rather than those of others. Additionally, those who initiate a program of high intensity exercise are less likely to continue with their program than those who train at a moderate level. Elders are similar to younger individuals in offering a wide variety of reasons for terminating an exercise program: difficulty in arriving to class on time, too expensive, inconvenient location, parking problems, insufficient staff attention, and belief that exercise had little value.

Social support can increase adherence to an exercise regimen. Individuals who exercise in a group are less likely to drop out than those who exercise alone. Spouses are also an important variable in exercise persistence.

Those most likely to begin and maintain an exercise program are internally motivated: they gain enough pleasure and reinforcement from the physical activity itself. Others may need external reinforcement, such as support from their physician, noticeable weight loss, attention from staff,

or socialization from peers to maintain their physical fitness program.

A shortage of appealing facilities and programs may contribute to low rates of exercise participation among elders, although this is changing in many communities. The decor of a facility, type and volume of music, age of other participants, and type and difficulty level of programs play a role in whether elders are attracted to exercise participation. Just as younger people, elders are different—some like to exercise in a group; others pursue solitary physical activity. Some prefer to exercise with others their own age; others prefer a facility with mixed ages. Some older people prefer same-sex facilities; others prefer to exercise with both men and women. If possible, financial costs should be minimal or free as many elders have limited reserves for recreation. Ideally, a variety of programs for older people would be available in a community, using effective marketing techniques so that elders are aware, and encouraged to participate in them.

To accommodate frail elders, the facility must be physically accessible (within easy walking distance, adequate parking nearby, or serviced by public transportation) because transportation problems

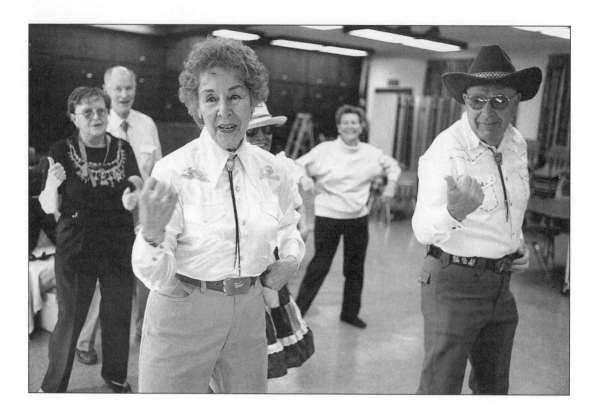

prohibit many from participating in programs. However, it is important to realize that the most widely recommended form of physical activity is walking. It can be done almost anywhere and has no equipment or dress requirements, except a well-fitting pair of shoes.

Support from the health professional also motivates a client to continue an exercise regimen. Clients respond well to individual attention from the staff and adhere to an exercise program more readily when the professional and client mutually agree on an exercise contract, including objectives of the exercise program, specific instructions, time frame, and goal setting. All clients should be counseled to engage in a program of regular physical activity tailored to their health status and personal lifestyle. Elders should be provided with information on the benefits of physical activity in maintaining health and well-being, its role in disease prevention, treatment, and rehabilitation, and effective exercises for cardiac fitness, muscle strength and endurance, flexibility, and coordination that are geared to their abilities.

SUMMARY

Regular physical activity can slow many physiological changes associated with age as well as prevent or reduce deterioration caused by chronic illness. A number of positive health benefits result from regular physical activity: reduction of body fat, increased cardiovascular efficiency, decreased fat in the bloodstream, and increased bone mass and joint mobility. Psychological and intellectual benefits have also been noted. Physical activity plays a significant role in the prevention and treatment of a number of chronic illnesses (including obesity, heart disease, hypertension, pulmonary disease, osteoporosis, lower back pain, and depression). The negative effects of physical inactivity are significant and affect many body systems. The physician plays a significant role in directing people to exercise. However, the individual's motivation to begin and continue in an exercise program is the final indicator of success.

ACTIVITIES

1. If you plan to work with elders, you will be a better role model if you are physically fit and have a positive attitude about exercise. To better understand your own fitness level, monitor the amount and type of exercise you engage in for one week using the following chart:

   A.

   Type of exercise: Intensity:

   Duration: Frequency:

   Is this usual?

   B.

   Do you feel you get enough exercise per day?

   If not, what is keeping you from exercising more?

   What activities could you add to your schedule?

   What other activities might you omit to make room to exercise?

   Which exercise activities may you carry on through old age?

2. Interview five elders regarding their exercise beliefs and practices. Ask them to compare the amount and type of physical activity they currently undergo with what they did ten, twenty, and thirty years ago. Has their activity level changed? What are their reasons for changing their activity level?

3. Visit four places where you can observe individuals of all ages participating in physical activities (e.g., tennis court, swimming pool, health club, bowling alley, jogging or bike trails, or aerobics class). What is the proportion of elders present? What factors might prohibit their participation? How might participation be encouraged in those locations? Ask about special programs for seniors. What types of activities are offered? Does the facility keep statistics on participation and dropout rates? How do they characterize participants?

4. Visit a local nursing home. What physical activity programs does it offer? Who attends? How might attendance be increased?

5. Visit a local convalescent hospital. Find out how much time is spent per day per resident in physical activity. You may wish to compare the activity programs in several convalescent hospitals.

6. Using references given in this chapter, design an exercise program for a group of elders in a community setting that improves endurance, strength, flexibility, balance, coordination, and agility. Do you have variety in the program? How much can be done in a social setting? How would you motivate elders to continue the program? How does it differ from an exercise program in which you would be willing to participate?

7. Design a thirty-second television or radio spot to encourage exercise in elders. What approach do you take? Who might sponsor such an advertisement?

8. Discuss exercise concepts with people of different ages: a child, a teenager, a young adult, and an older adult. Compare their perceptions of how much exercise is enough, what exercises are effective, and how much they do.

9. Create a fifteen-minute educational module to educate elders in a community setting about the value of exercise for older people. Develop objectives, outlines, and methodology.

10. Find out if a local hospital offers a postcoronary exercise/rehabilitation program. Interview staff to determine the clientele, kinds of exercises, dropout rate, and ways professionals motivate clients to stay in the program.

11. Talk to a nurse or a physician in a local hospital or nursing home and find out the protocol for treatment and rehabilitation of bedridden patients. Outline a plan to improve their care, keeping in mind the resources available at the site.

12. You have just been hired by a local fitness center to develop a fitness program for older adults. What type of program will you design? How will you

motivate elders to join and continue with the program? What types of advertisements will you use? What are some strategies you could use to motivate a chronically ill, postcoronary, bedridden, or sedentary elder to exercise?

13. What exercise programs does your community have for older adults?

Visit the programs and compare the type of exercise program, the population utilizing the program, and the cost. Talk to several individuals frequenting the programs.

BIBLIOGRAPHY

1. Caspersen, C.J., Powell, K.E., and Christenson, G.M. 1985. Physical activity, exercise and physical fitness. *Public Health Reports* 100:125–31.

2. McGinnis, J.M., and Goege, W.H. 1993. Actual causes of death in the United States. *Journal of the American Medical Association* 270:2207–12.

3. *Physical activity and health: A report of the Surgeon General.* 1996. Washington, D.C.: U.S. Department of Health and Human Services.

4. Blair, S.N., Kampert, J.B., and Kohl, H.W., et al. 1996. Influences of cardiorespiratory fitness and other precursors on cardiovascular disease and all-cause mortality in men and women. *Journal of the American Medical Association* 276:205–10.

5. Blair, S.N., Kohl, H.W., and Barlow, C.E., et al. 1995. Changes in physical fitness and all-cause mortality: A prospective study of healthy and unhealthy men. *Journal of the American Medical Association* 273:1093–98.

6. Kushi, L.H., Fee, R.M., Folsom, A.R., and Mink, P.J., et al. 1997. Physical activity and mortality in postmenopausal women. *Journal of the American Medical Association* 277:1287–92.

7. Hakim, A.A., Petrovitch, H., and Burchfiel, C.M., et al. 1998. Effects of walking on mortality among non-smoking retired men. *New England Journal of Medicine* 338:94–99.

8. Paffenbarger, R.S., Hyde, R.T., Wing, A.L., and Hseih, C. 1986. Physical activity, all-cause mortality and longevity of college alumni. *New England Journal of Medicine* 314:605–12.

9. Lee, I. M., Chung-Cheng, H., and Paffenbarger, R.S. 1995. Exercise intensity and longevity in men: The Harvard Alumni Health Study. *Journal of the American Medical Association* 273:1179–84.

10. Ballor, D.L., Katch, V.L., Becque, M.D., and Marks, C.R. 1988. Resistance weight-training during caloric restriction enhances lean body weight maintenance. *American Journal of Clinical Nutrition* 47:19–25.

11. Hartung, G.H. 1995. Physical activity and high density lipoprotein cholesterol. *Journal of Sports Medicine and Fitness* 35:1–5.

12. Paterson, D.H. 1992. Effects of aging on the cardiorespiratory system. *Canadian Journal of Sport Science* 17:171–77.

13. Sforzo, G.A., McManis, B.G., and Black, D., et al. 1995. Resilience to exercise detraining in healthy older adults. *Journal of American Geriatrics Society* 43:209–15.

14. Stofan, J.R., DiPietro, L., Davis, D., Kohl, H.W., and Blair, S.N. 1998. Physical activity patterns associated with cardiorespiratory fitness and reduced mortality: The Aerobics Center Longitudinal Study. *American Journal of Public Health* 88:1807–13.

15. Lane, N.E., Block, D.A., and Jones, H.H., et al. 1986. Long distance running, bone density and osteoarthritis. *Journal of the American Medical Association* 255:1147–51.

16. Aoyagi, Y., and Shephard, R.J. 1992. Aging and muscle function. *Sports Medicine* 14:376–96.

17. Skeleton, D.A., Young, A., Greig, C., and Malbut, K.E. 1995. Effects of resistance training on strength, power and functional abilities of women age 75 and older. *Journal of American Geriatrics Society* 43:1081–87.

18. Fiatarone, M.A., Marks, E.C., and Ryan, N.D., et al. 1990. High-intensity strength training in nonagenarians: Effects on skeletal muscle. *Journal of the American Medical Association* 263:3029–34.

19. Fiatarone, M.A., O'Neill, E.F., and Ryan, N.D., et al. 1994. Exercise training and nutritional supplementation for physical frailty in very elderly people. *New England Journal of Medicine* 330:1769–75.

20. Byrne, A., and Byrne, D.G. 1993. The effect of exercise on depression, anxiety and other mood states: A review. *Journal of Psychosomatic Research* 37:565–74.

21. Singh, N.A., Clements, K.M., and Fiatarone, M.A. 1997. A randomized controlled trial of progressive resistance training in depressed elders. *Journal of Gerontology* 52A:M227–M335.

22. McMurdo, M., and Rennie, L. 1993. A controlled trial of exercise by residents of old people's homes. *Age and Ageing* 22:11–15.

23. deVries, H.A., and Adams, G.M. 1972. Electromyographic comparison of single doses of exercise and meprobamate as to effects on muscle relaxation. *American Journal of Physical Medicine* 51:130–41.

24. King, A.C., Oman, R.F., and Brassington, G.S., et al. 1997. Moderate-intensity exercise and self-rated quality of sleep in older adults. *Journal of the American Medical Association* 277:32–37.

25. Emery, C.F., and Blumenthal, J.A. 1991. Effects of physical exercise on psychological and cognitive functioning of older adults. *Annals of Behavioral Medicine* 13:99–107.

26. Dustman, R.E., Ruhling, R.O., and Russell, E.M., et al. 1984. Aerobic exercise training and improved neurophysiological function of older individuals. *Neurobiology of Aging* 5:35–42.

27. Hill, R.D., Storandt, M., and Malley, M. 1993. The impact of long-term exercise training on psychological function in older adults. *Journal of Gerontology* 48:P12–P17.

28. Friedman, R., and Tappen, R.M. 1991. The effect of planned walking on communication in Alzheimer's disease. *Journal of the American Geriatrics Society* 39:650–54.

29. Asher, R.A. 1947. The dangers of going to bed. *British Medical Journal* 2:967–68.

30. Nakamura, E., Moritani, T., and Kanetake, A. 1989. Biological age versus physical fitness age. *European Journal of Applied Physiology* 58:778–85.

31. Lazarus, B.A., Murphy, J.B., and Coletta, E.M., et al. 1991. The provision of physical activity to hospitalized elderly patients. *Archives of Internal Medicine* 151:2452–56.

32. Centers for Disease Control. 1990. Coronary heart disease attributable to a sedentary lifestyle— selected states, 1988. *Morbidity and Mortality Weekly Report* 39:541-544.

33. Hambrecht, R., Niebauer, J., and Marburger, C., et al. 1993. Various intensities of leisure time physical activity in patients with coronary artery disease: Effects on cardiorespiratory fitness and progression of coronary atherosclerotic lesions. *Journal of the American College of Cardiology* 22:468–77.

34. Lavie, C.J., and Milani, R.V. 1995. Effects of cardiac rehabilitation programs on exercise capacity, coronary risk factors, behavioral characteristics, and quality of life in a large elderly cohort. *American Journal of Cardiology* 76:177–79.

35. Wenger, N.K., Froelicher, E.S., and Smith, L.K., et al. 1995. Cardiac rehabilitation as secondary prevention. Clinical Practice Guidelines. Quick Reference Guide for Clinicians, No. 17. Rockville, MD: U.S. Department of Health and Human Services, PHS, Agency for Health Care Policy and Research and National Heart, Lung and Blood Institute. AHCPR Publ. no. 96-0673, October.

36. Butler, R.M., Beierwaltes, W.H., and Rogers, F.J. 1987. The cardiovascular response to circuit weight training in patients with cardiac disease. *Journal of Cardiopulmonary Rehabilitation* 7:402–9.

37. Kasch, F.W., Boyer, J.L., and Van Camp, S.P., et al. 1990. The effect of physical activity and inactivity on aerobic power in older men (a longitudinal study). *The Physician and Sports Medicine* 18:73–78.

38. American College of Sports Medicine. 1993. Position stand on physical activity, physical fitness, and hypertension. *Medicine and Science in Sports and Exercise* 25:i–x.

39. Gardner, A.W., and Poehlman, E.T. 1995. Exercise rehabilitation programs for the treatment of claudication pain. *Journal of the American Medical Association* 274:975–80.

40. Manson, J.E., Nathan, D.M., and Krolewski, A.S., et al. 1992. A prospective study of exercise and incidence of diabetes among US male physicians. *Journal of the American Medical Association* 268:63–67.

41. Burchfiel, C.M., Sharp, D.S., and Curb, J.D., et al. 1995. Physical activity and incidence of diabetes: The Honolulu Heart Program. *American Journal of Epidemiology* 141:360–68.

42. Manson, J.E., Rimm, E.B., and Stampfer, M.J., et al. 1991. Physical activity and incidence of non-insulin-dependent diabetes mellitus in women. *Lancet* 338:774–78.

43. Kirwan, J.P., Kohrt, W.M., and Wojta, D.M., et al. 1993. Endurance exercise training reduces glucose-stimulated insulin levels in 60- to 70-year-old men and women. *Journal of Gerontology* 48:M84–M90.

44. Council on Exercise. 1990. Diabetes and exercise position statement. *Diabetes Care* 13:804–5.

45. Mayer-Davis, E.J., D'Agostino, R., and Karter, A.J., et al. 1998. Intensity and amount of physical activity in relation to insulin sensitivity. *Journal of the American Medical Association* 279:669–74.

46. Centers for Disease Control. 1996. Prevalence of physical inactivity during leisure time among overweight persons—Behavioral risk factor surveillance system, 1994. *Morbidity and Mortality Weekly Report* 45:185–188.

47. Nelson, M.E., Fiatarone, M., and Morganti, C.M., et al. 1994. Effects of high-intensity strength training on multiple risk factors for osteoporotic fractures. *Journal of the American Medical Association* 272:1909–14.

48. Gregg, E.W., Cauley, J.A., Seeley, D.G., Ensrud, K.E., and Bauer, D.C. 1998. Physical activity and osteoporotic fracture risk in older women. *Annals of Internal Medicine* 129:81–88.

49. Dekker, J., Mulder, P.H., Bijlsma, J.W.J., and Oostendorp, R.A.B. 1993. Exercise therapy in patients with rheumatoid arthritis and osteoarthritis: A review. *Advances in Behavioral Research and Therapy* 15:211–38.

50. Hochberg, M.C., Altman, R.D., and Brandt, K.D., et al. 1995. Guidelines for the medical management of knee arthritis. *Arthritis and Rheumatism* 38:1541–46.

51. Ettinger, W.H., Burns, R., and Messier, S.P. 1997. A randomized trial comparing aerobic exercise and resistance exercise with a health education program in older adults with knee arthritis. *Journal of the American Medical Association* 227:25–31.

52. Kover, P.A., Allegrante, J.P., and MacKenzie, R., et al. 1992. Supervised fitness walking in patients with osteoarthritis of the knee. *Annals of Internal Medicine* 116:529–34.

53. Dexter, P.A. 1992. Joint exercises in elderly persons with symptomatic osteoarthritis of the hip or knee: Performance patterns, medical support patterns, and the relationship between exercising and medical care. *Arthritis Care Research* 5:36–41.

54. Boulware, D.W., and Byrd, S.L. 1993. Optimizing exercise programs for arthritis patients. *The Physician and Sports Medicine* 21:104–20.

55. Bigos, S., Bowyer, O., and Braen, G., et al. 1994. Acute low back problems in adults. Clinical Practice Guideline, Quick Reference Guide Number 14. Rockville, MD: U.S. Department of Health and Human Services, Public Health Service, Agency for Health Care Policy and Research, AHCPR Pub. no. 95-0643. December.

56. Giovannucci, E., Ascherio, A., and Rimm, E.B., et al. 1995. Physical activity, obesity and risk for colon cancer and adenoma in men. *Annals of Internal Medicine* 122:327–34.

57. Thune, I., Breen, T., Lund, E., and Gaard, M. 1997. Physical activity and risk of breast cancer. *New England Journal of Medicine* 336:1269–75.

58. Cerhan, J.R., Chiu, B., Wallace, R.B., et al. 1998. Physical activity, physical function, and the risk of breast cancer in a prospective study among elderly women. *Journal of Gerontology* 53A:M251–56.

59. Shumway-Cook, A., Gruber, W., Baldwin, M., and Laio, S. 1997. The effect of multidimensional exercises on balance, mobility, and fall risk in community-dwelling older adults. *Physical Therapy* 77:46–57.

60. Province, M.A., Hadley, E.C., and Hornbrook, M.C., et al. 1995. The effects of exercise on falls in elderly patients. *Journal of the American Medical Association* 273:1341–47.

61. Centers for Disease Control. 1996. State-specific prevalence of participation in physical activity-behavioral risk factor surveillance system, 1994. *Morbidity and Mortality Weekly Report* 45:673–75.

62. Centers for Disease Control. 1997. Monthly estimates of leisure-time physical inactivity—United States, 1994. *Morbidity and Mortality Weekly Report* 46:393–97.

63. Williford, H.N., Barfield, B.R., Lazenby, R.B., and Olsen, M.S. 1992. A survey of physician's attitudes and practices related to exercise promotion. *Preventive Medicine* 21:630–36.

64. Centers for Disease Control. 1992. *Project PACE: Physician's manual: Physician-based assessment and counseling for exercise.* Atlanta, GA: Centers for Disease Control.

65. American College of Sports Medicine. 1990. The recommended quality and quantity of exercise for

developing and maintaining cardiorespiratory and muscular fitness in healthy adults. *Medicine and Science in Sports and Exercise* 22:265–74.

66. Pate, R.R., Pratt, M., and Blair, S.V., et al. 1995. Physical activity and public health. A recommendation from the Centers for Disease Control and Prevention and the American College of Sports Medicine. *Journal of the American Medical Association* 273:402–7.

67. Mittleman, M.A., Maclure, M., and Tofler, G.H., et al. 1993. Triggering of acute myocardial infarction by heavy physical exertion. *New England Journal of Medicine* 329:1677–83.

68. *Physical Activity and Cardiovascular Health. NIH Consensus Statement.* 1995 December 18–20;113:1–33.

Dietary habits of youth set the stage for health and disease in old age. The time to nourish your body for late life is now.

Alice Chenault

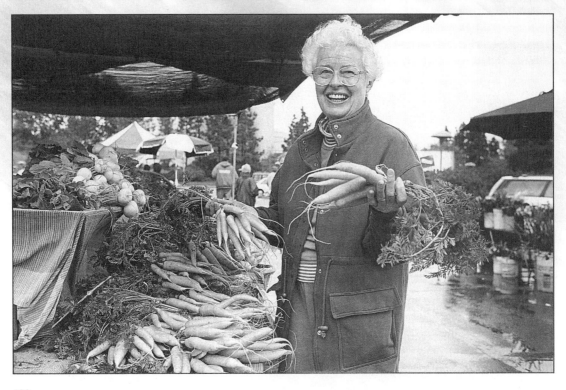

Our nutritional well-being plays a significant role in our state of health and quality of life, no matter what our age. While the same nutrients are essential for individuals of any age, changes accompanying aging may alter the amount of specific nutrients required by older people. Issues, such as obesity, cholesterol, saturated fats, and vitamin therapies, are often in the news, raising public consciousness of the importance of eating well. Furthermore, new understanding of the role of vitamins and minerals in health and disease is underscoring the importance of nutritional counseling as an adjunct to medical therapy. Poor eating habits accelerate many age-related decrements and increase the likelihood of several chronic illnesses in later life.

This chapter will examine the essential nutrients needed for all ages, strategies for choosing a healthful diet, the role of nutritional supplements, the effect of drug use on nutritional status, the nutritional status of elders, factors affecting food intake, and the relationship between nutrition and a number of chronic diseases. Programs to enhance nutritional status among elders will also be discussed.

THE STUDY OF DIET AND NUTRITION

Although there is widespread interest in the role of nutrition in health and disease, studying the complex role of diet and illness is quite difficult for many reasons. First, most Americans have access to a tremendously varied diet. We can eat a variety of foods year round, in and out of season, and often grown and packaged in different parts of the country or world. It is difficult to measure the nutrients found in a single food accurately (e.g., an apple), and this difficulty is compounded when a variety of different kinds of apples from different locations are consumed. Similarly, it is very difficult to determine the "average" diet of a person or a population. What is the average number of servings of fruits and grain you ate today, this week, this month, this year, or over your lifetime? If you cannot remember exactly, you are not alone. Most people are notoriously poor at remembering what they eat. Those responding to

food surveys may not tell the truth—they may underestimate the number of potato chips and overestimate the amount of broccoli they have eaten.

There are various ways researchers attempt to accurately determine what elders are eating; each method has its strengths and weaknesses. In an attempt to determine what people are eating and compare this to their risk of disease or blood levels of certain vitamins, surveys are conducted. The most common survey used is a twenty-four-hour *dietary recall.* In this method, individuals list the type and amount of foods they ate in the last twenty-four hours. Sometimes the period is extended beyond twenty-four hours. In this case, often a *food record* is used, where individuals are provided with a diary and asked to record the type and quantity of all foods they ate over a specified period, usually three days. In a *dietary history,* individuals answer a variety of questions regarding food they generally do or do not eat, the portion sizes, the frequency, and the method in which the foods are prepared. As an example, individuals may be asked to estimate whether they consume a certain portion size of yams, hamburger, corn oil, or eggs once daily, more than once daily, five to seven times weekly, two to four times weekly, or less than once a week. They may also be asked how long they cook their vegetables and how often they salt their food. Trained dieticians/nutritionists review the results of these surveys and calculate the amount of various nutrients, vitamins, and minerals consumed and then estimate the degree of nutrient deficiency or excess.

The above methodologies rely on self-report: elders are asked to remember or record foods eaten over a specified time period or estimate the frequency they consume certain foodstuffs. These methods are hindered by poor recall, lack of consistency in filling out the forms, overreporting nutritious foods to please the interviewer, and lack of information on portion size, quality of food, and method of preparation. The studies may be biased against ethnic elders who eat traditional foods not included on standard questionnaires. It may be difficult to estimate serving sizes or food composition when meals are delivered by Meals on Wheels, bought prepackaged, or served in a restaurant or food site. Finally, diet may change over time or vary by cohort or age.

Nationwide surveys, the most widely respected measures of adult nutrition, are periodically conducted to assess whether adults in the population are receiving adequate nutrition. These surveys use some of the same methodologies discussed above including twenty-four-hour dietary recall and dietary surveys; examples are the National Health and Nutrition Examination surveys (HANES) and the Nationwide Food Consumption Survey (NFCS). The U.S. Department of Agriculture's Continuing Survey of Food Intake by Individuals (CSFI) is also commonly used. Numerous smaller studies have examined the nutritional status of elder subgroups in community and institution settings. More details are provided in a later section.

Population studies of community elders may underestimate nutritional deficiencies because they exclude the bedridden, isolated, cognitively impaired, and homeless. Those with cognitive or memory impairment are less likely to be able to remember what they ate and to record their dietary intake. Additionally, population data tell little about individual variation. For instance, a study may show that, on the average, elders get enough protein, but, in fact, some may get too much and others too little.

When self-reported information is combined with physical assessment, such as weight, body fat, or blood levels of nutrients, nutritional status can be more accurately assessed. Measurements of weight, height, arm circumference, and skinfold thickness, when compared to population norms, can determine elders' level of malnutrition or obesity. A physical examination can also detect obvious signs of nutritional deficiency. Finally, laboratory tests on blood and urine can indicate current levels of essential nutrients.

One of the more accurate methods to determine food intake is to measure blood levels of vitamins. Researchers might measure the level of zinc or vitamin C in the blood to more accurately assess diet. Studies like this are commonly conducted to compare individuals with a particular disease to those without the disease.

The overwhelming majority of studies on nutrition are population-based, measuring the nutritional status of many individuals at one point in time, then determining if there is a relationship between blood levels of nutrients or dietary habits with the subsequent development of disease. For example, a study may find that those with higher levels of vitamin C have lower rates of cancer. Although these studies provide interesting leads, they are flawed in many ways. Most obvious, those with high vitamin C intakes are often the same people who are more likely to exercise, eat a wide variety of fruits and vegetables, be of normal weight, be health-conscious, and eat fiber. Thus, it is very difficult to separate out the "effect" of vitamin C from the other behaviors that likely reduce cancer risk.

We must be thoughtful as we interpret research reported in the popular press relating the effect of a particular nutrient on disease. To illustrate the complexity of such research, let us review the relationship of beta carotene intake and lung cancer. Multiple studies reported that individuals with lung cancer have lower levels of beta carotene in their blood than individuals without cancer. However, these studies are easily misinterpreted. Some may say, for example, that beta carotene protects against cancer, and individuals who have a high intake of beta carotene will be less likely to get cancer. However, this interpretation is wrong for a number of reasons. We cannot be sure that cancer itself is not altering the levels of vitamins and minerals in the blood. Thus it may be that those with cancer and those without had the same level of beta carotene in their diet and blood, but that the cancer has lowered the beta carotene levels in some way. Further, even if low levels of beta carotene are associated with cancer, this does not mean that dietary supplementation of beta carotene will reduce cancer risk. In fact, a study of male smokers given beta carotene supplements found no cancer reduction among those receiving supplements. It may be that some other component of food is more important than beta carotene, and the still-undiscovered component found in foods high in beta carotene is actually protective against cancer. Or, it could mean that the dosage of supplements were insufficient to cause change.

The "gold standard" to determine the benefits of various nutrients or nutrient supplements are randomized controlled double-blind trials. In these studies, individuals (called subjects) are randomly assigned to receive either a placebo (looks the same but has no active ingredient) or a nutritional supplement. "Double-blind" means that neither the subjects nor the researchers know who receives which pill. At the end of the study period, the subjects are evaluated for outcome (for example, number who had a heart attack). Statistical calculations are done to determine whether there is any association between the nutrient and the subsequent outcome. These studies allow researchers to "control" for all the other things that may cloud the true association between nutrition and disease.

THE SCIENCE OF NUTRITION

Food provides energy as well as other essential components for optimal body function. The body must have energy, or fuel, in order for it to survive. With the exception of diet sodas, black coffee, and tea, almost all food contains some usable energy in the form of protein, carbohydrates, or fat. The amount of energy contained in foods is measured in kilocalories (commonly referred to as calories) and represents the amount of energy required to heat 1,000 grams (about a quart) of water by 1° Celsius. Thus, if you burned the energy in a ten-calorie piece of candy, you could heat 1,000 grams of water 10° Celsius.

The burning of carbohydrates and protein yields about four calories per gram, while fat, a more concentrated energy source, yields nine calories per gram. Because fat is so concentrated, a relatively small portion contains more than twice as many calories as the same-sized portion of a food that is predominantly carbohydrate or protein. Some high-energy foods release as much energy as explosives in the body; for instance, a two-inch square of fudge (185 calories) releases as much energy as a small stick of dynamite, and a double-dip ice cream cone (334 calories) releases

energy equivalent to one-half cubic foot of natural gas. This huge amount of energy does not explode the body because it is released gradually by the enzyme-coordinated process of metabolism.[1]

For a number of reasons, individuals decrease daily caloric requirements as they age. The caloric requirements for the average man age twenty-five to fifty is 2,700 calories per day, which decreases to 2,400 at age fifty-one to seventy-five, and to 1,800 over age seventy-five. For women between ages twenty-five and fifty, the requirements are 2,000 calories per day, decreasing to 1,800 calories between ages fifty-one to seventy-five and to only 1,600 for women over age seventy-five.[2] Although there is a general decrease in caloric need, vitamin and mineral needs do not decrease proportionally. Because of decreased caloric need, elders should eat nutrient-rich foods and avoid high-calorie, low-nutrient foods such as processed foods and those high in fat or sugar.

Many factors contribute to elders' reduced need for fuel, or calories. With age, the proportion of body fat increases and muscle mass decreases. Furthermore, there is a small, progressive reduction in resting metabolic rate after maturity. Finally, as a group, elders are generally less physically active than younger adults, further reducing caloric needs. Although caloric need tends to decline with age, there may be as much as a 1,000-calorie variation among what individuals of the same age require, depending on their activity level and basal metabolic rate. Elders who are very physically active need more calories than those who are bedridden. Consumption of more calories than the body requires results in storage of that energy as fat deposits to be used in times of increased need.

DIETARY GUIDELINES FOR AMERICANS

Are you old enough to remember the "Basic Four" food groups? Most middle-aged and older adults recall this effort by the U.S. Department of Agriculture (USDA) to help Americans plan meals and eat more healthfully. Although "basic four" is forever a part of our lexicon, these groups are now

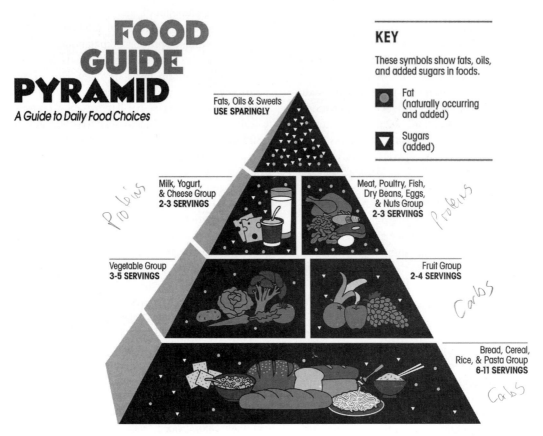

Figure 5.1
The Food Guide Pyramid
Source: U.S. Dept. of Agriculture. Human Nutrition Information Serices.

out of vogue, replaced by the Food Guide Pyramid (figure 5.1). The purpose of the Food Guide Pyramid is to help consumers make the best food choices for a healthier lifestyle. The pyramid provides a visual representation of a healthful diet. It is heavy on whole grains, fruits, and vegetables, and light on fat, oils, and sweets. Instead of four, there are now five basic food groups, but the amount of servings in each are not equivalent: the food group with the highest number of servings forms the base of the pyramid, and the foods to be eaten sparingly are at the top.

The Food Guide Pyramid emphasizes several important points that are consistent with an eating plan low in overall fat, saturated fat, and cholesterol. Health experts agree that it is important to eat a wide variety of foods to get sufficient nutrients and calories. The three food groups filling the largest space in the Food Guide Pyramid and with the most suggested servings are plant foods that naturally contain little or no fat or cholesterol: Bread, Cereal, Rice, and Pasta Group, Vegetable Group, and the Fruit Group. The pyramid includes fewer servings of the two food groups containing animal products—the Milk, Yogurt, and Cheese Group, and the Meat, Poultry, Fish, and Dry Beans, Eggs, and Nuts Group. Although animal products have traditionally been a major source of fat and saturated fat in the American diet, many lower-fat and fat-free products from these groups are now available. The USDA allowed the smallest space on the Food Guide Pyramid for the Fats, Oils, and Sweets Group, consistent with heart-healthy eating. These foods provide calories, but few vitamins and minerals. Further, it is important to be aware of sugars and fats added to foods in the other groups (e.g., French fries have a lot of added fat).

RECOMMENDED DIETARY ALLOWANCES

The human body requires more than forty nutrients to carry out its functions, including water, protein, fat, carbohydrates, vitamins, and minerals. The metabolism of protein, carbohydrates, and fat supplies the body with energy for growth and maintenance. Vitamins and minerals are needed to manufacture enzymes, needed for cell growth and maintenance. Water is perhaps the most essential element in the body. One can live for over a month without food, but only a few days without water. Even though dietary fiber is not a nutrient because it travels through the digestive system unchanged, it also plays an important role in physical health. These essential nutrients will be discussed more completely in the next section.

Each individual requires a different quantity of various nutrients, depending on activity and stress levels, drug use, age, gender, body size, and health condition. However, attempts have been made to standardize requirements to assist individuals to make good food choices. Perhaps the best-known standards are the Recommended Dietary Allowances, or RDA, developed by the Food and Nutrition Board of the National Academy of Sciences (table 5.1). As the role of diet in the onset of disease becomes clear, the RDA is continually modified. Whereas the RDA used to be simply the amount of nutrient necessary to prevent deficiency disease, it now focuses on levels sufficient to achieve health

TABLE 5.1	Daily RDA for Selected Vitamins and Minerals*		
Nutrient	**Age**	**RDA/day**	**Adequate Intake/day**
B vitamins			
Thiamine (B_1)	19+	1.1 mg	
Riboflavin (B_2)	19+	1.1 mg	
Niacin (B_3)	19+	14 mg	
Pantothenic acid (B_5)	19+		5 mg
Pyridoxine (B_6)	19–50	1.3 mg	
Pyridoxine (B_6)	51+	1.5 mg	
Biotin (B_7)	19+		30 µg
Folate (B_9)	19+	400 µg DFE**	
Cobalamin (B_{12})	19+	2.4 µg	
Magnesium	19–30	400 mg	310 mg
	31+	420 mg	320 mg
Vitamin D	19–50	5 µg	
	51–70	10 µg	
	> 70	15 µg	
Calcium	19–50		1,000 mg
	51+		1,200 mg
Phosphorus	19+	700 mg	

*Does not include pregnant or lactating women.
**1 DFE equals 1 µg of folate, 0.6 mcg of folic acid in food, or 5 µg on empty stomach.

benefits. In addition, guidelines are developed to suggest adequate intakes for nutrients where evidence is not sufficient to support a RDA. Because of a burgeoning interest and research in nutrition, this process has been very time-consuming, and their findings and recommendations are being issued little by little, accompanied by hundreds of pages of explanations. At the time of the writing of this book, recommendations were available for B vitamins, chlorine, calcium, vitamin D, fluoride, phosphorus, and magnesium. Because of increased focus on supplements and concern over how much might be "too much," the National Academy of Sciences Food and Nutrition Board is also in the process of releasing guidelines for tolerable upper limits of several vitamins and minerals. These numbers may provide guidance to those taking megadoses of vitamin and mineral supplements. Updated information is available on the National Academy Press web site at http://www.nap.edu/ readingroom/index.html.

Adult RDA guidelines for most nutrients are divided into subsections grouped by age and special guidelines are issued for pregnant or lactating women. In most cases, elders are grouped with other adults over age nineteen. Despite the vast differences in health status and activity level of adults of various ages, recommended allowance for nutrients is the same. Some experts assert that the RDA for some nutrients should be modified for older adults.[3] For example, they suggest that the RDA for vitamin A is likely too high, while that for riboflavin, B_6, B_{12}, and vitamin D are too low. The RDA values have also been criticized because their values are specified only for "healthy" adults. Elders with even one chronic disorder may require more than the RDA of many nutrients.

Because of the increased focus on the use of supplements and concern over how much might be too much, the National Academy of Sciences Food and Nutrition Board is also developing guidelines for Tolerable Upper Limits on several vitamins and minerals. They are being determined from research on animals and humans. For instance, at this printing, the Tolerable Upper Limit has been defined for the following: calcium, 2,500 mg/day; magnesium, 350 mg/day; phosphorus, 3,000 mg/day; vitamin

D, 50 mg/day; and fluoride, 10 mg/day. These numbers can provide some guidance to those taking megadoses of supplements. The status of the Board's work in this area can also be found at the website listed previously.

NUTRITIONAL DISEASES

Malnutrition

Malnutrition is caused when a person has an inadequate intake of energy-rich foods. *Kwashiorkor* is a syndrome of inadequate protein intake, while *marasmus* results from inadequate protein and calories. American elders who are malnourished generally have a combination of these two syndromes, called *protein-calorie malnutrition.* These individuals undergo complex changes in body function that allow them to break down body tissues for energy. At first, expendable tissues, such as fat stores, are mobilized. However, after prolonged malnutrition, muscle and even organ tissue must be utilized. Individuals who are malnourished also reduce their metabolic rate since they are trying to conserve energy. Further, both the function of the immune system and healing processes are reduced.

Those who are malnourished may display symptoms of mental illness. One classic study placed a group of healthy young men on a calorie-deficient diet for six months. The subjects lost weight and reported feeling insecure, irritable, moody, and depressed. They also had no emotional control, no interest in others, and were unable to make decisions.[4] Since these symptoms are similar to those with mental illness, it is important that nutritional inadequacies be ruled out before a diagnosis is made.

Malnutrition is not limited to the less-developed parts of the world. Some estimate that 10 percent of elders living in the United States are malnourished, while other studies estimate as much as 25 percent.[5] Malnourishment among older people in our country is likely due to a combination of factors: poor food choices, lack of appetite, inability to shop and prepare food, social isolation, and poverty. Malnutrition is much more common among hospital patients because illness can cause

Nutritional Supplements: Boon or Bust?

Increasingly adults of all ages are turning to liquid nutritional supplements to provide extra "nutritional assurance" or to substitute for a meal (e.g., Ensure, Boost). Available as beverages, powders, or puddings in an array of flavors, they were originally developed for people who are malnourished but are too weak to eat, who need to gain weight, who cannot prepare food for themselves, who have difficulty chewing and swallowing, and who are being fed through a tube. They used to be only available through hospitals but can now be purchased wherever food and drugs are sold.

The companies making the products have implemented extensive advertising campaigns to expand their sales to those adults who are well. The ads tout that these products can help lose weight, gain weight, maintain weight, boost energy, and save time. Consequently, the sale of these supplements is skyrocketing. Middle-aged adults, even young adults, are drinking them instead of lunch or a snack and are reassuring themselves that they are getting all the nutrition they need.

What are they? The formulas mix skim milk, sugar, oil, water, and generally soy protein with vitamins, minerals, and flavorings. One 8-ounce serving has about two dozen vitamins and minerals (15 to 50 percent of RDA for each), 10 to 16 grams of protein, 200 to 360 calories, 35 grams of carbohydrates, and 10 grams of fat. One serving costs $1 to $2. Some products are lactose-free, and a few have fiber. These drinks are advertised as nutritionally complete. Although they are not harmful, they do not provide the balanced nutrition that is claimed because they lack fiber and many of the other important nutrients found in fruits and vegetables. For this reason, healthy adults should not use them regularly as a meal substitute. Also, those people who drink them between meals will gain weight. It is better to eat a healthy snack that is more nutritious and less expensive than a supplement.

---

malnutrition, and malnutrition can cause illness. Those who are malnourished heal more slowly, have more frequent re-admissions to the hospital, and exhibit higher rates of infection, accidents, and death. Estimates vary widely, but it is agreed that malnutrition is a common and serious problem among nursing home residents. Federal legislation now mandates that elders' nutrition status and ability to feed themselves be assessed upon admission and periodically during their stay.

Weight Loss and Artificial Feeding

Although gradual weight loss should be encouraged in the obese, unexplained weight loss or weight loss that occurs without dieting and exercising should be promptly evaluated. Weight loss without dieting may be due to an undiagnosed cancer, thyroid disease, or heart or lung disease progression. Weight loss, especially if accompanied by anorexia or lack of appetite, may be due to severe depression, dementia, cancer, or the end stages of a terminal illness. Oral health problems may cause involuntary weight loss, especially among the frail.[6]

Because of the degree of malnutrition in institutionalized elders, individuals should undergo a thorough physical examination and a complete nutritional history when admitted to a hospital or nursing home. In addition, daily monitoring of weight and dietary intake is necessary, and nutritional supplements should be considered. These may include vitamin or mineral supplements, concentrated oral nutrition, intravenous nutrition, or feeding through a tube (either through the nose or through a tube inserted directly into the stomach). When weight loss is associated with anorexia, patients may be prescribed medications to stimulate appetite, such as marinol (a synthetic version of a chemical found in marijuana) or steroids. For individuals with a terminal illness, a focus on eating comfort and preparing appealing meals should be the goal.

Artificial feeding may be accomplished through tubes into the digestive system or into a vein. A tube placed through the nose into the stomach is called a nasogastric tube. A gastrostomy tube is placed through the abdominal wall into the stomach. A jejunostomy tube is placed through the abdominal wall into the small intestine. Intravenous feeding, called total parenteral nutrition (TPN), infuses a solution of sugars, fats, proteins, vitamins, and minerals directly into the blood stream to provide nourishment when natural eating is not possible.

Artificial feeding, either through a tube placed in the digestive system or through the vein, is appropriate for short-term use. These therapies may be used for elders who are malnourished to increase their stamina, for those undergoing cancer chemotherapy, or for those unable to eat after surgery. Those with cancer of the throat or stomach or those with severe bowel problems often must be fed through tubes (intravenous or into the intestine) for prolonged periods of time as they are unable to take oral nutrition. Likewise, those with neurological illnesses, such as strokes or end-stage dementia, are often unable to swallow and may be maintained by tube feeding for months or years.

Long-term use of artificial feeding must be carefully considered. It is unacceptable to many patients and families unless there is hope that the patient's functional status will improve. For instance, if an elder suffers a massive stroke that affects her ability to swallow, she might be kept on artificial feeding during rehabilitation attempts. However, if she remains unconscious, artificial feeding may be discontinued to allow her to die.

Artificial feeding is a medical procedure that is associated with risks and benefits. Benefits include improved nutritional status, improvements in immune system function and wound healing, and decreased risk of death. Risks include nasal irritation and sore throat (nasogastric tube), surgical complications (gastrostomy, jejunostomy, or permanent IV), and infections. Those with tubes in the digestive system may suffer from aspiration pneumonia brought about by breathing food particles

into the lungs. Those receiving TPN must often receive insulin as well as frequent blood tests to ensure the balance of nutrients is correct. Artificial feeding of any type may cause nutrient imbalances, fluid overload, or agitation related to being "hooked up" to tubes. There is some fear that nutritional supplementation in advanced cancer may increase metabolic rate and thereby "feed" the tumor, so artificial feeding is generally not recommended.

Obesity

Although undernutrition can be a problem for some frail elders, a much more common type of malnutrition in this country is overweight and obesity. Various measures have been used over the years to define obesity. Obesity used to be defined as being 20 percent or more above ideal body weight. Ideal body weight was determined from standardized tables, many of which were originally developed by life insurance companies in an attempt to price life insurance policies accurately.

In 1998, the National Institutes of Health released the first federal clinical overweight and obesity guidelines, using the body mass index (BMI), a ratio of height to weight, as a measuring tool. Although life insurance companies still use height/weight tables, the BMI is becoming more common since it is more strongly associated with total body fat content in adults. An adult with a BMI of 25 to 29 is considered overweight, and a person with a BMI of 30 and above is considered obese. According to these new guidelines, over half the adults in the United States are overweight or obese.

Multiple studies have documented adverse health effects from obesity. Those who are overweight have a higher risk of heart disease, some cancers, stroke, hypertension, gallbladder disease, osteoarthritis, and adult-onset diabetes. It is clear that being overweight is less harmful than being obese and that many risks increase sharply at a BMI of more than 30.

Many assertions about the hazards of obesity are based on studies of younger adults and may overlook the fact that those who are overweight often have other characteristics besides their

What's Your BMI?

Can you pinch an inch (of fat)? If you jump up and down in front of the mirror without clothes, do you see a lot of movement where you shouldn't? Have you gained more than 10 pounds—or added more than two or three inches to your waist—since you turned 21?

Over the years, experts have suggested a number of ways to help people figure out if they weigh too much. But the one *they* usually use—often along with other measurements—is the BMI, or body mass index.

It's a number, usually between 16 and 40, that's calculated from your height and weight. The beauty of the BMI is that researchers can use one number to describe the fatness of both a five-foot woman and a six-foot man.

The National Center for Health Statistics defines "overweight" as a BMI of 27.8 (for men) or 27.3 (for women). That's about 20 percent over "desirable weight." Using that cutoff, one out of three Americans is overweight.

According to the World Health Organization, people with a BMI between 25 and 29 are "over-weight." Those with a BMI of 30 or higher are "obese." (Fifty-nine percent of American men and 50 percent of American women have BMIs of 25 or higher.) Your body mass index (BMI) is your weight (in kilograms) divided by your height (in meters) squared. No, don't reach for your calculator. Below is a chart that does the work for you.

Just locate your height along the left-hand column. Then slide your finger to the right along that row until you come to the number closest to your weight. At the top of that column is your BMI.

For instance, if you're 5'5" and 140 pounds, your BMI is 23. If you're six feet tall and 210 pounds, your BMI is 29.

If your height or weight isn't listed, or if you want to compute your exact BMI, here's a shortcut: Multiply your weight (in pounds) by 703 and then divide it by your height (in inches) squared.

Copyright 1999 CSPI. Reprinted from *Nutrition Action Healthletter* (1875 Connecticut Ave., N. W. Suite 300, Washington, D.C. 20009-5728. $24 for 12 issues.)

Body Mass Index (BMI)

Height	19	20	21	22	23	24	25	26	27	28	29	30	35	40
							Weight (Pounds)							
4'10"	91	96	100	105	110	115	119	124	129	134	138	143	167	191
4'11"	94	99	104	109	114	119	124	128	133	138	143	148	173	198
5'0"	97	102	107	112	118	123	128	133	138	143	148	153	179	204
5'1"	100	106	111	116	122	127	132	137	143	148	153	158	185	211
5'2"	104	109	115	120	126	131	136	142	147	153	158	164	191	218
5'3"	107	113	118	124	130	135	141	146	152	158	163	169	197	225
5'4"	110	116	122	128	134	140	145	151	157	163	169	174	204	232
5'5"	114	120	126	132	138	144	150	156	162	168	174	180	210	240
5'6"	118	124	130	136	142	148	155	161	167	173	179	186	216	247
5'7"	121	127	134	140	146	153	159	166	172	178	185	191	223	255
5'8"	125	131	138	144	151	158	164	171	177	184	190	197	230	262
5'9"	128	135	142	149	155	162	169	176	182	189	196	203	236	270
5'10"	132	139	146	153	160	167	174	181	188	195	202	207	243	278
5'11"	136	143	150	157	165	172	179	186	193	200	208	215	250	286
6'0"	140	147	154	162	169	177	184	191	199	206	213	221	258	294
6'1"	144	151	159	166	174	182	189	197	204	212	219	227	265	302
6'2"	148	155	163	171	179	186	194	202	210	218	225	233	272	311
6'3"	152	160	168	176	184	192	200	208	216	224	232	240	279	319
6'4"	156	164	172	180	189	197	205	213	221	230	238	246	287	328
							OVERWEIGHT					OBESE		

Source: World Health Organization.

excess weight that may contribute to these problems. Overweight people are more likely to be poor, of lower socioeconomic status, and sedentary. They may have different diets (e.g., higher fat) or lower vegetable consumption. Obese people are more difficult to examine, have decreased mobility and increased accidents, and are more prone to surgical complications than those of normal weight. In addition, those who are obese may experience more stress manifested as depression, guilt, self-hatred, and anxiety because of our cultural dictum against fat. Further, the discrimination endured because of our society's hatred of fat might be influential in health states of the obese. Thus, it may be that being overweight it not as harmful to health as is eating a high-fat diet, being poor, and being sedentary. Each of these factors likely contributes to the high risk. However, these factors are difficult to separate and study.

The association between body mass index and mortality weakens with age and is no longer present after age seventy-five.[7] This means that older people who are obese do not have greater mortality than their thinner counterparts. In fact, some earlier studies show that in very old age, those who are thinner have higher mortality rates, although it is suspected this is partly due to disease. Studies among adults show that health risks begin to accrue at about BMI of 27 to 28 and preliminary studies in elders suggest that their risk only increases after a BMI of 30. If adults with a BMI in the intermediate range do not have diabetes or high cholesterol levels, the effect of their weight upon their health status is likely to be minor. Finally, there is not good evidence that weight loss enhances health for those with a BMI of less than 30.

It is somewhat difficult to determine ideal weight among elders because they manifest many chronic and acute illnesses that may profoundly affect weight and health. Thus, elders with depression, cancer, or advanced chronic illnesses such as dementia, congestive heart failure, or chronic obstructive pulmonary disease may lose weight as their health worsens. However, when studies look at healthy older people without chronic illness

who do not smoke, it seems that being thinner is associated with better health and lower death rates. In fact, lowest mortality rates for elder men are about 20 percent below the U.S. average, and for women about 15 percent below the U.S. average.[8,9] Studies show that those with body mass index values between 19 and 22 have the best health and the lowest mortality.

Not only is the amount of excess weight a person carries important, but also the pattern of fat distribution. Weight gain primarily on the abdomen and chest ("apple-shaped") is associated with an increased risk for many diseases, including heart disease, stroke, elevated cholesterol, poor glucose tolerance, high blood pressure, and death. Those who gain weight on the hips and thighs ("pear-shaped") are at lower risk of death and disease. The National Institutes of Health, in addition to their guidelines for BMI, also released guidelines on waist circumference, a variable strongly related to abdominal fat and consequent health problems. They recommend that men maintain a waist size of less than 40 inches and women maintain a waist size of 35 inches to keep health risks low. If the BMI is less than 25, waist size isn't as important, but if the BMI is over 25 and the waist is large, the risk of diabetes, stroke, and heart disease is higher.[10]

Although being lighter is associated with improved health, there is less evidence that weight loss and dieting are as effective as never gaining the weight in the first place.[11] However, weight loss can reduce the symptoms of existing chronic illnesses, such as diabetes, arthritis, and hypertension, and prevent development of other symptoms. Those who work with obese elders should help them to understand the value of losing weight and learn ways to change dietary and exercise habits to achieve a weight loss goal. In many cases, losing weight enables a disease to be controlled without using drugs.

As in other age groups, rational weight loss principles should be followed. A combination of increased physical activity, increased intake of complex carbohydrates, increased consumption of fruits and vegetables, and decreased fat intake is the preferred method of weight loss for all age groups.

(See chapter 4 for the benefits of exercise in weight reduction.) Although many approaches to weight loss have been promulgated, none is as effective or as inexpensive as a combination of reduced calorie intake and increased calorie expenditure (eat less, exercise more). In general, consultation with a nutritionist, either alone or in a group setting, is an important component of any weight loss program. Patients should be followed to ensure they follow a regular exercise program, and that their proposed diet includes essential nutrients and takes both food preferences and income into account.

Diet counselors can enhance the success and maintenance of a weight loss program in a number of important ways:

- Offer support to their clients as they alter their eating and exercise habits to achieve weight loss.
- Enlist the support of the client's friends and families to help change eating and exercising behaviors.

- Examine the "excuses" people make for not losing weight (fear of failure, fear of ridicule) to help the provider better support the lifestyle change.
- Identify the barriers to changes in diet and physical activity.
- Establish a plan with small, achievable, stepwise goals in conjunction with the patient's goals and interests.
- Build in positive reinforcement (rewards) and incentives.
- Keep track of the clients' improvement and give positive feedback.
- Focus on the positive effects of reduced weight rather than on the number of pounds lost is key to success.
- Reinforce that you are not just proposing a diet, but a permanent lifestyle change in eating and physical activity.

Self-help groups, such as Weight Watchers or Overeaters Anonymous, have had much success in

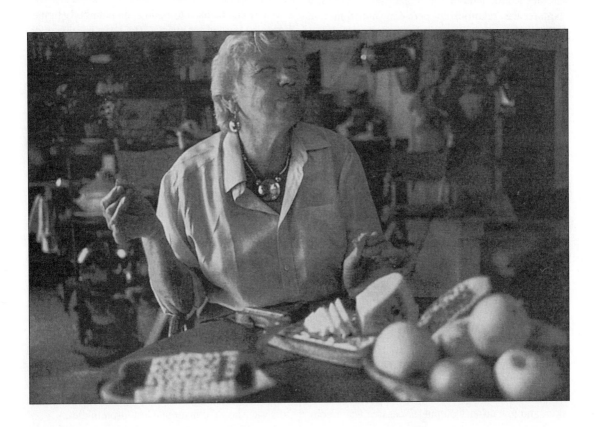

assisting individuals to follow through on a weight loss program. Weight loss programs are the most successful for those with a strong motivation to lose weight, such as cardiac patients and newly diagnosed diabetics.

ESSENTIAL DIETARY COMPONENTS

The human body requires a wide variety of nutrients to carry out its essential functions. This section discusses the essential components of a nutritious diet and common food sources for each nutrient. The response of the body to insufficient amounts of a particular nutrient will also be addressed.

Some nutrients are needed in large amounts, such as water, proteins, carbohydrates, and fat. Other nutrients, such as vitamins and minerals, while also essential, are needed in much smaller amounts. Although this section will mention the relationship of nutrition to some chronic illnesses, another section later in this chapter will more fully explore the relationship between nutrition and heart disease, cancer, and diabetes.

Water

Water is essential to most body processes, including swallowing, digestion, elimination, and regulation of body temperature. All chemical reactions within the body need water; even small changes in water balance can lead to metabolic problems. In addition, water, especially hard water, provides the body with needed minerals such as zinc, magnesium, calcium, and copper.

The healthy older person requires from one-and-a-half to two quarts of water each day, some of which is obtained from food. Elders have less body water than younger groups and are more susceptible to dehydration. Healthy older people are not as likely as younger people to complain of thirst and tend to drink less than younger people, suggesting that elders cannot rely totally on their thirst mechanism to determine needed water intake. Symptoms of mild dehydration include weakness, confusion, dry mouth, and flushed skin. Symptoms of more severe dehydration include sunken eyes, dry loose skin, and low urinary output. Excessive water con-

sumption can aggravate diseases, such as congestive heart failure. Thus, some elders require diets with fluid restriction.

Proteins

Protein is the main component of blood, skin, hair, muscles, and organs, and of enzymes that control the chemical processes within the cell that keeps us alive. Body tissues are composed of complex proteins built from combinations of building blocks called amino acids The instructions to make the proteins in our bodies are found in our genes, but the material needed to make those proteins have to come from the proteins from the food we eat.

Some amino acids are manufactured in the body from other dietary components, while others, called *essential amino acids,* must come from the food we eat. Proteins may come from vegetable or animal sources. Once ingested, proteins are broken down into amino acids in the intestines and absorbed so they can be used to build and repair body tissues, or to be burned for energy. The body requires more protein during periods of rapid growth, illness, and recovery from surgery or injury. Although older people may need less protein to maintain their declining muscle mass, the amount of protein recommended is the same for all individuals over age 25.

Many people from developing nations do not get sufficient protein in their diets. However, in the United States, many people consume an excessive amount of protein. The metabolism of excess protein, especially animal protein, can put a strain on the liver and kidneys and can deplete the bones of needed calcium. For most elders, protein should comprise only about 10 to 15 percent of their daily total caloric intake. It is estimated that elder men require about 93 grams of protein and elder women 73 grams of protein a day. Because protein needs are increased in times of stress or when recovering from a wound, those who are chronically ill, bedridden, or who have decubitus ulcers are at a high risk of protein deficiency and should increase their protein consumption to twice the Recommended Daily Allowance (RDA). On the other hand, those with osteoporosis and kidney disease should consume a low-protein diet.

Major dietary sources of protein are nuts, legumes, fish, meat, eggs, and dairy products.

Carbohydrates

Carbohydrates provide the major source of calories because they are inexpensive and easy to prepare, store, chew, and digest. Carbohydrates are easily broken down and provide an immediate source of energy. Foods classified as carbohydrates vary widely. Some are simple (sugars), such as sucrose, fructose (found in fruits), and lactose (found in dairy products). Others are complex (starches), which are more difficult to digest, but provide energy over a longer period of time. Carbohydrates are broken down into sugar by saliva and stomach enzymes, enter the blood stream as sugars, and the hormone insulin permits the sugar to enter each body cell to produce energy.

Sometimes carbohydrate-rich foods are commercially processed, altering it in some way (e.g., white rice and flour, refined sugar), and reducing its store of vitamins, minerals, and fiber. Manufacturers of processed foods often add back some of the vitamins, but the product remains low in fiber (figure 5.2).

Complex carbohydrates are becoming the chosen food of health-conscious eaters. Once avoided by dieters who thought complex carbohydrates were fattening, we now know that they are a good source of energy for those who want to lose weight since they are not high in calories. Complex carbohydrates are digested more slowly and therefore satisfy hunger longer while providing essential vitamins and minerals. Because carbohydrates are filling, daily caloric intake tends to decrease. They are also the main source of fiber. Complex carbohydrates should make up at least 55 percent of the calories in the diet. No deficiency disease of carbohydrates is known because complex carbohydrates are the most available and inexpensive of all the food groups.

Main sources of carbohydrates are whole-grain breads and cereals, rice, beans, pastas, fruits, and starchy vegetables.

Fats

Despite their negative press, fats are important: they provide energy, transport fat-soluble vitamins, insulate and cushion the body, and manufacture essential cell components. Fats also provide flavor to food and a feeling of fullness. All animal and plant foods contain fats; foods high in fats include dairy products, vegetable oils, and red meat. Fats can be synthesized by the liver or may be ingested in the diet.

There is little danger of insufficient fat intake; even if one ingests no visible fat, about 10 percent of all calories would still be derived from fat. On the average, Americans consume an average of 40 percent of their calories as fats. The American Heart Association recommends no more than 30 percent of caloric intake be composed of fat since excessive fat consumption is associated with obesity, heart disease, and some cancers. Some experts believe that 30 percent is still too high and Americans should aim for a diet containing only 15 to 20 percent. Excess fat intake is particularly harmful for elders since it provides calories in a concentrated form with few vitamins, minerals, fiber, or other nutrients. In addition, some elders have a reduced tolerance for fat due to digestive problems.

There are many different types and subtypes of fats. Two major types are triglycerides and cholesterol. *Triglycerides* are used predominantly for energy. These fats are made of two- or three-long chains of molecules called fatty acids connected to a short carbohydrate backbone. These long chains may be polyunsaturated (meaning they have a lot of sites available for other molecules to bond), saturated (no available sites), or monounsaturated (containing only one open site), depending on the type of bonds that chains the molecules together.

Saturated fats are generally found in animal products such as meat and butter, although vegetable shortening that is "hydrogenated" is also saturated. These fats are generally solid at room temperature. A diet high in saturated fats is strongly associated with an increased risk of atherosclerosis, elevated cholesterol, and heart disease. *Unsaturated fats* are generally liquid at room temperature, although they may solidify in the refrigerator. *Polyunsaturated fats,* such as margarine and most vegetable oils, protect against heart disease, but they may be associated with an increased risk of cancer. *Monounsaturated fats,* such as olive oil and fats found in avocados and nuts, are thought to be the healthiest type of fat (figure 5.2). *Trans fats,* reported to be associated with some

Kind of Fat	% Saturated	%Poly	%Mono
Canola oil	6	32	62
Safflower oil	10	77	13
Sunflower oil	11	69	20
Corn oil	13	62	25
Olive oil	14	9	77
Soybean oil	15	61	24
Margarine (tub)	17	34	24
Peanut oil	18	33	49
Cottonseed oil	27	54	19
Chicken fat	31	22	47
Lard	41	12	47
Beef fat	52	4	44
Palm kernel oil	82	2	11
Coconut oil	92	2	6

Figure 5.2

Kinds of fat and their composition

Source: *Compositions of Foods,* U.S. Department of Agriculture

cancers and heart disease, are formed by bubbling hydrogen atoms through vegetable oils. Known as partially hydrogenated oils, these are found in deep-fried foods, solid margarine, and are most common in packaged cakes, cookies, and crackers.

The common types of oil and their proportion of saturated, polyunsaturated, and monounsaturated fat are listed in figure 5.2. Most foods contain combinations of more than one type of fat. No one type of fat is "all good" or "all bad." It is recommended that the majority of fat intake come from monounsaturated and polyunsaturated fats. Package labels are the most reliable guides to the amount of various types of fat in foods. However, labels do not indicate the amount of trans fats; these are present if the words "partially hydrogenated" appear in the ingredient list.

Cholesterol is perhaps the most commonly discussed fat these days. It differs from triglycerides in both appearance and function. Cholesterol is a very complex molecule that resembles a steroid in appearance. It is needed to maintain cell membranes, and is essential for the manufacture of vitamin D. Cholesterol is only found in animal products. Even high-fat vegetables, such as avocados, have no cholesterol.

The body does not require cholesterol in the diet because the liver can make what it needs. When cholesterol is included in the diet, the cholesterol goes to the liver for distribution or excretion. In most people, the liver responds to high-cholesterol diets by reducing its synthesis and increasing its excretion. Many people can eat very high cholesterol meals and not have elevated blood cholesterol levels. However, for some, this compensation is inadequate; unless the cholesterol they ingest is kept low, they will have too much in their bloodstream. The cholesterol cycle is extremely complex, so only a simplified explanation is presented here.

The liver gathers the cholesterol from the blood and packages it in large molecules, which includes proteins and triglycerides, called LDL (low-density lipoprotein). LDLs then circulate through the bloodstream to release needed cholesterol to body cells. When there is a high level of LDL molecules in the bloodstream, some cholesterol may deposit in the walls of the blood vessels, creating atherosclerosis. When excess cholesterol needs to be returned to the liver, it travels in another type of molecule called HDL (high-density lipoprotein). In this form, cholesterol can be recycled or excreted. HDL is thought of as the "good" cholesterol because it is returned to the liver for disposal. High levels of HDL in the bloodstream, common among women and athletes, are thought to protect against heart disease. In contrast, LDL cholesterol is the "bad" cholesterol that contributes to atherosclerosis and heart disease. There are even subcategories of HDL and LDL that influence risk; however, discussing them is beyond the scope of this text.

The easiest and safest way to reduce cholesterol is through a low–animal fat diet. However, increasing numbers of adults are being prescribed cholesterol-lowering drugs. Their success in reducing heart disease death among elders has not been fully studied. See chapter 10 for a discussion of cholesterol-lowering drugs.

Major sources of fat are animal and vegetable oils, meat, fried foods, cheese, butter, ice cream, and whole milk.

Fiber

What grandma called "roughage" is now called "fiber," and health experts are encouraging people

This graph shows how much of 15 nutrients in whole wheat flour is left after being milled into enriched white flour.

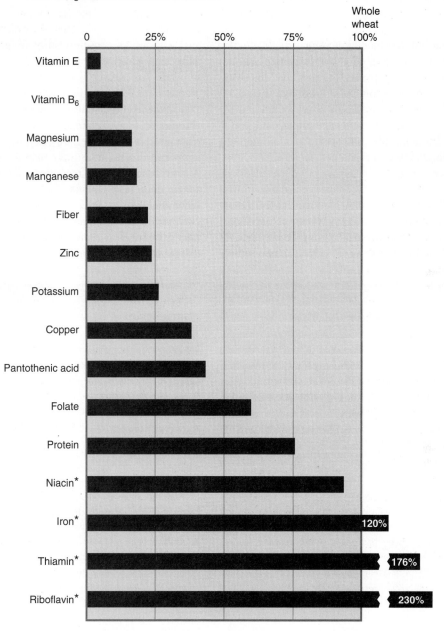

* = This nutrient has been added to enriched white flour.

■ = Enriched white flour.

Figure 5.3
Whole vs. Refined Flour
Source: USDA Nutrient Database for Standard Reference, Release 11 (www.nal.usda.gov/fnic/foodcomp).

to eat more of it. Fiber is the undigestible parts of plants. *Soluble fiber* (which gets sticky in contact with water) is found in oats, beans, barley, fruits, and vegetables. It is known to lower cholesterol levels and stabilize blood glucose levels. *Insoluble fiber* is known for its ability to absorb large quantities of water as it passes through the digestive tract. This creates a soft, bulky stool that is easy to pass. Foods rich in insoluble fiber include corn, wheat bran, fruit and vegetable skins, and leafy greens. Insoluble fiber is especially important in the prevention of constipation.

Fiber speeds the passage of digested food through the intestine and stimulates defecation. Fiber can add volume to foods, helping you to feel fuller after eating fewer calories, and prevents constipation. There are other benefits to increasing dietary fiber. A diet high in fiber is associated with decreased serum cholesterol and a decrease in blood pressure. Those who consume a diet high in fiber have lower risks of cancer (especially of the colon), diverticulosis, diabetes, and heart disease. High-fiber diets are associated with a high consumption of fruits, vegetables, and grains, which also enhance health.

The American Dietetic Association recommends 20 to 35 grams of fiber a day. In the United States, the average adult consumes about half that amount. Elders may tend to eat even less fiber since foods rich in fiber are often hard to chew. A high-fiber diet includes more than 35 grams a day. A high fluid intake is recommended as well. For some, fiber supplements, such as Metamucil, is recommended to relieve constipation or lower cholesterol. People should increase their dietary fiber slowly, as a rapid increase can cause gas, diarrhea, and abdominal cramping.

The New Artificial Food: Reduced-Calorie Flavor but not Without Risk

Concerns about cutting calories by reducing sugar and fat in the diet while maintaining flavor has spawned a new crop of artificial foodstuffs. Artificial flavoring and colors have been around for decades and are designed to make foods look and taste more appealing; however, these generally add no calories or nutrition to the food. Artificial sweeteners have fewer calories than sugar and are safer for diabetics, but provide a similar level of sweetness. Artificial sweeteners include saccharin (e.g., Sweet'N Low) and aspartame (e.g., NutraSweet). Although these sweeteners were originally developed for diabetics unable to tolerate conventional sugar, their appeal is widespread: almost all Americans consume some artificial sweeteners. Tea, yogurt, soft drinks, ice cream, and many other products are available sweetened with aspartame or saccharin. Although both boast fewer calories than sugar, studies find that consumption of these artificial sweeteners is not associated with weight loss. It is thought that people crave sugar calories and get them elsewhere instead. Saccharin has been found in animal studies to be associated with increased risk of cancer, however, it has not been taken off the market. Evidence is building that aspartame has a variety of side effects, from ringing in the ears to muscle spasms.

Sucrose polyester, also called olestra, is an artificial fat substitute that does not get digested by the body. It is now added to ice creams, potato chips, and other products to provide the sensation of fat without its caloric load. Many people find it tastes very much like "the real thing." However, olestra has its risks. Even moderate intake may be associated with symptoms of poor digestion such as bloating, gas, abdominal cramps, diarrhea, and rectal leakage. In addition, this artificial fat has been found to significantly reduce beta carotene absorption in the body. Although foods made with olestra are supplemented with these vitamins, elders should be careful because olestra may deplete body stores of important nutrients. Preliminary studies suggest that olestra may not be effective in weight loss. When olestra was substituted for regular fat in one trial, the men eating it reported more hunger and increased their dietary intake the following day, compensating for most of the previous day's energy deficit.[12]

Vitamins

Vitamins are a diverse group of chemicals needed in small amounts so the body can complete the chemical reactions that produce energy needed for growth, maintenance, and repair. Since vitamins are not made in the body in sufficient amounts, they must be included in the diet. Fat-soluble vitamins (A, E, D, and K) are stored in body fat and the liver. Excessive levels of these vitamins can be toxic. Water-soluble vitamins (carotenoids, vitamin C, and the B-complex vitamins) do not build up to toxic levels because they are regularly excreted in the urine. However, they need to be ingested more often and are more easily destroyed by cooking than the fat-soluble vitamins.

This section discusses each vitamin, its role in health, signs of deficiency, and common dietary sources. The role of specific vitamins in preventing and treating chronic diseases and disorders of elders will be discussed in a later section. See table 5.1 for the established dietary guidelines for vitamins and minerals.

Vitamin A

Vitamin A (retinol) can be ingested directly, or vitamin A can be made by ingesting carotenoids (the most prominent is beta carotene) that are converted to vitamin A by the liver. High doses of retinol are toxic, but carotenoids are safe, even in high quantities. Carotenoids are actually pigments and can cause the skin to turn orange if an individual eats a large amount of carrots or takes edible "tanning pills."

Vitamin A is essential for vision, skin, and mucous membrane function. It is also an antioxidant (see chapter 2). Vitamin A deficiency may be due to impaired absorption or storage as well as inadequate intake. Liver disease, reduced bile production, and antibiotics and laxatives can cause reduced absorption. A severe deficiency of this vitamin is first evident with reduced night vision and dry eyes, which can lead to blindness. Further vitamin A deficiency may cause rough and reddened skin, increasing infection susceptibility.

Studies have found a relationship between high amounts of vitamin A or beta carotene in the blood and increased immune cell function in healthy elders.[13] Those who have a high dietary intake of vitamin A or carotenoids have a lower risk of cancer, heart disease,[14] macular degeneration,[15] cataracts,[16] and other illnesses. Preliminary studies suggested that supplements of vitamin A or carotenoids reduce the risk of disease because of their antioxidant properties. However, studies using vitamin supplements have been less conclusive. A large randomized trial of elderly smokers found an increase in lung cancer among those taking beta carotene.[17] This study received a lot of attention and was criticized on many counts. Some suggested that smokers had too much preexisting lung damage to benefit from antioxidants, while others suggested that beta carotene obtained from supplements was not as effective at reducing cancer as beta carotene derived from foods.

Vitamin A derivatives (e.g., Retin-A and Accutane) are used to treat dermatological conditions including acne, facial wrinkling from sun damage, and precancerous lesions.

Animal products are a major dietary source of vitamin A. Major dietary sources of carotenoids are orange and yellow fruits and vegetables, especially apricots, cantaloupe, sweet potatoes, and carrots.

Vitamin B Complex

The vitamin B complex was originally thought to be one vitamin, but as more were discovered, subscripts one through twelve were added. There are eight B vitamins, each known both by a number and a chemical name. Each plays a role in cell reproduction or metabolism of proteins, fats, and carbohydrates.

Thiamine (B_1) enrichment of foods in our country has largely eliminated the dreaded disease beriberi, which leads to paralysis, heart failure, and death. However, between one-third and one-half of all Americans, particularly the poor and alcoholics, suffer from mild thiamine deficiency. Symptoms of a mild deficiency are appetite loss, nausea, depression, and mental confusion. Alcoholics are often deficient in thiamine, likely due to inadequate intake, insufficient absorption, and

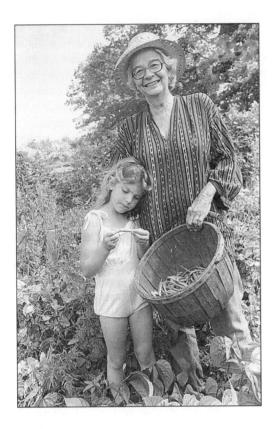

heightened need. Because of the prevalence of thiamine deficiency among alcoholics, some have suggested enriching alcoholic beverages with the vitamin.

Major dietary sources of thiamine are whole and enriched grains, legumes, organ meats, and green leafy vegetables.

Riboflavin (B₂) is essential for the action of other B vitamins. Deficiency is characterized by visual problems, cracking of the corners of the mouth, and scaly skin rashes. Strict vegetarians, alcoholics, and those who take estrogen supplements are at higher risk for riboflavin deficiency. Some believe riboflavin to be the most common marginal deficiency among elders and the poor.

Major dietary sources of riboflavin are liver, dairy products, and whole or enriched grain products.

Niacin (B₃) deficiency causes pellagra, characterized by the "four Ds": dermatitis, diarrhea,

dementia, and death. Pellagra used to be a widespread disease, but now that refined carbohydrates are enriched, this deficiency is uncommon except among alcoholics. Mild deficiencies may appear as depression and mental confusion. High doses of niacin are successfully used to treat high cholesterol levels and are much less expensive than the other cholesterol-lowering drugs. Excessive intakes of niacin are associated with liver damage. The body is able to make its own niacin if the amino acid, tryptophan, is ingested.

Major dietary sources of niacin are meat, poultry, and legumes.

Pantothenic acid (B₅) is found in a wide variety of foods and is manufactured by intestinal bacteria. Because of this, a deficiency state does not occur. However, marginal deficiencies may contribute to disease states.

Major dietary sources of pantothenic acid are vegetables, fruits, and meats.

Pyridoxine (B₆) is essential for antibody production and brain and nerve function. Deficiency of pyridoxine is rare. The need for pyridoxine increases for those who ingest high levels of alcohol or protein, use prescription medications such as levodopa, are heavy smokers, or use estrogen supplements.

Major dietary sources of pyridoxine are bananas, vegetables, meat, liver, whole grains, and egg yolks.

Biotin (B₇) is present in all foods; however, it is lost in food processing and refrigeration and is not added back during enrichment. Although not common, symptoms of deficiency are gastrointestinal distress, fatigue, and depression. Persistent diarrhea or long-term therapy with antibiotics or sulfa drugs can create a deficiency state.

Major dietary sources of biotin are organ meats, legumes, egg yolks, nuts, and whole grains.

Folate (B₉) is a plant-based vitamin that has received increased attention because of its role in prevention of neural tube defects when taken by pregnant women and its role in reducing risk of cardiovascular disease. Folic acid is a synthetic form of folate used in vitamin supplements and used to fortify foods, such as cereals and breads. Folic acid is about twice as potent as folate. Because of this confusion, the newest RDA refers to "dietary folate equivalents." Thus, to meet the RDA of 400 mcg of "dietary folate equivalents," one may eat 200 mcg of folic acid.

Homocysteine is the product of the breakdown on an important amino acid. It is now known that high homocysteine levels are associated with a high risk of cardiovascular disease and death in both men and women.[18] Some believe that homocysteine is even more important that high cholesterol in increasing heart disease risk. It is now known that folic acid, whether taken in food or as a supplement, acts to convert homocysteine back to another amino acid, thus reducing its level in the blood. Although there has not been a randomized controlled trial examining whether folic acid supplementation reduces death rates from heart disease or stroke, the possible connection is so strong that many are adopting a "just in case" attitude and urging folic acid supplementation.

Researchers estimate that if half the population in the nation began taking the RDA of 400 mcg of folate daily, there would be 28,000 fewer deaths from cardiovascular disease each year.[19] In 1998, the government required manufacturers to add folic acid to any foods containing enriched (white) flour. However, many believe the level of fortification is too low.

Low folate intake is relatively common in the population. Heavy alcohol consumption, estrogen therapy, chemotherapy, and some other drugs can deplete folate. Although folate is plentiful in foods, it is inactivated when cooked for even five minutes. Intestinal bacteria also synthesize this vitamin, but taking antibiotics can reduce the synthesis. Deficiency is most common among institutionalized elders and alcoholics. The first sign of folate deficiency is anemia.

Too much folate may have hazards as well. Excessive intake may mask deficiency of vitamin B_{12} (known as pernicious anemia). For this reason, it is recommended that elders do not take more than 1,000 mcg of folic acid daily and that they take supplements of B_{12}.

Major dietary sources of folate are cereals, lentils, beans, spinach, and pasta.

Cobalamin (B_{12}) is synthesized by bacteria found in the digestive tract. Other sources are meat, poultry, fish, and dairy products. Strict vegetarians may become deficient unless their intestinal bacteria produce sufficient quantities, however, rarely does anyone manifest vitamin B_{12} deficiency due to inadequate intake. Generally a deficiency results from inadequate absorption due to reduced stomach acid. This condition, called pernicious anemia, is most common in those over age fifty. Those at highest risk are individuals who had surgery on their intestines, who take drugs to neutralize stomach acid or dilantin for seizures, and who consume a lot of alcohol. These individuals develop confusion, dementia, loss of appetite, anemia, weakness, loss of sensation, and unsteadiness.

It is estimated that as many as 10 percent of the elderly have low vitamin B_{12} levels. Because of this, screening for vitamin B_{12} deficiency should be included any time an elder complains of a new neurologic symptom. The synthetic form of B_{12}, available in vitamin pills or fortified grains and cereals, is recommended for elders as their bodies may not fully absorb the natural form of the vitamin. Injections of the vitamin can rapidly correct the deficiency, and these may be followed by monthly B_{12} shots, nasal sprays inhaled weekly, or daily pills to keep levels in normal range.

Major dietary sources of vitamin B_{12} are meat, liver, kidneys, fish, yogurt, cottage cheese, and eggs.

Vitamin C

Vitamin C (ascorbic acid) is an important component of the structural proteins (e.g., collagen and elastin) that hold the body together. Additionally, it plays a role as an antioxidant and enhances the absorption of iron and calcium from the small intestine.

Severe vitamin C deficiency causes scurvy, characterized by a loss of appetite, irritability, and depression, followed by sore limbs and excessive bleeding from gums, bones, and joints. The disease was first noticed in sailors on long voyages without fresh fruits and vegetables. Although scurvy is now very rare, some experts believe that a mild deficiency can cause increased susceptibility to illness. Marginal deficiencies of vitamin C or the B vitamins may aggravate neurologic symptoms. Use of certain drugs affects the need for vitamin C. Those who take estrogen supplements or high doses of aspirin, smoke cigarettes, or drink alcohol heavily have an increased need for vitamin C.

The amount of vitamin C needed for optimal health is highly debated. Although only minimal levels of vitamin C are needed to prevent scurvy, some experts believe that higher levels of vitamin C in the diet prevent illness and enhance recovery. Studies show that vitamin C levels decrease during infection, surgery, or stress. Those with higher levels of intake of vitamin C (through food or supplements) and those with higher blood levels of vitamin C have a decreased heart disease risk, decreased serum cholesterol, reduced blood pressure, and increased longevity.[20] Vitamin C also may prevent cataract formation.[21] Elders with wounds, particularly decubitus ulcers, may benefit from vitamin C supplementation as it speeds healing.

There is no evidence to substantiate the claim that too much vitamin C can increase the incidence of kidney stones and gout in susceptible individuals. Any vitamin C not used is excreted in the urine. However, large doses may interfere with some diagnostic laboratory tests and cause diarrhea.

Major dietary sources of vitamin C are citrus fruits, cantaloupe, watermelon, strawberries, brussel sprouts, and broccoli.

Vitamin D

Vitamin D (calciferol) is not technically a vitamin, but a hormone because it is manufactured in one part of the body and affects another part. When skin is exposed to sunlight, vitamin D is activated in a complex chain of events that also involves the kidneys and liver. The end product, calciferol, increases the amount of calcium absorbed from the intestines: without it, calcium is poorly absorbed. Besides sunlight, some animal products contain vitamin D. In the United States, milk is

fortified with a form of vitamin D, called ergosterol. Because the body maintains a steady blood calcium level, when intake is low, calcium is extracted from the bones. Exposing the skin to sunlight for twenty minutes three times a week will meet the vitamin D requirement. However, sitting by a window is not sufficient since glass windows prohibit the sun's ultraviolet waves that act upon the skin to make vitamin D.

Vitamin D deficiency causes rickets in children and osteomalacia and osteoporosis in adults—diseases that severely weaken the bones and increase susceptibility to fractures. In addition, deficiency is implicated in the development of skin and colon cancers. Researchers estimate that as many as one-half of all elders have a marginal deficiency of vitamin D, and most commonly occurs among the bedridden, ill, and institutionalized. Even elders with adequate intake can exhibit a vitamin D deficiency.[22]

Individuals with kidney and liver disease are more likely to exhibit a vitamin D deficiency, as are people who take bulk laxatives, antacids containing aluminum, cholesterol-lowering drugs, mineral oil laxatives, and drugs for epilepsy. Elders may be at higher risk of vitamin D deficiency for several reasons: decreased efficiency at making this vitamin in the skin, insufficient sunlight exposure, reduced intake of milk, and decreased absorption. Vitamin D levels may vary seasonally with levels lower in the winter and higher in the summer. In the Northeast, many people get inadequate Vitamin D from the sun; they must rely on fortified milk or vitamin supplements

Vitamin D deficiency can be detected with a blood test, and can be remedied with oral supplements. Some experts recommend that all elders take a 400 IU daily supplement because the benefits of reducing fractures far outweigh the low risk of side effects. Those with osteoporosis who take calcium (1,200 mg/day in food and supplements) and vitamin D (600 IU) supplements have reduced rates of bone loss and lower incidence of fractures.[23] Exposing the hands, face, and arms to sunlight for fifteen to twenty minutes at a time two or three times a week can also raise levels. Sun exposure must be longer in the winter months when vitamin D production is less efficient.

Major dietary sources of vitamin D are oily fish, cod liver oil, eggs, liver, butter, and fortified milk.

Vitamin E

Vitamin E is an antioxidant that prevents and repairs free radical damage caused to cell membranes and other cell components as a result of normal cell metabolism. Studies show an association between high levels of vitamin E and reduced risks of many diseases. Daily vitamin E supplementation may reduce heart disease risk,[24] and tardive dyskinesia.[25] A randomized, placebo-controlled trial of vitamin E supplementation in healthy elders revealed a stimulatory effect on the immune system.[26] It also improved the action of insulin in healthy people and those with adult-onset diabetes.[27] Studies also show that patients with Alzheimer's disease who take vitamin E have slower declines in cognitive function.[28] In addition, vitamin E supplements may decrease cataract formation.[29] In high dosages, vitamin E also reduces blood clotting.

Even with sufficient intake of vitamin E, a deficiency may result in those who cannot absorb fat properly. Symptoms are serious and obvious and include anemia and nervous system abnormalities.

Major dietary sources of vitamin E are vegetable oils.

Vitamin K

Vitamin K is manufactured by bacteria in the large intestine. The main function of vitamin K is to promote blood clotting. Vitamin K deficiency is very rare in adults, but can occur in individuals on long-term antibiotic therapy because the antibiotics kill the colon bacteria. Additionally, those who have difficulty in absorbing fats or who take mineral oil are at higher risk of deficiency. Symptoms of deficiency include anemia, prolonged bleeding, and easy bruising.

Major dietary sources of vitamin K are leafy green vegetables.

Minerals

Minerals are inorganic substances needed in relatively small amounts for proper body function. Some are a necessary part of cell structure, body fluids, and tissues; others have very specific functions (e.g., iodine needed to make thyroxin; iron to produce hemoglobin) Some minerals, such as calcium, magnesium, phosphorus, sodium, potassium, and chlorine, are needed in amounts greater than 100 mg per day (macronutrients). Other minerals are needed in trace amounts such as iron, iodine, copper, manganese, zinc, chromium, fluorine, and selenium (micronutrients). In addition, trace elements, such as tin, vanadium, silicon, arsenic, nickel, and cadmium, may be important, but recommended doses have not been established. Furthermore, the quantity of each mineral needed is no measure of its relative importance in the body.

Mineral deficiencies are more common than vitamin deficiencies. Although vitamins are usually present in foods in similar amounts throughout the world, some areas are very poor in specific minerals and trace elements, predisposing residents of these areas to deficiencies. In elders, mineral deficiencies may be related to decreased absorption, marginal diets, medications, and disease states. This section will discuss the role of selected minerals in health and disease, signs of deficiency, and common food sources. See the section "Relation of Nutrition to Chronic Illness" later in this chapter for a discussion on the role of minerals in cardiac disease, cancer, and diabetes. Refer to table 5.1 for the RDA of several of the following minerals.

Calcium

Calcium is the mineral needed in the highest quantity by the body. It is crucial to bone formation, blood clotting, heartbeat regulation, muscle contraction, and neuron function. Dietary calcium is absorbed through the small intestine with the help of vitamin D. Blood calcium levels must always remain constant. Both high calcium intake and physical activity stimulate calcium to deposit in the

The Antioxidant Vitamins

A trio of antioxidants, vitamin C, vitamin E, and beta carotene, have received much media attention for their possible role in preventing heart disease, cancer, and other illnesses. These nutrients are believed to help the body protect itself from damage caused by free radicals formed from normal cell metabolism and from environmental damage, such as pollution and cigarette smoking. Cumulative damage from free radicals within cells is thought to be a major factor in the development of cancer, heart disease, and other conditions.

Many population-based studies have documented that those who eat a diet high in antioxidant vitamins, or those with high blood levels of these vitamins, have lower rates of cancer, hypertension, stroke, heart disease, and other conditions—even greater longevity. Studies also show that those who take vitamin supplements have a lower rate of many types of cancers. Because taking antioxidant vitamins may be effective, inexpensive, and risk-free, many believe that they may help and couldn't hurt. Sales of these vitamins have increased dramatically over the past few years.

It is still not clear whether the benefits of antioxidant vitamins shown in the studies are due to "confounding factors." For example, those who eat a healthy diet high in fruits and vegetables may engage in other healthy behaviors, which are the real reason they live longer. It is also unclear whether the same benefits could be realized from supplements as from whole foods. A few large-scale trials set out to answer this question.

Recent studies found that antioxidant supplements may not be as helpful as first believed, and, in some cases, may be harmful. One of the studies observed 29,000 middle-aged male smokers in Finland. One group was given beta carotene supplements, another group was given vitamin E supplements, and a third group was given a placebo (sugar pill). The researchers reported a significantly increased risk of lung cancer among the group taking beta carotene. Among those taking vitamin E, there was a lower rate of prostate cancer, but a higher rate of bleeding stroke.[30] Another large study of 18,000 healthy men and women also reported an increased risk of deaths from lung cancer and deaths overall among those taking supplements of beta carotene and vitamin A when compared to those who took none. The deaths occurred primarily among smokers, former smokers, and those with previous exposure to asbestos.[31]

Although other trials have shown positive effects of antioxidant supplements in preventing cancer and heart disease, the mixed findings reported in these trials are making researchers more cautious in recommending antioxidant supplements for everyone.

It may be that the specific vitamin may not reduce the risk of cancer and heart disease; rather, it may be the habit of eating a variety of fruits, vegetables, and whole grains that also happen to be high in antioxidants. While fruits and vegetables are rich in vitamins C, E, and beta carotene, they also contain literally hundreds of other compounds, many of which have not been fully characterized, that may be the "real" health-protective molecules. Beta carotene, for example, may be merely an "indicator" for a host of other chemical substances found in fruits and vegetables. Further research is attempting to isolate other helpful compounds that may influence the positive health effects. For instance, compounds called flavenoids, found in many fruits and vegetables, are associated with reduced cancer risk. The handful of antioxidants that have been isolated and packaged into pills are likely a very small component of the benefits from eating whole foods.

Even with the discovery of more important chemicals, it is unlikely that the short-cut approach of taking vitamins rather than eating a varied plant-based diet will be effective. It is more likely that combinations of these and other antioxidants are the most effective. At this point, many experts do not recommend daily uses of antioxidant supplements but rather encourage elders and others to eat a diet high in fruits and vegetables. However, some experts, including the Alliance for Aging Research, do suggest 4 to 16 times higher RDAs for antioxidant vitamins. They recommend, for example, that adults should consume 250 to 1,000 mg per day of vitamin C, 100 to 400 IU of vitamin E, and 10 to 130 mg per day of beta carotene.[32]

bones. Conversely, low intake gradually depletes calcium from the bones to maintain a constant blood level of calcium.

The RDA for calcium intake for adults over fifty is 1,200 mg, and 1,000 mg for those nineteen to fifty. According to the Osteoporosis Foundation, the average adult daily intake of calcium is between 500 to 700 mg. Low calcium levels in older people can be due to low calcium intake, reduced absorption in the intestine, or low level of physical activity. Furthermore, a high-protein diet, some soft drinks, and some drugs reduce blood calcium levels.

Low consumption of calcium has been associated with reduced bone density in normal men and women and increased susceptibility to fracture. Calcium supplements have been shown to increase bone mass and to reduce the risk of hip fractures among the elderly. Calcium deficiency has been linked to hypertension. Marginal calcium deficiency may be aggravated by low-cholesterol diets prescribed to manage hypertension, which discourage intake of calcium-rich dairy products.

Figure 5.4 lists those foods rich in calcium. Note that dairy products are by far the most effective dietary source of calcium. Further, milk is fortified with vitamin D to facilitate calcium absorption. Even though some green vegetables have calcium, many contain substances that reduce calcium absorption (e.g., the oxalic acid in spinach). A high-fiber diet is known to reduce calcium absorption, so vegetarians may need to increase overall calcium intake. Since it can be difficult to get enough calcium each day, supplements are suggested, particularly calcium carbonate (e.g., Tums), as they offer a high proportion of usable calcium. Also, cereals and orange juice are increasingly being fortified with calcium. It is recommended that no more than 2,500 mg be ingested in a day. There is little danger of taking too much calcium because the excess is excreted. It was once believed that kidney stones were caused by an excessive intake of calcium, but it is now known that kidney stones are related to low calcium intake.[33] For some people, supplements cause constipation.

Calcium is found in dairy products (yogurt, milk, and cheese), tofu (check label), sardines, and collard greens.

Sources of Calcium		
Food Item	Serving Size	Calcium Content/mg
Yogurt,		
plain, nonfat	8 oz.	452
plain, lowfat	8 oz.	415
Sardines (with bones)	3 oz.	326
Calcium fortified		
orange juice	8 oz.	300
Milk	8 oz.	300
Tofu, firm*	1/2 cup	278
Swiss cheese	1 oz.	270
Turnip greens	1 cup	249
Cheddar cheese	1 oz.	207
Salmon (w/bones)	3 oz.	180
Yogurt, frozen	4 oz.	155
Broccoli, cooked,		
fresh	1 cup	178
Ice cream, soft serve	1/2 cup	118
Almonds	1 oz.	75
Orange, medium	1	52
*with calcium sulfate		

Figure 5.4
Sources of Calcium

Chlorine and Sulfur

Chlorine works with sodium to maintain acid-base and fluid balance of the body and is part of the hydrochloric acid secreted by the stomach. Almost all chlorine is consumed in the form of sodium chloride (salt). Because salt is ubiquitous in our food, no dietary deficiency is known. However, chlorine may also be present in small quantities in drinking water to reduce the growth of bacteria. Research suggests that the chlorine in drinking water may be carcinogenic, leading to an increase in cancer risk, particularly cancer of the bladder. Although the health benefits of germ-free water outweigh the possible cancer risk, new methods to purify water are being developed.

Major sources of chlorine are salt and animal products. The major source of sulfur is animal products.

Chromium

Chromium is essential for body cells to extract glucose from the bloodstream when insulin is present. Long-standing chromium deficiencies may promote adult-onset diabetes. Chromium supplements have been reported to increase the cells' ability to retrieve glucose from the blood. Food processing drastically decreases the amount of chromium available in foods, and this mineral is not replaced by the enrichment process.

Chromium-rich foods include brewer's yeast, blackstrap molasses, pasta, potatoes, wheat germ, whole grains, and mushrooms.

Copper

Copper helps transport oxygen from the lungs to the body tissues. This mineral is also important in producing the structural fibers, collagen and elastin. Symptoms of copper deficiency include anemia, reduced immunity, loss of color in the skin and hair, and damage to the brain and spinal cord.

Major dietary sources of copper include shellfish, nuts, cocoa, dried beans, mushrooms, and whole grains.

Iodine

The main function of iodine is to make the thyroid hormone, thyroxine, which regulates metabolic rate. Iodine deficiencies result in hypothyroidism due to inadequate production of thyroid hormone and an enlarged thyroid (goiter). Radioactive iodine is used therapeutically to treat thyroid disease. Iodine deficiency is rare in the United States because iodine is routinely added to salt.

Major dietary sources of iodine, besides fortified salt, are saltwater fish, clams, oysters, and seaweed.

Iron

Iron is the key component of hemoglobin, which transports oxygen from the lungs to peripheral tissues, and of myoglobin, which transports oxygen to working muscle. Additionally, iron is needed to make several enzymes that convert nutrients into energy, helps produce elastin and collagen, maintains the immune system, and assists in nerve transmission.

Iron is continuously recycled by the body and is only depleted through blood loss. Iron-deficiency anemia is common among elders and may result from impaired iron absorption, or blood loss due to disease, injury, or ingestion of drugs such as aspirin. Insufficient iron causes a shortage of red blood cells, reducing the amount of oxygen available to the tissues.

Symptoms of iron-deficiency anemia are weakness, headache, and heart palpitations. Those who have a vitamin C deficiency may also be more susceptible to iron deficiencies because vitamin C enhances absorption of dietary iron. In a disease called hemochromatosis, individuals are not able to excrete iron normally, and iron builds up in the liver causing cirrhosis: these individuals should eat low-iron diets and require periodic blood draws to reduce their iron level. There is also some suggestion that high iron stores may be associated with an increased risk of cardiovascular disease.[34] Those taking supplements often have constipation. Iron levels in the blood are easily tested, and an iron supplement should not be used unless it is indicated by a simple blood test.

Major dietary sources of iron are liver, dried beans, raisins, prunes, shellfish, and some meats.

Magnesium

Magnesium is required for every major biological process, including glucose metabolism, energy production, DNA and RNA synthesis, nerve cell function, and muscle relaxation. Magnesium also lowers blood lipid concentrations, stabilizes the heart beat, and decreases blood clotting.

Marginal magnesium deficiency is extremely common in the U.S. population; the majority of Americans fall short of the RDA of magnesium, most consuming less than two-thirds of the RDA. Magnesium deficiency is particularly common among elders. Magnesium deficiency may be caused by a low-calorie diet, diabetes, alcohol use, heavy exercise, excessive diarrhea and vomiting, and use of diuretics or digitalis. Symptoms of magnesium deficiency are nausea, diarrhea, tremors, and loss of appetite or coordination. Magnesium deficiency occurs after long-term dietary deficiency when the body uses up its stored magnesium. Occasionally blood tests will be normal, even though the body is dangerously low in magnesium stored inside the bones and cells. Detecting these types of deficiencies requires more sophisticated tests of blood and urine.

Dietary magnesium can have an important effect on glucose metabolism and risk of diabetes. Two large studies showed that those who consume low levels of magnesium in their diet are more likely to develop adult-onset diabetes.[35] In addition, those who already have diabetes have lower-than-expected levels of magnesium. As of yet, it is unclear whether magnesium supplements improve insulin sensitivity. Some studies report that a low magnesium level is associated with high blood pressure. However, magnesium supplements have not been shown to lower high blood pressure. Magnesium deficiency contributes to calcium deficiency as well and may play an important role in the development and treatment of osteoporosis.[36]

Dietary sources of magnesium include whole-grain cereals, black, navy, lima and pinto beans, lentils, almonds, and spinach.

Phosphorus

Phosphorus is crucial for every cell reaction that releases or uses energy. This mineral is also an important part of DNA and RNA, cell membranes, and bones, and helps balance blood acidity. Vitamin D regulates the levels of phosphorus in the blood by controlling the rate at which it is absorbed and excreted. A phosphorus deficiency is rare because it is abundant in all proteins and is used as an additive in processed foods such as soft drinks. However, excessive phosphorus intake (soft drinks and meat contain high quantities) may predispose an individual to osteoporosis by increasing the rate of bone demineralization and increasing calcium excretion.

Dietary sources of phosphorus are red meats and many soft drinks.

Potassium

Potassium is involved in nerve conduction, muscle contraction, regulation of heart beat, and body fluid balance. Diarrhea, the use of diuretics, excessive sweating, or fasting can cause potassium deficiencies. Symptoms of deficiency are rapid heartbeat, muscle weakness, nausea, and vomiting.

High potassium intake has been associated with a decreased risk of hypertension. Thus, those who eat diets rich in fruits and vegetables containing potassium have lower blood pressure. Some hypertension medications deplete potassium, and supplementation is needed to maintain blood potassium in the normal range. Most individuals taking these medications are prescribed daily doses of potassium to prevent deficiency. A low potassium intake is also correlated with increased stroke mortality.

Potassium supplementation can also have side effects: potassium can be dangerous for those with kidney disease or those on potassium-sparing diuretics, and potassium overdose at five times the RDA can be fatal. The best way to increase potassium intake is through increased dietary consumption of foods high in potassium.

Major dietary sources of potassium are potatoes, raisins, bananas, avocados, cantaloupe, orange juice, sardines, and skim milk.

Selenium

A trace mineral that was once believed to be poisonous, selenium is now known to be a strong antioxidant. It works with vitamin E to protect the immune system by preventing the formation of free radicals. Selenium and vitamin E act synergistically to help produce antibodies. It is necessary for the pancreas to function and tissue elasticity.

Dietary sources of selenium vary, depending on where the foodstuff is grown. Meat and grains are a good source, as is brewer's yeast.

Sodium

Sodium is necessary for nerve transmission and muscle contraction, and helps maintain the acid-base balance of the blood. It also works with potassium and chloride to affect how much water is retained and eliminated in the body. Sodium deficiencies are rare as the body needs only about 200 mg per day (the amount in one-tenth of a teaspoon of salt). In our country, sodium excesses are common because most processed foods are high in sodium. In fact, the average woman consumes about 3,000 mg of salt a day, and the average man ingests 4,000 mg. It is recommended that salt consumption remain below 1,800 mg per day. Excess sodium in the body is eliminated in the urine.

The greatest danger of a high-sodium intake is high blood pressure. About half of those with hypertension cannot effectively eliminate sodium, and are called "salt-sensitive." For them, consumption of excess salt will raise their pressure further. The excess sodium in the blood pulls water into the bloodstream from the tissues—water that would ordinarily have been excreted. This excess volume in the blood causes blood pressure to rise. If the arteries are not flexible enough to accommodate the increase, a stroke, congestive heart failure, build-up of fluid in the lungs, or kidney disease can occur. There is no easy way to determine who is salt sensitive except by long-term monitoring. Salt-sensitive people need a more restricted salt diet. Elders are more often salt-sensitive than younger individuals because sensitivity to sodium increases with age.

Cutting back on sodium reduces high blood pressure. One study reported that among the elderly, a low-salt diet can decrease blood pressure, and when combined with weight loss, may reduce it sufficiently to stop blood pressure medication.[37]

Those with congestive heart failure are also sensitive to salt intake because sodium causes fluid retention, which leads to more stress on the heart. These individuals are often prescribed a low-sodium diet and may need to use more diuretics if they eat too much sodium. In addition, a high-sodium diet has been associated with excessive calcium loss in the urine, which can aggravate osteoporosis among postmenopausal women.[38]

Food high in sodium include sausages, cured hams, hot dogs, fast foods, canned soups, salad dressing, ketchup, mustard, pickles, cheese, chips, and pretzels.

Zinc

Zinc is an essential chemical in more than 300 metabolic enzymes. It plays an integral role in the synthesis of DNA and in proteins involved in immunity. It is also essential for night vision. Zinc deficiency is characterized by decreased sense of smell, delayed wound healing, and increased susceptibility to infection. Although severe zinc deficiency is rare, marginal zinc deficiencies may be common among elders, especially the poor and hospitalized. Progressive zinc deficiency may play a role in the gradual, age-related decrease in immunity. Multiple studies find zinc supplementation increases immune response in elders, even in doses of 15 to 30 mg per day.[39]

Zinc may also play a role in preventing upper respiratory infections. Zinc lozenges, taken at the first sign of a cold, have been shown in some studies to reduce the duration of cold symptoms.

Major dietary sources include oysters, other seafood, and red meat. Nuts and legumes contain high levels of zinc, but also high levels of compounds that reduce its absorption in the body.

VITAMIN AND MINERAL SUPPLEMENTS

It is now generally agreed that supplementing the diet with vitamins and minerals can promote health, especially among groups of people who are at higher risk for specific health problems. The general population is not waiting to hear from their doctors on what supplements to take or not take. As evidence is accumulating regarding the protective value of many vitamins and minerals, the public is responding by buying and using a variety of supplements. Currently, more than one-third of the nation's population is taking a vitamin or mineral supplement, to the tune of almost $6 billion a year.

A growing body of evidence suggests that some people might benefit from supplementing their diet with vitamins and minerals from a bottle. Supplements of folic acid, vitamin B_{12}, calcium, vitamin D, vitamin E, magnesium, and zinc may be helpful for some elders.

Many elders already take a multivitamin supplement that provides the RDA of most essential

What Is Your Opinion? To Supplement or Not?

"Yes," states Jeffrey Blumberg, Chief of the Anti-oxidant Research Laboratory at Tufts University, Boston. "I take four hundred international units of vitamin E every day. For me as a scientist, it means getting comfortable with uncertainty. I can't provide promises or guarantees or say the data are perfectly clear. I don't know what the exact dose should be, how long you have to take it before it takes effect, or what all the interactions are between vitamins. That's why we need more studies."

"But in this country we have hundreds of thousands of people dying from heart disease and cancer. I think the evidence suggesting vitamin E can reduce the suffering and costs of these diseases is very strong, and there appears to be no downside. Vitamin E doesn't even cost much. Are there other healthy behaviors you can engage in to lower your risk? Yes. Does taking vitamin E substitute for them? Of course not."

"A perfectly reasonable person could look at the data today and decide to take a supplement. Another equally reasonable person could choose to wait."

"No," feels Julie Buring, Epidemiologist at Harvard University and principal investigator for the Women's Health Study.

"I currently don't take vitamin E supplements because the health claims haven't been substantiated. When you ask scientists who take vitamin E if it will reduce the risk of heart disease and cancer, they reply, 'I don't know, but why not take it?' It's a strange argument. They don't take it because it works but because they can't think of any reason not to."

"Even the wildest proponents of vitamin E, when pressed, admit that what they really believe is that a diet rich in antioxidants is good for you, that it may not necessarily be vitamin E behind the benefits but a combination of antioxidants. In fact, it may not be antioxidants at all but other nutrients."

"Look, if someone says to me, 'I'm taking vitamin E. Do you think it will help?' My answer is, 'I don't think it will hurt. But can I just run through your list of risk factors? Because, for God's sake, don't tell me you're still smoking, or that you're not watching your fat or exercising, or you're not eating lots of fruits and vegetables.' Because all those things are much stronger at raising risk than vitamin E is at lowering it."

vitamins and minerals. There are many brands of multivitamins on the shelves, some of which are specifically geared for older people.

Several studies have attempted to assess the value of a multivitamin supplement upon an elderly population. The most important effect of multivitamin supplementation for elders according to one study is enhanced immune functioning.[40] In another study, each elder patient was tested for nutritional deficiencies then prescribed an individualized regimen of nutritional supplements. After 6 months, each elder improved on several measures of immune functioning.[41] In a landmark study, elders taking a multivitamin and mineral supplement plus vitamin E and beta carotene had half the number of colds, flu, and infection-related illnesses than the control

group without the supplements. And when they got sick, they got better in half the time. Further, the study reported that those who were taking the supplements had a better antibody response than the group not taking the supplement. This was accomplished with rather low levels of supplements.[42]

There are some problems with using megadoses of vitamins and minerals. Individuals who are taking one vitamin or mineral for a perceived imbalance may take too much of one mineral, which may interfere with the absorption of another; they may rationalize the consumption of a poor diet because they "took vitamins." One study found deficiencies of vitamins E and A, calcium, and zinc in a sample of elders, and many of these elders were taking dietary supplements. These elders had adequate or excessive intakes of some vitamins, but remained deficient in others.[43] Physicians are seldom consulted about vitamin and mineral supplements and seldom prescribe them, even when they may be beneficial. Furthermore, because of a lack of nutrition education in medical schools, physicians are not the best source of information. Finally, vitamin supplements should not replace a balanced diet; there are likely many more essential nutrients in food besides those recognized by the Food and Nutrition Board.

RELATION OF NUTRITION TO CHRONIC ILLNESS

Inadequate nutrition is known to contribute to a number of degenerative diseases and disorders common to older people. There are diseases that are made worse when particular types of foods are eaten (e.g., diabetes and gout). In these cases, dietary modification reduces the symptoms. Other diseases respond to particular vitamin or mineral supplements. Multiple explanations have been proposed for this phenomenon. A nutrient deficiency may have predisposed the patient to illness in the first place. Or, the disease process may have created an increased need for some nutrients. Furthermore, some diseases associated with old age may actually be caused by nutrient deficiencies.

Good eating habits have the potential to prevent and reduce the progression of many of these diseases. The exact role that proper nutrition or dietary supplementation can play in the prevention and treatment of chronic conditions is the subject of many research studies and is still poorly understood. The pivotal role of calcium and vitamin D in osteoporosis has already been discussed. This section will discuss relevant research on three other chronic illnesses that are significantly influenced by nutrition—cancer, diabetes, and heart disease.

Cancer

It is generally agreed that about one out of three cancer deaths is due to diet. Several nutrients are hypothesized to play a role in the prevention of cancer. Multiple population-based epidemiological studies have suggested that diets rich in fruits and vegetables, high in fiber and low in fat, are associated with reduced risk of many cancers, including colon, breast, and prostate. These studies suggest that both whole foods and particular nutrients may play a role in the development of cancer. Whereas some nutrients (e.g., beta carotene, vitamin C, or calcium) are thought to protect against the development of cancer, others (e.g., food additives and fat) may actually promote cancer.

Cancer comprises a heterogeneous group of diseases, each with varied risk factors and patterns of occurrence. However, most cancers share some etiologic aspects. Namely, most cancer is likely caused by an interaction between genetics and environment, causing damage to cellular DNA and allowing unchecked cellular growth. It is thought that dietary components may work by repairing cellular damage caused by free radicals, may modify hormones in the blood, or may impact immune system function.

Deficiencies of several vitamins have been associated with cancer. Low levels of antioxidant vitamins (vitamin E, vitamin C, beta carotene) in the diet or the bloodstream are associated with increased risks for many cancers, including gastrointestinal cancers, lung cancer, breast cancer, and prostate cancer. However, not all studies find consistent results. In the Nurses' Health Study, more than 88,000 women have been followed for twenty years. The researchers found that those who have been taking a multivitamin containing folate for fifteen years had one-quarter the risk of colon cancer of those who didn't take multivitamins.[44]

Minerals have also been associated with altered cancer risk. Calcium and vitamin D have been inversely associated with colon cancer development in many studies. Those with colon cancer have a lower intake of calcium and lower serum levels of vitamin D and calcium than the controls. Additionally, calcium supplements given to those at high risk for developing colon cancer slowed the progression of abnormal cell growth.[45]

Low blood levels of selenium, a trace mineral, may increase cancer risk, especially lung and skin cancers. Selenium supplementation has potential to reduce some cancers. A randomized placebo-controlled trial of selenium supplementation (200 μg per day) in those aged eighteen to eighty years found the risk of death from lung, colon, and prostate cancer was cut in half among those taking selenium compared to those taking a placebo.[46] The magnitude of reduction of lung cancer attributed to selenium supplementation was greater than that attributed to cigarette smoking! These unique and exciting findings need to be verified with more studies before selenium can be recommended for cancer prevention.

High dietary consumption of fruits and vegetables has been linked to reduced risks of many cancers; however, recent research has found that some specific types of foods may play a role in preventing tumors. Cruciferous vegetables (broccoli, cabbage, and brussel sprouts) may protect against tumor formation by releasing a chemical that helps to detoxify carcinogens. These vegetables are more effective if eaten raw. Compounds found in garlic, chili peppers, and onions may protect against cancers. Consumption of cooked tomatoes, in pasta or pizza sauces, has been linked to lower rates of prostate cancer. Consumption of green and black teas that contain antioxidants are also associated with reduced cancer risk. Tofu has been linked to lower risk of breast cancer, as has a diet high in berries. In addition, a meta-analysis of thirteen studies showed strong evidence that high fiber intake is associated with a decreased risk of colorectal cancer[47] and breast cancer.[48]

A high-fat diet is related to the development of breast, prostate, and colon cancers in animal and epidemiological studies; however, the association is not strong and not consistent because it is unclear if a high-fat diet predisposes one to develop cancer or accelerates the growth of an existing cancer. It is also not clear which types of fats are the most harmful, although animal fats, trans fats, and polyunsaturated fats have been implicated. Some suggest that monounsaturated fats may protect against cancer.[49] Studies are currently underway to assess whether reducing fat in the diet reduces risk of cancer or its recurrence.

Some additives and preservatives are converted to carcinogens during digestion. Sodium nitrate, used to preserve meats, is converted into nitrosamine, a cancer-causing agent. Vitamin C can neutralize nitrosamines in the body and is sometimes added to foods containing nitrates to prevent toxin formation. Saccharin, an artificial sweetener, is known to cause cancer in laboratory animals. Salted and pickled foods are related to the development of stomach cancer.. Some preservatives (e.g., BHT) act as antioxidants and may be protective against cancers.

Cancer increases the need for certain nutrients, but the disease and its treatment often diminish the ability or desire to eat. Lack of appetite occurs in many cancer patients at the time of diagnosis and during advanced illness. *Cachexia,* characterized by anorexia (loss of appetite), weight loss, and weakness, is common in advanced cancer victims and is caused by diversion of nutrients to support cancer tissue. Dietary proteins are needed for tissue growth, and if insufficient protein is ingested, the tumor cannibalizes muscle and other tissue to maintain its rapid growth. Cancer patients need adequate nutrients to increase their tolerance to therapy and to prevent starvation. Often cancer patients are prescribed high-nutrient liquid beverages (e.g., Boost, Ensure), in addition to meals, to maintain caloric intake. Sometimes tube feeding or IV feeding (TPN) is prescribed to improve nutrition, particularly early in the disease. However, it has not been established whether nutritional support offered in late-stage cancer prolongs survival. It may even accelerate tumor growth rate.

Cancer therapies can alter nutritional status by reducing food intake or absorption. Radiation therapy can irritate the small intestine, causing diarrhea and chronic nutrient malabsorption. Those undergoing chemotherapy may experience nausea, vomiting, a full feeling, and changes in smell and taste perception. Both radiation and chemotherapy are associated with oral pain, which may reduce nutrient intake.

Diabetes

A poor diet and obesity contribute to the development of adult-onset diabetes. Most adult-onset diabetics in the United States are obese: those who are overweight have an increased risk of developing the disease, especially those who have a large waist. For instance, a woman who has a 32-inch waist has four times the risk of a woman with a 28-inch waist. A woman with a 38-inch or larger waist has a diabetes risk six times higher.[50]

For the vast majority of diabetics who are overweight, weight loss is the only treatment necessary. Weight loss has also been shown to correct abnormal glucose tolerance, a common prediabetic condition. A diet high in complex carbohydrates and fiber improves all aspects of diabetic control in both types of diabetes. In addition, preliminary studies indicate that zinc and chromium supplements, minerals associated with insulin action, may also play a role in diabetes management.

Heart Disease

A wealth of epidemiologic, clinical, and laboratory studies link saturated fat and cholesterol to the incidence of atherosclerosis and coronary artery disease. There has been much research and discussion in the past few years on the role of dietary fat, particularly saturated fat, in promoting heart disease. Although most experts agree that saturated fats should be reduced in the diet, there is a controversy about whether polyunsaturated fats or monounsaturated fats are safer substitutes. Current recommendations are to reduce all dietary fat to below 30 percent, with less than 10 percent of all fat to be derived from saturated fats. A decrease in dietary fat reduces morbidity and mortality from atherosclerosis and heart disease, as well as some cancers. In the last two decades, there has been a slow decline in heart disease in the United States, which experts attribute to the public's reduction of fat in the diet.

An interesting study on over 80,000 middle-aged women reported that total fat intake was not related to the risk of coronary disease, but instead to the type of fat. The women who reported high intake of monosaturated and polyunsaturated fat had a lower incidence of heart disease than those who reported high intake of saturated and trans unsaturated fats. The study suggested that it is more important to replace the type of fat than reducing overall fat intake.[9]

A person's total cholesterol (LDL, HDL and triglycerides), easily measured by a blood test, is evidence of the degree of cardiovascular risk. Total cholesterol that is too high, HDL cholesterol that is too low, or an unhealthy ratio of total cholesterol to HDL is associated with an increased risk of atherosclerosis and heart disease. Reducing levels of blood cholesterol or increasing levels of HDL cholesterol seems to decrease risk. The best way to reduce cholesterol is to increase exercise, lose weight, and reduce dietary consumption of all fats, but in particular saturated fats and trans fats. Medications can also help some people lower their cholesterol levels. Because of the media's coverage of cholesterol, many people have changed their eating habits in order to reduce cholesterol and subsequent risk of heart disease. In general, the lower the level of cholesterol, the lower the risk of heart disease. However, the relative proportion of different kinds of cholesterol, particularly HDL and LDL, is also important. Thus, having a low total cholesterol level with a low HDL is predictive of higher heart disease risk than having a higher cholesterol with more HDL. There are some risks of low cholesterol as well, however, as very low levels may be associated with serious illness, such as cancer.

Low blood levels or low dietary intakes of several vitamins, minerals, and fiber intake have also been associated with heart disease. One large-scale study found that those with low levels of beta carotene, vitamin E, and vitamin C in their blood had increased incidence of angina.[51] Beta carotene supplements may also reduce incidence of strokes and heart attacks in susceptible individuals. Folate in diet or supplements is associated with reduced risk of heart disease[52] as is vitamin E.[24] Additionally, megadoses of niacin are used to decrease cholesterol and triglycerides and reduce the recurrence rate of heart attacks. Low blood levels of several minerals seem to increase heart disease risk: calcium, copper, potassium, magnesium, and selenium. There is also evidence from two large cohort studies of middle-aged and elder males that a high-fiber diet is associated with a reduced risk of heart attack.[53,54]

Minerals, especially sodium, potassium, and magnesium, are related to blood pressure, a major risk factor for heart disease. In addition, weight loss and a low-fat diet may also reduce blood pressure. A recent clinical trial suggests that the initiation of a diet high in fruits and low in fat lowered blood pressure in normal people, and for those with hypertension, the reductions were similar to drug therapy.[55]

EFFECT OF DRUG USE ON NUTRITIONAL STATUS

Many prescription and over-the-counter drugs affect nutritional status. Some irritate the stomach, cause nausea, vomiting, diarrhea, or alter the absorption or excretion of nutrients. Others alter electrolyte balance, carbohydrate or fat metabolism, or levels of healthful bacteria in the digestive tract. Drugs that alter taste perception can either drive people to overeat in search of satisfaction or to lose their appetite. Appetite may be increased directly by some drugs or indirectly by improving mental status. Current diet, other drugs taken concurrently, and presence of chronic illness must be taken into account when analyzing the effect of drug intake on nutritional status. Table 5.2 illustrates a few of the more common interactions.

The drug that causes the most nutritional problems is alcohol. Those who drink heavily have reduced appetites, may not select nutritious foods, and may consume a large proportion of their calories as alcohol. When those who drink heavily do not eat, weight loss and nutritional deficiencies develop. In addition, alcohol affects food absorption and utilization by damaging the stomach, liver, and pancreas. Excessive alcohol consumption can lead to deficiencies in proteins, water-soluble vitamins, magnesium, potassium, and zinc. Zinc absorption is decreased, and excretion is increased. Magnesium is excreted in abnormal amounts in alcoholics and excessive iron is absorbed, causing liver damage. Heavy drinkers often have inadequate vitamin D production, resulting in calcium deficiency and osteoporosis.

Some vitamins and minerals are needed in higher amounts in alcoholics to repair the damage caused by alcohol. Thiamine, and to a lesser degree other B complex vitamins, are particularly subject to depletion since they are needed to metabolize alcohol.

Cigarette smoking also increases the need for particular nutrients. The Food and Nutrition Board recommends that smokers get more vitamin C (100 mg compared to 60 mg). In addition, deficiency of B complex vitamins, especially B_{12} and folate, may act synergistically with cigarette smoking in the development of lung cancer. Although cigarette smoking is traditionally associated with weight loss, it may actually result in weight redistribution with more fat concentrated in the midsection, a weight pattern associated with increased mortality.

NUTRITIONAL STATUS OF ELDERS

Major changes have occurred in the average American diet over the lifetime of the current elder population. Historically, individuals probably ate a similar diet throughout their lifespan. However, the current cohort of elders was likely the first to see radical changes in diet and food choice throughout their lifetime. Growing up in a time when everything was made from scratch, they are aging with microwaves, fast-food restaurants, prepackaged dinners, and a dizzying array of produce, ethnic food, and choices that were unheard of in the past.

Today, there is increased reliance on prepackaged foods, frozen foods, and eating out. Within the last few decades, as a nation, we are eating more fat, salt, and sugar and fewer whole grains. There has been a small reduction of fat consumption in the past few years, particularly animal fat, spurred by research linking dietary fat and heart disease. Although consumption of fresh vegetables has been increasing over the last quarter century, Americans still eat far too little produce and an inadequate amount of whole grains. Consumption of sugar is rising annually, and the consumption of sodas has been skyrocketing,

TABLE 5.2	Nutrient-Drug Interactions

Alcohol: Can lead to deficiencies in all nutrients, especially the B vitamins, zinc, and iron. Can replace nutritious eating.

Antacids: Magnesium salts can cause diarrhea, which can impair intestinal absorption. Reduces acidity of stomach, perhaps altering protein digestion.

Antibiotics: Tetracycline can block absorption of iron, magnesium, and calcium salts. Other antibiotics can impair folic acid action in the body.

Anticoagulants: Can cause vitamin K deficiency. When taken with vitamin E supplements, may cause excessive blood thinning.

Anticonvulsants: Can induce folate and vitamin D deficiencies.

Antidepressants: Can accelerate breakdown of vitamin D.

Antidiabetics agents: Some inhibit absorption of B_{12}.

Aspirin: High doses may cause gastrointestinal bleeding, which can result in anemia. Can increase requirements for vitamin C, K, and folic acid. Can cause nausea and vomiting. When taken with vitamin E supplements, may cause excessive blood thinning.

Barbiturates: Can speed breakdown of vitamin D. Excessive sedation may cause missed meals. Can impair absorption of folic acid.

Cancer chemotherapy: Causes nausea and vomiting. Impairs appetite and absorption.

Colchicine: Can inhibit secretion of enzymes needed to break down complex sugars.

Corticosteroids: Can decrease pancreatic enzymes and cause stomach irritation. Can impair absorption of vitamins C, A, and D, folic acid, and potassium.

Digoxin: Can cause nausea and vomiting.

Diuretics: Can cause loss of potassium in the urine. Low levels of potassium in the blood can cause mental confusion and high blood pressure. Long-term use may cause calcium and magnesium deficiency.

Estrogen: Extended therapy can result in deficiencies of folic acid and vitamin B_6.

Ibuprofen: Can cause stomach irritation.

Laxatives: Can cause diarrhea-like effects whereby food passes through the intestines too quickly to be totally absorbed. Mineral oil binds fat-soluble vitamins, impairing their absorption.

MAO inhibitors: Cannot eat foods containing tyramine (wine, hard cheeses, chocolate, beef, or chicken livers).

Opioids: Can cause nausea and vomiting unless taken with food.

taking the place of milk and juices. Americans consume more than enough calories to keep them overweight, while still suffering from deficiencies in many nutrients. This trend is even more widely noted among elders whose increased nutrient requirements (related to aging and disease) combined with diminished caloric intakes conspire to increase the risk of nutritional deficiencies.

Overall, surveys reveal that a significant proportion of American elders suffers from insufficient calorie intake and other nutrient deficiencies. In general, the data from national surveys indicate that the older people interviewed did not consume sufficient calories to meet energy and nutrient rec-ommendations. Further, a substantial proportion of older people had vitamin and mineral intakes below two-thirds of the RDA.

Institutionalization and hospitalization can have profound effects on nutritional status. Hospitalization exposes elders to the stresses of disease, surgery, and diagnostic and treatment procedures that further deplete their nutritional stores. Many elders lose weight during hospitalizations, especially those requiring surgery and bedrest. Because those elders who are the most frail and the most ill are in hospitals and nursing homes, multiple studies report a high rate of nutritional inadequacy.

Studies and anecdotal reports suggest that the quality of food served in hospitals and nursing homes can be poor, and meals may not be appropriately balanced. One study of university teaching hospitals found that only 7 percent of the hospitals studied met requirements for calories, fat, cholesterol, sodium, calcium, fruits and vegetables, grains, and fiber. In general, these diets were too high in fat, and too low in fruits, vegetables, and grains.[56] Additionally, the food served in institutional settings is often unappealing. Although these elders may benefit the most from nutritional supplements, they are seldom prescribed.

Factors Affecting Nutritional Status

A number of variables profoundly affect food selection and consequent nutritional status. A sample of physiological, psychological, educational, socioeconomic, cultural, and environmental factors influencing food selection are discussed in the following pages.

Physiological Factors

Disability from chronic illness can severely affect mobility, energy level, and visual acuity, which decrease interest in eating and ability to shop for and prepare food. Visual decrements can make it difficult for elders to read labels, comparison shop, and cook. Reduced mobility may force an elder to shop only at nearby stores, which may be expensive or offer little selection. Disabled elders may overuse prepackaged foods. Medication-related problems in taste or smell acuity, lack of appetite, dry mouth, and nausea affect the ability and motivation to eat. Further, dental problems, such as ill-fitting dentures, lack of teeth, and poor oral hygiene, can make chewing difficult and reduce motivation to eat. Food intolerances and the necessity of following a prescribed diet can also affect interest in food and narrow food choices. Alcohol misuse is a very common cause of lack of interest in food and subsequent malnutrition.

Psychological Factors

People's emotional state can have profound consequences on motivation to shop for and prepare nutritious meals. Anxiety and depression can cause either a diminished appetite or overeating. Elders who are lonely or grieving may be less likely to cook for themselves and may depend on processed snack foods. Those who are depressed or who have low self-esteem may not want to leave the house to shop or may be too lethargic to cook.

Educational Factors

Level of education and knowledge about nutrition affects people's food choices and methods of meal preparation; elders with a high education level generally have fewer nutrient deficiencies than those with less education. For instance, elders with a low educational level may fry foods whereas those with more education may steam or broil their foods. Elders who are illiterate, who have a minimum of nutrition education, or who speak English poorly may be unable to read and understand product labels. Also, elders who are less educated may select foods based on advertisements or coupons. Finally, those with severe cognitive deficits may be incapable of shopping or preparing meals for themselves.

Economic Factors

Financial status influences the quality of food purchased and motivation to eat healthfully. Income is related to diet quality; elders who are poor are less likely to have an adequate diet since many high-nutrient foods are expensive. Elders who rely on economic assistance programs are more likely to have poor nutritional intake. In poor areas, there are often no large grocery stores, and elders may have to rely on convenience markets near their house for overpriced, processed foodstuffs. Those with higher incomes can afford to spend more on food. However, a high income does not ensure nutritional adequacy.

Living Arrangements

Social interaction patterns affect food intake and nutritional status. Those living alone have the poorest diets. Social isolation can also affect the motivation to shop, prepare meals, or eat well. Many elders do not like to prepare and eat a meal alone or go out to eat alone. Older men living alone have poorer diets than those living with a spouse; however, this same trend is not noted among older

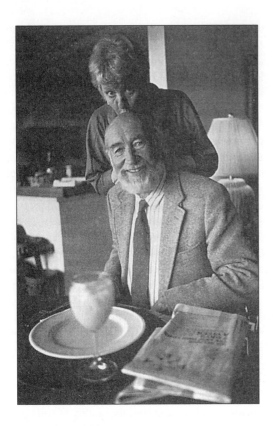

studies show that elders are open to trying new foods and that eating patterns may change dramatically with age. For instance, one longitudinal study found that elderly men decreased dietary fat over approximately twenty years, during which public education campaigns were aimed at encouraging them to make these very changes.[57]

Environmental Factors

The availability of community nutrition programs, distance from shopping facilities, transportation availability, and geographical location can also affect food choices and nutritional status. Elders in the inner city may have reduced access to supermarkets, and often small grocery stores close to home are expensive. Inner-city elders, especially women and those with mobility decrements, may be reluctant to shop because they are afraid of being crime victims. Fresh fruits and vegetables are more available and less expensive in some areas than others. Climate may affect food choices because winter snows and excessive heat may confine some older people to their homes. Additionally, elders in rented rooms or hotels have limited access to cooking or refrigeration facilities.

women. Elder women tend to eat a greater variety of foods than men and are more likely to choose fresh fruit, vegetables, and milk products, while men eat more meat. Also, older people who live alone may have physical or mental problems that make food preparation difficult. Other variables might reduce the ability to shop for food: living in a high-crime area, inability to drive a car, and lack of access to public transportation.

Cultural Attitudes and Behaviors

Differences in eating patterns among age groups are common because each generation grew up in a different cultural milieu. For instance, many elders associate white bread with wealth and beans with poverty. Elders from varied ethnic backgrounds may limit food choices to those traditional foods that are available locally.

Food consumption habits established early in life may be hard to break. However, numerous

Assessment of Inadequate Nutrition

Physicians need to be alert to signs and symptoms in elderly patients suggesting poor nutrition. Malnutrition and dietary inadequacies generally develop gradually, and manifestations are subtle. Nonspecific symptoms may be attributed to age changes or chronic illnesses and be ignored by both the elder and the physician. Nutritional status is notoriously difficult to evaluate and may not be seen as a priority for elders or their physicians.

Assessment and treatment of inadequate nutrition is an important part of medical care. Federal regulations now specify that nutritional screening be included when elders are provided with home health services and in hospitals and nursing homes.

Assessment should include measures of weight taken over long time periods to document weight gains or losses that may have been missed by the elder or family. In addition, assessing dietary intake

The Functions of Food in American Culture

Food is an important part of living. Attitudes and behaviors surrounding food and eating are learned and shared. Each culture imparts its own meaning to food and eating. In the United States, food may serve a number of psychological, social, cultural, and even economic functions.

Food may be a manifestation of friendship. Most social events include food and drink, and some—picnics, dinner parties, Thanksgiving, cocktail parties, coffee breaks—center around eating and drinking. Individuals seldom prefer to eat alone. Dinner is the focal point for interaction in many American families.

Food and drink can also serve as status symbols. Filet mignon is more prestigious than macaroni and cheese. For some, the offer of food—a special dessert, a candlelight meal, or an invitation to dinner—is a way to show love. Conversely, refusal to eat what another has cooked may be a sign of rejection. Eating can also serve as an outlet for boredom, unhappiness, loneliness, or stress. Nursing home personnel can often detect a resident's stress level by the amount of wasted food and complaints about the food.

People may use food as a reward for self or others. We are all familiar with such statements as, "You mow the lawn and I'll take you for an ice cream," or "I deserve this piece of cake, I worked so hard today."

Food can express individuality, and many people are proud of their secret recipes. Some get attention by eating uncommon food combinations, while others get attention by not eating at all. Vegetarians may use their food preferences as a political statement or as evidence of their health concerns. Some food habits, such as fasting or avoiding certain foods, may reflect spiritual beliefs.

Food consumption is an important source of ritual and security. Most of us know the rules governing American eating: main course comes before dessert, three meals a day, no alcohol before noon, and cereal is a breakfast food. Members of various populations, such as children, vegetarians, teenagers, and ethnic groups, have certain food preferences that establish them as part of a group. Certain foods impart security because of long-standing habit.

Finally, food serves an economic purpose in America because the provision of foods in supermarkets and restaurants is a profit-making venture. Millions of dollars are spent yearly on advertising that encourages us to buy particular food products even when we are not hungry and the food is not healthful. A disproportionate amount of advertising money is targeted for junk or convenience foods rather than nutritious foods.

(including level of appetite, number of meals per day consumed, and patient recall of foods eaten) is important. Accounts from reliable witnesses are very helpful. For example, discussion with a family member may provide additional information. Physical complaints that may be related to food should be followed up: constipation, stomach upset, anorexia (lack of appetite), and functional status (particularly ability to shop and prepare own meals) are important. An important component of the nutritional assessment is an evaluation for alcoholism, as well as alterations in psychosocial status (e.g., recent bereavement), depression, and medications used.

A physical examination can give important information about dietary practices; for example, many oral and dental problems are associated with poor nutrition. During a physical exam, it is important to evaluate whether an elderly patient can swallow well—coughing after taking in liquids, for example, may signify that the elder is aspirating food into the lungs. Muscle wasting, reduced cognitive skills, and clinical signs of dehydration are important clues that malnutrition may be present.

Several instruments have been developed to facilitate nutritional screening. One project, the Nutritional Screening Initiative, is a collaborative

The Warning Signs of poor nutritional health are often overlooked. Use this checklist to find out if you or someone you know is at nutritional risk.

Read the statements below. Circle the number in the yes column for those that apply to you or someone you know. For each yes answer, score the number in the box. Total your nutritional score.

DETERMINE YOUR NUTRITIONAL HEALTH

	YES
I have an illness or condition that made me change the kind and/or amount of food I eat.	2
I eat fewer than 2 meals per day.	3
I eat few fruits or vegetables, or milk products.	2
I have 3 or more drinks of beer, liquor or wine almost every day.	2
I have tooth or mouth problems that make it hard for me to eat.	2
I don't always have enough money to buy the food I need.	4
I eat alone most of the time.	1
I take 3 or more different prescribed or over-the-counter drugs a day.	1
Without wanting to, I have lost or gained 10 pounds in the last 6 months.	2
I am not always physically able to shop, cook and/or feed myself.	2
TOTAL	

Total Your Nutritional Score. If it's—

0-2   **Good!** Recheck your nutritional score in 6 months.

3-5   **You are at moderate nutritional risk.** See what can be done to improve your eating habits and lifestyle. Your office on aging, senior nutrition program, senior citizens center, or health department can help. Recheck your nutritional score in 3 months.

6 or more   **You are at high nutritional risk.** Bring this checklist the next time you see your doctor, dietitian or other qualified health or social service professional. Talk with them about any problems you may have. Ask for help to improve your nutritional health.

These materials developed and distributed by the Nutrition Screening Initiative, a project of:

AMERICAN ACADEMY
OF FAMILY PHYSICIANS

THE AMERICAN
DIETETIC ASSOCIATION

NATIONAL COUNCIL
ON THE AGING, INC.

Remember that warning signs suggest risk, but do not represent diagnosis of any condition. Turn the page to learn more about the Warning Signs of poor nutritional health.

**The Nutrition Checklist is based on the Warning Signs described below.
Use the word <u>DETERMINE</u> to remind you of the Warning Signs.**

DISEASE

Any disease, illness or chronic condition which causes you to change the way you eat, or makes it hard for you to eat, puts your nutritional health at risk. Four out of five adults have chronic diseases that are affected by diet. Confusion or memory loss that keeps getting worse is estimated to affect one out of five or more of older adults. This can make it hard to remember what, when or if you've eaten. Feeling sad or depressed, which happens to about one in eight older adults, can cause big changes in appetite, digestion, energy level, weight and well-being.

EATING POORLY

Eating too little and eating too much both lead to poor health. Eating the same foods day after day or not eating fruit, vegetables, and milk products daily will also cause poor nutritional health. One in five adults skip meals daily. Only 13% of adults eat the minimum amount of fruit and vegetables needed. One in four older adults drink too much alcohol. Many health problems become worse if you drink more than one or two alcoholic beverages per day.

TOOTH LOSS/MOUTH PAIN

A healthy mouth, teeth and gums are needed to eat. Missing, loose or rotten teeth or dentures which don't fit well or cause mouth sores make it hard to eat.

ECONOMIC HARDSHIP

As many as 40% of older Americans have incomes of less than $6,000 per year. Having less—or choosing to spend less—than $25-30 per week for food makes it very hard to get the foods you need to stay healthy.

REDUCED SOCIAL CONTACT

One-third of all older people live alone. Being with people daily has a positive effect on morale, well-being and eating.

MULTIPLE MEDICINES

Many older Americans must take medicines for health problems. Almost half of older Americans take multiple medicines daily. Growing old may change the way we respond to drugs. The more medicines you take, the greater the chance for side effects such as increased or decreased appetite, change in taste, constipation, weakness, diarrhea, nausea, and others. Vitamins or minerals when taken in large doses act like drugs and can cause harm. Alert your doctor to everything you take.

INVOLUNTARY WEIGHT LOSS/GAIN

Losing or gaining a lot of weight when you are not trying to do so is an important warning sign that must not be ignored. Being overweight or underweight also increases your chance of poor health.

NEEDS ASSISTANCE IN SELF CARE

Although most older people are able to eat, one of every five have trouble walking, shopping, buying and cooking food, especially as they get older.

ELDER YEARS ABOVE AGE 80

Most older people lead full and productive lives. But as age increases, risk of frailty and health problems increase. Checking your nutritional health regularly makes good sense.

The Nutrition Screening Initiative, 1010 Wisconsin Avenue, NW, Suite 800, Washington, DC 20007
The Nutrition Screening Initiative is funded in part by a grant from Ross Laboratories, a division of Abbott Laboratories.

project of more than twenty-five professional organizations committed to identifying and getting services to those with the greatest nutrition risk. The project includes an initiative to increase screening of elders in the community and to improve nutrition counseling and education. The consortium developed a screening tool for elders to be self-administered and scored by older persons, family members, caregivers, or physicians. This brief ten-item checklist is easily scored and can accurately identify noninstitutionalized older persons at risk for low nutrient intake and dietary health problems. The group also identified several warning signs of poor nutrition to accompany the questionnaire to educate the elder and those who care for them. Initial testing of the screening tool found it simple to use and accurate in predicting nutrient deficiencies; in one study of elder Medicare beneficiaries, 25 percent were determined to be at high nutritional risk. One of four elders at risk had dietary intakes below 75 percent of the RDA for three or more nutrients.[58]

The Clinton administration has required that all health plans that receive Medicare monies must assess the nutritional status of each new Medicare member within 90 days of enrollment, and many programs are using the checklist developed by the Nutrition Screening Initiative. In July 1998, over 1 million Medicare members had completed the checklist, and about one-third exhibited signs of nutrition and health risk. In addition, this questionnaire is used to screen elders applying for federal food programs.

For more information, contact the Nutrition Screening Initiative, 1010 Wisconsin Ave. NW, Suite 800, Washington D.C. 20007; 202-625-1662.

NUTRITION EDUCATION AND COUNSELING

Nutrition education and counseling is indicated for the one in three elders identified to be at risk of nutritional deficiencies, and some suggest all elders can benefit. As a group, elders know very little about the science of nutrition. Since elders were school children, there have been major changes in how we think about diet and nutrition—a move away from the "Basic Four" to the Food Guide Pyramid, and an increased focus on dietary specifics such as trans fats, artificial sweeteners, and specific antioxidants.

Nutritional education and counseling can prevent or reduce the progression of disease and improve general health and well-being. Physicians may provide dietary counseling, however, they are inadequately trained in this area and nutritional counseling can be time-consuming. Therefore, it is often preferable for a trained nutritional counselor to provide counseling and education to elders in assessing dietary deficiencies, setting goals to improve diet, and monitoring progress. Nutritional counselors, generally registered dieticians, help clients to modify their diets to improve nutritional quality, decrease fat, or increase fiber. To be effective, nutritional counselors must consider the multiple factors that affect nutritional status—food preferences, economic status, and health condition—when advising clients on dietary practices and be trained to facilitate behavior change.

Nutritional counseling and education may include simple interventions, such as the distribution of pamphlets or other materials. Individual sessions with elders and their families may discuss nutritional problems and develop acceptable solutions. Elders may be invited to classes focusing on particular nutritional needs (such as "cooking nutritious meals for one" or "rational weight loss"). They may receive information about community services offering meal programs. Elders may be encouraged to use nutritional supplements (either pills or high-protein beverages).

Other types of nutritional education may include: discussion groups on nutrition-related topics at senior centers, nutrition sites, apartment complexes, cooking classes, potlucks, large-print nutrition newsletters in simple language, nutrition column in local newspaper, public service announcements on radio or television regarding nutrition education, community garden programs, food cooperatives, or programs where elders are trained as peer nutrition outreach counselors. Studies show that nutritional counseling is more

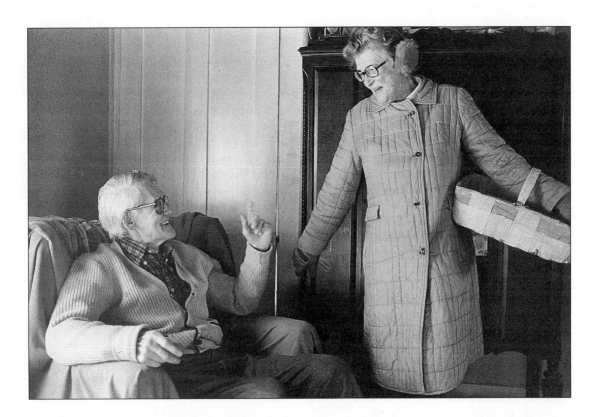

effective when continued over a long period of time. The counselors and clients can regularly review and adapt the diet regimen to the clients' changing needs or wants. Success is also increased if spouses or friends attend the counseling sessions to give support to the clients. These individuals may be counseled on ways to assure that elders under their care are receiving adequate nutrition. Finally, topics should be geared to the desires and experiences of the participants. Educational activities for elders may need to be adapted to geographical location, varied cultures, and education level. Special efforts should be directed toward low-income, uneducated, isolated, and minority elders.

Health professionals also need to be educated about the importance of nutrition in the health in older adults, the importance of nutrition and supplements in the prevention and treatment of chronic diseases, as well as important interactions between drugs and diet. Although most doctors

believe that diet is important in disease, few take dietary histories or prescribe nutritional interventions to their patients.[59] An important component of the Nutrition Screening Initiative is the education of physicians and other professionals about the importance of good nutrition, strategies to screen for nutritional risk, techniques to ascertain etiology of risk, and methods to improve patient's nutritional status through education and counseling.

NUTRITION PROGRAMS

A number of federal, state, and local intervention programs have been developed to meet nutritional needs and to promote nutrition education among elders. In addition, private organizations and the food industry have taken an interest in this topic and have developed health education materials.

The Older Americans Act allocates federal monies to each state to provide lunch programs and nutrition education to elders. This federal nutrition program provides both meals and social support to homebound elders who are unable to cook for themselves. Most communities participate in this program of public-private partnerships, allowing them to serve diverse elder populations. A recent evaluation revealed that these programs are quite successful and cost-efficient.[60] Elders served by these programs often are at high risk for nutritional deficiencies. They are likely to be either over- or underweight, have physical impairments, be poor, or live alone. New federal guidelines require states to screen potential clients for these nutritional programs with the questionnaire developed by the National Screening Initiative mentioned above.

Congregate meal services may be offered at churches, senior centers, or schools, or they may deliver meals to a person's home. They generally ask the older person for a small donation, and most of them pay a little to defray the costs of the meal. All programs provide nutritious meals that contain at least one-third the RDA, although these meals may constitute one-half to two-thirds of an elder's daily food intake. These programs strive to improve elders' nutrition and reduce their isolation. Elders served by the programs had lower rates of nutritional deficiency for many vitamins and minerals compared to those who do not use the programs. These programs have been found to be effective at serving isolated, poor, and minority elders who are referred to the program through hospitals or nursing homes.

In 1994, 127 million meals were provided to 2.3 million people at community-based sites, and 113 million meals were provided to 877,000 homes with federal funding estimated at about $470 million. However, many eligible elders remain unserved; almost half of all programs have waiting lists. Many social service experts are frustrated at the limitations of these feeding programs and at the number of elders who still go hungry.[61] Most programs offer only one meal a day and many serve only on weekdays. The people served, and those waiting for food, are often very ill, very poor, and very old.

The federal Food Stamp Program supplements the food budget of almost 2 million low-income elders. However, this figure represents less than half of those who are eligible to receive the support. Perhaps many elders fail to take advantage of the service because they are unaware of the program, lack transportation to the stamp distribution site, or do not want the stigma of applying for and using the coupons. Federal and state modifications of the Food Stamp Program have included providing cash to recipients to use for food or providing debit cards that work at grocery stores. Welfare reform policies have affected the availability of food stamps.

A number of feeding programs are financed locally, either by churches, United Way funds, private organizations, local taxes, or other means. Free dinners, soup kitchens, and home-delivered meals for the homebound are fairly common in some communities. Many restaurants and cooperative grocery stores offer discounts to older people. The number and types of programs vary tremendously among communities. Expansion of current programs and the development of new programs are needed to provide quality nutrition to special groups of elders, especially rural, inner-city, ethnic, socially isolated, homebound, and the poor. Adequate financial support and effective publicity are two variables that increase the effectiveness of such programs.

SUMMARY

Nutrition is an important aspect of health throughout the lifespan. The Recommended Daily Allowance (RDA) is the recognized standard of nutritional requirements for healthy people; however, these recommendations may have to be modified for elders, due to their changing physiology and health status. In general, elders' reduced metabolic rate causes a decreased daily caloric requirement making it harder to ensure adequate levels of essential nutrients. Vitamin and mineral supplements are commonly used among some elderly groups.

National studies show that some groups of American elders are malnourished—especially in total calories and certain vitamins and minerals, while others suffer from obesity. The Nutrition Screening Initiative was developed to identify and treat nutritional problems among our nation's elders. Individual nutrition assessments should be a part of routine medical care. Nutrition has an impact on a number of chronic illnesses common among elders. In some cases, poor food choices encourage the disease process; in others, the disease may cause an increased need for some nutrients. The progression of cancer, diabetes, osteoporosis, and heart disease are strongly influenced by diet. Nutritional counseling and education, as well as community nutrition programs, are effective ways of increasing elders' knowledge and motivation to eat healthfully.

ACTIVITIES

1. Record what, when, and why you ate each item for at least three days. Compare the nutritional value and caloric intake with the RDA. What type of foods are you eating in excess? Are there some nutrients you are lacking? What psychosocial factors affected your food intake?

2. Eat all meals alone for three to four days. How was your food intake affected? Keep a daily journal to record your feelings.

3. Attend a lunch at a local nutrition site for elders. What is the menu? Describe the associated educational or recreational activities. If you have the opportunity, visit two different sites and compare them.

4. Question an elder regarding his or her dietary intake in the last twenty-four hours and analyze nutritional value and caloric intake. What problems do you see with this approach?

5. Design a pamphlet to inform elders about a particular aspect of nutrition.

6. Develop objectives, and outline the content of a twenty-minute educational program on some aspect of nutrition for a group of independent elders.

7. What educational programs does your community offer to elders on nutrition? What meal programs are offered?

8. Design a day's menu that includes the RDA for all vitamins and minerals staying within the caloric requirements for an adult age twenty-two to fifty. Now modify it for someone over age fifty.

9. Ask five friends or relatives the following questions to determine what information they have about vitamins and minerals: Do you take vitamin or mineral supplements? How often? Which ones? Who told you to take them? What do you believe each does for you? What foods contain high values of these supplements?

BIBLIOGRAPHY

1. Chenault, A. 1984. *Nutrition and health.* New York: Holt, Rinehart & Winston.

2. National Research Council. Subcommittee on the Ninth Edition of the RDAs. 1980. *Recommended dietary allowances.* Washington, D.C.: National Academy Press.

3. Russell, R.M., and Suter, P.M. 1993. Vitamin requirements of elderly people: An update. *American Journal of Clinical Nutrition* 58:4–14.

4. Keys, A., Brozek, J., and Henschel, A., et al. 1950. *The biology of human starvation* vol. II, Minneapolis: University of Minnesota Press.

5. Peter D. Hart Research Associates, Inc. 1993. *National survey on nutrition screening and treatment for the elderly.* Washington, D.C.: Peter D. Hart Research Associates, Inc.

6. Sullivan, D.H., Martin, W., Flaxman, N., and Hagen, J.E. 1993. Oral health problems and involuntary weight loss in a population of frail elderly. *Journal of the American Geriatrics Society* 41:725–31.

7. Stevens, J., Cai, J., and Pamuk, E.R., et al. 1998. The effect of age on the association between body mass index and mortality. *New England Journal of Medicine* 338:1–7.

8. Lee, I. M., Manson, J.E., Hennekens, C.H. 1993. Body weight and mortality. *Journal of the American Medical Association* 270:2823–28.

9. Hu, F.B., Stampfer, M.J., and Manson, J.E., et al. 1997. Dietary fat intake and the risk of coronary heart disease in women. *New England Journal of Medicine* 337:1491–99.

10. National Institutes of Health. 1998. *Clinical guidelines on the identification, evaluation, and treatment of overweight and obesity in adults.* Washington, D.C.: National Institutes of Health.

11. Kassirer J.P., and Angell, A. 1998. Losing weight—an ill-fated new year's resolution. *New England Journal of Medicine* 338:52–54.

12. Cotton, J.R., Westrate, J.A., and Blundell, J.E. 1996. Replacement of dietary fat with sucrose polyester: Effects on energy intake and appetite control in nonobese males. *American Journal of Clinical Nutrition* 63:891–96.

13. Watson, R.R., Prabhala, R.H., Plezia, P.M., and Alberts, D.S. 1991. Effect of beta carotene on lymphocyte subpopulations in elderly humans: Evidence for a dose-response relationship. *American Journal of Clinical Nutrition* 53:90–94.

14. Morris, D.L., Kritchevsky, S.B., and Davis, C.E. 1994. Serum carotenoids and coronary heart disease. *Journal of the American Medical Association* 272:1439–41.

15. Seddon, J.M., Ajani, U.A., and Sperduto, R.D., et al. 1994. Dietary carotenoids, vitamins A, C, and E and advanced age-related macular degeneration. *Journal of the American Medical Association* 272:1413–20.

16. Jacques, P.F., and Chylack, L.T. 1991. Epidemiological evidence of a role for the antioxidant vitamins and carotenoids in cataract prevention. *American Journal of Clinical Nutrition* 53(1 suppl.):3525–55.

17. Albanes, D., Heinonen, O.P., and Taylor, P.R., et al. 1996. Alpha tocopherol and beta carotene supplements and lung cancer incidence in the alpha tocopheral, beta carotene cancer prevention study. *Journal of the National Cancer Institute* 88:1560–70.

18. Morrison, H.I., Shaubel, D., Desmeules, M., and Wigle, D.T. 1996. Serum folate and risk of fatal coronary heart disease. *Journal of the American Medical Association* 275:1893–96.

19. Boushey, C.J., Berresford, S.A.A., and Omenn, G.S., et al. 1995. A quantitative assessment of plasma homocysteine as a risk factor for vascular disease: Probable benefits of increasing folic acid intakes. *Journal of the American Medical Association* 274:1049–57.

20. Enstrom, J.E., Kannim, L.K., and Klein, M.A. 1992. Vitamin C intake and mortality among a sample of the United States population. *Epidemiology* 3:194–202.

21. Taylor, W.C., Pass, T.M., Shephard, D.S., and Komaroff, A.L. 1997. Cholesterol reduction and life expectancy: A model incorporating risk factors. *Annals of Internal Medicine* 106:605–14.

22. Thomas, M.K., Lloyd-Jones, D.M., and Thadhani, R.I., et al. 1998. Hypovitaminosis D in medical inpatients. *New England Journal of Medicine* 338:777–83.

23. Dawson-Hughes, B., Harris, S.S., Krall, E.A., and Dallal, G.E. 1997. Effect of calcium and vitamin D supplementation on bone density in men and women 65 years of age or older. *New England Journal of Medicine* 337:670–76.

24. Stampfer, J.M., Hennekens, C.H., Manson, J.E. et al. 1993. Vitamin E consumption and the risk of coronary disease in women. *New England Journal of Medicine* 328:1444–49.

25. Egan, M.F., Hyde, T.M., and Albers, G.W., et al. 1992. Treatment of tardive dyskinesia with vitamin E. *American Journal of Psychiatry* 149:773–77.

26. Meydani, S.N., Meydana, M., and Blumberg, J.B., et al. 1997. Vitamin E supplementation and in vivo immune response in healthy elderly subjects. *Journal of the American Medical Association* 277:1380–86.

27. Paolisso, G.P., D'Amore, A., and Giugliano, D., et al. 1993. Pharmacologic doses of vitamin E improve insulin action in healthy subjects and non-insulin-dependent diabetic patients. *American Journal of Clinical Nutrition* 57:650–56.

28. Sano, M., Ernesto, C., and Thomas, R.G., et al. 1997. A controlled trial of selegiline, alpha-tocopherol, or both as treatment for Alzheimer's disease. *New England Journal of Medicine* 336:1216–22.

29. Robertson, J., Donner, A.P., and Trevithick, J.R. 1991. A possible role for vitamins C and E in cataract prevention. *American Journal of Clinical Nutrition* 53(1 suppl.):346S–351S.

30. Albanes, D., Heinonen, O.P., and Taylor, P.R., et al. 1996. Alpha tocopherol and beta carotene supplements and lung cancer incidence in the alpha tocopherol, beta- carotene cancer prevention study. *Journal of the National Cancer Institute* 88:1560–70.

31. Omenn, G.S., Goodman, G.E., and Thornquist, M.D., et al. 1996. Risk factors for lung cancer and for intervention effects in CARET: The Beta-Carotene and Retinol Efficacy trial. *Journal of the National Cancer Institute* 88:1550–59.

32. Voelker, R. Recommendations for antioxidants: How much evidence is enough? *Journal of the American Medical Association* 271:1148–49.

33. Curhan, G.C., Willett, W.C., Rimm, E.B., and Stampfer, M.J. 1993. A prospective study of dietary calcium and other nutrients and the risk of symptomatic kidney stones. *New England Journal of Medicine* 328:833–38.

34. Salonen, J.T., Nyyssonen, K., and Korpela, H., et al. 1992. High stored iron levels are associated with excess risk of myocardial infarction in eastern Finnish men. *Circulation* 86:803–11.

35. Salmeron, J., Manson,, J.E., and Stampfer, M.J., et al. 1997. Dietary fiber, glycemic load, and risk of non-insulin dependent diabetes mellitus in women. *Journal of the American Medical Association* 277:472–77.

36. Sojka, J.E., and Weaver, C.M. 1995. Magnesium supplementation and osteoporosis. *Nutrition Reviews* 53:71–74.

37. Whelton, P.K., Appel, L.J., Espeland, M.A., et al. 1998. Sodium reduction and weight loss in the treatment of hypertension in older persons. *Journal of the American Medical Association* 279:839–46.

38. Devine, A., Criddle, A., Dick, I.M. 1995. A longitudinal study of the effect of sodium and calcium intakes on regional bone density in postmenopausal women. *American Journal of Clinical Nutrition* 62:740–45.

39. Bogden, J.D., Olkske, J.M., and Munves, E.M., et al. 1987. Zinc and immunocompetence in the elderly: Baseline data on zinc nitriture and immunity in unsupplemented subjects. *American Journal of Clinical Nutrition* 46:101–9.

40. Bogden, J.D., Bendich, A., and Kemp, F.W., et al. 1994. Daily micronutrient supplements enhance delayed-hypersensitivity skin test responses in older people. *American Journal of Clinical Nutrition* 60:437–47.

41. Roebothan, B.V., and Chandra, R.K. 1994. Relationship between nutritional status and immune function of elderly people. *Age and Ageing* 23:49–53.

42. Chandra, R.K. 1992. Effect of vitamin and trace element supplementation on immune responses and infection in healthy subjects. *Lancet* 340:1124–27.

43. Ryan, A.S., Craig, L.D., and Finn, S.C. 1992. Nutrient intakes and dietary patterns of older Americans: A national study. *Journal of Gerontology* 47:M145–M150.

44. Giovannucci, E., Stampfer, M.J., and Colditz, G.A., et al. 1998. Multivitamin use, folate, and colon cancer in women in the Nurses' Health Study. *Annals of Internal Medicine* 129:517–24.

45. Rozen, P., Fireman, Z., and Fine, N., et al. 1989. Oral calcium suppresses increased rectal epithelial proliferation of persons at risk for colorectal cancer. *Gut* 30:650–55.

46. Clark, L.C., Combs, G.F., and Turnbill, B.W., et al. 1996. Effects of selenium supplementation for cancer prevention in patients with carcinoma of the skin. A randomized controlled trial. *Journal of the American Medical Association* 276:1957–63.

47. Howe, G.R., Benito, E., Casteletto, R. et al. 1992. Dietary intake of fiber and decreased risks of cancers of the colon and rectum: Evidence from the combined analysis of 13 case-control studies. *Journal of the National Cancer Institute* 84:1887–96.

48. Howe, G.R., Hirohata, T., and Hislop, G., et al. 1990. Dietary factors and risk of breast cancer: Combined analysis of 12 case-control studies. *Journal of the National Cancer Institute* 82:561–69.

49. Trichopoulou, A., Katsouyanni, K., and Stuver, S., et al. 1995. Consumption of olive oil and specific food groups in relation to breast cancer risk in Greece. *Journal of National Cancer Institute* 87:110–16.

50. Carey, V.J., Walters, E.E., and Colditz, G.A., et al. 1997. Body fat distribution and risk of non-insulin-dependent diabetes mellitus in women. The Nurses' Health Study. *American Journal of Epidemiology* 145:614–19.

51. Riemersma, R.A., Wood, D.A., and MacIntyre, C.C., et al. 1991. Risk of angina pectoris and plasma concentrations of vitamins A, C, and E and carotene. *Lancet* 337:1–5.

52. Rimm, E.B., Willett, W.C., and Frank, B.H., et al. 1998. Folate and vitamin B6 from diet and

supplements in relation to risk of coronary heart disease among women. *Journal of the American Medical Association* 279:359–64.

53. Rimm, E.B., Ascherio, A., and Giovannucci, E., et al. 1996. Vegetable, fruit, and cereal fiber intake and risk of coronary heart disease among men. *Journal of the American Medical Association* 275:447–51.

54. Pietinen, P., Rimm, E.B., and Korhonen, P., et al. 1996. Intake of dietary fiber and risk of coronary heart disease in a cohort of Finnish men. *Circulation* 94:2720–27.

55. Appel, L.J., Moore, T.J., and Obarzanek, E. 1997. A clinical trial of the effects of dietary patterns on blood pressure. *New England Journal of Medicine* 336:1117–24.

56. Singer, A.J., Werther, K., and Nestle, M. 1999. The nutritional value of university hospital diets. *New England Journal of Medicine* 335:1466–67.

57. Hallfrisch, J., Muller, D., and Drinkwater, D., et al. 1990. Continuing diet trends in men. The Baltimore Longitudinal Study of Aging (1961–1987). *Journal of Gerontology* 45:186–91.

58. Posner, B., Jette, A.M., Smith, K.W., and Miler, D.R. 1993. Nutrition and health risks in the elderly: The nutrition screening initiative. *American Journal of Public Health* 83:972–78.

59. Levine, B.S., Wigren, M.M., and Chapman, D.S., et al. 1993. A national survey of attitudes and practices of primary care physicians relating to nutrition: Strategies for enhancing the use of clinical nutrition in medical practice. *American Journal of Clinical Nutrition* 57:115–19.

60. Voelker, R. 1997. Federal program nourishes poor elderly. *Journal of the American Medical Association* 278:1301.

61. Lieberman, T. 1998. Hunger in America. *The Nation* (March 30):11–16.

6

SEXUALITY

I think sex should be confined to one's lifetime.

Woody Allen

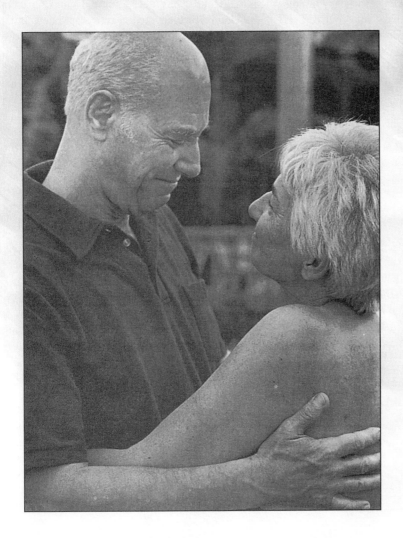

Sexuality encompasses a wide range of sensual or erotic feelings or behaviors, including sexual fantasy, affectionate hugs among friends, flirtatious glances, and genital intercourse among lovers. Attitudes and behaviors regarding sexuality are an integral part of one's personality. Early sexual attitudes and experiences significantly affect our expression of sexuality at all ages. The views of families, peers, and culture also tremendously influence sexuality by defining which behaviors are acceptable and which are not.

While most people have little trouble understanding that young adults have sexual needs, their stereotypical view of the older adult does not include sex. However, elders do have sexual desires and the capacity to enjoy sexual intercourse. This chapter discusses misconceptions of elder sexuality and explores the gamut of sexual behavior in later years, including variations in sexual behavior among subgroups. Sexual dysfunction, its causes, diagnosis, and treatment will also be addressed. Accurate information about sexuality in later life will enable professionals to better provide an accepting atmosphere. Such knowledge also facilitates a realistic perspective of sexuality in our own later years.

STEREOTYPES OF ELDER SEXUALITY

The topic of elder sexuality is wrought with misinformation and bias, which, in turn, affects our attitudes toward older people, and ultimately our own sexual feelings and behavior in later life. These myths also add to our fear of losing sexual function with age. A discussion of some of the more common misconceptions about aging and sexuality follows.

"Sexuality is reserved for the young."

Americans generally associate sexuality with the physical characteristics of youth: beautiful young women with firm and shapely bodies, and muscular slim-hipped men are the archetypes of sexual attractiveness. To a much larger extent than we may realize, images on television, motion pictures, and magazines both shape and reflect our impressions of what is beautiful or sexy. Because older persons (and most of the younger population) do not conform to the popular conception of sex appeal, nobody wants to look old. The cosmetic industry takes advantage of this fear of growing old by turning our trepidation into its profit. A preponderance of products—face creams, age spot removers, hair dyes to cover the grey—reinforces our fear of aging and consequent loss of sexual attractiveness.

The belief that only the young are sexually appealing damages young and old alike. The prejudices of the young against growing old will continue as the young age, eventually making them the victims of their own negative attitudes. Older women seem to be especially affected by society's narrow image of female sexuality. Revised definitions of sex appeal that can withstand the physical changes of age (e.g., grace, competence, sexual energy, playfulness) are necessary to ease the fear of the inevitable changes in appearance that accompany aging.

"Elders' sexual needs are amusing or insignificant."

Elder lovers expressing affection in public are often described as "cute" and commented on as if they were children—amusing, but not to be taken seriously. Physicians may also consider elder sexuality inconsequential; few take a sexual history or discuss sexual concerns with older patients. They may brush off patients' concerns about sexual dysfunction saying that sex is not that important at their age, or the dysfunction is just part of growing old. Since sexual dysfunction may be a symptom or consequence of disease or a medication side effect, the discussion of sexual issues is critical to accurate diagnosis and treatment.

Early studies of sexuality did not give elders adequate attention. Alfred C. Kinsey and his colleagues, among the first human sexuality researchers, devoted only three of 1,700 pages to describe the sexuality of those over age sixty.[1,2] Later, William Masters and Virginia Johnson's classic work[3] elucidated the physiology of the

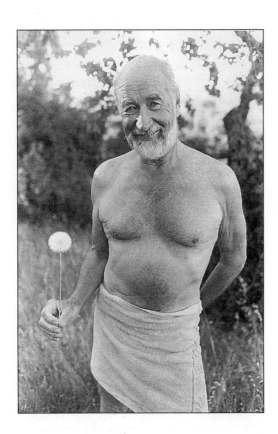

married, when the students' estimates of frequency of sexual intercourse of their parents were compared to Kinsey's data, the students consistently underrated their parents' sexual activity.[4] Most likely the inconsistency between the expected and actual sexual frequency of their grandparents is even greater.

Young people may underestimate the frequency that older people have intercourse because they find sexual intercourse among older people to be immoral, disgraceful, or distasteful. Adult children often have difficulty seeing their parents as adults with sexual feelings. This belief is especially common among adult children with a sexually active parent who is divorced or widowed.

"Older people can't perform sexually."

The misconception that elders have a diminished ability to have sexual relations is often promoted on television and in the print media. For instance, the joke book *Sex over Sixty,* has nothing but hundreds of empty pages, implying that older people don't have sex—or any sex worth writing about. Verses in birthday cards also perpetuate the view that sex and age are mutually exclusive. The following are only a few of the many light-hearted, but insidious, verses describing sexual inactivity in the later years:

human sexual response, but only thirty-one of a total of 694 subjects were over age sixty. These scholars admitted that more studies needed to be conducted on elders. Nevertheless, little subsequent research has expanded or replicated their preliminary impressions.

"Older people don't enjoy sex.
If they do, it's abnormal."

Many younger people find it difficult to accept that older people engage in sexual intercourse. There is something sinister about elder men who are interested in sexual matters; they are "dirty old men," and "grandma" couldn't possibly be interested any more. Perhaps the young unconsciously envision the old as an extension of their parents. Some years ago, a large group of college students were requested to estimate the frequency of sexual intercourse of their parents. Even though 90 percent of those students believed their parents to be happily

- A birthday riddle for your 50th birthday:
  Q. What do you call a 50-year-old with a good sex life? A Liar

- New research indicates that old folks have sex just as often as younger people. They just can't remember it.

- You know you're getting older when a beautiful woman pops out of your birthday cake—and your first thought is "Gee, does this mean the cake's not real?"

- Remember birthdays of years past? When doing it three times a night didn't refer to getting up to go to the bathroom?

- We used to have bodies that wouldn't quit! Now they won't even start!

- At our age, sex is like birthdays, it happens once a year.

- Don't worry about another birthday: you're not old until your whoop-de-doo turns to whoop-de-don't.
- Don't worry about being a year older. You still know where it's at—the hard part is remembering what it's for.
- On your birthday, remember: you're never too old to do it. 'Course you may be too old to survive the experience.
- Can older people really enjoy sex? Of course, but not with each other!

A common misconception about aging and sexual activity is that older men can't have intercourse even if they want to because impotence is a natural part of growing older. In fact, impotence is not a result of the aging process but is due to factors that can happen at any age. Studies consistently show sexual activity is not only possible but practiced by elders into their eighties and nineties. The belief that sexual ability is lost with age is harmful because it may act as a self-fulfilling prophecy. If sexual activity is expected to decline, it probably will.

SEXUAL ACTIVITY IN LATER LIFE

For many elders, interest in sexual activity, intercourse, and other forms of sexual expression persist into later life. Frequency of intercourse may decline, especially among those who are widowed and lack a partner, or among those with chronic illnesses or use of medication, that affect performance. However, interest in sex, desire for physical affection, and sexual fantasy persist into the later years.

Sexual Interest

Data from the classic study by Starr and Weiner contradict the attitude that older people do not think about or enjoy sex.[5] When over 800 elders aged sixty to ninety-one were asked if they liked sex, 96 percent of the women and 99 percent of the men answered affirmatively. Eighty-four percent of both men and women believed touching and cuddling to be very important in their lives.

Come to Me
by Sue Saniel Elkind

Come to me looking
as you did 50 years ago
arms outstretched
and I will be waiting
virgin again
in white that changes to spashes of roses
as we lie together
Come to me smiling again
with your mortar and pestle
and vitamin pills
because I am given to colds
and coughs that wrack us both
Oh come to me again
and I will be there
waiting with withered hands
gnarled fingers
that will leave their marks
of passion on your back.

(from *When I Am Old I Shall Wear Purple: An Anthology of Short Stories and Poetry;* (ed.) S. Martz. Manhattan Beach, CA: Papier-Mâché Press.)

Seventy-five percent of men and 55 percent of women reported that they became excited by sexy pictures, books, and movies. Another survey of healthy elders aged eighty to 102, found 88 percent of men and 71 percent of women still fantasize about being affectionate and intimate with their partner. However, in this population, 25 percent of the men and almost half the women surveyed reported no interest in sex.[6]

Intercourse

Although the majority of men and women retain the capacity to become sexually excited and orgasmic, studies consistently report a gradual decline in the frequency of intercourse with advancing age. Sexually active couples have intercourse less frequently, and the proportion of couples who are sexually active diminishes in all cultural groups studied. However, there is great variability among elders, and those who are active in their younger years are more likely to maintain higher levels in their later years. In general, both men and women wish they were even more sexually active and cite impotence (men) and relationship problems (women) as key reasons for a decline in frequency.[7] In general, men are more likely to curtail or discontinue sexual activity than women—possibly secondary to illness, and widowhood is the most important factor cited for decreasing frequency among older women.[8]

The first systematic study of intercourse frequency was conducted by Kinsey and colleagues.[1,2] They studied elder males and reported a gradual decline in intercourse frequency with age: 20 percent were inactive by age sixty and by age eighty, 75 percent were sexually inactive. However, more recent studies report a higher frequency of intercourse among elders. The Starr-Weiner Report sampled elder participants at senior centers between the ages of sixty and ninety-six.[5] They reported that, elders who were sexually active had intercourse an average of 1.4 times a week. Almost 7 percent of their male sample was sexually inactive; almost 30 percent of their female sample was inactive. Although the percentage of both men and women who were not sexually active increased with advancing age, more women were inactive than men at every age. Seven percent of males in their sixties were inactive, compared to 22 percent of females; 15 percent of men in their eighties were inactive, compared to 57 percent of females. Elders of both sexes reported, on average, that they would like intercourse twice weekly. Three-fourths of respondents reported that sex felt as good or better than when they were younger.

A study of white elders aged 80 to 102 found that two-thirds of the men and one-third of the women engaged in sexual intercourse at least occasionally.[6] About half the men and one-fourth of the women had regular sex partners, and, in about half of the cases, the partner was not a spouse. One-quarter of the men and 10 percent of the women

reported intercourse several times monthly to several times weekly. Of these, over three-fourths of the men reported enjoyment, compared to less than half the women. A high frequency of intercourse in the later years in this study was associated with having engaged in extramarital sex in younger years, being married, and the importance of sex to the subjects. In this study, there was no association between past and present frequency of sexual intercourse.

A study of blue-collar elderly men reported about one-half engaged in intercourse.[9] The National Survey of Families and Households reported that 24 percent of those age seventy-six and older report sexual intercourse in the last month (compared to 53 percent of those age sixty and older), with an average frequency of four times a month.[8]

Interpretation of studies on intercourse frequency is difficult for a number of reasons. Studies may be hindered by a "cohort effect." For instance, if a study finds that elders age sixty and older report less frequent intercourse than younger adults age thirty to forty, there are several ways to interpret the information. The elders studied may have engaged in intercourse less frequently when they were in their thirties, or they may be more reticent about reporting their sexual practices (especially regarding extramarital sex or masturbation). Every decade, a new group of elders enters their "senior years," and studies on the sexual activities of the previous generation are less applicable. This effect is reduced with longitudinal studies as the same group of people are followed over a long time period.

Studies of sexual practices among elders have a "volunteer bias." People who are willing to participate in studies about their sex lives may not be representative of others in their age group. They may be more open about talking about sexuality, may engage in more frequent sexual activity, or have a higher interest than the general population. Men may be more inclined to overestimate their sexual activity—it is a measure of virility for some. But women may underestimate sexual activity for fear of being judged "unladylike." Whether individuals are truthful in answering questions about their sexuality is unknown.

Multiple factors influence the frequency of intercourse. The most obvious is the availability of a partner, especially for women. The combination of women's longer life expectancy and the tendency for women to marry men older than themselves adds up to a large proportion of older widows. Older women are less likely to have intercourse if they are unmarried. Health problems or medication use by one or both partners can also contribute to a decline in intercourse frequency, either by diminishing interest or ability. Finally, the same psychological factors affecting intercourse frequency among younger populations are also important in the elderly. Masters and Johnson attribute decreased frequency in all age groups to six variables: boredom with partner, preoccupation with career or economic pursuits, mental or physical fatigue, overindulgence in food or drink, physical and mental infirmities of individual or partner, and fear of impotence.[3]

The frequency of sexual intercourse has a strong cultural component. For instance, a study of the sexual activity of Mangaian men in Polynesia reported the average number of orgasms decreased from three per night in eighteen-year-old males to once a night in males in their late forties. Even with the drop in frequency, the average frequency of sexual intercourse among elder men was still significantly higher than their North American counterparts.[10] Another study reported coital frequency of the Mayurbhanj Santal of India to be once a day for males at age sixty, often maintaining that frequency at age seventy. The average sexual frequency of young males was reported to be two to four times a day.[p] As in other studies, the relationship between truth and fiction is unknown.

Even if the frequency of intercourse diminishes somewhat with advancing age, its quality may remain as good or improve for many. The Starr-Weiner study reported that about 40 percent of females over age sixty found sexual activity to be better than when they were younger. Almost half said it was the same and less than one-tenth said it worsened.[5] Both men and women retain the capacity to become sexually excited and orgasmic throughout life. Lack of a partner and cultural constraints affect frequency of intercourse much more than physiological changes due to age.

Dear Ann Landers: Love and Sex in Late Life

I read the various letters you printed in response to "sexless in Canada," who found sex unhygienic and degrading. A woman from Virginia said that, in her opinion, there is no connection between love and sex.

I am 78 years old and my wife is 61. Making love is a very important part of our relationship. To me, it is a demonstration of the love and affection I feel for my spouse. I call her my spouse; because she is much more than a wife. She is my mate, my comforter, my companion and my lover. While walking alone or in a crowd, we hold hands or lock arms. It's obvious to anyone who sees us that we belong to each other. Even while sitting on the couch and watching TV, we search for each other's hands.

To the lady from Virginia who thinks there is no connection between love and sex, I can only say it's a shame for a person to have to go through life denying herself the tremendous pleasures and spiritual warmth one derives from a complete relationship.

I know this may sound like something out of a "B" movie, but it's not. To look at us, you would see two over-the-hill, middle-class senior citizens—a tall, skinny guy and a dumpy little gal. But we have found something very special in each other. We have cast aside religious hang-ups and do what comes naturally, as God created us. The rewards have been enormous. We are not just "going through life," we have life flowing through us.—Harvey in Orlando, Fla.

Permission granted by Ann Landers and Creators Syndicate.

Masturbation

Although the vast majority of men and women have masturbated some time in their life, there are severe prejudices against it. Masturbation has been considered a sin throughout Christian history, and many religious groups still believe it to be immoral. Because it is such a sensitive topic, it is difficult to obtain accurate information about elders' masturbatory practices. Only during the last few years has masturbation been acknowledged as a normal and even beneficial activity for all age groups.

In general, studies report that those who are married are less likely to practice masturbation than those who are not. Starr and Weiner reported in their sample of over 800 elders that 43 percent of the men and 47 percent of the women had masturbated. Of those men and women who masturbated, over half reported that they engaged in the activity once a month or more. Among men, masturbation occurred in 40 percent of the married group, 44 percent of those widowed, 57 percent of those divorced, and 69 percent of those who were never married. For women, masturbation was practiced in 39 percent of those who were married, 47 percent of those widowed, 66 percent of those divorced, and 81 percent of those who were never married.[5]

Masturbation can be beneficial both physiologically and psychologically. It maintains the elasticity and lubrication of the vagina for women and preserves erectile ability for men. Orgasms, with or without a partner, are known to reduce stress and induce sleep. Masturbation enables individuals to have control of their own sexuality. It also stimulates sexual appetite and is a way to enjoy sexuality without relying on a partner. Despite its benefits, masturbation is rarely discussed, even among good friends.

Other Sexual Behaviors

Although sexual behavior encompasses more than intercourse and masturbation, these behaviors capture researchers' attention because they are more easily measured. However, numerical data on frequency of sexual intercourse and masturbation present a limited view of sexuality. Sexual behav-

iors such as oral stimulation, fantasy, mutual masturbation, cuddling, and kissing are also important. One study of healthy elders aged eighty to one hundred two found that touching and caressing without sexual intercourse was the most common activity, engaged in by 82 percent of men and 64 percent of women.[6] Another large-scale study found that upper and middle-class elders with decreased erectile capability were likely to substitute mutual masturbation and oral sex for intercourse, while lower-class elders were not.[9]

CHANGES IN SEXUAL RESPONSE WITH AGE

Physiological changes in the genital system with age are minimal, and do not significantly affect sexual capacity in either gender (see chapter 3). However, preliminary studies by Masters and Johnson (1966) in a very small sample of older adults suggested minor changes in sexual response in the later years.[3]

Researchers Masters and Johnson pioneered the study of human physiological sexual response through direct observation. They brought subjects of various ages into the laboratory and quantitatively measured sexual response. As part of their study, Masters and Johnson studied twenty males and eleven females over age sixty and made preliminary comparisons in sexual response between their young and old subjects.

Although the classic work of Masters and Johnson greatly expanded knowledge of human sexual response, their work on describing changes in sexual response in older men and women cannot be considered conclusive. Their data should not be used to generalize about elder sexuality because of their small sample size, scarcity of other corroborative research, effects of a laboratory setting on normal sexual response, and the unknown health status of participants. Despite the preliminary nature of their data, the results of Masters and Johnson's studies have been repeatedly cited as definitive. Until collaborating studies are reported, age-associated changes in sexual response are unknown.

Masters and Johnson identified four distinct phases of sexual response in both males and females: (1) excitement—the development and increase of sexual tension in response to stimulation, (2) plateau—sexual tension is intensified and subsequently reaches the extreme level, (3) orgasm—those few seconds of sexual release with primary focus on the pelvic area, and (4) resolution—the move from the height of orgasmic stimulation to the resting state. Among the twenty men over age sixty who were observed, sexual excitement developed more slowly, the intensity of penile sensation was lessened, and increased time and more direct stimulation were needed to achieve an erection when compared to younger men. The plateau period was longer in older men, allowing them to maintain an erection longer before the need to ejaculate. Often a full erection was not achieved until ejaculation was imminent. Ejaculatory force was reduced and orgasm intensity and length was shorter in older men. During orgasm, elder men also had fewer pelvic muscle contractions, diminished sexual flush, and less nipple and testes engorgement with arousal than younger subjects. After ejaculation, the erection subsided more rapidly, and a longer time was needed to achieve another erection. Older men also frequently went from the plateau phase to the resolution phase without ejaculation.

"Aging makes sex less imperative. You can take it or leave it, and that uncovers something that is precious. I can report that women look better to me now than they did when I was young because when I was young, sex was demanding. It was ego; I could be attracted to a woman that I despised, and then not feel good about myself. Now it seems possible to admire only women whom I like, which feels good. It feels cleaner and purer."

Abraham Maslow

Among the eleven older women observed, Masters and Johnson reported decreased vaginal lubrication and expansion with stimuli when compared to the younger women. However, nipple erection and clitoral responses to stimulation were no different than in younger women. Both the orgasmic and resolution phases were shorter in older women. However, the capacity to achieve orgasm, even multiple orgasms, did not change with age. Among the women in the sample who had intercourse at least twice weekly, age-associated changes in sexual response were reduced or absent. This finding of reduced age changes in women who were more sexually active has been confirmed by more recent research. Bachmann reported that among fifty-nine healthy women age sixty to seventy years, those who remained sexually active had increased vaginal lubrication, elasticity, and vaginal depth compared with those who were inactive.[12] Just as in other body systems, the "use it or lose it" phenomenon seems to play a role in sexual functioning.

SEXUALITY IN SPECIAL ELDER POPULATIONS

Although statistics can be helpful in gaining a general picture of elder sexuality, many ignore the sexual needs of special elder populations. This section will examine the sexual practices of older unmarried women, elder homosexuals, and institutionalized elders.

Older Unmarried Women

Women without spouses comprise a large proportion of the elder population and include the never-married, divorced, and widowed. Older women are less likely to have a male partner than women of other age groups. The fact that women live longer than men accounts for a great deal of this imbalance. Women outnumber men at all ages, and the gap widens with advancing age. There are eighty-four men for every 100 women between ages sixty-five to sixty-nine. But, by age eighty-five to eighty-nine, there are only forty-three men for every 100 women. Because women live longer than men and they usually marry older men, the probability of widowhood is high.

Older men are nearly twice as likely to be married as older women. There are almost four times as many older widows as widowers. African American women are even more likely to be widowed. The average age of widowhood in our country is fifty-nine. Because of this sex differential, older men are eight times more likely to remarry than older women, usually to younger women.

Societal attitudes are also responsible for the lack of male partners for older women. Older men are more likely to seek relationships with younger women than those their age or older. This has been attributed largely to our cultural attitude that a man's value is determined more by career or financial success, but a woman's value is determined by how young she looks rather than what she does. Although there are many advantages of older women–younger men relationships, the trend in that direction is not significant and is unlikely to affect those already in their later years.

As heterosexual relationships may not be a viable alternative for many older women, they may explore other avenues of sexual satisfaction to increase control of their sexuality. The alternatives include a range of physical and emotional expressions, such as expanding affectionate relationships with men and women, exploring sexual fantasy, erotic books and movies, and masturbation.

Elder Homosexuals

Because homosexuality is still unacceptable to many in our society, it is difficult to accurately estimate how many Americans are homosexual. Estimates also vary because of the difficulties in defining homosexuality—is one same-sex sexual contact enough to define someone as a homosexual? What about a married individual who prefers same-sex contact but is not currently engaged in it? What about those who enjoy sexual expression with both men and women? It is thought that the percentage of homosexuals in the older population is similar to that of younger age groups—about 10 percent. Because taboos against homosexuality

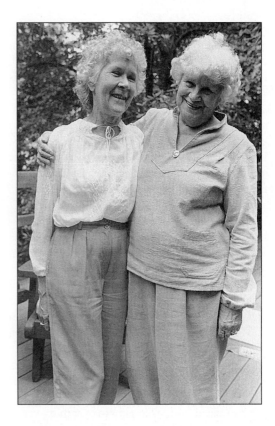

were stronger in the past, many older people are even less likely to identify themselves as gay or lesbian than their younger counterparts.

Prejudices and stereotypes about older gays (male homosexuals) and lesbians (female homosexuals) abound in our culture. The image of older lesbians is that they are a lonely, pathetic, and troubled group that somehow missed having a relationship with "a good man," "the right man," or just "any man."[13] For gay males, the stereotype persists that they are unhappy and have no close relationships. Although research on elder homosexuals is sparse, evidence is accumulating to dispute those stereotypes. However, most studies are limited by small sample size, nonrandom approach, and poor response rates. In addition, studies in this area are limited by cohort effects. Because there may be stark differences among generations and from year to year (depending on the societal climate toward gays and lesbians), results in one study are often not relevant to elders of other ages or studies conducted in different years. More large-scale research is needed to better define the changing needs of this segment of society.

In general, women's goals in intimate relationships are thought to be similar whether their partners are males or females. They look for personality, hygiene, intelligence, and manners. One researcher asserted that lesbian relationships resemble close friendships with the added component of romantic and erotic attraction.[14]

One study of mainly white middle-class lesbians conducted in the early 1980s, explored the lives of seventy-four lesbians over age fifty. Almost half had been married, and one-third had children; over half reported themselves to be in excellent mental health (only 2 percent felt unstable or unhappy). Lesbians in this sample were likely to practice serial monogamy—a series of long-term, committed relationships with other women throughout their lives. About three-fourths of the sample had five or fewer serious lovers in their lifetime. Almost half were currently in relationships that had lasted from six months to over thirty years; most had been in the same relationship for five years or more, and half had relationships that had lasted at least fifteen years. About one-third reported they had no sex partners within the past year, although a small proportion reported multiple partners.[13]

In a similar study of mostly college-educated lesbian women over age fifty in 1986 to 1988, Deevey reported that about 40 percent were formerly married, and 31 percent had children. Most reported excellent mental health. Almost all were still sexually active.[15] A later study reported that more than half of all lesbian women and gay men had children, and most reported high levels of life satisfaction.[16]

Research on elder gay men is also sparse. A large study questioned 112 highly educated homosexual men between the ages of forty and seventy-nine.[17] The men reported levels of life satisfaction comparable to older men and women in the general population. Three-fourths of the men were at least somewhat satisfied with their sex lives. Older gay men seemed less anxious about their sexual orientation when compared to younger gays. Most men in the study (86.6 percent) rated themselves as exclusively homosexual. Almost three-fourths of the men in Berger's study never married. Over 60 percent of homosexual men in the study lived with other people. Most lived only with their lovers, although combinations of lover, roommates, and family were reported. Most elder gay men in this study continued to engage in a high level of sexual activity. However, the group was very diverse. Over 60 percent engaged in same-sex relations at least once weekly; only 6 percent reported no sexual activity within the past six months. The number of same-sex partners reported within the past six months varied considerably. Although over half limited their activity to one partner, almost one-fourth reported three or more partners within the six-month period. Most were not currently in an exclusive relationship, but had been in the past. Older gays generally maintain their frequency of sexual activity through their later years, but with fewer partners than when young.[17]

Data on sexual activity from studies on gay men conducted in the early 1980s probably do not reflect their behavior in the 1990s. The advent of the HIV epidemic significantly impacted the gay male population in the United States and resulted in multiple health behavioral changes among older gay men. The focus of many relationships was shifted from sexual satisfaction to caregiving as an entire generation of men cared for friends and lovers who were dying of AIDS. Those who survived often dramatically changed their sexual practices—either reducing the number of partners or practicing safe sex. As a whole cohort of men lost their primary partners, more men practiced abstinence than before. Further, society as a whole became much more interested in the sexual practices of gay men, more studies were conducted, some prospective/longitudinal, to better characterize this population in order to target public health resources toward containing the AIDS epidemic.

The AIDS epidemic also affected the sensitivity of health and social service workers to the presence of gay and lesbian couples who demanded "family" status in visitation rights and health care decision making. Gay and lesbian couples encountered legal obstacles to obtaining these rights, and learned to complete advance directives, durable power of attorney for health care or finances, and other legal documents specifying their relationship and the rights of their partners. Many support groups emerged for gay partners involved in caregiving or dealing with the loss of their loved ones. In larger cities, a number of services for gay and lesbian elders have been initiated (e.g., services to homebound elderly gays, hospice programs, housing programs, and information and referral services). Although some agencies have initiated services specifically for elder homosexuals, other existing agencies (e.g., the YMCA and Senior Multipurpose Centers) have expanded their services to meet the needs of elder homosexuals.

The Gay and Lesbian Association of Retired Persons (10940 Wilshire Blvd, Suite 1600, Los Angeles, CA 90024, phone 310-966-1500) is an organization to assist older gays and lesbians with housing and other issues.

Institutionalized Elders

Institutionalized elders are often seen as asexual, and their needs for closeness, sexual release, and physical attractiveness are not considered. Staff often respond in a paternalistic way to the sexual behavior of elders in nursing homes and are uncomfortable when the institutionalized masturbate, flirt, or talk of sexual topics.[18] While it is true that most institutionalized elders report little interest in intercourse, a few are interested. A larger proportion are interested in other forms of sexual expression, such as caressing, kissing, masturbation, or improving their appearance. A study of institutionalized elders reported 91 percent of the respondents had neither masturbated nor had sexual intercourse in the month prior to the interview.[19] However, one-sixth of the inactive group reported that they would be interested, but lacked the opportunity (e.g., had no willing or desirable partner or lacked privacy). A more recent study on male nursing home residents with good mental function found that half of the sixty-one men interviewed had sexual partners. During at-home visiting periods, 17 percent had sexual intercourse with their partners at least once a month, and 73 percent engaged in hugging, kissing, and other sexual behavior. The majority of sexually active men said they felt sexually satisfied. However, most sexually inactive men without partners also said they were sexually satisfied, perhaps because of their lower expectations or masturbatory practices.[20]

It is unrealistic to expect that all, or even most, institutionalized elders have the interest or capacity for genital sexuality. The majority of the residents have a number of serious disabling illnesses and treatments that impact their sexuality. Most are more concerned with the day-to-day living, eating, and body care than sexual thoughts. It is important to remember, however, that not all nursing home residents are permanent—some will recuperate and will return to their homes. Nevertheless, more institutionalized elders might participate in a broader range of sexual activity if provided with a supportive environment.

Regardless of age, keeping up one's appearance is a strong contributor to feeling attractive and sexual. This need continues in the later years, whether sick or well. Nursing home residents report that remaining physically attractive is the most important and acceptable way for them to express their sexuality. Institutionalized women unanimously report they felt unattractive to the opposite sex.[19] It is important to assist nursing home residents to be clean and well-dressed, with attention to face, hair, nails, and skin so they can maintain their feelings of sexual attractiveness and sexual identity. This may be especially important for older women.

The nursing home setting itself can deprive elders of their sexual rights. Lack of privacy commonly influences sexual activity in nursing homes.

Few places offer privacy for married couples, and even fewer attend to the needs of the unmarried. Privacy is created in some homes by setting aside a room in the facility for couples. Privacy can also be increased by allowing the doors of residents' rooms to be closed and by lifting restrictions on personal visits. Segregation of men and women residents by wings or floors reduces the amount and kinds of sexual expression among residents. One study reported that in one nursing home when men and women were no longer isolated from one another, the residents became more socially adjusted, improved their grooming, reduced their use of profanity, and increased sexual relations and contact between the sexes.[21]

The attitude of nursing home staff toward elder sexuality has a strong influence upon sexual expression among the residents. Even though staff may voice their acceptance of elder sexual expression, their actions may not be as supportive. Staff may help meet elders' sexual needs in a number of ways. Perhaps the most important is to touch elders gently and with affection when accomplishing daily tasks of moving, transferring, and bathing. Providing opportunities for both sexes to mingle, discussing with families the sexual needs of their older rela-

They'd Never Tell
Laura Goodwin, R.N.

He came to her every Wednesday,
after he had his tub bath, with his best black suit on
   that the nurse's aides had helped him with,
his hair all slicked back (the few strands he had left
   which encircled his head like a halo),
he shuffled over to her room in his oversized thick-
   soled shoes,
a big smile on his face.

She, in turn, was waiting for him in her room,
her hair all freshly done in a beehive by the beauty
   parlor,
with her best pink dress on,
sitting in her easy chair with a smile on her face, too.

She was allowed to have eight ounces of whiskey at
   bedtime,
which, after the nurse gave it to her, she kept on her
   bedside table,
waiting for their meeting.

She had asked the administrator of our nursing home
   for a double bed,
when he refused, we nurses pushed both of the twin
   beds together in her room,
after he went home for the day.

He would look back and forth before he knocked on
   her door,
and she would make him wait for a few seconds
   before she said,
"Who is it?,"
As if she didn't know.
When he replied, she let him in.

The nurses always placed an invisible "Do not disturb" sign on the door.

He always left at seven a.m.,
blew a kiss to her, and said, "I love you."
She always said, "I love you too."

The nurses then would all hurry up to rearrange the
   room,
before the administrator got in for the day,
giggling with excitement the whole time at our
   deception.
None of us would ever tell.

Now they are both just memories I carry with me,
happy memories that make me smile,
and I wonder if someday I'll be living in a nursing
   home,
and need someone not to tell.

tives, and allowing privacy for sexual activities, either alone or as a couple, can be effective. Educating the staff can alter negative attitudes toward sexuality and aging.[22]

THE EFFECT OF CHRONIC ILLNESS ON SEXUALITY

Sexuality may be compromised by physical problems accompanying chronic disease or by psychological reactions to being ill. Some symptoms associated with chronic illness can cause discomfort during intercourse. Skeletal pain, angina pain, or breathing difficulty during intercourse tends to make the individual hesitant about the sexual act. Chronic illness also has a significant emotional component. The illness may cause an individual to feel tired, depressed, and uninterested in sexual activity. Furthermore, chronic illness may alter personal appearance, which may affect body image and self-esteem. However, intercourse can provide intimacy and relaxation, reduce isolation and depression, take attention from physical problems, and help the person to feel "normal." The degree to which chronic illness affects sexual capacity and interest is highly dependent upon the extent of disability, and the elder's coping skills, attitude towards sexuality, and motivation for sexual activity.

Couples vary in their support for one another during periods of illness and disability. The degree that they accept changes in sexual activity is related to the strength and previous communication patterns of the marriage. The well partner may lose sexual interest because of concern of causing more pain to the mate, lack of interest by the ill partner, or fear of contracting the disease. Chronic illness also promotes dependence. If the ill person was traditionally the initiator of sexual activity, subsequent sexual activity may be affected. Those who work with older people need to be cognizant of the effects of various diseases upon sexuality.

Certain general guidelines are helpful in maximizing sexual activity among elders with chronic illness. Changing medications or reducing the dosages of those medicines that affect sexual performance should be considered if possible. Medications can be prescribed to reduce symptoms associated with sexual activity (e.g., medications for joint pain in a patient with arthritis or nitroglycerine in a patient with chest pain). Elders can be counseled on alternative sexual positions or alternative means of sexual expression. Although such information should be shared with the patient and partner, it is seldom offered.

Selected chronic illnesses that have a significant impact on elders' sexuality follow. Although not discussed, other diseases and conditions such as obesity, arthritis, and lower back pain may also be significant.

Heart Disease

Elders who have had a heart attack are often cautious about resuming intercourse because they have the misconception that sexual activity will bring upon another heart attack. Whether emotionally or physiologically based, a number of studies report that up to 75 percent of couples significantly decrease or eliminate intercourse after the husband experiences a heart attack. The most commonly reported reason for reduced sexual activity is decreased ability and lowered satisfaction. It is not clear whether the decrease in performance and interest is due to drugs, organic problems, or psychosocial considerations. When the heart attack is accompanied by smoking, the likelihood of impotence increases significantly. In studies of women, heart attacks cause a similarly reduced level of sexual activity and fear of resuming sexual activity.

Despite the fears of those who have had a heart attack, the physical demands of intercourse are minimal, and sexual activity may be both physically and psychologically beneficial: it reduces tension, aids sleep, increases self-esteem and self-image, and is an enjoyable, low-level physical activity that serves to normalize their lives. The physical demands of intercourse are no greater than walking around the block or up a staircase and can be resumed eight to twelve weeks after a heart attack. Intercourse can be assumed to be safe if

Sexuality and Parkinson's: A Spouse's View

In any relationship between a man and a woman, whether there is a disability or perfect health, there is a need for loving, caring, and sharing, and what more perfect way is there than through our sexuality?

As in all aspects of our life together, I have learned to accommodate Sid's parkinsonism, just as he has, and to make the necessary adjustments. But I have never given up on showing my love for him, either by voice, touch, or in our sexual relationship.

When Sid and I first started dating, his parkinsonism was already well advanced, but somehow it didn't prevent our love for one another from growing and ripening into a lifetime commitment to one another. From the very beginning, I realized that there would have to be careful timing and flexibility on my part to respond to the moment. I learned to adjust to sexual experiences at any hour of the day and in any part of the house. Instead of making it awkward and embarrassing, it made it more exciting. I learned that sometimes I would need to be the aggressor. I found it fun to dress in very feminine attire and to make myself as attractive as possible with makeup and scent. Sid's appreciation makes it worth the effort.

Each of us brings to a relationship all of the feelings and attitudes we have developed over the years of our lives. Sometimes these include some myths and misconceptions. Included is the myth that sexuality and feelings of love are for the young and beautiful people as portrayed by the mass media.

Another misconception is that disabled people can't and shouldn't have a full and satisfying sexual life. Neither of these wrong ideas should be perpetuated by the parkinsonian or the spouse.

In coping with a chronic illness, there is a delicate balancing act of adequate rest, exercise, diet, positive emotions, controlling of stress, and, most important of all, giving and accepting love. I have found that there is no more satisfying way of giving and accepting love than through sexual expression. This doesn't necessarily mean that you have to experience a mutual orgasm. It can be cuddling and fondling as a daily routine. One of my favorite times of the day is our afternoon rest period when cuddling is an important part. Sometimes it leads to a relaxed nap, and other times it can result in a fuller sexual expression.

Even when the sex act can't be completed, we both gain a sense of being loved and secure in the knowledge that the next time will be better. I have found it elating to realize that sex doesn't have to cease to exist as one grows older and has to deal with health problems. In fact, it can be the best time of your life. You certainly have more freedom when you are older, and there are fewer distractions and interruptions.

If you have the right attitude, the sexual relationship with your Parkinson partner can become one of the most rewarding in your life.

Reprinted from *Patient Perspectives on Parkinson's* by Sid and Donna Dorras, 1997. National Parkinson Foundation.

the individual passes an exercise treadmill test. Although it is true that sexual activity can trigger a heart attack, the risk is extremely low (less than twenty chances in a million in those with heart disease) and is reduced further in those who get regular physical exercise.[23] Since masturbation is less taxing, one investigator suggests that this activity substitute for sexual activity soon after the attack until intercourse can be resumed.[24] If chest pain usually occurs during intercourse, physicians generally prescribe nitroglycerine to be taken immediately before sexual intercourse.

Perhaps the greatest contributor to diminished sexual activity after a heart attack is inadequate information. Those who had a recent heart attack are frightened and are very motivated to "follow doctor's orders" in diet and activity programs for recovery. However, they seldom receive information on sexual activity from their physicians, and are hesitant to bring up their questions in this area. Studies indicate that up to four-fifths of male heart attack patients receive no sexual information from their physicians. In one study of female patients, almost half received no information. Further, any discussions between the patient and the physician are more likely to be initiated by the patient.[25]

Hypertension

Hypertension can accelerate atherosclerosis and increase incidence of vascular erectile dysfunction. Although many elders who are hypertensive are impotent, most are not impotent from the disease but rather from the medications used to treat it. Thiazide diuretics are the most commonly prescribed drugs used to treat high blood pressure because they are inexpensive and safe and cause few side effects. However, complaints of decreased desire, difficulty in maintaining an erection, and difficulty with ejaculation are common among those who take diuretics. But, all side effects could be reduced by using lower doses of the diuretics. Beta blockers most often reduce sexual performance; newer drugs or lower dosages are less likely to cause problems. Alterations in drug prescription or reduction in drug dosages should be considered.

A high level of total blood cholesterol and a low level of "good" cholesterol or HDL is associated with an increased risk of erectile dysfunction in men. It is believed to be due to the narrowing of the blood vessels of the penis from cholesterol deposits (atherosclerosis).[26] In addition, some medications used to treat elevated cholesterol may reduce sexual functioning.

Cancer

The effect of cancer upon sexual interest and function depends on the location and extent of the cancer as well as the type of treatment. Sexual interest and activity may be impaired because of the patient's physiological reactions to the cancer or treatment, such as nausea from chemotherapy, incision pain, and fatigue, or because of psychological factors—depression, fear of death or disfigurement, or fear of losing one's spouse.

The importance of sex in a person's life should be considered in the decision regarding the type of therapy to be prescribed. For instance, radiation treatment for prostate cancer for a sexually active man may be more desirable than a prostectomy, not because of success rate, but the latter may significantly affect his ability to perform sexually.

Although being able to be sexual after cancer treatment is an important part of the recovery process, partners of those with cancer may worry whether their partners are well enough for sexual activity or they may be uncomfortable with their lover's altered appearance. Furthermore, the well partner may fear that the cancer is contagious or feel guilty about having sexual interest since the ill partner may feel sick or depressed. Also, couples may not have privacy for sexual expression when one partner is hospitalized. While sexual activity may have to be put on hold temporarily, restoring a sex life is a key part to feeling healthy and normal again.

Both those with cancer and their partners need support and education to better understand the effect of the disease and its treatment on sexuality. Physicians rarely discuss sexual performance with their cancer patients, either before or after surgery. It is important that a physician discuss the effects of radiation and chemotherapy on sexual desire and performance, tips on lovemaking after therapy, and how to deal with the feelings of seeing a partner with a surgically altered body.[27] Self-help groups are excellent ways for those with cancer to share information and gain support for sexual concerns. The American Cancer Society has initiated self-help groups for those who have undergone mastectomies or ostomies. Cancer treatments have a significant effect on elder sexuality and will be discussed under "Surgery" in the next section.

Diabetes

Diabetes, especially type I or juvenile-onset diabetes, is the most common organic cause of erectile dysfunction, and the proportion of older diabetics who are impotent increases with advancing age. Studies report as many as three-fourths of insulin-dependent diabetic males become impotent as their disease progresses. Impotence can occur in those with type II (adult-onset) diabetes as well. In both cases, ten to twenty years of the disease usually precede erectile dysfunction. Researchers generally agree that the dysfunction is caused by destruction of the nerves that open the penile arteries to permit the blood to enter. Although erectile function is lost, sensation, orgasm, and ejaculation may remain unaffected. Among diabetic males, the loss of erectile function may be more threatening than blindness or the loss of a lower extremity, which may also accompany diabetes.

Tight diet and drug control can reduce the risk of erectile dysfunction in both type I and type II diabetics. A diabetic should be screened carefully to determine if impotence is drug-induced or due to other physiological or psychological causes. If impotence occurs even when diabetes is controlled, the chance of recovery is unlikely, and penile implants may be considered.

Few studies have been conducted on the sexual problems of diabetic women, perhaps because women can still participate in sexual intercourse even when nonorgasmic. Some experts believe that the sexual problems of diabetic women are underdiagnosed as a result. The main complaint of diabetic women is insufficient lubrication, and consequently, painful intercourse.

Arthritis

Arthritis may make sexual activity painful or more difficult because of joint stiffness. As in other chronic conditions, elders need education and counseling to cope with the sexual consequences of arthritis. Education should include a discussion of alternative sexual positions to reduce pain, varied forms of lovemaking, the value of a warm bath and analgesics before sexual activity, and plans for sexual activity during times when pain levels are low. Those with hip replacements need special advice on when intercourse can be resumed and which positions decrease danger of dislocation.

OTHER FACTORS INFLUENCING SEXUAL FUNCTION

Sexual function can be profoundly influenced by a number of factors other than chronic illness: medication, alcohol and tobacco use, surgery, extended sexual inactivity, and psychosocial variables. This section will discuss the effects of these variables upon sexual interest and activity in the later years.

Medications

Elders take a greater proportion of prescription drugs than any other age group, and these medications, in combination with cognitive deficits and disease, can cause or aggravate sexual difficulties.[28] It is estimated that a significant proportion of sexual dysfunction can be attributed to medication use.[29] Over-the-counter medications can also affect sexual drive or performance among both men and women. The adverse reaction of a drug upon sexuality depends on the dose, duration of therapy, other drugs taken at the same time, psychological factors, and the state of the circulatory, hormonal, and nervous systems. Drugs can interfere with nerve or blood vessel function, dry out mucous membranes, or affect sex hormone levels. The patient should be educated about possible alterations in sexual function and, if the side effects are unacceptable, alternative therapy should be considered. Sexual dysfunction may cause an individual to stop taking a necessary medication, sometimes without consulting the physician.

Alcohol and Tobacco

Alcohol has a negative effect on sexual potency in both men and women. The validity of Shakespeare's words, "[alcohol] provokes the desire, but takes away the performance," is well-documented. Although low blood levels of alcohol may accelerate sexual arousal by reducing inhibitions, increased blood alcohol levels diminish performance. The use of alcohol over the long term can cause problems with vascular insufficiency— insufficient blood supply to the organs. This has a significant effect on the ability to achieve and maintain an erection. There is also decreased nerve sensitivity that varies with the individual. In men, excessive alcohol ingestion can cause temporary impotence, and long-term abuse causes irreversible loss of erectile function, even if drinking is stopped. About three-fourths of alcoholic men are impotent. Chronic alcohol use has been documented to cause reduced testosterone levels and reduced testicular size.[30] Alcoholism is the most common cause of impotence among men in their middle years. Women alcoholics also suffer from decreased libido and have difficulty achieving orgasm.

Long-term smoking causes an impeded blood flow to the organs, primarily because of the development of atherosclerosis in the vessels, including those in the penis. Preliminary studies suggest a higher rate of impotence among smokers.[31] In the Massachusetts Male Aging Study, it was found that smoking combined with heart disease resulted in a high incidence of impotence. Heart patients who smoked were almost three times as likely to suffer total impotence as heart patients who didn't smoke.[32] Although there is improvement when smoking is stopped, some of the damage may be irreversible.[33]

Surgery

Whether surgery causes sexual dysfunction depends upon the extent of nerve and blood vessel destruction in the genital area. Although all pelvic surgery is associated with an increased risk of impotence or other sexual dysfunction, some operations are more destructive than others. Additionally, there is a psychological component to postoperative sexual problems.

In men, prostate cancer surgery is the most common pelvic surgery affecting erectile function. Many of the treatments of prostate cancer (e.g., radiation, testosterone-blocking medications, castration, or prostatic removal) carry a risk of sexual dysfunction. Castration (removal of the testes), the most radical treatment, causes significant impairment of sexual desire and erectile capacity. Furthermore, castrated men commonly report their partners to be less sexually responsive after the operation, indicating that the change in body image may also have a great effect.[34] Testicular prostheses are available to normalize appearance after castration.

Radical prostatectomy, when the prostate gland is removed through the abdomen, commonly caused impotence in the past. Newer methods that attempt to save the major nerves in the area have substantially increased the chances of continued erectile function. Even if erection capacity is lost, penile sensation and ability to reach orgasm will usually be unimpaired, although there may be a decrease in orgasm intensity.

Another common surgery, the transurethral resection procedure (TURP), is performed to reduce the effect of the enlarged prostate on urinary function. The procedure, which is much more common than the radical prostatectomy, removes portions of the prostate gland through the urethra so that urinary flow can be increased. The TURP is also much less likely to affect erectile capability. However, after the operation, about half the men will no longer ejaculate outside the body; the ejaculate flows into the bladder to be excreted during urination (called retrograde ejaculation). If men are thoroughly educated about the changes in sexual function expected with surgery, the incidence of erectile dysfunction is reduced.

Another type of pelvic surgery that may affect sexual function in males is removal of the bladder. The percentage of sexual impairment caused by this surgery is similar to radical prostatectomy.

Among women, pelvic surgery can also affect sexual function. A hysterectomy, or removal of the uterus, is the second most common operation performed on women (cesareans are first). Data on the effect of hysterectomies upon sexual interest and activity are conflicting. Some studies indicate that a hysterectomy results in no change or an increase in sexual response, while others reveal a significant number of women who report diminished desire or lack of orgasm. It is difficult to study how much of the change is due to physiological causes and how much is psychological. The chances of sexual dysfunction seem to increase when the ovaries are also removed, probably due to a decrease of estrogen and consequent thinning and drying of the vaginal wall. After a hysterectomy, the physical changes resulting from surgery may reduce sexual pleasure by increasing vaginal dryness and pain during intercourse, and decreasing genital sensation.

Some hypothesize that the uterus plays an important role in orgasm; its rhythmic contractions enhance orgasm, and the pressure of the penis against the cervix is one trigger for orgasm. On the other hand, many assert that sexual dissatisfaction may have been present before the operation. Education and counseling have been reported to prevent potential psychosexual problems.[35]

Psychological effects are common after a woman has a mastectomy. The breast is a symbol of femininity in our culture and is a significant part of a woman's sexual identity. The loss of a breast may alter a woman's sex role, sexual image, and sexual relationships. Reduced sexual activity and orgasms are reported consequences of mastectomy. However, older women generally rate their sexual adjustment after mastectomy more positively than younger women.

The sexual interest of both men and women can be affected by the creation of an artificial opening (stoma) in the abdominal wall. In general, these openings are created to reroute the excretion of urine or feces due to obstruction, inflammation, or cancer. Multiple types of stomas are possible.

Other openings may be created to provide an avenue for artificial feeding—for example, a tube is placed through the abdomen into the stomach to allow feedings when a person cannot eat due to throat cancer. Adjustment to a stoma can cause anxiety, alteration in body image, and anxiety about leakage or odor, all which can impact sexual

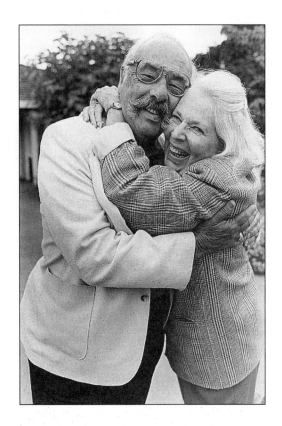

interest and desire in the patient or partner. Specialized nurses can assist in stoma management, and support groups are available to help their adjustment.

Widower's or Widow's Syndrome

If an older man attempts sexual intercourse after being sexually inactive for a year or more, he may be unable to achieve an erection. This phenomenon is called the widower's syndrome. The initial trauma of impotence may become chronic unless the man has a sensitive partner or therapy is initiated. A similar phenomenon may occur in older women, called the widow's syndrome.[36] A year or more of abstinence from sexual activity may reduce the elasticity of vaginal walls and reduce the production of vaginal lubrication. Normal vaginal function usually returns within six weeks to three months after resumption of sexual activity. Masturbation reduces the likelihood of these syndromes.

Psychosocial Considerations

Sexual difficulties at any age are likely combinations of biologic, attitudinal, and situational problems. Just as in other age groups, sexuality of elder men and women is highly influenced by their psychosocial adjustment and health. The quality of the relationship is one of the most crucial aspects influencing desire and satisfaction with sexuality.[37] Many long-term couples have unresolved resentments, anger, and stereotypical patterns of communication or sexual intimacy that impact their ability to adjust their sexual routine to changing physical or emotional circumstances. Although the media is saturated these days with talk about improving communication and fulfillment in marriage and relationships, today's elders grew up in a time when this was not so. They more often believed that marriage was "for life," whether the couple was compatible or not, and they had more rigid sex roles. It is likely that they focused more on the day-to-day tasks of raising a family and earning a living than on improving their communication or maximizing their sexual inventiveness. Despite a lifetime of marriage and sexual activity, they may not have the strong communication skills needed to adjust to the changes that accompany aging.

Just as in other age groups, elders are influenced by the societal attitude that older people are not masculine or feminine, but neuter, or asexual. As we grow older, if we are not recognized as masculine or feminine, a degree of self-identity is lost.

If an older woman accepts the widely held belief that a youthful and firm body is necessary for sexual attractiveness, she will be less likely to initiate or encourage sexual interaction, feeling that she doesn't measure up. Similarly, older men are victimized by the emphasis on physical performance. They may focus on the act of ejaculation itself rather than a range of sexual expression. They may judge their sexual adequacy by comparing the frequency of intercourse, the rapidity in attaining an erection, and the firmness of their erection with their performance in their younger years. Focusing upon the decrements are likely to set up a vicious cycle of impotence and strained relationships.

SEXUAL DYSFUNCTION

Sexual dysfunction is a physiological impairment in sexual response that prevents sexual arousal or orgasm. Sexual dysfunction is not a normal accompaniment to old age. However, sexual dysfunction is more common among elders because they use more prescription drugs and have more illnesses that affect desire and performance. Although some sexual problems can be easily reversed, others cannot. Lack of sexual interest and enjoyment may occur in either sex. It is considered a dysfunction to be treated only if it is seen as a problem by the individual or the partner.

The most common sexual dysfunction for men is erectile dysfunction (commonly called impotence), or the persistent inability to achieve or maintain an erection sufficient for satisfactory sexual performance. Occasional failure to achieve or sustain an erection is normal for men of all ages and does not qualify as erectile dysfunction. Men with erectile dysfunction may maintain sexual desire and even the capacity to reach orgasm. Four factors are needed for potency: normal male sexual organs, normal levels of testosterone and other hormones, an adequate nerve and blood supply to the penis, and a healthy psyche. Any one missing factor may result in partial or complete erectile dysfunction.

Studies vary widely in the extent of erectile dysfunction in the population. It is common for men to report more difficulty with erections with advancing age. Studies report that from one-half to three-fourths or more of elderly men have some erectile difficulties at least some of the time.[37] In the Massachusetts Male Aging Study of men ages forty to seventy, 52 percent were impotent, with the number of those with complete impotence tripling from forty (5 percent) to seventy (15 percent).[32] Other experts estimate that about 40 percent of men are impotent by eighty. Because of the sensitivity of the subject, differences in definitions of impotence, and the fact that most samples consist of elders with medical problems, these figures may not accurately reflect the prevalence of impotence among older men.

Contrary to popular belief, 80 to 90 percent of all erectile dysfunction is due to a physical problem, and only about 10 percent is psychogenic.[38,39] Psychologically based dysfunction may be intermittent, it often has a sudden onset, and erections are occasionally attained. In contrast, the problem is likely to be of organic origin if it progressively worsens, and a decrease in erections in the early morning and during sleep is noted. Approximately half the cases of impotence are reversible or treatable. The most common causes of impotence among elderly men are due to damage to the nerves and blood vessels from diabetes and atherosclerosis.[40] See table 6.1 for an overview of the possible causes of erectile dysfunction.

Fears regarding erectile dysfunction can be debilitating to both partners, and fear itself can impede sexual satisfaction. In some cases, a vicious cycle is initiated whereby the couple is trapped in a pattern of fearing impotence, which decreases the quality of the sexual interaction. In turn, this results in higher rates of erectile dysfunction, which can cause irritability, insecurity, blaming, and more fear, further decreasing sexual interaction and satisfaction.

Premature ejaculation is another sexual dysfunction that may occur in elder males. It is generally psychological in origin. Although it is more common in young, inexperienced males, premature ejaculation may also accompany a new relationship in later life.

Women also suffer from sexual problems that impair their enjoyment of sexual intercourse. Dyspareunia (pain during intercourse) may be due to reduced lubrication and elasticity of the vagina or a local infection that causes painful uterine contractions during orgasm. A related disorder is

TABLE 6.1	Possible Causes of Erectile Dysfunction

ENDOCRINE

Diabetes
High estrogen
Low testosterone

BEHAVIORAL

Alcohol use
Marijuana, other illicit drug use
Tobacco use
Prescription drug use

NEUROLOGICAL

Stroke (including TIAs)
Parkinson's disease
Alzheimer's disease
Multiple sclerosis
Neuropathy
Spinal cord injury

VASCULAR

Atherosclerosis
Coronary bypass surgery
High total cholesterol and low HDL

PENIS

Trauma
Peyronie's disease

PROSTATE

Prostate cancer surgery and radiation
Prostatitis

PSYCHOLOGICAL

Anxiety
Depression
Marital discord
Stress

(Adapted from Ackerman, Montague, Morganstern, 1994 p. 32.)

vaginismus, the involuntary constriction of the lower third of the vaginal muscles when intercourse is attempted. Vaginismus may be due to the woman involuntarily trying to protect herself from painful stimulation associated with intercourse. *Primary orgasmic dysfunction* implies that a woman has never been able to achieve an orgasm through intercourse or masturbation. In contrast, *situational orgasmic dysfunction* is the inability to reach orgasm consistently enough to satisfy self and partner.

Unlike primary orgasmic dysfunction, situational orgasmic dysfunction infers the woman has achieved orgasms in the past. Experts generally believe situational dysfunction to be psychologically based. Lack of knowledge and sensitivity of the partner may play a role. There is very little research on the diagnosis and causes of sexual dysfunctions in women. Some studies suggest that sexual dysfunctions are relatively common among women; one study found over half had admitted to sexual difficultiies when asked by the clinician.[41]

Diagnosis of Sexual Dysfunction

Elders are often reluctant to volunteer information regarding sexual behavior to a physician, but are more likely to need help than younger clients. They may consider their problems to be due to the normal aging process, minimize the importance of their sexual needs and desires, or be embarrassed to broach the topic. To make matters worse, health professionals may lack training in taking a sexual history or feel there is a lack of time, may be uncomfortable initiating discussions with a person who is older than themselves, or have inadequate knowledge of the sexual needs of the chronically ill.

When physicians do ask patients if a sexual problem exists, many will volunteer significant concerns. In one study, only six of the forty men suffering from impotence raised the problem to their physician. However, twenty of those who were impotent were interested in receiving treatment for their problem when asked.[42]

The following considerations have been suggested as important in taking a sexual history from elders:[43]

Assure a private interview space,

Allow adequate time,

Pay attention to responses,

Project a nonjudgmental, unassuming attitude,

Use lay language, simple descriptions, and diagrams,

Use open-ended questions,

Do not hurry the interview.

Diagnosis of sexual dysfunction, similar to that of other diagnosis, requires thorough medical history (including psychosocial factors), physical examination, and laboratory testing to pinpoint the cause of the problem and to help select an effective treatment. The medical history should include a thorough listing of diseases and their treatment, family disease history, alcohol and prescription drug intake, and a sexual history.

A sexual history gathers information to aid in diagnosis and can serve as a vehicle for patient education. Often in conducting the sexual history, the practitioner can uncover misconceptions or misinformation about sexuality that serve as the basis for sexual disatisfaction. Additionally, the practitioner can use this opportunity to discuss the impact of drugs or illness on sexual function. A sexual history includes the following:

- frequency, duration, and turgidity of erections,
- number and gender of sexual partners,
- desired level of sexual activity,
- satisfaction with frequency and variety of sexual activity,
- quality of erection, ejaculation, and orgasm,
- history of present relationship with partner,
- level of communication with partner about sexual matters,
- use of alcohol or other recreational drugs,
- physical demands of intercourse,
- social situation, including other life stressers,
- how illness affects sexuality (desire, attitude, and activity),
- presence of pain during sexual activity (genital or other),
- practice of safe sex.

Information obtained from the sexual history can be combined with physical examination findings and diagnostic tests to determine the cause of erectile dysfunction or other sexual difficulties.

A physical examination is important to uncover possible contributors to sexual problems. For instance, a pelvic examination can uncover the presence of vaginal infections or atrophic vaginitis (a condition resulting from low levels of estrogen), which can be the root of the problem.

Laboratory evaluations, including measurement of hormones, cholesterol level, blood pressure, and liver function tests can be important in identifying contributing causes for sexual dysfunction. If the doctor suspects problems in the blood supply to the penis, the blood vessels in the penis can be evaluated by ultrasound or arteriography techniques (where dye is injected into blood vessels and an X-ray is taken). Taking a penile blood pressure can help evaluate impotence; a low penile blood pressure is associated with vascular disease and an increased risk of heart attack or stroke. Other diagnostic tests include intrapenile injections and nerve conduction studies. The American Foundation for Urologic Disease has launched a toll-free hotline to dispense free information on impotence (1-800-473-0616).

Treatment of Sexual Dysfunction

Depending on its origin, a sexual dysfunction can be treated in a variety of ways. Many medical conditions and prescription drugs can cause sexual dysfunction, and treating the medical problem or changing the medication type or dosages may be all that is needed to remedy the problem. When a sexual dysfunction is psychological in origin, the patient and partner are generally referred to a sex therapist. If the problem is due to chronic illness or a hormone deficiency, drugs, injections, or implants might be prescribed. If erectile dysfunction is caused by a problem with the veins or arteries in the penis, surgery can be performed.

The health professional should understand that not all elders want their sexual problems treated. One study showed almost one-half of the men who reported impotence declined to have the problem examined. These men tended to be older and sicker than the rest of the sample.[42]

The overwhelming majority of treatments for sexual dysfunction focus on restoring male erectile function, even though a significant proportion of women cannot reach orgasm. Is it because most researchers are men, and impotence is of greater interest to them? Or, is it because women can participate in the sex act and satisfy men without excitement and orgasm? Are data on women more difficult to gather? Medical treatments to restore sexual functioning are discussed in the following paragraphs. Sex education and counseling, mentioned in the next section, are also appropriate treatments.

Medications and Hormones

The search for aphrodisiacs is probably as old as civilization itself. Oysters, chocolate, ginseng, rhino horns, and Spanish fly are only a few of the many potions claiming to enhance sexual desire. However, they are not without risk. Spanish fly, made from a species of European beetle, is perhaps the most dangerous. It irritates the urinary tract as it leaves the body, causing blood to rush to the sex organs. It is a poison that can burn, leading to scarring, infections, and even death. Preliminary studies suggest that yohimbine, synthesized from a tree in West Africa, may increase sexual desire and erectile capability; however, the medication is most effective in psychogenic impotence.[28]

By far the most talked about medication is the pill that came on the market in 1998, Viagra (sildenafil). In order to understand how Viagra works, it is necessary to know the mechanism of a normal erection. An erection begins in the brain when a stimulus (vision, touch, smell, even a thought) stimulates a particular set of nerves that send messages down the spinal cord, around the prostate gland, and into the penis, where they direct cells to produce a chemical called cyclic GMP. The chemical relaxes muscles in two spongy cylinders of the penis, allowing them to fill with blood, ultimately stiffening the penis. The expanding spongy tissue then squeezes veins that normally drain blood from the penis, trapping the blood inside. Viagra works by blocking the enzyme that breaks down the cyclic GMP. As a result, the cyclic GMP accumulates in the penis and gradually results in an erection.

Although Viagra doesn't work for everyone, research confirms it is an effective treatment for many men with erectile dysfunction. One study confirmed its effectiveness on two-thirds of the subjects' attempts at intercourse.[44] However, the study excluded men with various common medical conditions (high blood pressure, peptic ulcer disease, angina, or alcohol abuse) and those using

Patients Clamor for Impotence Drug; Supply Can't Meet Demand

New York (AP)—Duke University Medical School urologist Craig Donatucci has given up answering calls on the new pill for impotence.

Patients asking about Pfizer Inc.'s drug, Viagra, now get a recorded message: "because of the volume of patient calls for Viagra, Dr. Donatucci is unable to take phone calls concerning this new drug."

Although the drug started hitting pharmacy shelves earlier this month, many druggists haven't gotten their first shipment and doctors are still evaluating the latest impotence treatment. But patients aren't waiting to get in line.

Viagra captured a whopping 79 percent of the market from rival impotence drugs during its second week of sales, through April 10, according to IMS America, a research information company that reported the figures April 20.

The drug had 5 percent of the market during limited availability the previous week.

The drug's popularity more than doubled the total number of impotence prescriptions patients filled in the United States, from a total of 20,106 in the week ended April 3 to 54,000 in the week ended April 10.

Atlanta urologist John Stripling wore out his hand writing 500 prescriptions in two weeks. Now he's using a rubber stamp to prescribe the pill.

"I've never seen such interest in a prescription drug in all of my years of medicine," said Sterling, who had 300 people waiting for the drug to become available and is getting 25 calls a day from interested patients.

Donatucci said he's written 150 prescriptions and is scheduling appointments for those who get his message.

Doctors and drug industry analysts expect Viagra to eclipse competing impotence nostrums within months.

The drug owes its popularity less to what it does than to what it doesn't do: make strong men wince. Existing impotence drugs must be either injected into the penis or inserted into the urinary tract.

Two men in five have problems getting an erection at age 40. Nearly 7 do at age 70. Pfizer estimates the number of men coping with impotence worldwide at 140 million.

The drug should bring Pfizer $300 million in sales during the rest of the year, said Mariola Hagger, an analyst with Deutsche-Morgan Grenfell. Many analysts expect it to bring in more than $1 billion in annual sales after 2000.

"It doesn't make you 21 again, but it does solve the problem," said Robert W. Shay, a 70-year old Los Angeles resident who took part in clinical trials of the drug from 1996 to 1997.

Shay, who used to take performance-boosting injections, said Viagra works about as well as the shots but is less painful.

The drug was originally intended as a treatment for angina. It was supposed to increase blood flow to the heart. But the rush of blood filled another organ instead. Pfizer decided that one man's side-effect was another man's cure and developed it as an impotence treatment.

Unlike the injections, which can leave the user erect for an hour without outside stimulation, Viagra allows the user to react normally to sexual stimulation.

Some doctors say they're worried that sexually potent men will use the drug as a performance booster—a kind of sexual steroid. A 52-year-old Viagra user in Atlanta who spoke on condition of anonymity said that's what he'd do if he didn't already need Viagra.

"If I was 16 or 17 and I could get hold of the stuff, I would," he said.

—Chico Enterprise Record, April 26, 1998, p. 5B.

aspirin or any other nonsteroidal anti-inflammatory drugs and blood thinners. Viagra does not work as well as injections or suppositories but is more comfortable and easier to use.

There are many caveats to the use of Viagra. First, the pill should be taken one hour before an erection is desired. Also, it is not an aphrodisiac: it doesn't increase sex drive and works only when a man is sexually stimulated. And the side effects may be significant: headaches, upset stomach, and vision abnormalities. Further, the drug is incompatible with nitrate drugs commonly used for heart problems. Both Viagra and nitrate drugs lower blood pressure: combining the two drugs causes blood pressure to drop dangerously low.

The Public Health Research Group is concerned that the drug hasn't been researched sufficiently, especially with those with heart and circulatory conditions and those taking high blood pressure medications. The researchers chose only study participants who did not have certain medical conditions or were not taking certain medications because of fear that the participants might be at increased risk for side effects. However, as of this writing, the FDA-approved labeling of Viagra does not list those conditions and drugs as being contraindicated. Thus, many men who would not be permitted in the study are getting prescriptions for Viagra, without any research to document their safety. Viagra may have contributed to the deaths of some men who died after taking the drug. The group is also requesting that drugs that commonly cause impotence be listed in the package insert to alert consumers that eliminating that drug may be all that is needed to solve the problem.[45]

Although there is some evidence that the drug can help women, as of this writing, studies have only been conducted with men. Finally, it is

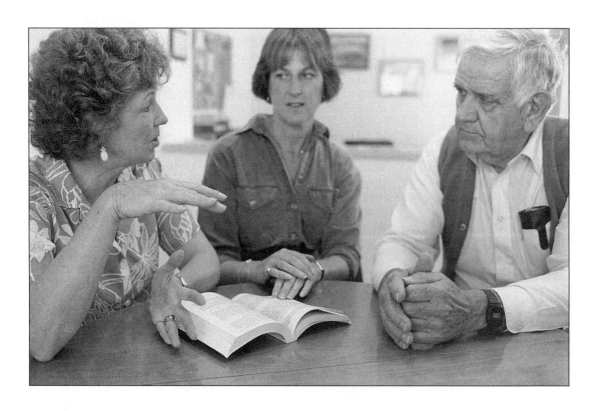

expensive, costing about $10 a pill. There have been very interesting debates regarding the number of pills that health insurance companies should reimburse the insured per month. Since many health insurance policies do not cover the cost of prescription contraceptive methods for women, many people think this is a discriminatory practice.

For those men who do not desire penile implants, a medication may be injected directly into the penis prior to intercourse to induce an erection. These medications include paraverine, phentolamine, and alprostadil (prostaglandin E). All are effective, and widely used. Prostaglandin E seems to cause the fewest side effects.

Prostaglandin E is a hormone that naturally occurs in semen that widens the arteries. These medications produce an erection within five to ten minutes of the injection and last thirty minutes to an hour, even in the absence of stimulation. Each injection costs about $2 to $4 and its use is restricted to no more than three times weekly or once in a 24-hour period. The most common side effect of the medications is penile pain, occurring in about one in ten men. Prostaglandin E may also be prescribed as a suppository that can be inserted into the urethra by a slender plastic tube.

Hormonal therapy can increase sexual desire in both men and women. Men with inadequate testosterone production can be prescribed injections of this hormone to increase sexual interest. It is believed that testosterone injections are ineffective (and may be dangerous) for men with normal testosterone levels. Some physicians are prescribing testosterone therapy to menopausal women to increase their energy and sexual drive. However, patients on this therapy should be carefully monitored because the drug can increase harmful blood cholesterol, facial hair in women, and growth of the prostate in men. Physicians widely prescribe estrogen replacement therapy for menopausal and postmenopausal women, either as a vaginal cream or a dermal patch or pill (in combination with progesterone in most women), to maintain vaginal lubrication and tone after menopause.

Dihydroepiandrostenedione (DHEA), an androgen produced naturally by the body that declines with age, is also under investigation for its ability to increase libido and sexual functioning.

Mechanical Aids

Penile prostheses are useful for men with erectile dysfunction that is caused by an irreversible physical problem. These implants have high patient satisfaction rates. Two major types of permanent implants are commonly used to make the penis rigid enough for intercourse. One type consists of plastic rods implanted into the penile shaft. These create a permanent erection, and athletic supporters may be worn so the erection is not detectable in street clothes. The second major type is an inflatable implant that creates an erection when fluid is pumped from an implanted reservoir into two cylindrical chambers implanted in the penile shaft. The fluid pump is activated when a bulb in the scrotum is squeezed, causing the cylinders to expand. When the need for an erection is over, a valve is pressed, allowing the fluid to flow from the cylinder back into the reservoir. The advantage of the inflatable implant is a natural appearance of the penis. However, neither type will restore arousal or orgasm if these capacities are lost. The cost of a semirigid or malleable penile prosthesis is about $3,000; inflatable prostheses cost about $9,000.

Another treatment for erectile dysfunction is the *external vacuum device,* which uses suction to draw blood into the penis; back-flow of blood is prevented with a tight band at the base of the shaft. A clear plastic device is placed over the penis and pressed firmly against the pelvic area, then a hand pump creates suction that draws blood into the penis. Erection occurs in three to five minutes and lasts up to thirty minutes. These patients achieve orgasm, but will not ejaculate. The band should not be worn for longer than thirty minutes. The cost of the vacuum device ranges from $200 to $400. Men who can achieve but not sustain erection may benefit from the tight band alone. A splinted condom worn on the outside of the penis, after an erection is achieved by vacuum, may also be used. Although these devices are available from sex supply stores, health professionals recommend that they be used under medical supervision to minimize adverse effects.

Sex Therapy

Most models of sex therapy have developed from the work of Masters and Johnson[46] and are based on the assumption that sexual problems arise because normal sexual response is blocked by anxiety or fear of failure. They assert that both partners are responsible for the sexual dysfunction. Generally, a male-female cotherapist team provides education, counseling, and daily assignments to the couple that involve progressive exercises in mutual pleasure along with verbal feedback. The goal of the mutual pleasure-giving exercises is to learn that sexual contact should not be goal-oriented (orgasm); lovemaking should be pleasurable in itself. The therapists request that the clients refrain from intercourse for a time to reduce performance anxiety. This type of therapy is the most effective in cases of impotence and premature ejaculation. Modifications of this model include the use of a single therapist instead of a team, less frequent sessions, and individual rather than couple counseling.

A different counseling approach may be used when the problem extends to other aspects of the relationship. Long-standing dissatisfaction with both the sexual and nonsexual aspects of the relationship or lack of communication skills indicate a need for more general counseling. In addition, learning to cope with sexual problems created by chronic illness and developing alternative ways to express sexuality call for other counseling approaches. No matter what the method, the goal of sex therapy should be to increase sexual satisfaction and fulfill needs for intimacy, acceptance, and love.

SEX EDUCATION

Masters and Johnson believe ignorance to be the greatest deterrent to sexual function for all ages. This statement seems to be especially applicable to elders who are less knowledgeable about sexuality than any other age group because they had little or no sex education in their earlier years. Although most older people have had a lifetime of sexual experience, attitudes of the older generation reflect a restrictive view of sexuality. Some people believe the primary reason for sexual activity is to bear children and that sex is appropriate only for married persons in their childbearing years. Self-pleasure or masturbation is unacceptable to many, even though commonly practiced. Studies show a high rate of sexual misinformation among elders, which may adversely impact their sexual satisfaction.

Sex education for middle-aged and elder adults is rare, and teaching materials are sparse. This may be due to the belief that elders have other priorities and are neither sexually active nor interested in learning about sexuality. Alternatively, many believe that older people already know what they need to know. However, one survey of 378 middle-aged and older adults who were being evaluated for sexual problems suggested a high prevalence of misconceptions about sexual functioning. Many of those questioned did not know: (1) a woman could be sexually satisfied even if her partner could not maintain an erection, (2) the role of hormones in erectile dysfunction, and (3) older women may require a longer time to become sexually aroused and may require a lubricant for sexual intercourse.[47]

Another reason for the lack of sex education courses and accompanying materials for elders is the widespread belief that older people do not want to discuss sexual topics. Those who have asked elders have reported otherwise.[5] One study reported a 90 percent response rate when community elders were issued written invitations to attend a sex education class in a clinic setting.[48] The following is only a sample of sexual issues that might be addressed in sex education classes for older people:

- physiological changes accompanying aging that may affect sexual interest and activity,

- effects of illness and surgery on sexual interest and activity,
- alternative sexual expression, including masturbation,
- dealing with sexual repression in our culture,
- maintaining a healthy sexual identity,
- effects of drugs on sexuality,
- counteracting myths of sexuality and aging,
- communicating with partner about sexual needs, and
- communicating sexual problems to the health professional.

Sex education for elders has been reported to be highly successful in increasing elders' knowledge and changing their sexual attitudes and behaviors. In one study, elders reported a 400 percent increase in intercourse and masturbation.[22] Another study reported similar positive results.[49]

Family members and those who work with elders also benefit from education about elder sexuality. The White and Catania study[22] reported significant gains in knowledge and sexual permissiveness toward elders as a result of sex education classes for families and nursing home staff.

The attitude of the health professional is an important variable in the educational process for any age group. An older person's willingness to discuss sexual concerns depends upon the educator's openness and comfort with the topic. A health professional needs to be accepting of an elder's sexuality, whatever this might entail. Just as professionals should not be judgmental of sexually active elders, neither should they pressure the older person to conform to sexual norms of younger adults. Health professionals need to take elders' educational level and cognitive ability into account when developing programs. Just as in other types of health education, sex education is more successful if elders are involved in the planning, topic selection, publicity, and group facilitation.

SUMMARY

Studies clearly show that sexual interest and activity continue into old age. However, a number of stereotypes about elder sexuality continue to persist. Research on sexuality reflects this bias because studies on elder sexuality are sparse and generally have small sample sizes and other methodological problems. Although sexuality encompasses a number of behaviors, most studies have concentrated on intercourse and masturbation. Preliminary work shows that these behaviors tend to decrease slightly with age. However, intercourse frequency is highly dependent on the presence of a partner. The classic work on sexuality by Masters and Johnson shows some alterations in sexual response with age in both men and women; however, their small sample size precludes generalizing about their findings. Evidence seems to indicate that those who continue sexual activity throughout life have little alteration in sexual response.

It is difficult to make generalizations about elder sexuality because there are a number of elders with different needs and concerns regarding sexuality, such as unmarried women, homosexuals, and the institutionalized. Furthermore, some chronic illnesses, including arthritis, heart disease, cancer, and diabetes, are likely to affect elders' sexual interest and ability. Other factors that influence sexual interest and activity are testosterone deficiency, prescription drugs, overuse of alcohol, extended sexual inactivity, and psychosocial factors.

Sexual dysfunction, an impaired ability or interest in sexual activity, can occur among men and women. Types include erectile dysfunction and premature ejaculation in men, and dyspareunia, vaginismus, and orgasmic dysfunction in women. These dysfunctions may be caused by drug reactions, psychological effects, or physiological factors and may be treated with sex therapy, drugs, penile implants, or hormones. Although sex education for elders is uncommon, it has been shown to be highly successful.

ACTIVITIES

1. Ask ten individuals of different ages these three questions:
   a. What is your age?
   b. At what age do you think sexual activity ceases?
   c. At what age do you think sexual interest ceases?

   Compare your responses with others in the class. How do the results differ among age groups? What informal conversations did your questions stimulate?

2. Interview five students regarding their estimates of sexual activity between their parents and grandparents. How do they compare to average frequencies discussed in the chapter?

3. Visit a local skilled nursing facility and question both an administrator and an aide regarding the sexual life of the residents. Have the administrator describe regulations regarding sexual activity in the home. Is the right to privacy part of the patients' rights? Is sexual activity considered as part of the right to privacy? Notice the physical layout of the home. How does it discourage or encourage sexual intimacy?

4. Develop model guidelines for expressions of sexuality in a nursing home. Include guidelines for gay, unmarried, and married couples; the severely demented; privacy for masturbation; sex education; and maintaining personal appearance.

5. Collect cartoons and greeting cards that address sexuality in the later years. Analyze them in terms of the image they project about older people and the myths perpetuated about sex and elders.

6. Develop an instructional program to teach a group of community elders about an aspect of sexuality. Include objectives, methods, teaching materials, content outline, and discussion questions.

7. Develop an educational campaign to educate older adults about safe sex practices.

BIBLIOGRAPHY

1. Kinsey, A.C., Pomeroy, W.B., and Martin, C.R. 1948. *Sexual behavior in the human male.* Philadelphia: W. B. Saunders.

2. Kinsey, A.C., Pomeroy, W.B., Martin, C.R., and Gebhard, P. 1953. *Sexual behavior in the human female.* Philadelphia: W. B. Saunders.

3. Masters, W.H., and Johnson, V.E. 1966. *Human sexual response.* Boston: Little, Brown.

4. Pocs, O., Godow, A., Tolone, W.L., and Walsh, R.H. 1977. Is there sex after 40? *Psychology Today* (June):54–56, 87.

5. Starr, B.D., and Weiner, M.B. 1981. *The Starr-Weiner Report on sex and sexuality in the mature years.* San Francisco: McGraw-Hill.

6. Bretschneider, J.G., and McCoy, N.L. 1988. Sexual interest and behavior in healthy 80- to 102-year-olds. *Archives of Sexual Behavior* 17:109–29.

7. Wiley, D., and Bortz, W.M. 1996. Sexuality and aging—usual and successful. *Journal of Gerontology* 51A:M142–46.

8. Marsiglio, W., and Donnelly, D. 1991. Sexual relations in later life: A national study of married persons. *Journal of Gerontology* 46:S338–44.

9. Cogen, R., and Steinman, W. 1990. Sexual function and practice in elderly men of lower socioeconomic status. *Journal of Family Practice* 31:162–66.

10. Marshall, D.S. 1971. Sexual behavior in Mangaia. In *Human sexual behavior. Variations in the ethnographic spectrum,* D.S. Marshall and R.C. Suggs, eds. New York: Basic Books.

11. Winn, R.S., and Newton, N. 1982. Sexuality in aging: A study of 106 cultures. *Archives of Sexual Behavior* 11:283–98.

12. Bachmann, G. 1990. Coitus promotes older women's genital health. Reported in January at the ACOG annual clinical meeting.

13. Almvig, C. 1982. *The invisible minority: Aging and lesbianism.* Syracuse, NY: Utica College of Syracuse.

14. Peplau, L.A. 1981. What homosexuals want. *Psychology Today* (March):28–38.

15. Deevey, S. 1990. Older lesbian women—an invisible minority. *Journal of Gerontological Nursing* 16:35–39.

16. Quam, J.K., and Whitford, G.S. 1992. Adaptation and age-related expectations of older gay and lesbian adults. *The Gerontologist* 32:367–74.

17. Berger, R.M. 1982. *Gay and gray.* Chicago: University of Illinois Press.

18. McCartney, J.R., Izeman, H., Rogers, D., and Cohen, N. 1987. Sexuality and the institutionalized elderly. *Journal of the American Geriatrics Society* 35:331–33.

19. White, C.B. 1982. Sexual interest, attitudes, knowledge and sexual history in relation to sexual behavior in the institutionalized aged. *Archives of Sexual Behavior* 11:11–22.

20. Mulligan, T., and Palguta, R.F. 1991. Sexual interest, activity and satisfaction among male nursing home residents. *Archives of Sexual Behavior* 20:199–204.

21. Silverstone, B., and Wynter, L. 1975. The effect of introducing a heterosexual living space. *The Gerontologist* 15:83–87.

22. White, C.B., and Catania, J.A. 1982. Psychoeducational intervention for sexuality with the aged, family members of the aged, and people who work with the aged. *International Journal of Aging and Human Development* 15:121–38.

23. Muller, J.E., Mittleman, M.A., Maclure, M., Sherwood, J.B., and Tofler, G.H. 1996. Triggering myocardial infarction by sexual activity. *Journal of the American Medical Association* 275:1405–9.

24. Bohlen, J.G., Held, J.P., Sanderson, M.O., and Patterson, R.P. 1984. Heart rate, rate—pressure product, and oxygen uptake during four sexual activities. *Archives of Internal Medicine* 144:1745–48.

25. Papadopoulos, C., Beaumont, C., Shelley, S.I., and Larrimore, P. 1983. Myocardial infarction and sexual activity of the female patient. *Archives of Internal Medicine* 143:1528–30.

26. Wei, M., Macera, C.A., Davis, D.R., Hornung, C.A., Nankin, H.R., and Blair, S.N. 1994. Total cholesterol and high density lipoprotein cholesterol as important predictors of erectile dysfunction. *American Journal of Epidemiology* 140:930–37.

27. Schover, L.R. 1997. *Sexuality and fertility after cancer.* New York: John Wiley and Sons.

28. Deamer, R.L., and Thompson, J.F. 1991. The role of medication in geriatric sexual function. *Clinics in Geriatric Medicine* 7:95–111.

29. Morley, J.E. 1986. Impotence. *American Journal of Medical Education* 80:897–905.

30. Ackerman, M.D., Montague, D.K., and Morganstern, S. 1994. Impotence: Help for erectile dysfunction. *Patient Care,* March 15, pp. 22–56.

31. Mannino, D.M., Klevens, R.M., and Flanders, W.D. 1994. Cigarette smoking: An independent risk factor for impotence? *American Journal of Epidemiology* 140:1003–8.

32. Feldman, H.A., Goldstein, I., and Hatzichristou, D.G., et al. 1994. Impotence and its medical and psychosocial correlates: Results of the Massachusetts Male Aging Study. *Journal of Urology* 151:54–61.

33. Ackerman, M.D., Montague, D.K., and Morganstern, S. 1994. Impotence: Help for erectile dysfunction. *Patient Care,* March 15, pp. 22–56.

34. Bergman, C., Damber, J.E., and Littbrand, B., et al. 1984. Sexual function in prostatic cancer patients treated with radiotherapy, orchiectomy or oestrogens. *British Journal of Urology* 56:64–69.

35. Bachmann, G. 1990. Psychosexual aspects of hysterectomy. *Women's Health Institute* 1:41–49.

36. Masters, W.H., and Johnson, V.E. 1981. Sex and the aging process. *Journal of the American Geriatrics Society* 29:385–90.

37. Wiley, D., and Bortz, W.M. 1996. Sexuality and aging—usual and successful. *Journal of Gerontology* 51A:M142–46.

38. Williams, G. 1987. Erectile dysfunction: Diagnosis and treatment. *British Journal of Urology* 60:1–5.

39. Johnson, L.E., and Morley, J.E. 1988. Impotence in the elderly. *American Family Physician* 38:225–40.

40. Mulligan, T., and Katz, P.G. 1989. Why aged men become impotent. *Archives of Internal Medicine* 149:1365–66.

41. Ende, J., Rockwell, S., and Glasgow, M. 1984. The sexual history in general medical practice. *Archives of Internal Medicine* 144:558.

42. Slag, M.F., Morley, J.E., and Elson, M.K. et al. 1983. Impotence in medical cinical outpatients. *Journal of the American Medical Association* 249:1736–40.

43. Harward, M.P. 1991. Evaluation of sexual dysfunction in women. *Hospital Practice* 26:53–54, 56–57.

44. Goldstein, I., Lue, T.F., Padma-Nathan, H.L., and Rosen, R.C., et al. 1998. Oral sildenafil in the treatment of erectile dysfunction. *New England Journal of Medicine* 338:397–404.

45. Sidney Wolfe, MD, ed. 1998. Public Citizen's Health Research group petitions the FDA about sildenafil (Viagra). *Health Letter,* Public Citizen Health Research Group. (August):1–2.

46. Masters, W.H., and Johnson, V.E. 1970. *Human sexual inadequacy.* Boston: Little, Brown.

47. Adams, S.G., Dubbert, P.M., Chupurdia, K.M., Jones, A., Jr. Lofland, K.R., and Leermakers, E. 1996. Assessment of sexual beliefs and information in aging couples with sexual dysfunction. *Archives of Sexual Behavior* 25:249–60.

48. Salaman, M.J., and Charytan, P. 1984. A sexuality workshop program for the elderly. *Clinical Gerontology* 2:25–34.

49. Salaman, M.J., and Charytan, P. 1984. A sexuality workshop program for the elderly. Clinical Gerontology 2:25–34.

MENTAL HEALTH
AND ILLNESS

Why is it good to be old? Because I am more myself than I have ever been.

Mary Sarton

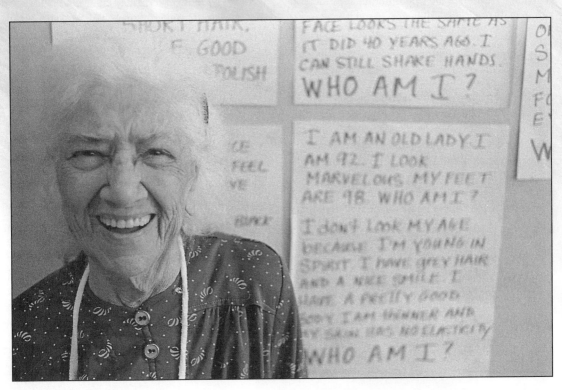

Most older people continue to function well and lead meaningful lives, just as they did in their younger years. However, they must deal with multiple age-associated losses, including the loss of employment, the loss of health, the deaths of loved ones, and their own future mortality. The ability of a person to adapt and be fulfilled in later life is related to a number of physical, psychological, and situational variables. Failing to adapt to change and loss can result in physical and emotional illness. Although most older people can adjust without help, a few require extra support or assistance. Friends and relatives offer help and support, while mental health services provide more formal assistance.

This chapter will discuss the life transitions commonly faced in old age and the multiple factors that influence successful adjustment. The nature, prevalence, and treatment of mental disorders common in the later years will also be addressed. Finally, the variety of community mental health services and mental institutions and the barriers that reduce the opportunities for elders to effectively use them will be discussed.

MENTAL HEALTH

What characteristics are associated with good psychological health? Is there a set of "ideal traits" or are many combinations acceptable? Are any particular characteristics necessary? What kind of balance between positive and negative traits is consistent with mental health? Are any traits really "all good" or "all bad"? When examining seemingly opposite traits, such as independence and dependence or introversion and extroversion, is one extreme better than the other, or is it "best" to be somewhere in the middle? Although we may say it is mentally healthy to be independent, how do we characterize those who express this trait to an extreme, remaining socially isolated, and refusing needed help? Conversely, what about those elders or disabled individuals who are fully dependent yet mentally healthy? To what extent are our definitions of mental health culturally or situationally determined?

Behaviors that are normal or adaptive in one situation may be abnormal in others. For instance, sadness or melancholy following the death of a friend is quite different from severe, prolonged depression. What constitutes abnormal or normal behavior also depends on the individual's personality and past actions. Lethargy may be normal in an elder who has always moved at a slow pace, but abnormal when suddenly appearing in another elder who usually is self-motivated and energetic. Finally, healthy behavior is culturally defined. For example, Asian cultures place more importance on the family and one's responsibilities to its members, stressing interdependence within the family. In contrast, American culture puts more emphasis on the desires and rights of the individual to achieve success and independence.

Psychologist M. Jahoda suggested six criteria necessary for positive mental health: positive self attitude, growth and self-actualization, integration of the personality, autonomy, reality perception, and mastery of one's environment.[1] However, what is meant by these criteria may change with advancing age or disability. Some believe "successful aging" is the ability to maintain low levels of disease and disability, high cognitive and physical functional capability, and active engagement with life, including maintaining interpersonal relationships and sustaining productive activity.[2]

The disabilities associated with aging may reduce an older person's ability to meet either of these definitions. A bed-bound frail elder with severe heart disease living in an institution has little opportunity to experience interpersonal growth as we might define it. Does this mean this elder is not mentally healthy? When poor health, disability, or financial circumstances force one to give up activities that formerly fulfilled the needs for autonomy and self-esteem, individuals must satisfy this need through a more restricted set of alternatives. Perhaps, then, mental health is best defined as maximizing satisfaction and future potential in the face of changing strengths, abilities, challenges, and resources.

Clearly, what constitutes mental health varies throughout the life cycle as individuals have different priorities to accomplish. Although each individual's life is unique, psychologists suggest that there are certain patterns and needs that are universal for each period of the life cycle. Whereas young adults look toward their future possibilities, elders may look more at the past and what they have achieved.

One critical developmental task of old age is acceptance: accepting changes in ideals and self-esteem resulting from advancing age, accepting one's own death and that of loved ones, and accepting physical and psychological decline. Elders must modify previous goals and accept the limitations of an aging body. They must also accept, without shame, their increased passivity and dependence, decreased physical health, and increased spectator role. However, they must also continue to develop and master new goals to maintain self-respect and self-esteem. Psychologist E. H. Erickson describes old age as ushering in the culmination of the life cycle, a time when the individual develops "ego integrity," mature judgment and satisfaction with a life well-lived. Poor adjustment is characterized by despair, the fear of death, and dissatisfaction with one's life.[3]

Psychological Changes with Age

While old age is associated with declines in cognition and memory, few elders would trade the wisdom they have accumulated from life's experiences for a second youth. This section will briefly discuss changes in cognition, memory, and personality in the later years.

Cognition

It is difficult to measure intelligence in any age group and especially difficult to measure changes in intelligence or cognitive ability with age. Most studies rely on standardized tests, such as IQ (intelligence quotient) tests. Scores are reported in comparison to others of the same age.

Multiple studies, both cross-sectional and longitudinal, show that most aspects of intelligence, as measured by these standardized tests, decline with advancing age. The Seattle longitudinal study

reported that intelligence increased over adulthood, remained stable in middle age, then evidenced declines in all areas measured by standardized tests.[4] Tests usually have sections on verbal, problem solving, mathematical, and memory skills. On almost every measure of intelligence, there is some age-associated decline. However, there are large variations: some individuals have greater losses in cognitive abilities than others, and some exhibit gains as well. Any one individual is likely to show declines in only one area, while remaining stable or even improving on other measures of intelligence.[5] However, some psychologists believe these tests to be inaccurate in assessing intelligence, particularly in assessing age-associated changes, because of their general nature. Many researchers have attempted to test other types of intelligence besides that measured by standardized tests.

Despite some cognitive losses, elders still maintain high levels of performance in activities of living. In general, elders can continue performing well in their occupation, reading, learning, and solving problems. Perhaps this is because experience can compensate for some of the decline in rapid problem-solving skills. One novel study compared young and older adults on their skills in food service. They found that younger adults scored more highly on tests of intelligence, but older food servers actually performed better on the job.[6]

Some elders suffer more losses in cognitive function than others. Cognitive losses are accelerated in those who are ill, those who are depressed, and those who do not receive stimulation from their environment. Studies have also reported that there is a significant drop in intelligence prior to death called "terminal drop,"[7] and long-term cognitive losses among one of four elders undergoing surgery.[8] Studies also suggest that elders who engage in reading, crossword puzzles, debates, or other stimulating activities score higher on intelligence tests than those with a more monotonous life. Researchers have also found that elders can improve their performance on intelligence tests (and likely intelligence) with training and education.[9]

Many researchers have attempted to test other types of intelligence besides that measured by standardized tests. No scale is perfect, and many intelligence tests are criticized for being "culturally specific" or incompletely measuring its complex dimensions. Research is ongoing to determine the physiological mechanism for the decline in intelligence. It is postulated that the decline may be associated with atherosclerosis and decreased circulation to the brain, death of neurons and altered neuronal connections, or cerebral atrophy from disuse.

Memory

It is true that some memory loss is a normal part of growing older. Both cross-sectional and longitudinal studies confirm this; however, only certain kinds of memory seem to be affected. Older people are more likely to perform poorly on memory tests requiring speed or a high degree of focused attention.[10] In addition, they are less likely to perform well on tests requiring them to recall or process new information compared to previously acquired information or skills. However, vocabulary generally improves with age, and the ability to reason and solve problems does not decline. Studies seem to suggest that episodic memory, the ability to remember specific ongoing events (e.g., what I ate for dinner yesterday), is most affected by the aging process.

Some anxious and depressed older people tend to be unduly concerned about minor memory lapses, which worsens the problem. When a memory lapse occurs, it is probably due to anxiety, lack of sleep, and drug side effects. The drugs that are most likely to cause memory problems are insulin, antianxiety and antidepressant medications, antihypertensive agents, and stomach acid supressants. Some chronic illnesses also affect memory, particularly hypertension. If an older person is concerned about memory loss and the onset of dementia, sometimes a simple medical examination may be all that is needed to reduce their concerns. This should include checking for drug interactions and underlying illnesses, and a discussion of lifestyle problems that might affect memory.[11]

The type of memory least affected by aging is the ability to recall events in the personal past, called reminiscing. Particularly for institutionalized elders, reminiscence may be the only pleasure left in their lives, a reminder of the "good old days" when they were not sick. Many psychologists believe that encouraging reminiscence in elders is an effective way to increase self-esteem and decrease depression.

Ways to prevent memory loss include maintaining good emotional and physical health and living in a stimulating environment. Many techniques have been developed to improve memory, called mnemonics. One popular way is to put what has to be remembered into smaller, more manageable units that can be more easily remembered (e.g., dividing the grocery list into smaller categories, such as fruits and vegetables). Another is to visualize what needs to be remembered (envisioning what will be in the grocery bags). Probably the best technique is to write things down, whether it is a grocery list, phone number, name, or when medicine was taken last. Linking something known with what is to be remembered, such as making up a song about a name, is also helpful.

Personality

Personality is a collection of distinct individual traits, qualities, and attributes that, when considered together, describe the essence of a person. Although there are many views on the traits that personality includes, one popular view is that of Costa and McCrae.[12] They distilled the major dimensions of personality into five groupings:

1. *Neuroticism* defines the continuum between mental health (stable and happy) and maladjustment (hostile, depressed, prone to break down).
2. *Extraversion* describes those who are warm, friendly, social and outgoing compared to those who are introverted and have solitary tendencies.
3. *Openness to experience* relates to the willingness to take risks and try new things compared to those who are more cautious and comfortable with the status quo.

4. *Conscientiousness* encompasses traits of organization, efficiency, and dependability compared to traits of irresponsibility, inconsistency, and unreliability.
5. *Agreeableness* relates to interpersonal qualities such as caring, empathy, cooperation, and lovingness, compared to scornful, rude, or unpleasant behaviors.

Each grouping represents a continuum with behaviors and characteristics at two extremes, one of which is "positive" and one "negative." However, in many cases, it is difficult to determine which traits are more positive or desirable than others, as much depends on the culture and the situation. Studies on personality types have shown that some particular combinations of personality traits are more common among those who are better adjusted, and some are more associated with poorer adjustment. For example, people who are more introverted or rigid have higher rates of depression and criminal activity. New evidence also suggests that personality traits may not be wholly determined by our living environment and previous experiences; rather, they may be inherited and mediated through our genes, brain chemicals, and hormones.

There are many instruments that measure personality. Independent of the measures used, multiple studies suggest that personality remains remarkably stable over time. However, these studies mainly consisted of upper-middle class whites who grew old during the mid-1900s. Other studies suggest that there are some differences with age. For example, some experts observe that both men and women grow more androgenous with age. This means that women exhibit more traditionally masculine traits (such as assertiveness) and men exhibit more traditionally feminine traits (such as nurturing).[13] Although some assert that these are psychological changes, still others suggest that the move toward androgeny may be biologically based as women have reduced estrogen production and men have reduced testosterone production.

It has been reported that older adults exhibit more mature coping styles than younger adults. Elders are less prone to angry outbursts or escaping into fantasy to cope with stress[14] and are less likely to be hostile and self-blaming.[15] The Grant longitudinal study of Harvard undergraduates reported that older men develop more mature coping techniques: they are more likely to use humor, cope with hardship by appreciating what one has, or attempt to "look on the bright side."[16] Others have not found a difference in coping styles among adult age groups.

TRANSITIONS IN LATER LIFE

Growing old in a youth-oriented society that places primary value on independence, competence, energy, and productivity is not easy. It is the primary adaptive task of old age to find satisfaction and self-esteem when role loss, social status loss and physical ailments are more noticeable and decrements more likely than ever before.

Iris Winogrond

Just as any other period in life, old age is accompanied by transitions that require adaptation. However, the transitions faced by each age group differ. In general, the young are preparing for employment, finding a mate, and setting up a home; the middle-aged are raising children, maintaining a job, and caring for aged parents. In the later years, many of the transitions are characterized by loss, such as:

- **Physical losses:** chronic illness and increasing disability, the loss of previous strength and endurance, and the loss of youthful appearance.
- **Psychological losses:** forgetfulness, impaired cognitive ability, reduced status, reduced independence, loss of control, facing one's own mortality.
- **Social losses:** changing residences, loss of job status, loss of driving abilities, loss of social status.
- **Economic loss:** loss of employment, reduced income from retirement, living on a fixed income despite increased costs of medical expenses and inflation.
- **Interpersonal losses:** death of spouse, friends, and family members.

Warning

When I am an old woman I shall wear purple
With a red hat which doesn't go, and doesn't
suit me.
And I shall spend my pension on brandy and
summer gloves
And satin sandals, and say we've no money for
butter.
I shall sit down on the pavement when I'm tired
And gobble up samples in shops and press
alarm bells
And run my stick along the public railings
And make up for the sobriety of my youth.
I shall go out in my slippers in the rain
And pick the flowers in other people's gardens
And learn to spit.

You can wear terrible shirts and grow more fat
And eat three pounds of sausages at a go
Or only bread and pickle for a week
And hoard pens and pencils and beermats and
things in boxes.
But now we must have clothes that keep us dry
And pay our rent and not swear in the street
And set a good example for the children.
We must have friends to dinner and read the
papers.
But maybe I ought to practice a little now?
So people who know me are not too shocked
and surprised
When suddenly I am old, and start to wear purple.

Reprinted from *When I Am An Old Woman I Shall Wear Purple,* ©
Papier-Maché Press.

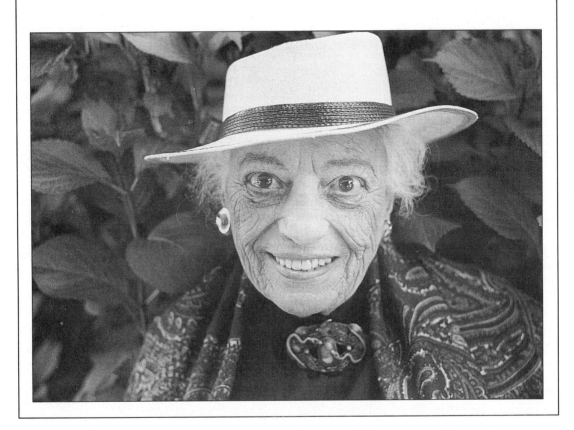

Whereas the possibilities in young adulthood were endless, old age has limited possibilities, decreased personal resources, and diminished health. Even though old age is accompanied by multiple losses, most elders adjust effectively and report high levels of life satisfaction and happiness.

The later years also has its benefits. Many older people experience the joy of seeing their children grow up into healthy successful adults. Many elders have grandchildren, and, if bumper stickers and T-shirts are any indication, they are an important part of their identity and happiness. For those who are still in good health and can afford it, travel opportunities provide an important part of their later years, especially among the young-old. And, although retirement is a loss for some who have not developed social networks or hobbies, for those who have many interests, retirement finally gives them the free time to read, garden, socialize, and volunteer. For some, it is the beginning of a new career. Good health, sufficient income, and a network of family and friends can truly make the later years "golden."

Retirement

The elderly used to be the most vulnerable segment of our society. When they were no longer able to work because of physical disability or illness, they had to rely on charity or their families for help. The Social Security Act of 1935, enacted during the Great Depression, provided a universal, stable income for retiring elders starting at age 65. These Social Security benefits were increased in succeeding years, and medical care benefits were added through Medicare. During this same period, more employers began to offer pensions, and individuals began saving for retirement through individual retirement accounts (IRAs). These changes completely revolutionized the financial situation of elders, transforming retirement, and fewer elders

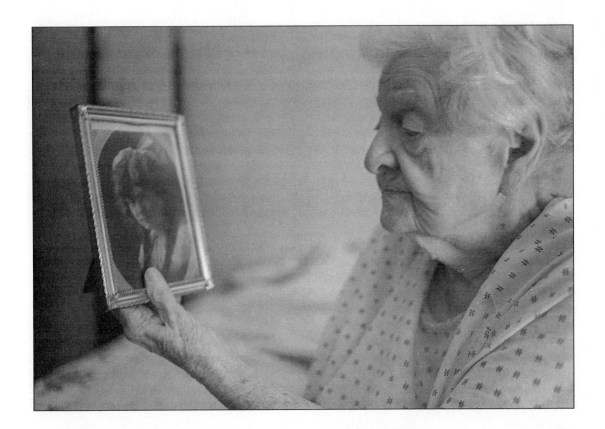

are poor in their later years. Now, for a good proportion of older people, retirement symbolizes an achievement and the beginning of the "golden years" of pleasure, traveling, and recreation.

Although many people look forward to retirement, it is a major transition and all changes engender conflict. The majority of elders cope very well with this transition, reporting high levels of life satisfaction. However, a few elders have difficulty coping. Those with poor health or lower incomes may realize that they are not able to do all they had hoped in retirement. Retirement can cause emotional stress on marriages as roles change and couples spend more time together.

There are vast differences in what older people do after retirement. Some travel, go back to school, volunteer their time, begin new hobbies, and spend time with grandchildren. However, others, particularly women living alone, minorities, and the very old, may have no pensions, are in poor health, and are likely to live in poverty. Many will not have the opportunity to experience the freedom of the "golden years."

New Relationships with Adult Children and Grandchildren

In general, elders derive much strength and support from relationships with adult children. Studies show that many elders live near adult children and visit frequently. One study found that one in three adults visits an aged parent daily or every other day and two-thirds report seeing that person once or twice in the past week.[17] Elders and their adult children may communicate through telephone calls, visits, and written communication. However, the amount of contact is not necessarily predictive of the quality of the relationship. In fact, contact may increase in times of trouble (such as the divorce of the adult child or the illness of the aged parent).

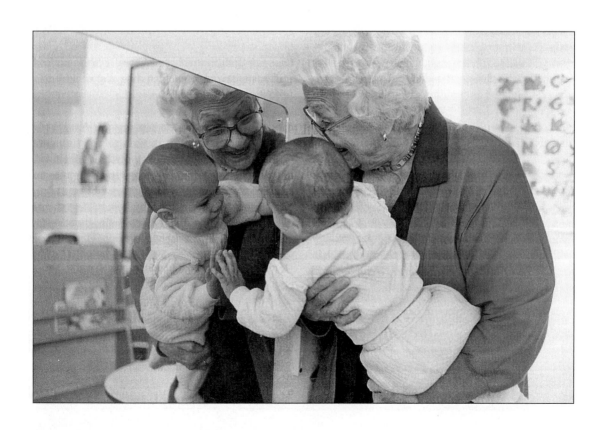

The quality of interaction between older adults and their children is important. With age, the relationship between adult parents and their children may change. Instead of parent-child interaction, many elders and their adult children are more akin to friends. In contrast, those parent-child relationships focusing on economic dependency are not as satisfying. With advanced age and increased disability, there is often a change in roles as adult children attempt to "parent" their parents. For example, an adult daughter, recognizing that her mother is no longer able to care for herself, may attempt to pressure her mother to move in with her family or to a nursing home.

In addition to alterations in relationships with their adult children, elders may also experience new or different relationships with their grandchildren. Grandparenting can be a source of joy and satisfaction to elders in their later years. Adult grandchildren can become friends to elders, or even provide caregiving. Elder grandparents may provide child care for their grandchildren when their own children are employed. At times, elders may unexpectedly be called upon to care for their grandchildren in their later years, due to the death or illness of the adult child.

Marital Transitions

Marital transitions are also common in later life. Relationships between partners evolve over the years, some becoming more dissatisfied with the relationship, others becoming more satisfied. Coping with the illness of a spouse is also a considerable transition, especially if the illness is prolonged and the spouse needs constant care. Adjustments to widowhood, divorce, and remarriage are also commonly experienced.

Changes in Relationship Satisfaction

In the 1800s, couples had children early in a marriage; therefore, many had very little time as a couple before the first child arrived (generally less than two years). Further, they were often widowed before their children were grown. These days, more couples delay having their first child, some

have none at all, and people are living longer. The combination of these trends means that about one-third of married life is spent simply as a couple.[18] As is clear, many couples cannot tolerate this much togetherness, leading to divorce. However, a good number of marriages last for decades.

Most studies of educated elders report a high degree of marital satisfaction as well as fewer arguments and more shared activities than younger couples.[19] However, studies analyzing the characteristics and success of older marriages rely on self-report rather than observation and do not take into account the changing expectations of marriage over the years. It is clear that expectations of marriage vary by generation. Many of today's elders look at marriage differently than young adults. They are more likely to believe that divorce is not an option. Further, there are obvious cohort differences. Those who are currently old may be satisfied that their spouse engages in traditional sex-specific roles and is a "good wife" or "good provider." Many do not expect their spouse to be their best friend, lover, and partner. It will be interesting to study how the marital relationship of those who are old now compares with the marital relationship of the baby boomer generation when they grow older.

Spousal Illness

Illness can prompt many changes in the relationship, and most of these are negative. When one partner becomes ill, the other must adapt to more responsibility, altered relationship roles, and less personal time. The well spouse often must assume intense care-giving responsibilities, while simultaneously receiving less support and encouragement. Illness may also impact elder sexuality and the ability to engage in other activities that the couple has enjoyed. The following vignette illustrates some of the changes that can occur in a relationship with illness.

> Mrs. Smith had always been known to their friends and their two daughters as "the strong one" who took care of everything. She was the hub around which the family revolved; she arranged social interactions, cooked and cleaned and shopped for her spouse, Mr. Smith. She was on the phone frequently

with the couple's daughters, assisting them with their problems. When Mrs. Smith suffered a stroke that left her unable to speak and paralyzed on one side of her body, Mr. Smith was abruptly cast into a caregiving role. First, he lived alone for almost a month while Mrs. Smith was in the hospital and then in a nursing home for rehabilitation. When she came home, she was unable to do any of her normal activities and required assistance in eating, bathing, and dressing herself. Mr. Smith threw himself into the role of caring for his wife, but found that he missed all the things she used to do. Now he felt he had to do his old jobs and hers as well. He missed the affectionate banter that was so characteristic, the sexual relations, and the easy way she had with their daughters. Sometimes Mr. Smith felt more like his wife's nurse than her husband and he longed to talk about his troubles, but the only person he was used to talking to about these things was his wife.

Despite its stresses, most elder spouses do not shy away from the strains of caregiving, and some elders report that the experience heightens their sense of love and commitment.[20] This commitment is evidenced by the estimate that of all those who are frail, 80 percent of them are cared for at home, mostly by the spouse.

Widowhood

Often the most traumatic death elders must face is the loss of a spouse. Not only is there a loss of a long-time companion, but also there is a change in their social and financial situation, a loss of someone to care for them when illness strikes, and additional responsibilities. A wife who has never paid the bills must take on that responsibility, and a husband who has never cooked now must feed himself. The loss of a spouse prompts grief and mourning reactions, termed bereavement.

Most studies suggest that women adapt better to the loss of a spouse than men. Although both men and women experience psychological distress, newly widowed men have a significantly higher rate of death and illness compared to their married counterparts. A widowed man maintains a higher risk of dying than a married woman throughout his life, but his risk drops if he remarries. This same trend is not apparent in women.

One possible explanation for this differential is that women's role in relationships is to watch over the physical, emotional, and social well-being of both partners. Others suggest that this is because women, in general, maintain closer and wider networks of social support, whether through friends, family, or coworkers, whereas men rely on their spouse much more for social support. Although there are clear differences in physical health, some studies suggest that men and women's psychological responses following the death of a spouse are relatively similar. Women generally suffer more of a decline in financial status than men upon widowhood and must cope with those associated stresses.

Support groups for widowed persons are helpful to aid in the transition; however, one study showed these groups were only effective for those with low self-esteem and poor mental health. Those of higher functioning reported increased depression after attending such groups.[21]

Widowhood can be associated with other transitions. For example, the type of friendships may change, including those sustained by the partner who subsequently died or those with a couple focus. Often friendships broaden and deepen with other widows, widowers, or adult children. Widowhood may also result in a change in living situation. The majority of widows and widowers do not elect to move in with their adult children, although some do. Often an adjustment must be made to a change in financial status. Finally, widowhood can have dramatic impact on sexual expression. Depending on their past sexual and marital satisfaction and present mental state, widowed men and women adapt by increasing the frequency of sexual fantasies and autoeroticism, developing an interest in seeking out a future partner, channeling sexual energy into other pursuits, or losing interest in sexual activities altogether.

Elderly Lovers and Newlyweds

Many usually assume that elder couples have been married for decades, but elders are often involved in new love relationships. One sample of elderly lovers found that there was no difference in report of passion compared to college students. In general, however, elder lovers advanced more quickly to commitment in their associations. Sexuality was a part of most relationships with elders reporting that sex was better. However, elders had more ambivalence about their decision to become sexual in a relationship. A final finding of this study was the reluctance to get married among older women. The reasons given were a fear the romance would end, a desire to avoid nursing an ill husband, and a lack of necessity to remarry.[22]

Elders get married for different reasons than young people.[23] Many elders report that they never intended to remarry after divorce or widowhood and are surprised that they met someone they cared about enough to remarry. The most common reason cited for marriage was companionship, with love as the second most common reason. Most elder remarriages were successful, with a majority reporting they were happier in the second marriage compared to the first. They attributed this difference to their maturity and the reduced stresses in their lives now that children were grown. Likewise, the survey by *Consumer Reports* of sexual behavior over age fifty reported the highest marital satisfaction among elders married less than five years, and the group almost as satisfied was that group married more than fifty years.[24]

Factors Affecting Adjustment

Coping successfully with the losses accompanying old age depends on multiple factors, such as past coping success, presence of support systems, personality, and personal reserves.

Personality traits profoundly influence how one adapts to the physical and social transitions that occur with advancing age. Those who are more extroverted, more flexible, and more expressive of their feelings generally cope better than those who are more introverted and inflexible. One personality trait, a sense of control or mastery over one's environment, is associated with positive physical and mental health in all age groups.[25] One classic study on institutionalized elders found that those given control over their daily schedule were more alert, happier, and lived longer than elders who were told

the staff would "take care of them."[26] When this study was repeated on community elders, similar results were obtained.[27]

Health status may affect ability to cope with the aging process, both physiologically and psychologically. When elders suffer reduced energy, diminished mobility, sensory decrements, and increased dependence and disability, they may also suffer from reduced ability to handle stress and adapt to changes. Both the symptoms of illness and the treatment regimen strain adaptive capacity. The illness and the pain, debilitation, and dependence that often accompany it, have a tremendous effect on elders' lifestyle and emotional health. Because many chronic illnesses worsen over time, elders are fearful of pain, progressive debilitation, and dependence. Physical illnesses are often accompanied by mental distress, especially anxiety and depression. Furthermore, the treatment of physical problems may cause feared mental symptoms (e.g., depression, insomnia, and hallucinations) and may restrict one's former lifestyle. Even the age-related decline in sensory abilities, especially vision and hearing, can result in withdrawal from social contacts, confusion, depression, and impaired orientation and mobility if not corrected.

Oftentimes, however, it is the elders' *perception of their health status* that is a more important predictor of coping ability than their actual health. In fact, elders' perception of their physical health is one of the strongest correlates with life satisfaction, adjustment, self-esteem, and mental health. A large-scale survey found that elders who believed themselves to be in good health used fewer health care resources, had a decreased mortality, and aged more "successfully" than those who ranked their health as poor.[28] Despite their physical decrements, the majority of elders think their own health is better than others their age.

Financial situation can also affect psychological health. Those with sufficient income are able to have their food, shelter, recreational, and health needs met. In contrast, those who are poor have the additional stress of maintaining their health with limited resources. As income generally declines after retirement, many elders must deal with poverty and its associated problems for the first time. Poverty and the fear of poverty affect the sense of security and increase anxiety and depression at any age.

It is well established that the presence of *social support* promotes health. Isolated adults have a significantly higher death rate than those with social ties; the more ties, the lower the death rate. As mentioned earlier, married men have less physical and psychological distress than single men. The presence of social supports not only buffers stress, but may reduce the symptoms of physical illness. Pets may provide social support, which improves coping ability. Pets often lavish their owners with attention, stimulate laughter, encourage regular exercise, and make owners feel safe and needed. Studies report that pets serve to buffer their owners from stress and illness.[29]

The *ability to cope with stress* is an important factor in determining successful adaptation to old age. Stress is any physiological or psychological situation that challenges the individual's capacity to adapt. For instance, extreme temperatures, radiation, noise, and starvation cause physical stress, while life events such as death of a loved one, change in residence, and retirement cause psychological stress. An individual's response to stress is more important than the amount of stress experienced. Certain personality types are able to adapt more easily to stress than others: some people are debilitated by it, while others are challenged.

Even though older people experience a number of life changes, they report less stress than any other adult age group. It is difficult to imagine, however, that with their multiple health problems and the associated losses of old age, that elders feel less stressed than younger groups. Perhaps elders do not identify feelings of worry, frustration, irritability, isolation, or anxiety as stress. On the other hand, elders may cope more effectively with stress for a variety of reasons: they have learned to anticipate the changes, allow themselves more time to adapt to their stressors, minimize the total number of stressors to those they can control, or adapt effective coping strategies. It remains to be seen what the reported stress level of today's baby boomers may be when they reach their later years, after growing up during the decades where "stress" has become a household word.

At any age, stress demands adaptation, and adaptation demands energy. Stress-management techniques such as relaxation, meditation, supportive counseling, social interaction, exercise, good diet, humor, and setting new goals may help people cope more effectively with their emotional and physical stressors. When the stress becomes unmanageable, temporary mood disturbances or even more serious mental illness may result.

MENTAL ILLNESS

Mental problems in older people may begin in their younger years or may appear for the first time in later life. If such problems appear for the first time in the later years, they are generally due either to an inability to adapt to stresses or to a physiological disorder in brain function that may have taken years to develop. Elders who have sustained multiple losses over a short time period, have little or no social support, or have adapted poorly to stress in the past are particularly vulnerable to the onset of mental disorders in later life.

It is estimated that 10 percent of persons in the United States have a disability from a diagnosed mental illness, and one in four people have experienced a mental disorder in the previous year.[30] Contrary to popular belief, elders do not have a higher rate of mental illness than younger age groups. In one national survey of adults, about 9 percent reported that they experienced frequent mental distress for at least two of the previous four weeks. The rate was highest among young adults eighteen to twenty-four and lowest among those sixty-five and over.[31] Many mental illnesses common to the general population (depression, schizophrenia, alcohol or drug abuse, or anxiety) are not as commonly reported among older people. However, the prevalence of severe cognitive impairment increases with age. One multicity study reported that only 1 percent of younger adults reported a cognitive impairment, by age sixty-five to sixty-nine, 5 percent reported having

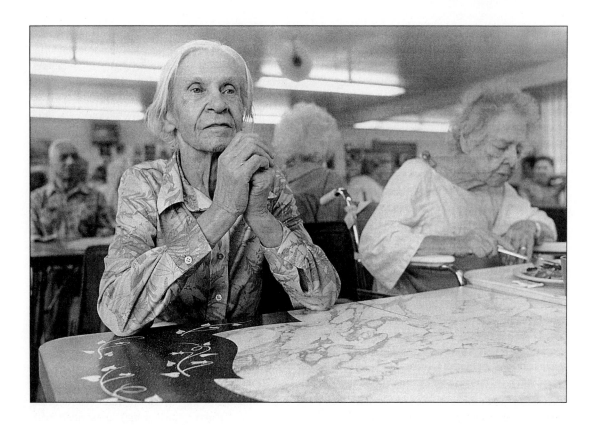

such a condition, and by age eighty-five and older, 16 percent reported being impaired. Drug abuse was almost nonexistent among the 65-plus age group. Women had a slightly higher incidence of mental disorders than men, with more affective disorders, anxiety disorders, phobias, and cognitive impairment. Men had a higher incidence of alcoholism than women.[32]

Elders in nursing homes have a much higher rate of mental illness than those living in the community. In fact, advanced mental illnesses (particularly dementia) are often the impetus for institutionalization. Numbers vary, but it is estimated that from 65 to 80 percent of nursing home residents have a mental illness, and from 60 to 75 percent of those have dementia.[33, 34]

Through the years psychiatrists and other mental health professionals have attempted to classify and define mental health and illness. Mental illness classifications vary over time—new illnesses are added or deleted under various classification systems. The most widely recognized classification schema recognized by mental health professionals is the *Diagnostic and Statistical Manual of Mental Disorders,* Vol. 4 (DSM-IV) developed by the American Psychiatric Association and is continually being revised.[35] The manual defines a mental disorder as a behavior or syndrome associated with distress or impairment in function. Each illness is clearly defined, and a list of criteria follows that characterize or diagnose that illness. The following section gives a brief overview of the most common mental disorders among elders.

Anxiety Disorders

Anxiety may be classified as a symptom or a mental disorder, depending upon the appropriateness of the response, the severity of the symptoms, and the degree to which it affects daily living. Transient anxiety can be a person's normal state of tension in response to a stressful situation. Whereas transient anxiety generally occurs in response to a specific environmental signal, such as an upcoming test, anxiety disorders occur without a specific external trigger. Because anxiety is a normal, and even a positive, reaction to many of life's stressors, it can be difficult to determine if it is severe enough to warrant a psychiatric diagnosis. For example, it is normal to be somewhat nervous when climbing up a high ladder, but the feeling is different with a phobia of heights. Likewise, determination of exactly when a normal behavior (such as checking the doors to be sure they are locked at night) becomes abnormal (repeatedly checking the doors each night) can be difficult for both patients and professionals. For anxiety to be considered a disorder, the symptoms must significantly affect social functioning, interpersonal relationships, or work effectiveness.

Regardless of the cause, anxiety is characterized by a combination of psychological symptoms, such as excessive worry, sense of foreboding and doom, or nervousness and physical symptoms such as dry mouth, restlessness, sweating, upset stomach, heart palpitations, insomnia, diarrhea, hyperventilation, shortness of breath, faintness, obsessive eating, or loss of appetite. Individuals may report a sense of dread or fear they are dying, losing control, or going crazy.

Anxiety is perhaps the most common of all mental disorders, affecting 23 million Americans. Nevertheless, most individuals with anxiety disorders are not diagnosed or treated. Diagnosing any of the anxiety disorders in elderly patients is difficult since it may occur in normal individuals or those with other disorders such as depression, dementia, or alcoholism. Furthermore, symptoms of anxiety mimic symptoms of illness: heart palpitations, shortness of breath, weakness, and appetite changes. For this reason, a comprehensive examination is necessary to determine if the person's anxiety is caused by disease, drug reactions, psychological problems, or transient life events.

Both transient and chronic anxiety should be treated because they increase feelings of helplessness and isolation, raise susceptibility to several illnesses, and decrease ability to withstand stress. Anxiety can be treated with relaxation or meditation techniques, psychotherapy, or medications. See the section on antianxiety drugs in chapter 10 for details.

The following section discusses the six most common anxiety disorders: generalized anxiety disorders, panic disorders, phobic disorders, adjustment disorders, post-traumatic stress disorders, and obsessive-compulsive disorders

Generalized anxiety disorders generally start early in life and pursue a chronic remitting and relapsing course. Individuals with this disorder are constantly worried or anxious that something terrible will happen, such as a natural disaster, financial peril, or harm to themselves or someone they love. They may know that their worry is out of proportion to the situation, but are unable to control it. Commonly, they experience physical symptoms such as muscle twitching, restlessness, tiredness, shortness of breath, dry mouth, dizziness, insomnia, and frequent urination. To meet the criteria for the diagnosis, these symptoms must persist for at least six months. This syndrome rarely starts in the later years. Buspar (busipirone), prescribed with cognitive-behavioral therapy, can assist persons to learn new ways to cope with anxious thoughts. Relaxation techniques, meditation, imagery, stress management, and biofeedback may also be helpful (discussed in chapter 12).

Panic disorders generally appear before the age of thirty and are characterized by brief, recurrent attacks of intense anxiety. Sufferers may believe they are having a heart attack, and professionals may concur, because they experience sweating, pounding heart, a sense of chest pressure, shortness of breath, and fear they are dying. If these symptoms occur for the first time in an elderly individual, other conditions, such as cardiac arrhythmias, medication reaction, or pulmonary disease should be considered. Panic attacks can lead to phobias as individuals try to avoid situations that may lead to another attack. The majority of individuals with panic disorder can be treated with cognitive-behavioral therapy. Antidepressants and antianxiety medications are also effective.

Phobic disorders are characterized by irrational fears that result in avoidance of particular situations or objects. These illnesses may be some of the more common in the elderly. For instance, agoraphobia is an irrational fear of open spaces, social phobia is a fear of interactions with others, and claustrophobia is a fear of closed spaces. These also generally begin in middle age; thus, the onset of a phobia in an older person should prompt the search for a functional limitation. For instance, an elder suddenly afraid of heights may actually be suffering a problem with balance. Cognitive-behavioral therapy, antidepressant medications, or beta blockers to slow the heart rate are effective treatments. Desensitization therapy, which involves gradually increasing exposure to the object of fear, can also be effective.

Adjustment disorders with anxiety occur following a stressful occurrence, for instance hospitalization or the diagnosis of cancer or Alzheimer's disease. Individuals with adjustment disorders manifest both physical and psychological symptoms of anxiety; however, their symptoms are often transitory as they adjust to the changes in their lives.

Exposure to a trauma or terrifying event can precipitate *post-traumatic stress disorder.* In this syndrome, individuals who have suffered a traumatic event (e.g., falling and not being discovered for hours or days) continue to relive the tragedy while awake and asleep. The illness occurs within three months of the event; some individuals recover within a year; in others, it becomes chronic. These people try to push the terrifying thought out of their mind, but repeatedly reexperience the event in flashbacks, nightmares, or memories. They may also suffer from depression, severe guilt or angry outbursts, and suicidal tendencies. Antidepressant medication and psychotherapy are effective.

People with *obsessive-compulsive disorders* have recurring uncontrollable thoughts, fears, and urges and have a need to ritually perform behaviors to reduce anxiety (e.g., continually checking locks on the door or ruminating on a past mistake). For the compulsion to be a true mental disorder, the ritual must consume at least one hour daily and interfere with daily life. This disorder responds well to psychotherapy and antianxiety and antidepressant medication.

Mood or Affective Disorders

Classification of mood disorders can be complicated because these illnesses run the gamut from normal sadness associated with bereavement to depression severe enough to result in admission to a psychiatric hospital. Matters are complicated further by the common usage of the word "depression" to encompass everything from transitory feelings of sadness to incapacitating despair resulting in suicide. Mood disorders include both depressive disorders (such as major depression or dysthymia) and the bipolar disorders, which are characterized by fluctuations between extreme excitability (mania) and depression.

Depression

Clinical depression is probably the most common psychological disorder among older people. Although studies suggest that the rate of major depression is lower among elders, many suspect that these low figures are due to underreporting. Depression in the elderly often goes unrecognized as neither the elder, the family, nor the physician realizes its presence.[36]

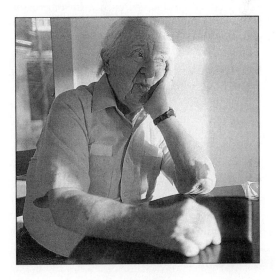

Because of the multiple physical problems associated with chronic illness in later life, elders, and those who care for them, often attribute symptoms of depression (such as lack of appetite, sleeplessness, loss of energy, and loss of pleasure) as normal accompaniments of old age. However, late-life depression causes much suffering to those who are undiagnosed and untreated, burdening families and institutions by having to care for those who otherwise would be able to care for themselves. Depression has been found to be a risk factor for the development of heart disease and cancer and contributes to a higher mortality rate from these and other diseases, particularly among men.[37,38]

Clinical depression, or major depressive disorder, is distinctly different from transient feelings of unhappiness or sadness following a loss. To meet the criteria for major depression, an individual must experience several of the following symptoms all day every day for at least two weeks: sadness, lack of enjoyment of activities previously found pleasurable, feelings of uselessness, and impaired ability to think clearly or concentrate. They may be unable to sleep, awaken too early in the morning, or suffer from excessive tiredness and sleepiness. Depressed individuals may complain of aches and pains, visit doctors frequently, and cry easily. They may experience thoughts of suicide, weight loss, sexual dysfunction, or feelings of hopelessness. They generally lack an appetite and energy. In some cases, depressed individuals also experience symptoms of anxiety, such as restlessness and panic.

Older people who are depressed may withdraw from social participation, refuse to speak, and become unable to care for themselves. In addition, depressed elders commonly manifest cognitive impairment, disorientation, slow speed of movement, angry outbursts, and shortened attention span. Some elders exhibit depression, but also symptoms of psychosis, such as loss of contact with reality or hallucinations. This condition is called psychotic depression.

Depression in old age may be a recurrence of depression from earlier years or it may appear for the first time. Those with the first onset of depression in their later years often suffer more severe depression, involving cognitive disturbances and abnormal brain patterns, These individuals may be more likely to develop Alzheimer's or other dementias in the future.

Depression commonly appears with other medical illnesses, such as heart disease, diabetes, dementia, or cancer. Depression, like all mental illnesses, is even more common among those residing in nursing homes.

There are other depressive disorders besides major depression. Dysthymia is a low-grade form of depression. People with dysthymia have long-standing symptoms of inadequacy and unhappiness that are not severe enough to meet the criteria for major depression. Individuals with *seasonal affective disorder* have depressive symptoms only during certain times of the year, most commonly the winter in northern latitudes. These individuals may be especially sensitive to lighting patterns so they are often treated by extended exposure to bright lights during winter days. *Reactive depressive disorders* describe symptoms of depression that follow a loss, such as the death of a loved one.

Depression is most often diagnosed by the patient's primary care physician. The presence of depression can be ascertained by several screening instruments. However, depression is underdiagnosed in all age groups, especially among older people. Further, depression may go unrecognized in the older population because its symptoms are mistaken for physical illness, medication reactions, "old age," or dementia. Loss of appetite, sleep disturbances, and fatigue are common in those who take multiple medications for their health problems. However, in elders, depressed mood may be less common than other symptoms, such as sleep and appetite disturbances. Elders may be less likely to see symptoms of depression as something to discuss with their physician and instead feel that they should "buck up."

In evaluating a patient for depression, the physician should first rule out other conditions that may cause or aggravate depressive symptoms: some diseases, medications, and excessive alcohol use. Differentiating between dementia and depression can be particularly difficult as severe depression can mimic dementia, and the two diseases often coexist. In general, dementia has a gradual onset, whereas depression develops more rapidly.

Studies seem to suggest that many bouts of depression lift spontaneously after a few months; however, treatment speeds recovery. Treatment of depression may be accomplished through individual or group psychotherapy, medications, or, in severe cases, electroconvulsive therapy. If depressed elders present a danger to themselves or others (e.g., they have a plan for committing suicide), then medical professionals are legally obligated to place the depressed patient in a secure hospital setting for twenty-four to seventy-two hours until treatment can be initiated and the danger is resolved.

Psychotherapy and medication is the most common treatment for depression. (See chapter 10 for details on antidepressants.) Light therapy, dance therapy, reading self-help materials, improving social supports, exercise therapy, and dietary supplements have all been proposed as alternative treatments. Antidepressant medications generally do not work immediately; usually they must be taken for three to six weeks before full symptom relief is noted.

An herbal remedy called St. John's wort has been shown in multiple small studies to be useful in treating mild to moderate depression. This herb can interact with other antidepressants, and those taking it should avoid foods rich in tyramine such as aged cheeses and red wine. In addition, because supplements are not regulated by the FDA, the quality and purity of this herb purchased over the counter may be highly variable.

The most controversial and misunderstood therapy for major depression is electroconvulsive therapy

What Is Your Opinion? Overselling Depression to the Old Folks

Stanley Jacobsen, age 70, a clinical psychologist

Depression in older men and women is a hot topic in the world of mental health. The dominant mental health experts say that too many older men and women are sad without reason—depressed and in need of professional help. I say the experts are missing the point. Oldness itself is a reason to be sad if you dwell on it, and it is in any event a matter of life and death to contend with. The remarkable fact is that most older people learn how to contain their oldness, and they are not depressed. Those who are slow to absorb the lesson can easily be confused and disheartened in a world that tells them they are losing their relevance and are likely to become a burden to family and society before they die, but not to worry, be happy. If they do worry, and look for help, they may well encounter a professional who is uncomfortable with the awesome incurability of oldness.

Health professionals want to reduce the struggle of the old to an illness. They label it "depression," search for a biological explanation of the "disease" and call the psychological, spiritual and social aspects of the conflict mere "risk factors." Unfortunately, by collud-ing in the denial that the fact of our mortality is significant to our mental health in later life, they contribute more to the prevalence of depression than its cure. Failure to credit the resilience and resourcefulness that successful aging requires (and that most people find within them) is a more significant public health problem than late-life depression.

My mind tells me that we cannot both love life and be indifferent to dying. If we mourn our decline toward death or, fearing it, overreact to an illness, perhaps our first need is simple, compassionate acceptance of the reality of our plight. If we resist admitting to unhappiness, as many older men and women are said to do, perhaps it is because the mood will be mistaken for pathology and we will find ourselves in the hands of a clinician who, defining the reaction as "a depression" and the depression as medial, will prescribe the pills. . . . I will not yield to the professionals' insistence that my being sad about being old is a disease.

Excerpted from Jacobsen, S. Overselling depression to the old folks, *Atlantic Monthly,* April 1995, pp. 46, 48, 50–51

(ECT), also called shock therapy. Studies continue to show it is an effective treatment for major depression. It has been endorsed by the National Institutes of Health as effective when antidepressants have not helped or cannot be given for a medical reason. It is especially useful for those who are suicidal or not functioning, because antidepressants take weeks for a full effect. Many experts assert it is at least as good, if not better, than drug therapy.

ECT is painless and safe. After receiving a short-acting anesthetic and a drug to prevent muscle contractions, the patient receives a weak electrical stimulus to the brain through small electrodes placed on the head. This produces a small, controlled seizure that lasts for about a minute. Most people are confused after the treatment and suffer short-term memory loss, but the side effects clear up quickly (about an hour). The benefits usually outweigh the risks. The usual course of treatment is three times a week for three to four weeks. It has been shown to have an eighty to ninety percent success rate and is safe even for frail elders.[39]

Bipolar Disorder

Bipolar disorder (formerly known as manic-depressive illness) occurs in 1 to 2 percent of the population, runs strongly in families, and can be quite difficult to diagnose and treat. Classically, individuals with bipolar disease manifest periods of depression interspersed with periods of heightened activity, irritability, poor judgment, and excessive energy called mania. The length of these cycles vary: some individuals rapidly change from excitable to depressed, others have long periods of relatively stable mental status, and still others are mainly depressed with occasional bouts of mania.

With age, periods of mania become less common and depression predominates. Bipolar disorder is a lifelong condition with a varying course that requires continual monitoring. Medications are used to stabilize mood, prevent mania, and treat symptoms of both mania and depression. The most commonly used medication is lithium, which has been used to treat this disorder for over forty years. Although lithium remains effective, drug dosages and blood levels must be carefully monitored in older people who have a higher rate of lithium toxicity. Anticonvulsant medications, antidepressants, and ECT are also used. Individual and group psychotherapy are important treatment modalities.

Somatoform Disorders

This cluster of disorders is characterized by multiple physical complaints without an identifiable cause. Contrary to popular belief, there is no evidence to support the idea that older people are more apt to suffer from somatoform disorders.[40] Two types, somatization disorder and hypochondriasis, will be described.

Somatization Disorder

This disorder is characterized by an excessive preoccupation with bodily function and complaints of pain and other problems affecting virtually every organ system. Generally, this disorder develops in adolescence and persists, with similar preoccupations and complaints, throughout life. These individuals tend to seek care from multiple physicians, and often undergo multiple diagnostic tests and even surgeries in an attempt to treat their innumerable problems. This disorder is more common in women, particularly women who report a history of childhood physical or sexual abuse. It seems to run in families and may be associated with other mental illnesses such as depression and alcoholism.

Hypochondriasis

This disorder is an unrealistic preoccupation with the body leading to preoccupation or fear of having a serious illness. For example, a woman with this disorder may be preoccupied with a fear of breast cancer and may seek care from multiple physicians and receive mammograms, but still be unconvinced that she does not have cancer. Hypochondriacs may also receive unnecessary diagnostic tests, drug treatment, or even surgery. Hypochondriasis is equally common among men and women and peaks in middle age. It may be difficult to differentiate this illness from normality because worry and preoccupation with health and illness are common among healthy Americans.

Paranoia in the Elderly

Mildred S. is a 76-year-old woman who lives alone in a small apartment in a neighborhood that has fallen into disrepair. She has lost her ability to hear well, and requires a cane to get around. Her son lives nearby and visits a few times a week, helping her to do her shopping. She doesn't have many friends in the neighborhood. She talks to her son often about the conspiracy in her neighborhood to get her to move out of her apartment and to get her money. Neighborhood residents harass her by peering into her windows, knocking at her door then running away, telephoning then hanging up when she answers the phone, and spying on her through high-technology lasers. When her son has questioned her neighbors about these activities, they have commented that she is a little eccentric, and deny any "spying activities" or really much interest in her at all.

Paranoid individuals have delusions that they are being persecuted by others for a perceived wrong-

doing. A delusion is a false belief based on mistaken assumptions about external reality that is not changed by obvious evidence to the contrary. Paranoia can occur alone in relatively high-functioning individuals, or may occur as part of another mental illness such as schizophrenia, depression, delirium, or dementia. In its milder forms, paranoia is characterized by rigidity in thought, unwarranted suspiciousness, hypersensitivity, exaggerated self-importance, and a tendency to blame others and attribute evil motives to them. Intellectual functioning is often normal. Paranoid individuals are seldom seen by mental health workers because they are secretive, or merely viewed as eccentric or senile by those around them. It can be difficult to determine whether or not the elder has a real reason to be fearful. In elders, most reactions are brief with only slight alterations in behavior, mood, and reasoning.

Family therapy is helpful for paranoid disorders; the family can be trained to listen and offer support to counteract the individual's fears, increase the elders' social interaction, and provide a stable environment to reduce paranoid incidents. Drugs, mainly minor tranquilizers, are effective in some cases.

Before diagnosing somatoform illnesses, physicians must rule out medical problems that may cause the vague constellation of symptoms. Individuals may be treated with minor tranquilizers, placebo medications, or harmless home treatments (such as warm baths) to assure the client that the physician is attempting to relieve the symptoms. Psychotherapy is usually unacceptable to the persons with somatoform disorders as they believe they have a real physical illness.

Schizophrenia

Schizophrenia is one of the most serious of all mental illnesses, and one of the most difficult to treat. Schizophrenia is characterized by delusions (false beliefs), thoughts of persecution, auditory hallucinations, and

illogical thoughts. People with schizophrenia hear voices, most often angry voices, which may command them to harm themselves or others. They may also harbor delusions about their body or religion (e.g., that one has a special religious mission or that one is the devil and condemned to burn in hell), or have grandiose (that they are an unrecognized, but very important person) or persecutory thoughts (that someone is after them). They may believe that the FBI is after them or that Martians are attempting to contact them through antennae on their heads. Individuals with schizophrenia may speak without emotional inflection, and their sentences may wander and not make much sense. They may express inappropriate emotions, for instance laughing when discussing the death of their spouses. In addition, they may dress or behave in a bizarre fashion.

Generally schizophrenia occurs first in late adolescence, although some people may acquire it in middle age. Most elders with schizophrenia have suffered the illness from a very young age and must contend with reduced intensity of symptoms coupled with side effects from long-term use of antipsychotic medications. Occasionally, schizophrenia has a first onset in old age, especially among women. It is associated with the following factors: paranoid symptoms, increased rate of hearing and visual problems, and a history of other members of the family who acquired the disease late in life. Most older schizophrenics need a structured environment for survival. Unfortunately, those placed in nursing homes are less likely to get adequate treatment because staff have neither the time, interest, nor training to respond to their needs.

An individual diagnosed with schizophrenia is never considered cured; interludes of sanity are assumed to be temporary remissions. However, the symptoms of schizophrenia are variable: some individuals are totally incapacitated, while others are able to function in society with medication. Those with schizophrenia have a high rate of suicide; one in ten schizophrenics commit suicide.

The mainstay of treatment is antipsychotic medications, usually for life (see chapter 10). However, a common side effect of long-term antipsychotic drugs is *tardive dyskinesia,* a syndrome of irreversible involuntary movements that resembles Parkinson's disease. Elderly patients are more susceptible to tardive dyskinesia than younger groups, especially elder women, and the incidence rises with length of treatment. Saltz and colleagues report that almost one of three elders who were prescribed antipsychotic medications had tardive diskinesia within a year.[41] Some suggest that the effect could be minimized if doses are reduced gradually to determine the lowest effective dose for each individual.[42]

Sleep Disorders

There are at least ninety known sleep disorders, and about two-thirds of them are associated with insomnia. Insomnia is defined as the inability to achieve and sustain restful sleep. Insomnia is an extremely common condition, affecting about one-third of all adults, although most never seek medical care for this condition. Many times, sleep disorders are no more than irritants, but when severe, mental health and immune functioning may be affected, possibly increasing infection risk.[43]

Elders report more sleep complaints than any other age group: difficulty falling asleep, periods of wakefulness in bed, restless sleep, and early morning awakening. It is estimated that up to one-half of all elders living in the community and two-thirds of elders in nursing homes have sleep disturbances.[44] Insomnia at night can lead to sleepiness during the day. Those who report sleep disturbances have a higher rate of auto accidents, reduced ability to concentrate, memory impairment, interpersonal problems, decreased immune function, and an increased risk of serious illness compared to those who sleep well. Despite these consequences, most sleep disturbances are not diagnosed or treated.

Insomnia can be transient, short-term, or chronic. Transient insomnia lasts at most a few nights and is generally associated with a specific stressful event (e.g., anxiety regarding the results of a medical test). Short-term insomnia lasts from days to months and is often precipitated by a more significant life stressor (e.g., death in the family). Chronic insomnia persists for longer than a month and is generally related to an underlying medical or psychological condition.

Some of elders' sleep complaints are due to age-associated changes in sleep patterns. With advancing age, the time it takes to fall asleep lengthens. Older people spend more time in light sleep and less time in deep-sleep stages. Although the number of times an individual awakens at night increases with age, elders are generally able to fall back to sleep. Sleeping becomes less efficient with age (that is, more time is spent in bed for less actual sleep).

Besides age, sleep disturbances can have a number of physiological and psychological causes. For example, sleep problems are commonly associated with depression, dementia, anxiety, heart disease, urinary problems and alcoholism. Many medications cause insomnia.

Caffeine in coffee, tea, soft drinks, and some over-the-counter medications can also have a significant effect.

When an elder complains of insomnia, a thorough history should be undertaken to determine whether an underlying cause of the problem can be treated. If the sleep disorder is severe, observation of sleep/wake patterns in a sleep laboratory provides further information.

Many sleep disorders can be improved by changing personal habits. If the sleep disorder is not improved with such behavioral changes, psy-chotherapy or drugs may be in order. Refer to chapter 10 for effective drug therapy for insomnia (sedatives/hypnotics).

Melatonin, a hormone found in the brain that regulates the body's internal clock, may help people with sleep problems to fall asleep more quickly and to stay asleep longer. However, further studies are needed to determine proper dosages and side effects. Melatonin is already available over the counter as a dietary supplement, but there is concern about its purity and potency because it is not regulated by the FDA.

Methods to Improve Sleep Habits

1. Try to establish a regular rising time in the morning and bedtime in the evening. A regular sleeping pattern strengthens the sleep/wake cycle and promotes a regular sleep onset time.
2. Avoid caffeinated beverages (coffee, tea, cola) and chocolate after the evening meal. Avoid high-calorie evening meals. A light snack, warm milk, or a banana before bedtime may promote sleep. Bananas and milk contain tryptophan, which helps induce sleep.
3. Wind down for a period before sleep. Quiet activities such as reading, relaxing in a hot bath, or meditating help promote sleep.
4. Avoid using the bedroom for watching television, doing paper work, eating, or other activities. Bedrooms should only be used for sleep and sexual activity.
5. Sexual activity is an effective method to induce sleep, practiced alone or with a partner.
6. Avoid stimulating thoughts, conversations, and activities around bedtime.
7. Make sure mattress, pillows, sheets, and blankets are comfortable. Wool or egg crate mattress covers can minimize tossing and turning.
8. Go to bed only when sleepy. If sleep does not occur after twenty minutes in bed, get up and engage in a relaxing activity until you feel tired.
9. Check the bedroom environment. When temperatures are too hot or too cold, it interferes with sleep. Reducing the noise level also helps create an environment conducive to sleep. If you cannot control the noise, earplugs or a white noise machine is helpful. Make sure the room is as dark as possible.
10. Engage in gentle exercise to produce fatigue before sleep. A daily brisk walk or other aerobic activity at least three hours before bedtime is helpful.
11. Restrict fluids in the evening and before retiring to help reduce the frequency of awakening to go to the bathroom.
12. Try relaxation techniques. Think of pleasant thoughts and images. If it works for you, try it the next time you have problems getting to sleep.
13. Avoid taking stimulating medications before bedtime, such as albuterol inhalers for asthma, Prozac, or beta blockers (propanolol). Avoid taking over-the-counter sleep medications. Have the pharmacist check any drugs you take to be sure they do not contain caffeine or any other stimulants.
14. Resist using alcohol or sedating drugs to get to sleep. Although they serve as short-term fix for insomnia, in the long run, it is better to develop good sleep habits.
15. Avoid taking naps during the day.

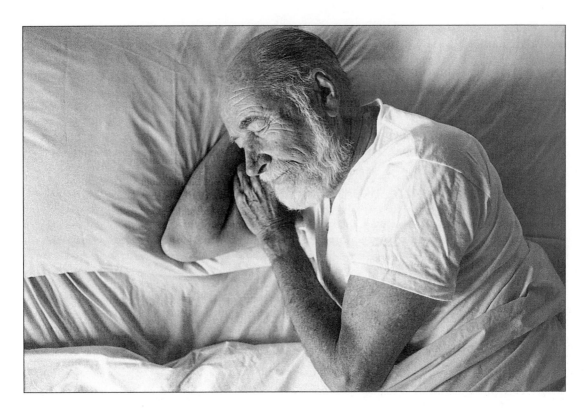

One reason for insomnia among older people could be a condition known as *restless legs syndrome*. Individuals with this syndrome experience rhythmic leg movements during sleep, which cause discomfort that can only be relieved by movement or stimulation of the legs. Unfortunately, the symptoms recur when the individual goes back to bed. Thus, elders may experience discomfort (often described as "crawling") in their legs, may wake up from sleep, get up and shower, apply ointments, rub their legs or walk, only to have the symptoms return when they try again to fall asleep. In rare cases the arms are affected or the individual has symptoms at other times, such as during a car trip. It is thought that 5 to 10 percent of the population has restless legs syndrome, with incidence increasing with advancing age. The problem is treated with medications for Parkinson's disease, long-acting benzodiazepines in low doses given at bedtime, or opioid painkillers (such as codeine), or combinations of these agents. Tricyclic antidepressants, Prozac, or lithium can worsen the symptoms.

Many elders suffer from *sleep apnea,* brief periods during sleep when breathing stops. Cessation of breathing may last from seconds to more than one minute and may occur hundreds of times a night. Each time the breathing is cut off, the elder awakens to breathe. Although this awakening is life-preserving, it is also a severe disrupter of sleep. Thus, those who suffer sleep apnea are generally very sleepy during the day. They may also suffer headaches or personality changes. The lack of oxygen at night puts these individuals at a higher risk of cardiac arrhythmias and sudden death from heart disease. In addition, these individuals suffer significant cognitive decline[45] and an increased risk of auto accidents from falling asleep while driving.

Sleep apnea may be caused by problems in the part of the brain that regulates breathing, but it is more often due to mechanical problems related to excess fat and tissue in the throat, cutting off breathing during sleep. Most of those who suffer from sleep apnea are middle-aged overweight men. Those who snore are also at higher risk because snoring is often related to excess fatty tissue in the throat. Diagnosis of sleep apnea may require time in a sleep laboratory. Treatment may include weight loss, surgery, or the use of a nasal device to increase oxygenation at night. Alcohol and sedatives worsen sleep apnea.

Substance Use Disorders

The major substance abuse problems among elders are the overuse of and dependence on prescription tranquilizers and alcohol; illicit drug use is exceedingly rare. Although it is thought that older people, particularly women, have high rates of abuse of prescription drugs (e.g., sedatives, painkillers), there are very few data to support or refute this stereotype. However, there is ample evidence regarding abuse of alcohol among elders, and this will be the focus of this section.

Alcoholism, also called alcohol dependence, is the excessive use of alcohol despite problems with work, family, or health. It is considered to be a progressive, debilitating chronic illness. The disease is often fatal and can cause health problems in virtually every organ system. Alcoholism is associated with multiple physical and psychological problems. Studies show that excess alcohol consumption shortens life expectancy, contributes to high suicide rates, worsens many chronic illnesses (especially diabetes), and creates nutritional deficiencies. Additionally, heavy alcohol use can induce dementia, cognitive deficits, depression, and psychosis. Alcohol affects muscular coordination, reaction time, and equilibrium, increasing susceptibility to accidents. Alcohol adversely affects the quality of sleep. Alcohol misuse is known to be associated with car accidents, suicides and homicides, and physical abuse of family members. Older alcoholics are also at high risk for adverse reactions when medications are mixed with alcohol.

Because of changes in the distribution and metabolism of alcohol with age, elders are more susceptible to intoxication by alcohol with advancing age. Older adults usually have a lower body-water content than younger adults, concentrating the alcohol, potentially causing more damage to organs and tissues. It is now known that older people break down less ethanol in the stomach, allowing a higher

How Much Alcohol is Too Much?

There has been much discussion in the medical literature about the value of "moderate alcohol use" in reducing the incidence of heart disease and death. But how much is too much? Because elders do not have the capacity of younger groups, the one to two drinks a day recommendation for the general population (one for women, two for men) is not suitable for the elderly, or even for women at any age. And how much is in a drink? One 4 oz glass of wine, a 12 oz glass of beer, and a 1.5 oz drink of 90 proof liquor are equivalent to one drink. For older adults, it is recommended that a maximum of one drink a day contributes to cardiovascular benefits. For some elders, even one drink is too much. Most studies indicate that the maximum benefit for men is two to six drinks per week.[47] The benefits for women at any age are not as well-studied and are less clear.

proportion of alcohol to circulate in the bloodstream. This occurs because they have a reduced amount of alcohol dehydrogenase, the enzyme in the stomach that breaks down alcohol, when compared to young men.[46] Also, elders often take medications that have a heightened effect when combined with alcohol.

The majority of elder alcoholics suffer from drinking problems throughout their entire life, but a few (less than 10 percent) begin drinking to excess later in life, generally after age sixty. It used to be thought that elders turned to alcohol later in life because of stressful, negative situations, but studies have never shown that to be valid. Most of the alcohol consumption among that group is social drinking.[48] It is now believed that elders continue their former patterns, and if anything, cut down on their drinking.

National surveys indicate a significant drop in heavy drinkers with advancing age and a higher percentage of abstainers among elders when compared to younger adult groups. Even older people who are alcoholics drink less than their younger peers; those who drink may drink only five or six days weekly and may consume less than four drinks daily.[49] Further, as many as half of all elders, and an even higher proportion of older women, abstain from alcohol completely.

Estimates vary, but it is generally agreed that the proportion of elder alcoholics is about 2 to 4 percent of the elder population, considerably lower that the 10 percent usually quoted for the population as a whole. However, the rates are higher among those who visit physicians and are admitted to hospitals. Alcoholism is more common among whites than African Americans and Hispanic Americans and those who are divorced, separated, and/or are living alone. Alcoholism is five times more common among elder men than among elder women.

There may be fewer elderly alcoholics for a number of reasons. Those who drank heavily in earlier life may have already died from alcoholism or its complications. Elders may have reduced alcohol consumption because they have become increasingly sensitive to the effects of alcohol. Or elder alcoholics may reside in sheltered living settings or institutions and are not counted in community studies. Experts predict that when the younger generation enters their later years, they will have a higher prevalence of alcohol use than those who are currently old.

Physicians seldom diagnose alcoholism in their patients, no matter what their age. Diagnosis of alcoholism is more complex in elders because alcoholism may have more subtle manifestations. Younger people who abuse alcohol are more likely to have visible signs of alcohol intoxication and withdrawal than elders. Additionally, the physical signs of alcoholism, such as depression, dementia-like reactions, poor grooming, incontinence, susceptibility to injury and falls, malnutrition, and general physical deterioration, may be attributed to chronic illness and old age. Further, elders' alcohol dependence is less likely to be detected by an employer or spouse, since many are already retired, live alone, and are not socially disruptive.

A variety of instruments have been developed to help doctors diagnose more cases of alcoholism in their practice. One of the simplest and most widely used is the CAGE questionnaire consisting of four items.[50] Answering yes to two of the questions is suspicious for alcoholism.

- Have you ever felt you should **C**ut down on your drinking?
- Have people **A**nnoyed you by criticizing your drinking?
- Have you ever felt bad or **G**uilty about your drinking?
- Have you ever had a drink first thing in the morning to steady your nerves or get rid of a hangover (**E**ye-opener)?

This screening instrument has been criticized because it may miss some elderly alcoholics. Instead, it has been suggested that the CAGE be combined with questions regarding quantity and frequency of drinking.[51] The Council of Scientific Affairs, part of the American Medical Association, has released guidelines for physicians to encourage them to be more active in preventing, diagnosing and treating alcoholism and alcohol-related problems in the elderly.[52]

Alcoholism can be treated. The first step is for physicians to advise elders to reduce or cease drinking because of adverse health effects. One study reported that just two 10- to 15-minute counseling sessions significantly decreased alcohol use and consequent physician visits among elderly men.[53] In contrast to young and middle-aged alcoholics, elder alcoholics do not generally need to be hospitalized and detoxified. If there are any symptoms of withdrawal, then cessation of drinking is often accomplished in a hospital or under close medical supervision at home with symptom-reducing medications (generally benzodiazepines such as librium). There are a number of treatment programs, and it is not clear which works best. One long and expensive study compared three methods, and all had the same success rate.[54]

Since no one treatment has been found to be better than another, Alcoholics Anonymous (AA) may be a good choice for elders because it is free, easily accessible, and is a way to be part of a social support

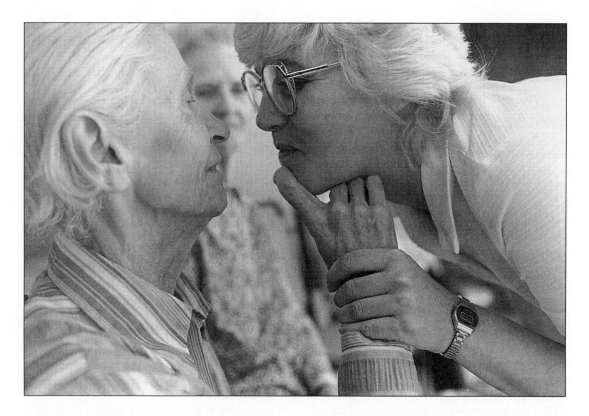

system. There are over 36,000 AA groups in the United States, and many are found throughout the world. Their theory of addiction is that alcoholism is a physical, mental, and spiritual disease that can only be conquered through lifetime abstinence and sustained participation in a recovery program. Usually the program includes other drug addictions besides alcohol. Meetings occur daily in many locations: schools, churches, community centers, and worksites. They generally begin with testimonials from those who are abstinent or trying to be, who talk about the negative effects of alcohol on their life and the positive effects of abstinence and the AA program. New members are assigned a sponsor who can provide support when cravings get strong. All members are unconditionally accepted, and there is support across class, gender, and ethnicity.

Psychotherapy and medication are also helpful. Two common program types for alcoholism treatment are cognitive-behavior therapy (developing coping skills to deal with situations that tempt one to drink) and motivational enhancement therapy (learn to identify and mobilize personal strengths and resources to reduce alcohol consumption). Drugs may also be prescribed as an adjunct to group work. Disulfiram, also known as Antabuse, is used to assist patients to maintain abstinence. When patients taking this drug drink alcohol, they become nauseated, flushed, and vomit or have diarrhea. Naltrexone (Revia) is a newer drug that blocks the opioid receptors in the brain, blunting the pleasurable effects associated with drinking, thus reducing cravings.

Dementia

Dementia is a progressive brain impairment that interferes with memory and normal intellectual functioning. Dementia can be caused by a number of factors: brain tumors, AIDS, trauma, environmental toxins, chronic lung disease, alcoholism, drugs, and multiple small strokes (multi-infarct dementia). The most common type of dementia,

Alzheimer's disease, is characterized by a gradual, irreversible, and progressive decline in mental functioning. In contrast, multi-infarct dementia is caused by multiple small strokes, each one causing more nerve damage. Symptoms are a sudden onset of dizziness, headaches, and decreased energy in addition to the classic dementia symptoms. The course of this type of dementia is erratic. Initially, individuals may recover lost function, but as more small strokes occur, the chance of recovery is low. Both Alzheimer's disease and multi-infarct dementia are irreversible and result in progressive, permanent mental impairment.

Other dementias are reversible: depression, hearing loss, thyroid disease, pneumonia, electrolyte imbalances, syphilis, and nutritional deficiencies (especially thiamine deficiency, which occurs in alcoholism). HIV/AIDS and certain drugs have been known to cause temporary dementia. A thorough medical evaluation is needed when symptoms of dementia occur. Generally, a sudden onset of symptoms signals a reversible drug reaction or treatable condition, while a progressively worsening deterioration that does not respond to therapy is more likely irreversible.

No matter what the type, dementia is characterized by a loss of cognitive skills, including memory, language, recognition, visual and spatial skills, and a change in personality. Elders with dementia are forgetful, have difficulty learning new things, and may try to minimize or deny their deficits. Short-term memory is much more affected than long-term memory, thus demented individuals may not be able to recall who made a visit earlier that day, but will be able to recall events in the distant past with clarity. They may have difficulty understanding directions, may get lost in previously familiar places, and their speech may become less coherent. Another common behavior is called "sundowning," a worsening of function in the evening hours. Dementia is also associated with physical declines, such as incontinence of bowel or bladder, inability to walk and, in the very end stages, inability to hold one's head up. The length of the disease is usually from eight to ten years after the onset of symptoms.

Although dementia can occur in midlife, the vast majority of cases are diagnosed after age seventy-five, and its incidence increases with age. It is estimated that over two million people in the nation have the disease, and two-thirds are women. The higher proportion of women is due to their longer life expectancy. The prevalence among seventy-five year olds is 4 percent, but by age ninety, the prevalence is 28 percent.[55] It is projected that as an increasing proportion of the population survives past eighty-five, the incidence of Alzheimer's dementia will skyrocket. Some degree of dementia is present in over half the nursing home residents and in one-third of all elderly residents of mental hospitals.[56]

By far the most common and most studied type of dementia is Alzheimer's disease. The cause of Alzheimer's disease is still a mystery. Age remains the strongest risk factor for Alzheimer's disease, although family history of the disease is also important. A history of a severe head injury where consciousness was lost is another major risk factor. Certain genes are associated with Alzheimer's disease. Those with a particular subtype of ApoE (ApoE4) a cholesterol-carrying blood protein, have a higher risk of Alzheimer's dementia, while those with ApoE2 seem to be protected from it. And, individuals with Down's syndrome (who have an extra copy of chromosome 21) have higher rates as well. Similarly, a chromosomal abnormality on chromosome 14 is common in those who develop Alzheimer's disease at a younger age. Some people who inherit the gene never develop the disease, and others without the gene do, so genetic screening is not recommended.[57]

Other risk factors for Alzheimer's disease have also been determined. African Americans and Hispanic American elders exhibit higher rates of Alzheimer's disease than whites. Those with lower educational attainment or occupational levels have at least twice the risk of developing Alzheimer's disease compared to those with more schooling.[58] A study of nuns found that those who had wordy, complex writing styles as young women were much less likely to develop Alzheimer's disease than those nuns who did not.[59] This may be because higher educational achievement allows elders to

Crumbs for my Heart
Loraine Bridge

I found her sitting in the lounge, in the spot we had shared so many times before. She wore a blue-and-green-plaid housedress, and as she sat there, her fingers traced the pattern over and over again. Once in a while her hand wandered to a small reveled spot, and a soft finger twisted itself through the loose thread. Her eyes met mine as I sat down.

"Hello," I said. "How are you?"

"Oh, pretty good," she replied. "And you?"

"Just fine," I answered. She hadn't visited with anyone for many days, and she seemed to enjoy my company.

"It's a lovely day," I said. "Cool but sunny."

"Is it? Where did all the leaves go?"

"Away," I replied. "It's fall now, and everything is getting ready for winter."

"I used to be so busy in the fall," she said, "but I haven't done anything at home yet."

"My garden was great this year. The strawberries were really nice," I replied.

Her eyes were so blue, so clear. Her face so pleasant. Her hair, always so well-groomed, fell in soft waves, pure white and soft as a thistledown.

I spoke again. "Let's go have some coffee. I brought some cookies Karen baked"

"Do you have a daughter?" she questioned.

"Yes, Karen is my daughter. She is 12 now."

"She bakes lovely cookies. You must always encourage her, even if they don't turn out just right. Otherwise she will lose interest in baking."

I crumbled a cookie. "Our boy is 16 now."

"What is his name?" she asked.

"Mark, and he's such a tall boy. Almost six foot four inches tall now."

"My that is big," she agreed. "I knew somebody called Mark, I think, but he was a little fellow."

And so we sat, talking of small things, common things. Once she mentioned "him," I didn't have to ask his name. I knew him well. He had been dead for many years.

Slowly the sun dipped behind the trees. It was time for dinner. Lights blinked on here and there. The nurse stood waiting at the door.

"I must be going," I said. "I have a long drive ahead of me."

"Do you live very far away?"

I answered slowly. "Almost 300 miles south of here."

She walked with me to the front door. "This has been nice," she said, "but I don't even know your name."

The words choked me. "It's Loraine . . ." I could say no more.

Then, for just one second, blinding recognition flashed across her face. Then shame. Then sorrow. Then nothing.

Softly she whispered, "Yes, my Loraine, and you are so pretty."

I turned and ran—the compliment clutched to my heart to ease its pain. I carried the words even more closely than I used to carry the cookies she handed out years ago, to ease my childhood hurt.

Dear Lord, thank you for letting Mother call me pretty.

compensate for the losses of Alzheimer's disease for a longer period of time.

Currently, the only sure way to diagnose Alzheimer's disease is to do an autopsy on the brain. When the brain is examined there are characteristic tangles of fibers within nerve cells, dead neurons, brain atrophy, and senile plaques (abnormal nerve cells wrapped with a waxy waste material). Thus, a probable diagnosis of Alzheimer's dementia must be made on an individual suspected of having the disease. When an individual shows signs and symptoms of dementia with a gradual onset, and other causes are excluded (such as multiple strokes, depression, AIDS, hypothyroidism, brain tumors), Alzheimer's disease is suspected. Generally, elders must undergo a thorough cognitive evaluation, blood tests, computerized tomography (CT) or other imaging of the brain, and physical examination.

There is currently no cure for Alzheimer's disease. However, several medications are shown to be helpful, at least for some. Cognex (tacrine), the first drug approved for Alzheimer's disease, improves cognitive function among those people with early signs of Alzheimer's disease.[60] However, tacrine is only a temporary stopgap: it delays the symptoms by about six months for one in four patients and has serious side effects. Nevertheless, it has been shown that those taking high dosages were significantly less likely to be placed in nursing homes than those with lower dosages.[61] Antidepressant and major tranquilizer drugs are often used to control the most troublesome behavioral disturbances that accompany dementia: sleeplessness, violent behavior, agitation, depression, and paranoia. Also vitamin E has also been shown to be effective in at least one controlled trial.[62] Gingko biloba, an herbal remedy, has shown some efficacy in a randomized, double-blind, placebo-controlled study in improving memory in patients with mild to moderate Alzheimer's disease.[63] Evidence is accumulating that hormone replacement therapy is associated with a lower risk and later onset of Alzheimer's disease among women.[64]

In the early stages of Alzheimer's disease, patients may need counseling to cope with stress and depression. For the later stages, providing a safe environment with adequate nutrition and body care is important. This may occur at home, in board and care homes, in nursing homes, or in specialized dementia care units.

Individuals with Alzheimer's dementia and other neurologic diseases often manifest behavioral problems. They may cry without stopping, become agitated and try to get out of bed even though they are too weak to walk. They may be verbally abusive or violent toward their caregivers, they may wander out of the house and get lost, or they may be very anxious and panicky, pacing or ruminating incessantly. Coping with these behavioral problems can be extraordinarily difficult for those who care for them. In many ways, the patient with Alzheimer's disease becomes a large child, dependent in many

activities of daily living, exhibiting poor judgment and needing constant supervision. Behavioral problems are a major impetus to institutionalize the elder with Alzheimer's disease.

Because of the length and severity of the disease, caring for an individual with Alzheimer's disease is exceedingly expensive, about $50,000 annually. From diagnosis to death (generally two to ten years), caring for one patient with Alzheimer's disease is more than $170,000. The total bill for care of Alzheimer's patients in the United States is more than $80 billion annually, with about half the costs financed by the federal government.[65]

Not only can the disease be financially devastating, but it can also be emotionally devastating. Family members must witness the slow, progressive physical and mental decline of a loved one with no hope of treatment or cure, often for several years. When the disease becomes advanced, patients cannot recognize family members, and cannot speak, walk well, or feed themselves.

The demented, and those who care for them at home, may receive assistance from a variety of health and social services in the community such as homemaker assistance, home health care, respite care, and adult day care. However, the presence of these services and the payment mechanisms vary significantly among communities so that formal assistance to remain in the home may not be available for many.

Many communities have organized support and education groups for families of those with Alzheimer's disease that have been reported to be effective in increasing the family's knowledge of the disease and their feelings of competence in caring for the health problems that accompany dementia. Family-based counseling and support can reduce the incidence of nursing home placement.[66] Many experts recommend psychotherapy or other support for caregivers of patients with Alzheimer's disease to reduce their own depression.

Delirium

Delirium is an acute, often reversible disorder of attention and concentration. The most common causes of delirium are infections (urinary tract infections or pneumonia), medications, or dehydration. However, there are multiple other causes including alcoholism, malnutrition, vitamin deficiencies, viral infections, abrupt drug withdrawal, fever, head trauma, heart attack, diabetes, or thyroid disease. Often, delirium is the result of a vulnerable patient dealing with many physical and environmental insults (such as medications, unfamiliar environment, infections and fear).

The symptoms of delirium are well-defined: agitation, confusion, disorientation, memory loss, decreased attention span, and insomnia alternating with excessive sleepiness. A hallmark of delirium is its constant fluctuation. One moment, an elder may be clear mentally and able to respond appropriately, and the next moment be quite confused or agitated. Or, they may be sleepy and difficult to wake up, then abruptly become agitated and excitable. Their days and nights may be mixed up, sleeping in the day and becoming agitated, fearful or anxious at night. Patients with delirium have difficulty concentrating even for a few moments, they may pick at the bedclothes and they often do not want to stay in bed. Visual hallucinations, such as seeing their dead father in the room, being paranoid, and refusing medications and food are other common symptoms.

Delirium begins much more abruptly and dramatically than dementia, often over hours to days. Delirium is a common occurrence among the elderly, especially after surgery and while in the intensive care unit.[67] Studies report that from 14 to 56 percent of elderly hospitalized patients experience delirium, resulting in longer, costlier hospitalizations, increased rate of nursing home placement, long-term cognitive defects and mortality rates of 10 to 65 percent.[68] One study of hospitalized elders showed that five factors were predictive of delirium onset: use of physical restraints, malnutrition, more than three medications, use of bladder catheter, and any other hospital- or doctor-caused adverse event.[69]

It is important that the patient be evaluated promptly when symptoms are observed because many cases of dementia are reversible, and prolonged delirium can lead to irreversible brain damage or even death. Treating the cause is the most effective way to correct delerium. Physical restraints should be kept to a minimum as these may increase fear and distress.

Prevention is better than treatment of delirium. Prevention includes reducing all medications to the bare minimum, maintaining a calm environment while hospitalized, encouraging family members to stay with confused elders, and providing medical treatment at home when possible. Having the elder visit a hospital or intensive care unit prior to hospitalization can reduce the risk of delirium.

ASSESSMENT OF PSYCHOLOGICAL VULNERABILITY

A thorough assessment of the impaired individual by a physician is necessary to accurately diagnose the cause and extent of mental dysfunction. The elder should be reassessed periodically to determine whether the treatments are working. A critical part of the assessment is to address the concerns and problems of family members. Medical history, physical examination and some laboratory tests (e.g., assessment of thyroid function) can assist in diagnosing factors that contribute to mental impairment. Many standardized forms have been developed to screen for various mental illnesses including alcoholism, depression, or dementia.

PSYCHOLOGICAL TREATMENTS

The mind is its own place, and can make a hell of heaven, a heaven of hell.

John Milton

Advances in psychoactive drugs have dramatically altered our understanding of the causes of mental impairments and have greatly improved the quality of life of those treated with them. Many illnesses that formally were thought to be amenable only to psychotherapy now can be effectively treated with medications. However, the increased reliance on medication should not replace "talk" treatments, particularly psychotherapy. Oftentimes, both are used to facilitate those with mental illness in living more functional and more fulfilling lives.

Psychotherapy is a type of structured relationship between a patient and professional with the purpose of improving the patient's mental health. There are a number of different types of psychotherapy, but most rely on structured conversation designed to facilitate change in the client's ways of thinking or acting. Clients may interact one-on-one with a psychotherapist or be part of a group. The techniques used depend upon the state of the impaired individual and the nature of the problem. With older people, as any other age group, the fit between client and therapist is crucial to the success of the therapy. Most therapists use a combination of approaches, focusing both on understanding the causes of behaviors and on offering strategies to alter unwanted behaviors.

Research documenting the effectiveness of various types of therapy has been limited and is almost nonexistent for elders, although it is generally believed they respond as well as other adult age groups. There are even fewer data on the optimal type, duration, and focus of therapy among the elderly.

What little research is available suggests that cognitive-behavioral approaches and interpersonal approaches are the most helpful. *Cognitive therapy* teaches people to recognize that their thought processes may cause psychological harm. To offer a simplistic example, depressed patients may be taught not to allow one negative experience to ruin their whole day and would be taught ways to focus on successes. Anxious patients might be taught to recognize when anxiety-producing thoughts enter their mind and learn ways to counteract them. *Behavioral therapy* teaches patients to increase certain behaviors through positive reinforcements and decrease other behaviors by being sure *not* to provide any positive reinforcements. For example, an elder who wishes to quit smoking may reward himself for each day without a cigarette. Another elder who wishes to get over a phobia of spiders may learn to relax at the thought of a spider or while looking at a spider in a book. Cognitive-behavioral therapy incorporates both cognitive therapy and behavioral therapy. *Interpersonal therapy* focuses on assisting elders to improve their

relationships with others by improving communication and interpersonal skills.

Many believe that therapy for elders should be shorter and more focused on problem solving using existing skills than on restructuring personality. Researchers Hayslip and Kooken have developed eight goals of therapy for elders: aid insight into behavior, provide symptom relief, provide relief to relatives, delay deterioration, aid in adaptation to the present situation, improve self-care skills, encourage activity, and facilitate independence. They assert that the most effective treatment a therapist can offer to alleviate a client's stress is to coordinate family, friends, and community resources to assist the client.[70] Because institutionalized elders commonly have cognitive deficits and physical and psychological limitations, the main goal of psychotherapy in that setting is to maximize physical and psychological function through environmental stimulation and to increase morale.

Psychotherapy can occur on an individual basis, through groups of individuals with similar problems who do not know each other, or with family members. In *individual psychotherapy,* a client and therapist work one-on-one focusing on elucidating, defining, and treating the client's problems. In *group therapy,* one or more counselors leads a group of clients, generally with similar problems or concerns. Group therapy is less expensive and can have the added benefit of facilitating social interactions. When there are difficulties within the familial or marriage relationship, family or marital therapy is indicated.

Family therapists attribute an individual's mental problems to a breakdown in the family's functioning. They assert that the family, not the individual, should be the treatment focus. As a result, all members of the family are convened, both as a group and individually, to work out the problem. This therapy can assist families in coping with the demands of the impaired family member or to work on relationships that are aggravating the older person's mental condition. *Marital therapy,* in which both partners receive counseling, enables them to better cope with life transitions that affect the marriage, including retirement, physical disability, or changes in sexual activ-

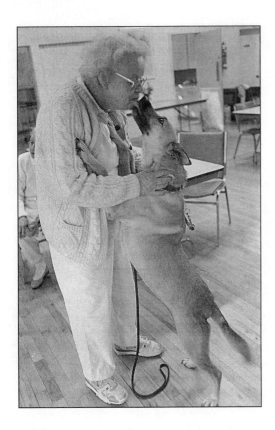

ity. Marital therapy for elders usually consists of short-term crisis intervention that focuses on a particular problem that has arisen or skill development in communication techniques. Elders are encouraged to develop new skills and to apply behavior that worked well in the past. Adult children may be brought in as necessary.

Alternative psychosocial approaches that do not use trained psychologists are commonly used among elder groups. Many of these encourage self-expression and social interaction. Some therapies involve the use of art, music, or dance to express deep-seated feelings and increase self-efficacy; others encourage elders to reminisce and review their life's accomplishments. For institutionalized elders, therapy may involve frequent reorientation to where they are and what is going on in the world, called *reality therapy,* or activities designed to facilitate social interaction. *Pet therapy* is gaining in popularity for its use among the elderly and disabled. In

nursing homes, pet visitation has been reported to expand conversation topics, increase sociability and animation, calm residents, and increase self-esteem.

Sometimes therapy is accomplished informally, through self-help groups or peer counselors. *Self-help or support groups* generally arise spontaneously in response to a specific need by persons who share mutual concerns. Typically, these groups are initiated by individuals who want them, although agencies and organizations may facilitate their formation. Most groups are formally organized and meet regularly. The meetings usually involve group discussions in which members learn from one another as they share experiences and give advice. The groups may invite professionals as guests when needed. Some groups publish newsletters, and many consider public education and advocacy part of their goal.

There are almost a million self-help groups in the United States, and the number is increasing. Self-help groups are available for a wide range of problems or situations. Some, such as Alcoholics Anonymous, stop-smoking, and weight-reduction groups, focus on controlling negative behaviors by working on techniques members can use to help themselves. Often groups bring together individuals who are in a similar situation, such as bereavement groups for those who have lost a spouse or support groups for those who are caring for a loved one with Alzheimer's disease. Some groups stress medical care or rehabilitation from a specific illness. For instance, there are groups for people with diabetes, people with colostomies, or people coping with the aftermath of breast cancer surgery. Finally, there are self-fulfillment and self-improvement groups designed to maximize personal potential.

Elder peer counselors offer informal, non-threatening interactions by establishing a personal relationship between the counselor and the elder in need. Elder peer counselors may work with individuals or groups of elders. They may visit elders in their own homes or in community centers or institutional settings. They may provide education, social support, counseling, and referral to appropriate community agencies. Peer counselors may be as effective as professional mental health workers in many instances. One study compared the effectiveness of

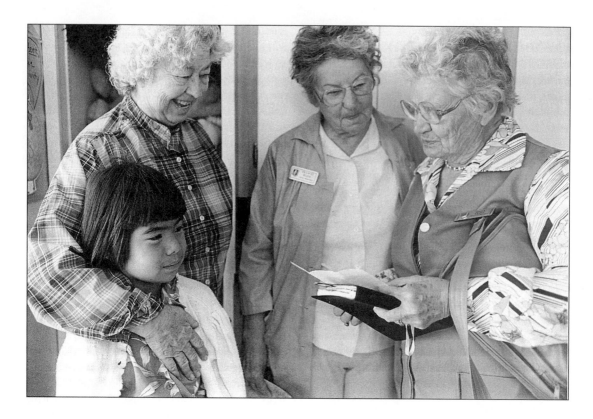

professionals with that of trained peer counselors in the delivery of an educational and therapeutic course on depression for elders. Participants reported reduced psychological distress after the course, and no difference was noted between those with a trained peer leader and those led by a professional.[71] Elder peer counseling can benefit both the trained elder and the client. Additionally, peer counselors are usually responsible and motivated workers, willing to become friends as well as helpers. This therapy reinforces the belief that elders are capable of solving their own problems.

MENTAL HEALTH SERVICES

History of Mental Health Reforms

Mentally ill elders have been affected by the changes in treatment philosophy and types of facilities over the years. The history of treatment for the mentally ill is one of many reforms but few suc-

cesses. Before the eighteenth century, the mentally ill were kept at home, allowed to wander around the community, housed in almshouses, or confined to jail with criminals. In the mid-1800s, reformer Dorthea Dix was instrumental in establishing institutions solely for the mentally ill. Although established with the belief they would provide more humane treatment for the mentally ill, these institutions became human warehouses where treatment was the exception. In the early 1900s, Clifford Beers, a Yale graduate who was institutionalized with bipolar illness, described the deplorable conditions in mental hospitals and launched the National Committee for Mental Hygiene.

In the 1950s, many reformers again called for a more humane treatment of the mentally ill. At that time, the number of persons confined to mental institutions reached half a million. The development of antipsychotic medications (also known as major tranquilizers) was the first really effective treatment for mental illness. The combination of an effective treatment and deplorable conditions in mental hospitals spurred legislative actions to reduce the number of mental patients by moving them into community settings where they would be better able to lead more normal lives. In the early 1960s, the Mental Health Act was passed to encourage the growth of community mental health centers that allowed mental patients to be treated with medication and therapy as outpatients. Currently, more individuals with mental illness are treated with medications as outpatients than are institutionalized.

However, the gains of deinstitutionalization have not been realized. Those with mental illnesses are seldom able to negotiate a complex mental health system. And, community resources have been inadequate to meet the needs of those who have been taken out of institutions because cost-cutting measures have forced communities to reduce the amount of services provided. Those with mental illness, particularly with schizophrenia or bipolar disease, are often isolated and seldom have an advocate to help them get treatment. Even when drugs are prescribed, the patient may not be compliant. Many community services focus on drug treatment, ignoring group or individual psychotherapy.

During the deinstitutionalization process, half the patients discharged were elders who had spent most of their lifetimes in a controlled environment. Many of these patients were "trans-institutionalized" from mental institutions into nursing homes, even though nursing homes were and still are not equipped to deal with mentally ill patients. Those mentally ill elders who were not moved into nursing homes have fallen through the cracks of the mental health system and live in single rooms in hotels or boarding homes. A few are homeless. Whether in the community or in a nursing home, the great majority of deinstitutionalized elders receive no care at all.

Providers of Mental Health Services

Many types of mental health professionals offer psychological services, whether in a private practice, clinic, or hospital setting. Although there is some overlap among services provided by various professionals, each has different training and expertise. Only psychiatrists can prescribe medications, although many other types of professionals and lay counselors can provide counseling services. With the advent of managed care and other measures to cut costs, there is increased reliance on therapists with fewer years of schooling to provide counseling services because these professionals are reimbursed at a lower rate than psychiatrists or clinical psychologists. Further, limits on number of visits per year have been initiated. Thus, a patient may seek care from a psychiatrist who will prescribe medications, but receive their counseling from a licensed clinical social worker.

Psychiatrists are medical or osteopathic physicians who are trained to diagnose and treat psychiatric problems with psychotherapy or medications. Most of these physicians practice psychiatry exclusively, but some are also trained as general medicine physicians. *Psychoanalysts* are psychiatrists who have received additional training in a psychoanalytic institute. These persons are trained to probe deeply into the client's unconscious. Therapy with these professionals is often long-term. *Clinical psychologists* have doctorates and are licensed to provide counseling and diagnostic testing for neurological and psychiatric illnesses. Other psychologists with master's degrees in counseling are trained in family therapy. *Clinical social workers* may have a master's or doctoral degree and can provide psychotherapy as well as make referrals to community resources. Social workers may work out of hospitals, community agencies, or may have private practices.

Clinical nurse specialists are registered nurses with special training in psychiatry. They may practice independently, but generally work through hospitals. *Occupational* or *recreational therapists* are trained to offer art, music, drama, vocational, play, or dance therapies. *Pastoral counselors* are clergy with specialized training in emotional disorders.

Types of Mental Health Services

Mental health services are of two types: institutional care and community-based care. Institutional care includes nursing homes, mental institutions, and mental wards of general hospitals. Community care encompasses community mental health centers, private psychiatrists and psychiatric outpatient clinics, halfway houses, and a variety of other support services that enable mentally frail elders to remain at home. Whether the individual is cared for in the community or in an institution depends on the extent of the mental problem, prognosis, physical status, current living situation, availability of community services, presence of social support, motivation to improve, and income.

Nursing Homes

Many mentally ill elders have traded the formal mental health system for custodial care in a nursing home. The process of deinstitutionalization and the advent of Medicare and Medicaid have inadvertently made nursing homes the primary place for mentally ill elders needing long-term care and supervision. One study found that about two-thirds of all elderly nursing home residents had a mental illness, but less than 5 percent of these had received any mental health treatment in the past month,[72] indicating significant neglect of the mental health needs of the residents.

Unfortunately, nursing homes have a deplorable reputation for diagnosing mental illness and providing mental health services to the residents who need them. The residents may be viewed as untreatable because of long-standing mental illnesses or because they have severe dementia with minimal cognitive ability. It is true that many in nursing homes are not in a position to have psychotherapy, as they are severely demented and minimally verbal. However, some would benefit from therapy. In addition, mental health professionals are less willing to come into the nursing home and care for these patients. Residents with behavioral problems may receive evaluations of medications, while those with less obvious mental illness, such as depression, are often undertreated. Even when treatment is initiated, generally there is a focus on medications instead of nondrug approaches that give stimulation and social support. The Nursing Home Reform Act implements monthly visits by physicians and close prescribing and monitoring of psychotropic drugs, which may ameliorate some of the current problems.

There is evidence that mentally ill patients transferred to psychiatric hospitals for treatment have better outcomes: reduced violence, depression, agitation, and, in some cases, may be able to return into the community.[73] Nursing homes may promote more dependence than psychiatric hospitals. One study reported that a year after transfer from a psychiatric hospital to a nursing home, schizophrenic patients had less ability to care for themselves than those who remained in the hospital. Those transferred who had organic brain syndrome were more depressed and less satisfied with their treatment than those who remained in mental institutions.[74] Chapter 13 will discuss nursing homes in more detail.

Public Mental Institutions

Even though the number of elders in state and county mental institutions has substantially declined in the last twenty-five years, these institutions still play a significant role in providing mental health care to this group. Older people comprise 30 percent of those residing in public mental health institutions; many have resided there since their early adult years. Half of those admitted to mental hospitals for the first time are over age sixty-five. The majority of institutionalized elders are schizophrenic, although a significant number are there for alcoholism and major depression.

Psychiatric Units of Acute Care Hospitals

Hospitals are the primary providers for those patients with acute mental problems or who are in a temporary crisis that needs to be managed. In addition to psychiatric intervention, a hospital can offer shorter stays, close supervision, high staff-per-patient ratio, and medical treatment in the patient's own community. The units are not designed for long-term treatment, counseling, or rehabilitation of chronically ill mental patients.

Inpatient geriatric psychiatric units began to appear about fifteen years ago at several teaching hospitals. As hospitals search for new opportunities to fill empty beds and generate income, the numbers of psychiatric units for geriatric patients in acute-care hospitals is increasing.

Community Mental Health Centers

These centers were federally legislated and funded by the Community Mental Health Centers Act in 1963. Community mental health centers have been set up in population centers of between 70,000 and 200,000. The centers offer five services: inpatient and outpatient care, twenty-four-hour emergency services, partial hospitalization, consultation, and education. Many provide additional services. The centers are available to all ages and have no restrictions regarding ability to pay or current and past health condition.

The centers are mandated to offer services to elders including diagnosis, treatment, liaison, and follow-up. About half the nation's older population has access to these facilities. However, elders comprise a small percentage of the patient load. Despite the mandate, these centers are not generally effective in meeting the mental health needs of elders. There is insufficient programming for this group and insufficient federal and state support for mental health programs for elders, as the services are seldom reimbursed by Medicare and Medicaid.

Private Therapists and Psychiatric Outpatient Clinics

Older people comprise less than 5 percent of the clients seen by private psychotherapists because these services are seldom reimbursed by Medicare and Medicaid, and the costs are prohibitive for many elders. Generally, elders who do participate are those in good health who are financially secure, highly educated, and have a positive attitude toward their treatment.

Halfway Houses

Psychiatric halfway houses provide a home environment for the mentally ill who can meet many of their own needs, yet need some support and supervision to be able to live in the community. These homes have great potential in serving the needs of mentally impaired elders since they prevent or postpone institutionalization for many. However, these facilities have many problems. Physical, mental, or financial abuse of residents may occur; cleanliness may be substandard; staff is poorly trained; and there are far fewer homes than are needed. Most elders rely on Social Security, Supplemental Security Income (SSI), or disability benefits to pay their bills. Homes located in community neighborhoods often face problems from neighbors who fear the mentally ill. Currently, board and care facilities and single-room-occupancy hotels house many mentally ill individuals. However, treatment, rehabilitation, or adequate supervision is rare.

Financial Reimbursement

In future chapters, Medicare, the federally funded insurance program for all over 65, and Medicaid, the joint federal and state funded program for the poor, disabled, and blind will be fully discussed. However, the following is a synopsis of the mental health benefits offered in each program.

Medicare

The Medicare program spends only 3 percent of its total dollars on mental health services. It is believed that the elderly underutilize Medicare-covered mental health services, probably because there are complex rules concerning coverage and reimbursement restrictions that are not found in the medical services of Medicare.

Four types of mental health inpatient services are covered under the hospital care category (Part A): psychiatric units in general hospitals, beds located in surgical or medical units in general hospitals, public psychiatric hospitals, and private psychiatric hospitals. There is a lifetime limit of 190 days in psychiatric hospitals. For general hospitals, there is a ninety-day limit per benefit period, with a sixty-day interval between benefit periods. For both psychiatric hospitals and general hospitals, the patient pays a deductible on first admission and pays a share of cost, depending on the length of stay. Mental health treatment in nursing homes is not covered under Part A.

For mental health needs, Part B covers physician and mental health provider services. This includes 80 percent of the approved charges for physician services for inpatient mental health care (in general hospital or psychiatric hospital), including monitoring of psychoactive medication, and 50 percent of approved charges for most outpatient mental health care, including evaluation of mental disorders and psychotherapy. The cap for reimbursement of mental health treatment services is $1,100 per year for treatment of medical disorders by all providers. However, psychotherapy and treatment of patients with Alzheimer's disease have no limit on treatment, but the 50 percent deductible still applies. To use Part B, the person must pay the premiums, the yearly deductible, and the coinsurance for each service. Those who need mental health services in nursing homes fall under Part B. For those who can afford a Medigap insurance policy, it covers what Medicare does not reimburse for both hospital and mental health personnel (details on this insurance are in chapter 12).

Medicaid

Although plans differ from state to state, the federal government mandates that states provide general hospital care, physician services, outpatient services in general hospitals, emergency room care, and nursing home care. Medicaid is the primary funding source for mental health care in nursing homes. Many states impose limitations on mental health care, including prior authorization requirements, physician supervision requirements, restrictions on the number of visits by providers, and special rate limits. Medicaid reimbursement rates to providers are 20 to 30 percent lower than the prevailing rates, discouraging providers from participating. Payment for psychiatric care is even lower than medical care. The pricing of care and the restrictions in the definition of services and providers are great, creating a tremendous barrier for nursing home residents to receive the care they need for mental illness.[75]

Financial considerations are perhaps the greatest barrier to availability of mental health services for older people. Although Medicare pays for half of all psychologic counseling, coming up with the other half puts the services out of reach for most elders. Further, because Medicare and Medicaid do

not offer full payment, there is a financial disincentive for mental health care providers to work with elders.

Elder Utilization of Mental Health Services

Despite the variety of mental health services available, older persons are underserved. In all age groups, only a fraction of those who need mental health services receive them. However, elders, especially ethnic elders, use these services the least. In general, adults of all ages, but especially elders, are more likely to visit their medical care provider than a mental health professional for both physical and mental illnesses. It has been suggested that the greatest obstacles to treatment is the failure of the medical provider to recognize mental illness in their older patients, perhaps taking a "back seat" to their more obvious physical problems. Experts have attributed low utilization to client factors, biases of the professionals toward treating elders, and barriers created by the mental health system itself.

Bias against the use of mental health services occurs among all age groups, but older persons are especially prone to resist psychological help from a stranger. Many believe that those who need a therapist are "crazy." Elders may not believe that mental problems are treatable, or may not admit that they have a psychological problem. Also, they may see the need for visiting a therapist as a weakness—an inability to solve their own problems. Further, the current generation of older people may not be comfortable talking about their feelings, but believe they should "tough it out" or "snap out of it" on their own.

Many older people attribute poor mental health to physical ailments or the aging process itself. Because of this, elders may be more likely to bring up their psychological concerns to their physician than to mental health professionals. On the other hand, some fear that if their mental disorders are fully explored, they may be stigmatized as mentally ill and institutionalized. Lack of awareness of available services may also play a role. When older people are educated about mental health services, they report an increased propensity to use such services.[76]

The negative biases of mental health professionals toward elders contribute to the low use of mental health services by older people. Some therapists may believe treating older individuals is not worthwhile because elders have only a few years left to live. Psychotherapists consistently rate older clients as having less chance of treatment success than younger patients, even though no research has documented this belief. Therapists also tend to attribute many symptoms of distress to organic symptoms or old age and may not treat them. Many of the therapists' biases may be due to a lack of knowledge about the characteristics, needs, and concerns of older people and the special considerations in dealing with an older client. Working with elders, particularly the sick or very old, may force therapists to confront the difficult, personal questions of their own aging, decline, and eventual death.

A limited supply of personnel skilled in geriatrics and the shortage of services geared to elders also serve as barriers to care. Many of the services are physically inaccessible to older people because outreach is seldom provided for those who are unable to get to the facility. Further, there is little cooperation and coordination among private medical providers, community agencies, and institutions. Because of this, the interdisiplinary approach to meeting the multiple needs of mentally ill elders is not an option in most communities.

Future Directions

Mental illnesses are a large and growing problem in our society, with little attention from the public. Private insurance plans continue to exclude mental illnesses from coverage or offer far too little in the way of benefits. Federal programs, including Medicare and Medicaid, reimburse mental health professionals at far less than the rates of medical professionals. Many elders go undiagnosed and untreated. It is feared that this problem may worsen with time as cost-cutting measures are implemented in an attempt to reduce climbing Medicare expenses. Concomitant with this decrease in funding is an increase in the aging population, creating a gap between need and availability of geriatric mental health services.[77]

A few novel ideas have been proposed to improve the delivery of mental health services to elders. Pilot projects have been funded to evaluate the use of familylike foster care arrangements for the elderly mentally ill with behavioral problems and to increase the availability of psychiatric and psychologic services in nursing homes. A comprehensive community-based mental health outreach program was designed in Maryland to seek out and treat elders with late-onset psychiatric disorders with provision of services in senior centers, in community mental health centers and in senior's homes using an interdisiplinary team approach.[79] Another program utilized drivers trained in mental health and other issues to provide a transportation service. While on their way to doctor's appointments, the driver informally assessed their need for mental health services, providing both referrals and transportation.[80]

The next few decades will witness the aging of the baby boomers, who are documented to have higher rates of mental illness, depression, drug abuse, anxiety, and alcoholism than any group previously measured.[78] This group is more "psychologically minded," having come of age during the time when mental illness was redefined in a more biological way. It is hoped that these aging baby boomers will demand better diagnosis and treatment strategies for mental illness and will advocate for fuller access to a variety of mental health services to maximize the quality of life in the later years.

SUMMARY

Mental health in elders can be defined as the ability to successfully adapt to the transitions of old age. This ability is related to a number of physical, psychological, and situational factors, such as personality, physical health, financial situation, availability of social support, and coping strategies. With age, there are some alterations in cognitive abilities and memory. Personality remains remarkably stable throughout the lifespan. Although most elders adjust readily to the stresses and transitions of old age, a few need outside assistance to deal with mental disorders.

In elders, mental disorders may appear for the first time during old age, but most commonly appear years earlier. Mental disorders include anxiety, depression and other mood disorders, somatoform disorders, schizophrenia, sleep disorders, alcoholism, delirium and dementia. Some mental disorders are underdiagnosed in the elderly because their symptoms may be mistaken for age changes or symptoms of chronic illness. Ongoing interdisiplinary assessments are important to diagnose and treat mental illness in the elderly. The common treatment for the majority of mental disorders is psychoactive medication, although some elders have access to psychotherapy and support groups.

Mental health services are available for elders in both community and institutional settings. These include public mental health hospitals, wards in general hospitals, nursing homes, community mental health centers, halfway houses, and individual and outpatient psychiatric services. However, these services are underutilized by elders for a number of reasons, including client factors, therapist biases, and system barriers.

ACTIVITIES

1. Develop your own definition of mental health, taking age and cultural background into account. Identify some behaviors that are universally healthy or unhealthy. Ask several individuals to characterize elders. Do their descriptions define a mentally healthy old age?

2. List the strategies you use to cope with stress, both those that are effective and those that are not. Which strategies work best for you?

3. Review the transitions associated with aging (e.g., widowhood, changes in marital relationships, change in relationship with adult children, retirement). Interview friends and families at different stages in their lives, including those without children. What are their hopes and plans for these transitions? If they have already experienced them, what was the overall effect on their lives? Do the experiences of those without children or those who are not married differ?

4. Conduct a life review with an older person. Tape the conversation (audio or video) and write a summary for the class. Be sure to give a copy to the person interviewed.

5. Seek out the mental health services in your community. Find out the percentage of clients who are over age sixty-five. Do they have any specialized services for elders? Do any have peer counselors? Do any have preventive programs?

6. Question elders about their attitudes toward mental illness and its causes and treatments and compare their views with your classmates. Do their views differ from younger groups?

7. Make a list of the self-help groups in your community. If possible, talk with a member to find out the percentage of participants over age sixty-five. Attend a support group session and report your response to the class.

8. Attend a meeting of Alcoholics Anonymous or Narcotics Anonymous. Be sure to identify yourself as a guest. What proportion of attendees appear to be elderly? Question some of the participants about the impact of various services on their sobriety and the role of AA or NA in their lives.

9. As people live longer, many younger elders spend their retirement years caring for their aging parents or spouse. How will this trend affect your plans for your old age?

10. Find out the number and percentage of persons age sixty-five and older who are patients in mental

institutions in your state. If possible, visit a facility, observe the patients, and find out the frequency and types of therapy utilized there.

11. Develop a group of programs to promote mental health and reduce mental deterioration in a nursing home.

12. Interview a nursing home administrator. What is the percentage of mentally ill elders in the facility? How are behavioral problems (e.g., wandering and disruptive behavior) managed? What therapy is available? What is the educational background of the therapist, if present?

BIBLIOGRAPHY

1. Jahoda, M. 1958. *Current concepts of positive mental health.* New York: Basic Books.

2. Rowe, J.W., and Kahn, R.L. 1997. Successful aging. *The Gerontologist* 37:433–40.

3. Erickson, E.H. 1982. *The life cycle completed.* New York: Norton.

4. Schaie, K.W. 1996. Intellectual development in adulthood. In *Handbook of the psychology of aging,* 4th ed., J.E. Birren and K.W. Schaie, eds. San Diego: Academic Press, pp. 266–86.

5. Schaie, K.W. 1990. Intellectual development in adulthood. In *Handbook of the psychology of aging,* 3rd ed., J.E. Birren and K.W. Schaie, eds. San Diego: Academic Press, pp. 291–309.

6. Perlmutter, M., Kaplan, J., and Nyquist, L. 1990. Development of adaptive competence in adulthood. *Human Development* 33:185–97.

7. Cooney, T.M., Schaie, K.W., and Willis, S.L. 1988. The relationship between prior functioning on cognitive and personality dimensions and subject attrition in longitudinal research. *Journal of Gerontology* 43:P12–P17.

8. Moller, J.T., et al. 1998. Long-term postoperative cognitive dysfunction in the elderly. *Lancet* 351:857–61.

9. Willis, S.L., and Schaie, K.W. 1986. Training the elderly on the ability factors of spatial orientation and inductive reasoning. *Psychology and Aging* 1:239–47.

10. Smith, A.D. 1996. Memory. In *Handbook of the psychology of aging,* 4th ed., J.E. Birren and K.W. Schaie, eds. San Diego: Academic Press, pp. 236–50.

11. Meharg, S., and Pankratz, L. 1996. The MILD interview: Evaluating complaints of memory loss. *American Family Physician* 54:167–72.

12. Costa, P.T., and McCrae, R.R. 1986. Cross-sectional studies of personality in a national sample: Development and validation of survey measures. *Psychology and Aging* 1:1140–43.

13. Helson, R., and Wink, P. 1992. Personality change in women from the early 40s to the early 50s. *Psychology and Aging* 7:46–55.

14. McCrae, R. 1982. Age difference in the use of coping mechanisms. *Journal of Gerontology* 37:454–60.

15. Irion, J.C., and Blanchard-Fields, F. 1987. A cross sectional comparison of adaptive coping in adulthood. *Journal of Gerontology* 42:502–4.

16. Vaillant, G. 1977. *Adaptation to life.* Boston: Little, Brown.

17. Crimmins, E.M., and Ingegneri, D.G. 1990. Interaction and living arrangements of older parents and their children: Past trends, present determinants, future implications. *Research on Aging* 12:3–35.

18. Aizenberg, R., and Treas, J. 1985. The family in late life: Psychosocial and demographic considerations. In *Handbook of the psychology of aging,* 2nd ed., J.E. Birren and K.W. Shaie, eds. New York: Van Nostrand Reinhold, pp. 169–89.

19. Carstensen, L.L., Gottman, J.M., and Levenson, R.W. 1995. Emotional behavior in long-term marriage. *Psychology and Aging* 10:140–49.

20. Fitting, M., Rabins, P., Lucas, M.J., and Eastham, J. 1986. Caregivers for dementia patients: A comparison of husbands and wives. *The Gerontologist* 26:248–52.

21. Caserta, M.S., and Lund, D.A. 1993. Intrapersonal resources and the effectiveness of self-help groups for bereaved older adults. *The Gerontologist* 33:619–29.

22. Bulcroft, K., and O'Connor-Rodin, J. 1986. Never too late. *Psychology Today* 20:66–9.

23. Pieper, H.G., Petkovsek, L., and East, M. 1986. Marriage among the elderly. Paper presented at the 39th Annual Meeting of the Gerontological Society of America, November 1986, Chicago.

24. Brecher, E.M., and Consumer Reports Book Editors. 1985. *Love, sex and aging.* Boston: Little, Brown.

25. Rodin, J. 1986. Aging and health: Effects of the sense of control. *Science* 233:1271–76.

26. Langer, E.J., and Rodin, J. 1976. The effects of choice and enhanced personal responsibility for the aged: A field experiment in an institutional setting. *Journal of Personality and Social Psychology* 34:191–98.

27. Slivinske, L.R., and Fitch, V.L. 1987. The effect of control enhancing interventions on the well-being of elderly individuals living in retirement communities. *The Gerontologist* 27:176–81.

28. Roos, N.P., and Havens, B. 1991. Predictors of successful aging: A twelve-year study of Manitoba elderly. *American Journal of Public Health* 81:63–8.

29. Siegel, J.M. 1990. Stressful life events and use of physician services among the elderly: The moderating role of pet ownership. *Journal of Personality and Social Psychology* 58:1081–86.

30. National Institute of Mental Health. Mental Illness in America: The National Institute of Mental Health agenda. WWW site: http://www.nimh.nih.gov/research/amer.htm. 1998.

31. Centers for Disease Control. 1998. Self-reported frequent mental distress among adults—United States, 1993–1996. *Morbidity and Mortality Weekly Report.* 47:325–31.

32. Regier, D.A., Boyd, J.H., and Burke, J.D., et al. 1988. One-month prevalence of mental disorders in the United States. *Archives of General Psychiatry* 45:977–86.

33. Burns, B.J., Wagner, H.R., and Taube, J.E., et al. 1993. Mental health service use by the elderly in nursing homes. *American Journal of Public Health* 83:331–37.

34. German, P.S., Rovner, B.W., and Burton, L.C., et al. 1992. The role of mental morbidity in the nursing home experience. *The Gerontologist* 32:152–58.

35. American Psychiatric Association. 1994. Diagnostic and statistic manual of mental disorders, 4th ed. Washington, D.C.: American Psychiatric Association.

36. Lebowitz, B.D., Pearson, J.L., and Schneider, L.S., et al. 1997. Diagnosis and treatment of depression in late life: Consensus statement update. *Journal of the American Medical Association* 278:1186–90.

37. Everson, S.A., Goldberg, D.E., and Kaplan, G.A., et al. 1996. Hopelessness and risk of mortality and incidence of myocardial infarction and cancer. *Psychosomatic Medicine* 58:113–21.

38. Penninx, B.W.J.H., Guralnik, J.M., and Mendes de Leon, C.F., et al. 1998. Cardiovascular events and mortality in newly and chronically depressed persons greater than 70 years of age. *American Journal of Cardiology* 81:988–94.

39. Cattan, R.A., Barry, P.P., and Mead, G., et al. 1990. Electroconvulsive therapy in octogenarians. *Journal of the American Geriatrics Society* 38:753–58.

40. Regier, D.A., Boyd, J.H., and Burke, J.D., et al. 1988. One-month prevalence of mental disorders in the United States. *Archives of General Psychiatry* 45:977–86.

41. Saltz, B.L., Woerner, M.G., and Kane, J.M., et al. 1991. Prospective study of tardive dyskinesia incidence in the elderly. *Journal of the American Medical Association* 266:2402–6.

42. Gilbert, P.L., Harris, M.J., McAdams, L.A., and Jeste, D.V. 1995. Neuroleptic withdrawal in schizophrenic patients. A review of the literature. *Archives of General Psychiatry* 52:173–88.

43. Irwin, M:., Mascovich, A., and Gillin, J.C., et al. 1994. Partial sleep deprivation reduces natural killer cell activity in humans. *Psychosomatic Medicine* 56:493–98.

44. Foley, D.J., Monjan, A.A., and Brown, S.L., et al. 1995. Sleep complaints among elderly persons: An epidemiologic study of three communities. *Sleep* 18:425–32.

45. Dealberto, M.J., Pajot, N., Courbon, D., and Alperovitch, A. 1996. Breathing disorders during sleep and cognitive performance in an older community sample: The EVA study. *Journal of the American Geriatrics Society* 44:1287–94.

46. Pozzato, G., Moretti, M., and Franzin, F., et al. 1995. Ethanol metabolism and aging: The role of "first pass metabolism" and gastric alcohol dehydrogenase activity. *Journal of Gerontology* 50A:B135–B141.

47. Camargo, C.A., Jr., Hennekens, C.H., and Gaziano, J.M., et al. 1997. Prospective study of moderate alcohol consumption and mortality in U.S. male

physicians. *Archives of Internal Medicine* 157:79–85.

48. Alexander, F., and Duff, R.W. 1988. Social interaction and alcohol use in retirement communities. *The Gerontologist* 28:632–36.

49. Schuckit, M.A., Atkinson, J.H., Miller, P., and Berman, J. 1980. A three-year follow-up of elderly alcoholics. *Journal of Clinical Psychiatry* 41:412–16.

50. Ewing, J.A. 1984. Detecting alcoholism: The CAGE questionnaire. *Journal of the American Medical Association* 252:1905–7.

51. Adams, W.L., Barry, K.L., and Fleming, M.F. 1996. Screening for problem drinking in older primary care patients. *Journal of the American Medical Association* 276:1964–67.

52. Council on Scientific Affairs. 1996. Alcoholism in the elderly. *Journal of the American Medical Association* 275:797–801.

53. Fleming, M.F., Barry, K.L., and Manwell, L.B., et al. 1997. Brief physician advice for problem alcohol drinkers. *Journal of the American Medical Association* 277:1039–45.

54. Project MATCH Research Group. 1997. Matching alcoholism treatment to client heterogeneity. *Journal of the Study of Alcohol* 58:7–29.

55. Brookmeyer, R., Gray, S., and Kawas, C. 1998. Projections of Alzheimer's disease in the United States and the public health impact of delaying disease onset. *American Journal of Public Health* 88:1337–42.

56. Moak, G.S., and Fisher, W.H. 1990. Alzheimer's disease and related disorders in state mental hospitals: Data from a nationwide survey. *The Gerontologist* 30:798–802.

57. American College of Medical Genetics/American Society of Human Genetics Working Group on APOE and Alzheimer's Disease. 1995. Statement on the use of apolipoprotein E testing for Alzheimer's disease. *Journal of the American Medical Association* 274:1627–29.

58. Stern,Y., Gurland, B., and Tatemichi, T.K., et al. 1994. Influence of education and occupation on the incidence of Alzheimer's disease. *Journal of the American Medical Association* 271:1004–10.

59. Snowdon, D.A. 1997. Aging and Alzheimer's disease: Lessons from the Nun Study. *The Gerontologist* 37:150–56.

60. Knapp, M.J., Knopman, D.S., and Solomon, P.R., et al. 1994. A 30-week randomized controlled trial of high-dose tacrine in patients with Alzheimer's disease. *Journal of the American Medical Association* 271:985–91.

61. Knopman, D., Schneider, L., and Davis, K., et al. 1996. Long-term tacrine (Cognix) treatment: Effects on nursing home placement and mortality, Tacrine Study Group. *Neurology* 47:166–77.

62. Sano, M., Ernesto, C., and Thomas, R.G., et al. 1997. A controlled trial of selegiline, alpha-tocopherol, or both as treatment for Alzheimer's disease. *New England Journal of Medicine* 336:1216–22.

63. Le Bars, P.L., Katz, M.M., and Berman, N., et al. 1997. A placebo-controlled, double-blind, randomized trial of an extract of Gingko biloba for dementia. *Journal of the American Medical Association* 278:1327–32.

64. Tang, M.X., Jacobs, D., and Stern, Y., et al. 1996. Effect of estrogen during menopause on risk and age at onset of Alzheimer's disease. *Lancet* 348:429–32.

65. Ernst, R.L., and Hay, J.W. 1994. The U.S. economic and social costs of Alzheimer's disease revisited. *American Journal of Public Health* 84:1261–64.

66. Mittelman, M.S., Ferris, S.H., and Shylman, E., et al. 1996. A family intervention to delay nursing home placement of patients with Alzheimer's disease: A randomized controlled trial. *Journal of the American Medical Association* 276:1725–31.

67. Jahnigen, D.W. 1990. Delirium in the elderly hospitalized patient. *Hospital Practice* 15:135–57.

68. Inouye, S.K. 1994. The dilemma of delirium: Clinical and research controversies regarding diagnosis and evaluation of delirium in hospitalized elderly medical patients. *American Journal of Medicine* 97:278:88.

69. Inouye, S.K., and Charpentier, P.A. 1996. Precipitating factors for delirium in hospitalized elderly patients. *Journal of the American Medical Association* 275:852–57.

70. Hayslip, B., and Kooken, R.A. 1983. Therapeutic interventions—mental health. In *The aged patient,* M. S. Ernst and H. R. Glasser, eds. Chicago: Yearbook Medical Publishers.

71. Thompson, L.W., Gallagher, D., Nies, G., and Epstein, D. 1983. Evaluation of the effectiveness of

professionals and nonprofessionals as instructors of "coping with depression" classes for elders. *The Gerontologist* 23:390–96.

72. Burns, B.J., Wagner, H.R., and Taube, J.E., et al. 1993. Mental health service use by the elderly in nursing homes. *American Journal of Public Health* 83:331–37.

73. Kunik, M.E., Molinari, V., and Orengo, C., et al. 1996. The benefits of psychiatric hospitalization for older nursing home residents. *Journal of the American Geriatrics Society* 44:1062–65.

74. Linn, M.W., Gurel, L., and Williford, W.O., et al. 1985. Nursing home care as an alternative to psychiatric hospitalization. *Archives of General Psychiatry* 42:544–51.

75. Lombardo, N.E. 1994. *Barriers to mental health services for nursing home residents.* Washington, D.C.: AARP Public Policy Institute, #9401.

76. Woodruff, J.C., Donnan, H., and Halpin, G. 1988. Changing elderly persons' attitudes toward mental health professionals. *The Gerontologist* 28:800–2.

77. Koenig, H.G., George, L.K., and Schneider, R. 1994. Mental health care for older adults in the year 2020: A dangerous and avoided topic. *The Gerontologist* 34:674–79.

78. Klerman, G.L., and Weissman, M.M. 1989. Increasing rates of depression. *Journal of the American Medical Association* 261:2229–35.

79. DeRenzo, E.G., Byer, V.L., and Grady, H.S., et al. 1991. Comprehensive community-based mental health outreach services for suburban seniors. *The Gerontologist* 31:836–40.

80. Gurian, B.S. 1992. Transportation as outreach, driver as mental health worker. *The Gerontologist* 32:561–62.

CHRONIC ILLNESS

If I'd known I was going to live so long, I'd have taken better care of myself.
Songwriter Eubie Blake, on approaching his 100th birthday

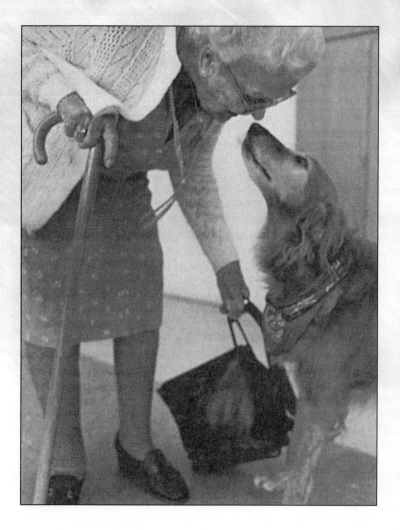

Chronic diseases are considered to be the most prevalent, costly, and preventable of all health problems. These illnesses are the leading causes of disability among adults. Chronic illness is a fact of life for many older people, with illnesses ranging from merely bothersome to severely disabling. In contrast to infectious diseases that are brief and curable, chronic diseases must be dealt with throughout life since they are frequently irreversible and progressive in nature. Thus, elders with chronic diseases often take multiple medications and visit a physician frequently to manage, rather than cure, their disease. Genetics plays a role in chronic disease. In addition, health behavior in early and middle adulthood influences the type and extent of chronic disease we endure in our later years.

Chronic diseases are often accompanied by long-term social and psychological consequences. The complex nature of chronic disease often requires cooperation among the individual, the family, and health and social service providers. This chapter will discuss the nature of chronic illness and provide an overview of the chronic diseases common in the later years. Although the biology of chronic illnesses may seem daunting, it is important for those in the health and human service field to be familiar with these illnesses in order to help older people minimize the impact of the disease upon their daily life. Understanding ways to prevent, treat, and manage chronic illness can help us to care for our aging relatives and teach us how we may reduce the risk of chronic disease in our own lives.

THE NATURE OF CHRONIC ILLNESS

In children and young adults, being sick is generally associated with conditions from which one expects to recover, such as the common cold, flu, strep throat, or pneumonia. These acute diseases have an abrupt onset and are generally caused by bacteria or a virus. They are generally self-limiting or easily curable with medication. With advancing age, however, the most troublesome health problems are due to chronic conditions such as arthritis, heart disease, stroke, and cancer. These conditions are generally incurable, progressive, and endure over many years, if not a lifetime. In general, the causes of chronic illness are multiple or unknown. Most are due to a combination of lifestyle or environmental agents (e.g., diet, cigarette smoking), heredity, and unknown factors. Physicians cannot cure chronic conditions, but can only reduce the symptoms and deterioration caused by the progression of the condition. Because chronic illnesses last a lifetime and require continuous medical supervision, the financial burden for care is considerable.

Although there are differences between chronic and acute illnesses, there are some similarities. An acute illness may be superimposed on a chronic one. In fact, the presence of chronic illnesses makes it easier for older people to contract an acute illness. For example, a heart attack or myocardial infarction appears to be an acute illness, but the underlying illness, coronary artery disease, is a chronic illness. Some complications of chronic illnesses are treated as acute illnesses; for example, an elder with diabetes may develop a urinary tract infection. Some chronic illnesses, such as a stroke, may seem to have a rapid onset, but it likely had been developing for years. Finally, with effective treatment, acute illnesses may become chronic. For example, AIDS is caused by a virus, and would be terminal were it not for effective antiviral therapy. Currently, adults with AIDS are living longer and must continue to deal with a variety of symptoms, much like controlling a chronic illness. Thus, the decision to call some illnesses acute and some chronic is somewhat arbitrary.

Chronic illnesses can occur at any age, but become more common in the middle and later years. More than 100 million Americans live with chronic conditions. Their direct health care costs account for over 75 percent of the health care expenditures in the United States. Chronically ill patients account for 80 percent of all hospital stays. In 1990, it was estimated that costs for treatment and medication for chronic illness was about $425 billion; costs were projected to increase to $798 billion in 2030 with 148 million individuals affected.[1]

Elders account for 40 percent of all chronic illness in the United States, even though they comprise only 13 percent of the population. More than four of every five elders have at least one chronic disease. The number of diseases per person increases with advancing age. Women report more chronic illness than men. In general, the greater the number of chronic illnesses an individual has, the greater the proportion of disability and dependence.

Chronic illnesses account for seven of the ten leading causes of death, or more than 90 percent of deaths among elders and a significant proportion of deaths among younger individuals as well (table 8.1). Even elders who die of an acute illness (pneu-

monia, urinary tract infection) likely suffered from one or more chronic illnesses that contributed to their death. The bill for treating chronic illnesses is enormous because chronically ill elders require frequent visits to the doctor and hospital and skilled nursing facility, utilize home health and rehabilitative services, and have a high bill for medications.

Chronic diseases among the elderly may be difficult to diagnose and manage. First, elders may report different symptoms than younger groups. They may feel less pain or have mental manifestations of physical problems (such as depression or confusion). They may not exhibit symptoms, or they may complain of multiple, nonspecific symptoms

TABLE 8.1	Ten Leading Causes of Death in Specified Age Groups: United States, 1996
15–24 Years	**45–64 Years**
1. Accidents and adverse effects	1. Malignant neoplasms (cancers)
2. Homicide and legal intervention	2. Heart diseases
3. Suicide	3. Accidents and adverse effects
4. Malignant neoplasms (cancers)	4. Cerebrovascular diseases (stroke)
5. Heart diseases	5. Chronic obstructive pulmonary diseases and allied conditions
6. Human immunodeficiency virus infection	6. Diabetes mellitus
7. Congenital anomalies	7. Chronic liver disease and cirrhosis
8. Chronic obstructive pulmonary diseases and allied conditions	8. Human immunodeficiency virus infection
9. Pneumonia and influenza	9. Suicide
10. Cerebrovascular diseases	10. Pneumonia and influenza
25–44 Years	**65 Years and Over**
1. Accidents and adverse effects	1. Heart diseases
2. Malignant neoplasms (cancers)	2. Malignant neoplasms (cancers)
3. Human immunodeficiency virus infection	3. Cerebrovascular diseases (stroke)
4. Heart diseases	4. Chronic obstructive pulmonary diseases and allied conditions
5. Suicide	5. Pneumonia and influenza
6. Homicide and legal intervention	6. Diabetes mellitus
7. Chronic liver disease and cirrhosis	7. Accidents and adverse effects
8. Cerebrovascular diseases (stroke)	8. Alzheimer's disease
9. Diabetes mellitus	9. Nephritis, nephrotic syndrome, and nephrosis (kidney disease)
10. Pneumonia and influenza	10. Septicemia (blood poisoning)

National Vital Statistics Reports, Deaths: Final data for 1996. November 10, 1998. vol 47(9).

such as weakness, dizziness, or lack of appetite. Secondly, because elders are likely to have more than one chronic disease, the symptoms of one disease may be mistakenly attributed to an already existing one and be ignored. Third, if they are taking medication for one condition, the side effects of medication may be misinterpreted as another condition. Finally, symptoms of chronic illness may be incorrectly attributed to normal age changes.

Management of chronic illnesses in elders can be complicated. Age changes in body systems reduce the ability to respond to the stress of illness. Additionally, elders often have more than one condition and require multiple medications and/or medical interventions. Because of this, they have an increased risk of medication side effects. Elders are less likely to tolerate a worsening of their disease. Some older people do not follow their physicians' directions for treatment and do not understand the cause of their condition. For these reasons, elders often exhibit more complications with chronic disease than younger groups.

Nevertheless, elders with chronic illnesses may have certain strengths that allow them to cope with the symptoms. There is a general expectation that old age is accompanied by illnesses of some sort, perhaps making elders accept disability more than a younger person. Because of maturity, or a fear of the consequences of poor health, they may be more likely to heed doctor's warnings and stop smoking or take their medications regularly. Elders with chronic illnesses, especially high blood pressure and arthritis, may be more likely to get support from their friends as it is very common in the elder age group. Because of Medicare, they are more able to maintain continuity with their medical providers and to seek specialist care when needed.

A discussion of the multiple chronic illnesses that affect older people is not intended to paint a portrait of debilitated, disabled old age. Although chronic disease and disabilities accumulate with age, most elders, especially the young-old, are in good health. Even among elders with chronic illness, most report their health to be excellent or good. Despite the high prevalence of chronic illness, these conditions do not usually restrict an older person's ability to complete daily tasks. Moreover, if a chronic disease is detected, the patient can start a treatment regimen to control many symptoms and reduce the progression of the disease. Finally, even though there is a high prevalence of chronic disease in the later years, it is not inevitable. Many can be prevented by changes in lifestyle such as improving diet, eliminating drug or tobacco use, losing weight, and increasing physical activity.

PSYCHOSOCIAL ASPECTS OF CHRONIC ILLNESS

When and if sickness does occur, some approach it with a determination and try to overcome it with all their power. Others greet it placidly, accepting treatment but making no effort on their own. Still another small group, believing it cannot be overcome, will themselves to die and accept nothing that would delay their death.

Eber Swope

Professionals who work with elders with chronic illnesses need both an understanding of their medical problems and an awareness of how the disease and symptoms impact everyday life. Although chronic illnesses affect individuals differently, those who are chronically ill share many of the same problems. A. L. Strauss, a sociologist, developed a framework to look at the psychosocial problems of the chronically ill and their families.[2] Although the same framework can be used for any chronic illness, some illnesses are complex, and coping with them takes up most of the day. Other diseases have little impact on a person's daily routine. Strauss asserts that, unless one understands how the chronically ill handle their illness on a daily basis, one cannot give effective care.

Because chronic illnesses are permanent and full recovery is not possible, elders with chronic illnesses should not be treated as if they are "sick." Concerned professionals and families may unconsciously promote dependence by allowing the chronically ill person to misuse the "sick role."

The sick role, developed by Talcott Parsons, a medical sociologist, is a phenomenon whereby a sick person is allowed to be dependent and is relieved of familial and societal responsibilities until she or he is well.[3] For example, the sick person does not need to do household chores and is allowed to take it easy. The ill person is not blamed for incurring the illness. However, it is understood that sickness is undesirable and deviant, and the sick person is obligated to do everything possible to get well. Usually family members are supportive, and the sick role is maintained until the individual is healthy enough to resume normal functioning. This model provides an excellent representation of what we do when we contract an acute illness, such as influenza. Luckily, the period of illness is rather short and, as soon as we are able, we resume our normal responsibilities and interactions with significant others at home and at work.

The sick role must be modified for the chronically ill because of the extended period of disability. When a chronically ill elder constantly assumes a dependent, egocentric role to cope with illness, both the chronically ill person and family suffer. The inability, or reduced ability, to participate in the daily activities in the home or at work removes the elder from those activities and roles that originally promoted self-esteem. Furthermore, preoccupation with the disease by both the elder and family may encourage dependence. Instead, elders should attempt to do the most they can despite their illness and go on with life as best as possible.

Although the sick role is sometimes appropriate for an elder who needs special care, health professionals and families should be wary of supporting overly dependent behaviors of chronically ill elders. Often family and professional caregivers inadvertently promote dependency by excessive care, which reduces coping effectiveness and encourages further decline in function. For example, a caregiver might dress and spoon-feed someone who can do it herself, albeit more slowly.

The term "miscarried helping" has been coined to describe a behavioral cycle of chronically ill individuals and their families. Miscarried helping occurs when well-intentioned attempts of support fail because they are excessive, untimely, or inappropri-

ate. This may begin at diagnosis, when expressions of empathy and affection dominate. Later, this optimism fades, and there is an increase in family anxiety as families struggle to accommodate the sick member's needs into their normal routines. Family members may neglect social engagements due to lack of time and energy, and lose the associated support. Increased isolation may occur, and caregivers may become drained and exhausted. The patient may suffer a loss of autonomy or feel guilty: "I am the reason my wife can't do the things she wants." As the two become more involved, they may begin to feel even more distress. The caregiver may begin to feel responsible for the patient's illness and become angry or frustrated. One family member may take on all the caring responsibilities causing tension in the family. When miscarried helping is observed by a health or social service professional, both the patient and caregiver need to be made aware of the pitfalls to each of them.[4]

Many other psychological factors may influence the severity of chronic illnesses. Elders differ in how they define and react to illness. For instance, one arthritic older woman may insist she is living well while another will constantly complain about her stiff joints. Some individuals become angry, deny they are ill, or become compliant and resigned to the patient role. Chronic illnesses can lead to mental health problems such as depression or anxiety. There is much variability in coping style and level of responsibility the elder assumes for the illness. Some people perceive every minor symptom as a worsening of the disease and seek frequent medical attention, while others take more responsibility upon themselves.

Caregiving extracts tremendous tolls from family members—financially, socially and emotionally (refer to chapter 14). Chronic illnesses that seriously impinge upon activities of daily living can often result in other social problems. A family member may have to quit work or move to care for a disabled elder. The monthly income or life savings of a couple may be depleted through medical expenses. The chronic illness of one member of a couple can severely impact the other. For example, if one spouse loses his sight and can

Problems of Daily Living for the Chronically Ill

1. *Preventing medical crises and managing them when they occur.*

   Some chronic diseases are characterized by potentially fatal medical crises (e.g., diabetic coma, heart attack, epileptic seizure, and stroke). To prevent a crisis, the person's life must be organized for crisis management—that is, the signs of impending crisis must be recognized and appropriate action is necessary when they occur.

2. *Controlling symptoms.*

   Although the physician prescribes a regimen intended to control symptoms, the individual must rely largely on personal judgment to control symptoms. The individual needs to be aware of the present capacity of his or her body and coming to terms with its reduced capability. Even minor symptoms may require a change in behavior, and major symptoms may call for redesigning daily life.

3. *Carrying out prescribed regimen and managing the problems associated with it.*

   The physician usually prescribes a treatment regimen to control the symptoms and progression of the disease, but the individual must learn the regimen, and to a greater or lesser degree, must organize the day around it. Some treatments are simple, such as ingesting a pill; others may take up a significant portion of the day. Whether or not a regimen is followed depends on a number of factors: Is the regimen easy to learn? How much time and energy does the regimen take? Is it painful? Are there side effects? Is it effective? Is it expensive? Does it lead to social isolation? When an individual has more than one chronic illness, the regimen often becomes more complicated and requires considerable juggling of time and energy.

4. *Preventing or coping with social isolation.*

   Many chronic illnesses are accompanied by lessened energy and mobility, impairment of sensory processes, visible physical disfigurement, or other deficits that may result in reduced social contact and isolation. The sick individual may withdraw from social activities, or former social contacts may withdraw. The more serious the disease, the more likely isolation will occur.

5. *Adjusting to changes in the course of the disease.*

   Both the sick individual and those close to him or her need to cope with the downward course of the illness. Every downward step requires the sick person to reassess health status and make arrangements to manage symptoms, social interactions, and activities of daily living. Those close to the sick person may also need to be involved in such arrangements since dependence increases as the illness progresses. The impact of the downward course of illness upon personal identity depends upon the illness. If the downward course is predictable, preparation is possible in advance of each new downward phase; if it is unexpectedly quick, then adjustment is more difficult.

6. *Attempting to normalize lifestyle and interaction with others.*

   The chief task of one who is chronically ill is to live as fully as possible despite the symptoms and the disease. How normal life can be depends on the extent of symptoms, disability, and the regimen required to keep the disease under control. The task of normalization is most difficult when the disease is fatal.

7. *Financing treatments and survival.*

   As chronic illness is usually life-long, it is nearly always accompanied by financial problems. One important characteristic of chronic disease is the cost of required treatment, especially drugs, machinery, physician visits, and home-based health services. Health problems can wipe out life savings rapidly, and the chronically ill have to seek other funding sources. The problem of seeking adequate funds for treatment and survival becomes more complex when one is also dealing with physical disability.

Adapted from Strauss, A.L. 1975. *Chronic illness and the quality of life.* St. Louis: C. V. Mosby Co.

no longer perform many activities of daily living, the other will have to take on more responsibility.

COMMON CHRONIC CONDITIONS AMONG ELDERS

The remainder of this chapter will discuss selected chronic conditions in middle-aged and older adults. Chronic mental disorders were discussed in chapter 7. Medications to treat these illnesses will be further discussed in the medication chapter.

The following descriptions do not detail the psychosocial effects of symptoms or treatment regimen because they are highly variable and depend on extent of illness, personality, coping skills, financial situation, and degree of social support. However, as you read about each of the chronic conditions, consider the impact of the illness on the affected elders and their families using Strauss's model as a framework. Some disease symptoms have little effect on lifestyle, while others may be so debilitating that institutionalization may result.

Cardiovascular Diseases

Cardiovascular diseases affect the heart and blood vessels and include heart disease and stroke, two predominant causes of death among the elderly. Heart disease is the number one killer, accounting for almost half of all deaths among elders, and stroke is number three (cancer is number two). The incidence of cardiovascular disease increases dramatically with age in both women and men. However, due to a number of factors, the incidence of cardiovascular disease is gradually declining in the United States. This section will discuss atherosclerosis, hypertension, coronary artery disease, congestive heart failure, arrhythmias, aneurysm, venous disease, and stroke. Although these various diseases are discussed separately, cardiovascular diseases share common causes and treatments.

Atherosclerosis

Atherosclerosis is a disease of the blood vessels. Atherosclerosis is the underlying cause of many diseases of the cardiovascular system, and pre-venting atherosclerosis would reduce much suffering from these diseases. In developed countries, it begins as early as childhood and slowly progresses throughout life. Affected arteries have fatty deposits in their walls that reduce the diameter of the artery, sometimes closing it altogether. These clogged arteries can occur anywhere in the body but are most dangerous in the coronary arteries (arteries supplying blood to the heart muscle) and blood vessels leading to the brain. Atherosclerosis should not be confused with arteriosclerosis, a general term referring to hardening of the arteries. Arteriosclerosis is a progressive, age-associated condition resulting in a loss of elasticity of the arterial walls.

Many people believe the development and progression of atherosclerosis is accelerated by the Western lifestyle: inactivity, smoking, obesity, and a diet high in fats. High cholesterol, diabetes, hypertension, and smoking all aggravate atherosclerosis. Treatment is focused in reducing dietary fat and lowering blood cholesterol levels, controlling diabetes and hypertension, and losing weight. Multiple studies show that a reduction in dietary fat, or in serum cholesterol, results in slowing of atherosclerotic plaque formation, or even reversal of plaque development. In addition, studies show that behavioral changes—such as modifying diet, quitting smoking, losing weight if obese, decreasing stress, and exercising regularly can delay the development of and even reverse atherosclerosis. A well-known program run by Dr. Dean Ornish combines a strict vegetarian diet with less than 10 percent of calories from fat, no smoking, an hour a day of yoga or meditation, and three hours a week of moderate exercise. He documents a significant reduction in atherosclerosis and heart attacks and an improvement in cardiovascular disease risk factors.[5]

A major contributor to atherosclerosis is elevated cholesterol, or hypercholesterolemia. It is known that an elevation in cholesterol (particularly the level of low-density lipoprotein, or LDL) is a significant risk factor for cardiovascular disease. A low level of HDL (high-density lipoprotein, the good cholesterol) is also associated with increased risk. Those with elevated cholesterol often have other cardiovascular risk factors including hypertension, diabetes, sedentary lifestyle, obesity, or tobacco use. High HDL levels are associated with being female and being physically active. However, the association between elevated cholesterol and cardiovascular disease is weaker among elders.

Experts recommend periodic measurements of cholesterol and HDL in men and women. Desirable cholesterol readings are less than 200 mg/dl, 200–239 mg/dl is borderline, and greater than 240 mg/dl is high. HDL cholesterol should be more than 35 mg/dl. HDL levels greater than 60 mg/dl reduce the risk of cardiovascular disease. If one has few risk factors for cardiovascular disease, there is less need for treatment. Dietary therapy (reducing dietary fat intake and dietary cholesterol) and exercise are the first type of treatment offered to those with elevated cholesterol, elevated LDL, or low HDL levels. If lifestyle modification fails to lower cholesterol, consideration is given to prescribing medications to lower cholesterol levels.

The more risk factors an individual has, the more likely he or she is to benefit from cholesterol lowering drugs. Those who are at highest risk for high cholesterol are males who have a family history of premature heart disease, are cigarette smokers, have hypertension, and have low HDL cholesterol and diabetes. However, the research conducted thus far has not found a significant association between high cholesterol readings and cardiovascular disease among men seventy-five and older or women over sixty-five. Interestingly, studies of elders eighty-five and over have shown that elders with the highest cholesterol levels have the lowest heart attack deaths, and those with the lowest cholesterol levels experience the highest heart attack death rate.[6] Another study reported that a low level of dietary fat was associated with a higher risk of stroke.[7] Obviously, more studies are needed to better understand this association.

Medication therapy for elevated cholesterol is controversial. Early studies suggested that lowering cholesterol was associated with increased death rates of accidents, suicide, and cancer.

However, evidence is mounting that lowering cholesterol levels with medications is effective at reducing heart disease morality in men up to age seventy-five and women up to age sixty-five.[8] However, medication may be very expensive and must be taken for life. For more detailed information on cholesterol-lowering drugs, refer to chapter 10.

When atheroslerosis occurs in the arteries of the legs, it may cause a condition called *intermittent claudication.* Elders with this condition complain of severe crampy pain in one or both legs whenever they walk a certain distance. This pain is due to insufficient blood flow to the exercising muscles. After resting briefly, the pain is relieved, but recurs upon walking. Some individuals may also experience numbness and coldness in their legs. There is no effective medication for this disorder. The best treatment is to exercise to the point of pain, rest, then continue to exercise, gradually building up circulation to the muscles. In severe cases, bypass surgery is performed where a vein from the lower leg is grafted to an artery above the site of narrowing.

Hypertension (High Blood Pressure)

Hypertension is known as "the silent killer" because most of the 50 million Americans with the disease (about one in four adults) have no symptoms. This deadly illness is a major risk factor for cardiovascular disease (especially heart attack), kidney disease, and stroke, especially among older people. Hypertension is most common among the elder population. Hypertension is defined as either a systolic blood pressure (the upper number) greater than 140, or a diastolic blood pressure (the lower number) greater than 90. The higher the blood pressure, the greater the risk of stroke, heart disease, and kidney damage.

Despite the lack of symptoms, high blood pressure may seriously damage body organs and blood vessels. Damage to the arteries increases the rate of atherosclerosis and strokes. Furthermore, the heart, by necessity, must become larger and thicker to pump blood through the narrowed vessels. A thickened left ventricle increases the risk of heart disease and irregular heartbeats (cardiac arry-

Blood Pressure: What is It and How is It Measured?

Blood pressure is the force exerted by the blood against the artery walls. When the heart contracts, a great volume of blood is forced into the arteries, and pressure reaches a maximum point (called systolic pressure). After the heart has contracted and pushes blood out, it pauses to refill. During this time, the pressure in the arteries is at its lowest point (called diastolic pressure). Readings are commonly expressed as a fraction; the top number is the systolic pressure, while the bottom is the diastolic pressure.

Systolic and diastolic pressure can be measured by an instrument called a *sphygmomanometer,* commonly known as a blood pressure gauge. The pressure the blood exerts on the arteries is measured as the amount of pressure able to fill a column of mercury in millimeters (mm). Thus, the average blood pressure would be reported as 120/80 mmHg (Hg is the chemical symbol for mercury). Low blood pressure is common, especially among women and athletes and is no cause for concern. Only when blood pressure becomes exceedingly low, or when blood pressure falls due to shock or blood loss is there cause for concern. On the contrary, high blood pressure is a medical condition that should be treated.

Blood pressure readings are highly variable. Anxiety, stress, physical activity, even giving a presentation, may elevate blood pressure. In addition, many borderline hypertensives exhibit a "white coat syndrome," in which their anxiety at seeing a doctor can increase blood pressure. One isolated high blood pressure reading should not be cause for treatment. To increase accuracy, at least three different readings should be taken at different visits and averaged. A more accurate alternative is using a mobile blood pressure instrument that is attached to the patient and automatically records hourly blood pressure throughout a twenty-four hour period.

thmias). When this compensation fails, congestive heart failure develops. Increased blood pressure also causes irreversible damage to the blood vessels in the kidneys and eyes, causing kidney failure and blindness. Hypertension can affect the brain and is associated with reduced cognitive function[9] as well as increased risk of strokes and associated dementia.

The major contributor to hypertension in the United States is obesity. Thus, weight loss is the single most important means to reduce hypertension. However, in many cases, the cause of hypertension is unknown. Experts postulate that many other factors play a role, including genetics, age, race, hormones, stress response, and excessive salt intake. Hypertension is more common among older people (especially women), African Americans, and the poor.

Blood pressure varies throughout the day, and several measurements of elevated blood pressure are required before treatment is initiated.[10] Those with hypertension need a thorough evaluation to rule out reversible causes and frequent follow-up to assure that blood pressure is normalized. These individuals also require more careful evaluation as they have an increased risk of other illnesses, particularly cardiovascular disease.

Some individuals do not have high blood pressure readings until they go into the doctor's office, called "white coat hypertension." Because of this, patients are encouraged to measure their blood pressure at home (with a calibrated cuff) or they might be given a portable monitor to wear at home that automatically measures blood pressure, usually over a twenty-four-hour interval. Automated blood pressure computers found in drugstores and supermarkets are not dependable: one study reported the pressure readings were inaccurate more than half the time.[11]

Many lifestyle modifications reduce hypertension; most of these also reduce other cardiovas-

TABLE 8.2	Recommended Treatments for Stages of Hypertension		
Blood Pressure Stages (Points)	Group A (No Risk Factors)	Group B (One or More Risk Factors*)	Group C (Certain Conditions**)
High normal (130–139/85–89)	Lifestyle modification	Lifestyle modification	Drug therapy
Stage 1 (140–159/90–99)	Lifestyle modification (up to 12 months)	Lifestyle modification (up to 6 months)	Drug therapy
Stages 2 and 3 (≥160/≥100)	Drug therapy	Drug therapy	Drug therapy

* Smoking, high cholesterol, age over 60, being male or postmenopausal female, or family history of heart disease.
** Diabetes, stroke, retinopathy, peripheral arterial disease, nephropathy, or clinical signs of heart disease.
Source: Sixth Report of the Joint National Committee on Prevention, Detection, Evaluation, and Treatment of High Blood Pressure. National Institutes of Health: Bethesda, MD.

cular risk factors. These include salt restriction, weight reduction, regular aerobic exercise, relaxation training, restricted alcohol consumption, reduction in dietary fat, and smoking cessation. Mineral supplements, such as calcium and potassium, are helpful in some cases. A randomized controlled trial in elders showed that sodium reduction and weight loss among obese individuals with hypertension reduced their need for medications.[12] Often programs that emphasize multiple positive lifestyle changes (including counseling, weight loss, diet, exercise, meditation, and drug therapy) are the most effective (see table 8.2).

Drug treatment of hypertension is somewhat controversial. Although there are a plethora of drugs available to lower blood pressure, only two of the oldest drugs (beta blockers and diuretics) have been shown definitively to reduce strokes and heart attack deaths. These also are the least expensive and have the longest track record on safety and efficacy. However, many elders require therapy with more than one medication for optimal blood pressure control. The medication chapter will provide more detail on the different types of hypertension drugs.

Studies of the elderly report that treatment of hypertension significantly reduces both heart attack and stroke deaths among elderly patients.[13] However, there is some suggestion that the bene-fits of treating hypertension among the oldest-old are not as clear. Despite the fearful and often deadly consequences of hypertension, about one-half of those with the disease do not manage to control their blood pressure with drugs or lifestyle modifications.

Coronary Artery Disease

Coronary artery disease is the biggest killer of adults and the most common type of heart disease in elders. The main contributor to coronary artery disease is atherosclerosis of the coronary arteries, the vessels that supply oxygen and nutrients to the heart muscle. A blood clot can more easily become lodged in a narrowed vessel, resulting in insufficient blood flow and oxygen to the heart. The reduction in blood flow may be temporary, as in *angina pectoris.* However, if a blood clot blocks nutrients and oxygen to the heart muscle, the part of the muscle that is deprived of oxygen and nutrients will die, causing a heart attack. The extent of the attack depends upon how much heart muscle is affected below the coronary artery blockage.

Risk factors for coronary artery disease are smoking, high blood pressure, high cholesterol, obesity, and a sedentary lifestyle. Although obesity is an important risk factor, it seems that the pattern of obesity is more important than the weight itself. Those with an abdominal and chest-area fat and larger waists (apple-shaped) have a higher heart disease risk than those who carry fat on their hips and thighs (pear-shaped).[14] Also, high levels of homocysteine, an amino acid in the blood common in those with low dietary intakes of B vitamins, are associated with a higher risk for heart attack deaths.[15,16] Triglycerides, another type of cholesterol, may also be important in predicting heart attack risk for both men and women. There is also some evidence that a hostile personality trait is a risk factor in coronary heart disease.

Older people have more than twice the incidence of heart attack than younger individuals. Men are more likely to die of a heart attack in their younger years than women. Women have a lower risk of cardiac disease until menopause, when their risk begins to increase until it approaches that of men. African Americans are more likely to die from a heart attack than whites, and they tend to have both a higher prevalence and increased severity of hypertension.

Because there are so many risk factors and because coronary artery disease is so prevalent, almost everyone is at risk. The risk of developing coronary artery disease can be reduced by positive lifestyle changes: reduce weight, increase physical activity, stop smoking, and reduce dietary fat. It is documented that the risk of heart disease and stroke may be minimized by taking low-dose aspirin (reduces blood clotting) or folate supplements (reduce homocysteine levels). Also, estrogen replacement in postmenopausal women reduces risk of cardiovascular disease, perhaps because it increases HDL levels.[17]

Angina pectoris occurs when the heart muscle needs more oxygen than is supplied by the coronary arteries because they are narrowed by atherosclerosis. The classic symptom of angina is a squeezing pressure under the sternum that may radiate to the arms or neck. Nausea, sweating, anxiety, and shortness of breath may accompany the pain. Anginal pain typically lasts a few seconds to a few minutes and may be relieved by rest or nitroglycerine tablets placed under the tongue to expand the coronary arteries. For most people, angina occurs only when the heart is under physical stress (exercise) or mental

stress. Although it has been known for a long time that physical stress could induce anginal symptoms, a recent study reported that the mental stress of daily life (tension, frustration, and sadness) can more than double the risk of anginal symptoms in the subsequent hour.[18] However, in severe forms, angina can occur at rest. Nitrites are commonly used (orally or as patches) to prevent and treat angina. Studies show that aspirin therapy can reduce risk and pain of angina and reduce risk of stroke. Other medications are detailed in chapter 10.

A heart attack, also called myocardial infarction, occurs when a blood clot blocks a vessel already narrowed by atherosclerosis. This completely cuts off circulation to all heart muscle beyond the clot. The following are classic heart attack symptoms: prolonged crushing chest pain radiating to the shoulder or arm, lightheadedness, shortness of breath, sweating, and nausea. In many cases, the pain may not be severe but does not disappear after ten minutes. Unfortunately, up to about one-fourth of all heart attacks are silent (no symptoms) or have only mild symptoms. These people may manifest only subtle mental changes such as confusion.[19]

The majority of heart attacks are not fatal. However, all heart attacks permanently damage heart tissue. This damage can result in cardiac arrythmias (such as irregular heart rate) or congestive heart failure. Fatal heart attacks are most common among younger people, the very old, and women.[20] Many studies have attempted to answer why women are more likely to die from a heart attack than men. Whether there are biological reasons, or whether it is the result of discrimination in diagnosis and treatment is not yet clear.

Anyone with chest pain for more than ten minutes should seek immediate medical care. If a heart attack is suspected, an aspirin should be taken immediately, and aspirin therapy should continue after the attack.[21] Almost half of all victims of a heart attack die before they reach the hospital.[22] The survival rate of a heart attack is doubled if hospitalization occurs within an hour of pain onset.

If victims seek care immediately, drugs can be administered to dissolve the clot, thus saving some heart muscle. Those who have had a heart attack require hospitalization to make sure muscle death does not progress, and congestive heart failure or life-threatening arrhythmias do not develop. The patient is generally sedated and given painkillers to reduce anxiety and subsequent stress upon the heart. After a few days of rest, the patient can gradually increase activity.

Generally, angiography, angioplasty, and/or bypass surgery is done one to two days after the heart attack. Angiography is a diagnostic procedure to determine the degree of narrowing in the coronary arteries. A thin tube is inserted into a vein and passed through the vein into the coronary arteries. A small amount of contrast dye is released and an X-ray taken as the contrast fills the arteries. This procedure localizes areas of narrowing in the artery that is at high risk of being totally shut off. These areas can then be treated with angioplasty, a procedure that widens the portion of the artery that has dangerously narrowed. Balloon angioplasty involves passing a deflated balloon into the artery, then inflating the balloon to widen the artery. Balloon angioplasty is a low-risk procedure. Another type of angioplasty is laser angioplasty, where a laser-tipped catheter vaporizes the plaque in the artery. Sometimes a tiny metal stent device is placed in the artery to hold it open.[23] Studies show little difference between angioplasty and clot-dissolving drugs in patient survival.[24]

In contrast to angioplasty, coronary bypass surgery is a lengthy surgical procedure that removes veins from the chest or leg and grafts them onto coronary arteries around the areas of narrowing. When you hear of triple bypass or quadruple bypass operations, you know that individual had three or four areas of narrowing in the coronary arteries that were grafted. Controversy surrounds the use of the bypass operation, especially among women and older people, because the risks may outweigh the benefits. Although studies comparing bypass operations to angioplasty are mixed, it is thought that people with severe disease benefit most from bypass surgery. Although there are higher risks of the surgery, those who undergo it often report better quality of life.[25]

People treated at hospitals where the doctors are more experienced in bypass operations or angioplasty have better survival rate[26] and people treated by cardiologists have a better survival rate than those treated by general practitioners.[27] Unfortunately, there is a wide variability in survival rates after a heart attack, which as of yet cannot be explained.[28]

Those who are recovering from a heart attack generally undergo a program of cardiac rehabilitation that combines exercise, diet, medication, and health education. Cardiac rehabilitation may be continued for months or even years. In cardiac rehabilitation programs, those who have suffered a heart attack are encouraged to begin a gradual, light exercise program, such as walking. One aspirin daily has been shown to reduce the recurrence of heart attack and the risk of death after a heart attack, even in the very old.[29] Beta blockers are extremely effective at reducing death and rehospitalization rates after myocardial infarction, but are underused in the elderly. One study found that only one in five elders who should have received beta blockers did, and many received calcium channel blockers instead, which were associated with a higher risk of death.[30]

Individuals may require further angioplasties, stent placement, or bypass surgery in the months following a heart attack. Depending on the amount of cardiac damage, these individuals may require therapy for congestive heart failure. Lifestyle modifications such as increasing physical activity, reducing stress, and following low-salt and low-fat diets may also lessen the threat of another myocardial infarction. Women may be prescribed hormone-replacement therapy.

Congestive Heart Failure

When the heart muscle is no longer able to pump blood effectively, that individual is said to have congestive heart failure (CHF). Although its name implies an abrupt heart stoppage, heart failure is generally a chronic condition of weakening ability of the heart muscle to pump effectively. Heart failure affects more than five million people in the United States, reducing their quality of life and limiting their activity. The incidence of heart failure increases with age. It is the most common reason for hospitalization of those over age sixty-five.[31] Congestive heart failure can range from a mild condition to a severely disabling condition of fatigue and breathlessness that requires multiple medications and oxygen. It can also be deadly: approximately half of those who are diagnosed with CHF will die within five years, and if severe, half will be dead in six months.[32]

There are multiple ways to classify heart failure. The heart may have poor output (called left heart failure), decreasing the blood supply to vital organs like the brain or kidneys. Alternatively, the heart may "back up" (called right heart failure), leading to excess fluid in the lungs and veins, and swelling of the ankles. This fluid retention is aggravated by hormones released by the kidneys. Since the kidneys are receiving less blood flow, they react as though the body is dehydrated; they release hormones to save salt and water, resulting in even more fluid back-up. The most common symptoms of congestive heart failure relate to poor output (decreased urine production, fatigue, and confusion) and "back-up" (shortness of breath and swollen ankles or fluid-distended abdomen).

The number one cause of congestive heart failure is hypertension. Because the heart has to work harder to pump blood through narrowed vessels, this creates a strain on the heart. The heart muscle enlarges with the increased workload, much like any other muscle that is stressed, but the heart tissue can only compensate so much. After prolonged strain, the heart muscle begins to fail as a pump. This results in both poor output and a backlog of fluid in the system. Other causes of CHF include single or multiple heart attacks that destroy heart muscle, diabetes, pulmonary diseases, heart valve disease, heart arrythmias, or other cardiac diseases. Risk factors include tobacco use, elevated cholesterol, elevated blood pressure, and diabetes.

Congestive heart failure must be carefully managed since any increase in symptoms may be life-threatening. Physicians may prescribe medications that increase the pumping ability of the heart, reduce the excessive fluid, and expand blood vessels to decrease pressure so blood can flow more easily. First, digitalis increases the pumping effi-

ciency of the heart. Second, diuretics help the body eliminate excessive water and salt. Diuretics also help mobilize the fluid from the ankles, lungs, and other areas where it accumulates. Third, vasodilators (ACE inhibitors) prevent certain hormones in the body from constricting blood vessels. Beta blockers may be prescribed to slow the heart rate and increase pumping efficiency. All of these medications have significant side effects and must be closely monitored.

In addition to drug therapy, counseling, education and lifestyle modifications can have significant impacts on quality of life. In particular, dietary sodium should be significantly reduced, alcohol use should be minimized, and an exercise program (e.g., walking) should be initiated.[33] The disease can worsen with excessive consumption of fluid or salty foods, not taking medications as prescribed, or other diseases such as a heart attack or pneumonia. A signal that the disease is worsening is shortness of breath or sudden weight gain indicating fluid retention. Because episodes of symptoms may be interspersed with periods without symptoms, elders may have difficulty complying with medical recommendations.

Cardiac Arrhythmia

A cardiac arrhythmia is an irregular heartbeat. Some arrhythmias have no symptoms and cause relatively few problems, others cause loss of consciousness or death. They may occur after years of other cardiac problems, such as congestive heart failure or heart valve disease, or they may occur after a myocardial infarction. Arrhythmias generally result from damage to part of the heart muscle that regulates heartbeat. Discussion of the multiple types of arrhythmias is beyond the scope of this text; however, two of the most common will be addressed.

Atrial fibrillation is a disorganized beat of the atrial heart chambers, preventing them from delivering blood efficiently to the ventricles. The elder may complain of palpitations, and the pulse is very irregular. This may be asymptomatic, or, if the person has cardiac damage, may cause problems. Atrial fibrillation is particularly dangerous if it is associated with a rapid heartbeat. If the beat of the heart has a tendency to change in and out of atrial fibrillation, the individual is at high risk of having a stroke. This is because blood pools in the atrial chambers of the heart during fibrillation and may clot. With the next beat, this clot could dislodge and travel to the brain. When this condition is detected early, sometimes medications or "cardioversion" (use of electric shock to the heart) can return the heart to normal. If this cannot be accomplished, the patient requires drugs to maintain the heart rate in the normal range (e.g., beta blockers, digoxin) and anticoagulants (coumadin or aspirin) to thin the blood and prevent strokes. Anticoagulants have been found to be effective in elders, but are too rarely prescribed in elders,[34] possibly because they require frequent dosage adjustments and medical visits, they interact with other medications, and they can cause a side effect of significant bleeding.

In contrast, arrhythmias of the heart ventricles are common following a heart attack and are a significant cause of death in the twenty-four to forty-eight hours following a heart attack. Ventricular fibrillation is a very disorganized rhythm of the ventricle where the muscle just quivers and cannot pump blood. This is a medical emergency, and the rhythm must immediately be converted to normal with electric shock or drugs or the person will die. If a person is at high risk of developing this condition, the physician may prescribe antiarrhythmic medications on a long-term basis.

Family members should learn cardiopulmonary resuscitation (CPR) and are often given a computerized defibrillator so they can administer electric shocks at home. A patient may also have an implantable defibrillator that senses the abnormal rhythm and delivers such a large shock to the heart that he or she loses consciousness. Sometimes a pacemaker can be used for this problem.

Stroke

Strokes are the third leading cause of death and the major cause of physical and mental disability among elders. *Ischemic strokes,* the most common type, result when a portion of the brain is suddenly denied needed blood. Most strokes are due to blood clots or clumps of cholesterol that break off inside a blood vessel in another part of the body. These fragments travel through the bloodstream to the brain where they lodge in a small blood vessel, cutting off blood supply to brain tissue beyond the blockage. The degree of damage depends on the area of the brain affected, the extent of brain tissue damaged, and the level of prior functioning. In contrast, *hemmorhagic strokes* result from bleeding in the brain caused by a burst blood vessel. This occurs primarily in those with severe hypertension.

A number of factors predispose individuals to strokes. The main risk factor is hypertension. Smokers have an increased stroke risk. Females are at higher risk than males. Several chronic diseases such as diabetes, heart disease, atherosclerosis, or atrial fibrillation also increase the likelihood of having a stroke.

Perhaps the most important warning sign for strokes are ministrokes or transient ischemic attacks (TIAs), which are caused by a temporary blockage of the arteries in the brain. They may result in transient or permanent motor weakness, blackouts, speech disturbances, or personality changes. The attacks may last from a few minutes to twenty-four hours. People who experienced a TIA are nine times more likely to have a stroke than the general population.[35] Warning signs of a stroke are as follows:

- sudden weakness or numbness of your face, arm, or leg,
- sudden dimness, blurriness, or loss of vision, particularly in one eye,
- sudden difficulty in speaking or understanding speech,
- sudden severe headache with no known cause,
- unexplained dizziness, unsteadiness, or sudden falls, especially accompanying other signs.

Although heart attack victims generally seek medical attention quickly, individuals who have suffered a stroke often delay seeking medical treatment. One study reported that less than one in four who had a stroke visit a physician within twenty-four hours.[35] This may be because the public (and particularly the elderly public) is unfamiliar with the symptoms.[36] New research is identifying clot-dissolving agents that can be administered immediately after a stroke to reduce the damage. However, medical care must be sought promptly (ideally less than one hour after the symptoms begin) for these to be effective.

The disabilities people suffer from strokes are highly variable and depend on the portion of the brain affected. Weakness or paralysis of the face, arm, or leg, or even the entire left or right side of the body is common. Many elders manifest alterations in thought patterns or speech (aphasia). They may lose their ability to comprehend speech, or to speak fluently. They may only be able to speak in obscenities, lose the ability to draw or write, be unable to read, or lose a portion of their vision. Some elders suffer seizures or hallucinations. They may lose sensation in parts of their body, experience lack of coordination or balance, or lose their ability to determine the position of their limbs.

The early signs of disability after a stroke are worse than during recovery. This improvement is partially due to a decrease in brain swelling over time and rehabilitation efforts. Sometimes when one part of the brain is damaged, such as the speech comprehension center, its functions are permanently lost; however, with some disabilities, other parts of the brain seem to accommodate by taking over the new task.

Strokes can be prevented by modifying stroke-related risk factors (e.g., normalizing blood pressure or achieving better diabetic control). People with atrial fibrillation suffer excessive stroke risk and must often go on long-term therapy with anti-coagulant drugs to reduce blood clotting. This medication may be most effective in elders over age seventy.[37] One extensive study reported that as little as one-tenth of an aspirin (30 mg) a day was sufficient to reduce the incidence of a heart attack or stroke among persons who previously had a stroke or a TIA.[38]

The major cause of a stroke is a blood clot that originates in the carotid artery because of atherosclerosis. Thus, intervention involves widening the carotid artery. The artery may be scraped out (cardiac endartectomy) or dilated with a balloon (balloon catherization). However, there is much controversy surrounding these procedures because they can cause strokes while trying to prevent them. Experts disagree under what circumstances these interventions are helpful.

The effectiveness of stroke rehabilitation depends on the type and extent of the stroke as well as the client's overall health status, motivation, personality, and financial resources. An extensive physical and mental assessment should be conducted as soon as possible after a stroke to determine sensory and motor loss, psychological state, and the patient's ability to speak and understand. As soon as possible, occupational, physical, and speech therapists should implement a rehabilitation plan. Almost 90 percent of all stroke victims have rehabilitation potential soon after a stroke, but this potential diminishes each day the stroke victims are not in a rehabilitation program. Some strokes, however, cause catastrophic damage, inhibiting elders' ability to be conscious, interact, or swallow. In these cases, family or other decision makers must decide whether to institute or continue artificial feeding, or whether to allow death to occur.

Because the emotional effects of a stroke are common (e.g., lack of motivation, depression, anxiety, or frustration) and can adversely affect recovery, psychological counseling and support are appropriate for both patient and family.

Aortic Aneurysm

Aneurysms are weakened areas in blood vessels that increase the propensity for the blood vessel to rupture or tear. The most significant type of aneurysm is the aortic aneurysm. In the United States, one in every 250 deaths among people over age fifty is attributed to ruptured aortic aneurysm. This diagnosis is frequently missed and even if surgery is undertaken immediately after rupture, about three-quarters of patients die. If these are detected early, before rupture, surgery can prevent complications, and carrying a death rate of less than 5 percent. These can be diagnosed during physical examination or radiological studies. Risk factors include hypertension, atherosclerosis, and cigarette smoking.

Venous Disease

Varicose Veins   With age, the veins in the body may lose their elasticity, their valves may not work properly, and they can become swollen and develop into varicose veins. These are more common in women than men and increase in incidence after age sixty-five. Varicose veins may ache, itch, swell, or bleed, and may be unattractive. Treatment includes compression stockings, surgical removal (stripping), or sclerotherapy, a procedure in which a chemical is injected into the vein to shrink it.

Deep Venous Thrombosis   A deep venous thrombosis occurs when a blood clot develops in a vein, generally in the deep veins of the legs or arms. These blood clots cause swelling, tenderness and localized redness, which may develop gradually. The blood clots can break off and travel to many other parts of the body. If they travel to the lungs, they are known

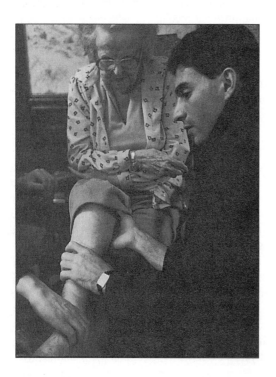

as pulmonary emboli, which are often deadly. Symptoms are sudden or gradual onset of shortness of breath, cough, and decreased exercise tolerance. People who are sedentary, who have broken or fractured bones, and who have cancer are at higher risk of deep venous thrombosis. Diagnosis is through ultrasound of the veins or through "venograms" where contrast material is injected into the vein. Blood clots are treated with anticoagulants. In general, an elder must be hospitalized and given intravenous heparin to dissolve the clot. Later the elder may be prescribed a blood thinner.

Cancer

Few words evoke such fear and anxiety as the word "cancer." Cancer is a general term that includes many different types of tumors that can affect nearly every body system. Cancers vary widely in their presentation, their symptoms, their treatments and their lethality. Some types of cancer are extremely rare, such as cancer of the heart, the small intestine, or muscles. Others are much more common, making cancer the second leading cause of death in the United States. Some types of cancer are almost universally and rapidly fatal (such as pancreatic cancer and some lung cancers), while others tend to grow more slowly (such as prostate cancer, skin cancers, and bladder cancer). Some cancers are increasing in number (melanoma), while others are decreasing (colon cancer, lung cancer).

A cancer is a group of body cells that, for an unknown reason, begins to multiply and grow out of control. It takes more than its share of nutrients and causes the body to produce new blood vessels to supply its voracious growth. Pieces of the tumor may break off and spread through the blood or lymph to other parts of the body (metastasize) and set up a new tumor site there. Not every tumor or mass is cancerous, but masses are a common symptom of cancer. The classic seven warning signals of cancer are:

- Change in bowel or bladder habits,
- A sore that does not heal,

- Unusual bleeding or discharge,
- Thickening or lump in breast or elsewhere,
- Indigestion or difficulty in swallowing,
- Obvious change in a wart or mole,
- Nagging cough or hoarseness.

In addition, overall system problems such as rapid weight loss without dieting, lack of appetite, and fatigue or weakness are ominous signs and should be evaluated promptly. Ideally, cancers should be detected before they cause symptoms through screening and early detection programs (e.g., mammography, rectal exams), which will be discussed more completely in chapter 11.

Cancer mortality is rising in the United States, despite decades of research and trials of new therapies.[39] Extensive research is being conducted to determine causes, prevention and treatment of various cancers, and much is being learned in these areas. Genetic factors, hormones, environmental toxins, cigarette smoking, radiation, and stress have all been implicated for some cancers. Despite advances in our understanding about the diverse group of illnesses called cancer, there is still no universal cure.

While many cancers can be very effectively treated if found early and still localized, most advanced cancers that have spread throughout the body cannot be cured with standard or alternative medical treatment. However, for some cancers, treatments may extend life, making "living with cancer" more common than "dying from cancer."

The risk of developing cancer increases significantly with age; more than half its victims are over age sixty-five. The most common cancer deaths among elders are lung, colon and rectum, prostate, and breast cancers. A number of factors may explain the increased cancer risk among older people. The aging process may reduce the ability of the immune system to reject abnormal growths. Some researchers hypothesize that elders lack sufficient DNA for the increased repair demands of an aging body, thereby allowing defective cells to grow unchecked. Another theory is that the elderly have had more time to be exposed to carcinogens such as cigarette smoke and environmental toxins.

Because cancer often has no specific symptoms, it may be difficult to diagnose in elders. In younger patients, cancer is usually the only disease condition present. However, in elders, cancer symptoms are often overshadowed by symptoms of other diseases. Furthermore, physicians may mistakenly attribute warning signals to diseases already present. For instance, the rectal bleeding characteristic of colon cancer may be attributed to long-standing hemorrhoids. Fatigue and weight loss may be attributed to "growing old."

Cancer is often found by the individual who notices a mass, has rectal bleeding, or "feels different." Cancers may be detected by a variety of screening tests, depending on the site. It is not reasonable to scan the entire body every year to assure no tiny cancers are growing. On the other hand, many simple screening tests are useful, especially among high-risk groups. These include rectal exams; colonoscopy; blood tests; breast, skin, or testicular self-exams; mammography; chest X-rays; and Pap smears. Physicians vary on recommendations for how frequently one should undergo these tests. Unfortunately, elders as a group are poorly informed about cancer and participation in cancer screening decreases rather than increases with advancing age.[40]

Generally, cancer is treated with surgery, chemotherapy, or radiation. Cancer treatments are riskier and have more side effects than almost any other type of medical treatment. Radiation and chemotherapy both inadvertently damage many normal cells in the process of killing the cancer cells, and treatment is very stressful for the body at any age. In addition, elders are generally less able to tolerate anesthesia or long surgical treatments and suffer more complications from surgery such as wound infections, postoperative heart attacks or strokes, and hospital-acquired infections such as pneumonia or urinary tract infections.

Age, rate of cancer growth, type and extent of treatment, health status, and the quality and the remaining length of life are important considerations when developing a treatment plan. Studies suggest that elders are more likely to develop cancer but are less likely to be treated for it. It is unclear how much of this differential is due to patient preferences, and how much is due to physicians not offering treatment to the elderly. While it is true that it may not be appropriate to treat cancer in a patient with advanced Alzheimer's disease, for example, studies suggest that elders tolerate surgery, radiation, and chemotherapy well. If treatment only increases the survival slightly, the procedure has a high complication rate, or cancer growth is slow, it may be better to limit treatment to symptom relief. However, in the majority of cases, elders can benefit from cancer treatments, even if they are very old and have other chronic illnesses, if it increases the quality of life in their remaining years.

Prevention of cancer is preferable to treatment. The single most effective way to prevent cancer is through cessation of cigarette smoking. Cigarette smoking is strongly implicated in cancer of the lung, head, and neck, among others. Multiple other lifestyle factors have been implicated in cancer prevention including diet, exposure to sunlight, environmental toxins, exercise, and medication use. Many believe there should be more money available for research to prevent cancer rather than to develop new treatment strategies. The goal of screening programs is to detect cancer at earlier stages, so treatment can be initiated, and ideally, reduce the death rate.

Lung cancer is the leading cause of cancer death in both men and women. In women, breast cancer is the second leading killer, while prostate cancer is second in men, and colorectal cancer is third in both genders. Cancer of the skin is the most common, but most cases are not deadly. These cancers will be addressed in more detail under the heading of the body system they affect.

Respiratory Diseases

The threat of both acute and chronic respiratory disease increases with advanced age. Experts attribute

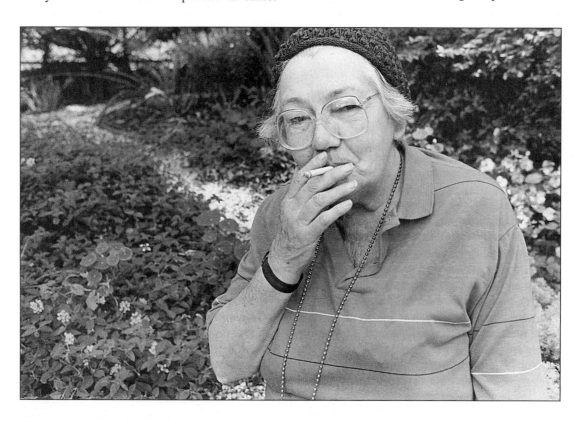

older people's increased susceptibility to respiratory conditions to many factors: decreased resistance to environmental contaminants and microorganisms, age-associated decrements that reduce pulmonary function, and length of exposure to carcinogenic substances.

Cigarette smoking is by far the prime cause of chronic bronchitis, emphysema, and lung cancer. Although rates of cigarette smoking are decreasing in the United States, the percentage of young women who smoke is increasing, and about one-fourth of the adult population smokes, an assurance that respiratory problems will continue to be significant.

Chronic Obstructive Pulmonary Disease

Chronic obstructive pulmonary disease (COPD) is an umbrella term for a number of chronic lung conditions including chronic bronchitis, emphysema, and asthma. In each condition, there is a chronic obstruction of air flow in the bronchi of the lungs that worsens over time. Although individuals may exhibit no symptoms early in the disease, abnormalities can be detected on tests of lung function. With time (and often more cigarette use), the disease worsens, causing debilitating breathlessness, cough, and weakness. Some individuals eventually need to carry supplemental oxygen.

COPD is the most rapidly increasing health problem in the United States. The percentage of deaths attributed to COPD has increased dramatically in the last twenty years, primarily because of cigarette smoking. Although cigarette smoking is implicated in about 90 percent of all COPD, frequent lung infections, pollution exposure, and second-hand smoke may also contribute. Men are more likely to suffer from COPD than women because a higher proportion of men smoke. The incidence of COPD also increases with age. The diseases and their associated disabilities develop gradually, sometimes taking twenty or thirty years to become serious or symptomatic. In general, COPD is caused by years of cigarette smoking, although its signs may appear after only a few years of smoking. Individuals with COPD may have emphysema, chronic bronchitis, or both.

Chronic bronchitis is the most common respiratory condition among elders. It is characterized by chronic cough and abundant sputum production for at least three months a year for two consecutive years. Chronic irritation by infections and/or environmental contaminants overwhelms the respiratory tract. Consequently the mucous cells produce excessive and thickened mucus, further decreasing the airway's ability to clear itself. Breathing becomes even more difficult as the number of mucus-producing cells thicken and narrow the bronchi. A persistent cough and expectoration occur as the body attempts to rid the airways of excessive mucus secretions.

Emphysema is an irreversible deterioration of the air sacs (alveoli) in the lungs that results in decreased oxygen consumption and carbon dioxide excretion. Air becomes trapped behind mucous plugs in the narrowed airways, causing prolonged inflation of the air sacs. This prolonged inflation of stale air reduces the amount of fresh air available for oxygen/carbon dioxide exchange. With time, the air sacs, which remain inflated by trapped air, eventually burst. Thus, the small separate air pockets merge to form larger sacs, which decreases the surface area available for oxygen/carbon dioxide exchange. Symptoms of emphysema include shortness of breath, difficulty in inhalation, and, in later stages, a barrel chest. Typically those with emphysema need to make a strong effort to exhale to rid themselves of trapped air.

Pulmonary function tests find signs of COPD in most smokers, even if they have no symptoms. To diagnose early COPD, many physicians use a spirometer to test patients' breathing capacity. Generally symptoms do not occur until a significant proportion of the lung tissue has been irreversibly damaged. With advanced COPD, frequent infections (pneumonia and bronchitis) may occur, and heart failure may develop.

Lung function can be improved with drugs that dilate (widen) the bronchi, steroids to decrease inflammation, and, as a last resort, portable oxygen. In recent years, research has shown that bronchodilators are very effective in chronic bronchitis, and one study reported that very few were being prescribed to patients who could be helped by them. Instead, the

Effects of Breathlessness on Lifestyle

A common symptom of emphysema and other COPDs is breathlessness. Coping with breathlessness and consequent lack of energy reserves is the central concern of the day for some individuals. The following two cases enable the reader to better understand the impact of breathing problems on everyday life:

One woman who becomes short of breath after a few steps requires two to three hours to get dressed. She arises from bed and goes to the bathroom, rests, washes sitting in a chair with frequent rest periods, walks back to the bedroom, rests, and dresses, always needing to rest every few minutes.

Another man worked out an elaborate routing pattern to mop his kitchen every week. He gathers the cleaning paraphernalia and puts it near a chair in the middle of the room—these motions requiring frequent periods of "getting my breath back." He mops a few strokes and rests, sitting in the chair.[2]

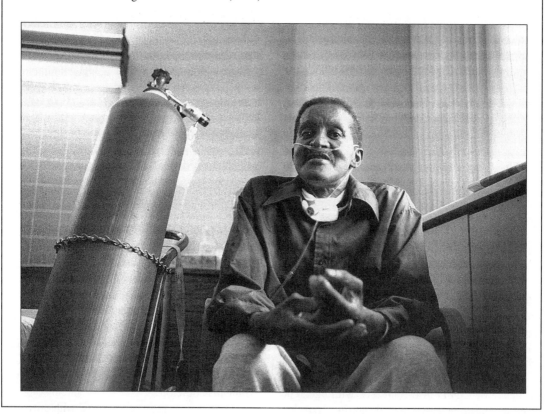

patients were receiving antibiotics. Those with COPD often require multiple courses of antibiotics to treat their recurrent infections. However, antibiotics are overused and should only be prescribed when there is a change in symptoms or when acute symptoms persist for more than two weeks. Elders with COPD can do breathing exercises or moderate physical exercises (such as walking) to reduce the symptoms. They often must learn energy-saving techniques for accomplishing daily activities.

Those who have COPD should eat a healthy diet and keep as physically active as possible to maintain muscle strength. If patients are still smoking, they should be strongly encouraged to stop to reduce further lung damage. Patients should learn which symptoms need medical supervision and ways to increase clearance of secretions. These include tapping on the chest to loosen secretions and lying on one side to help drain them. In rare cases, lung transplant or lung reduction surgery is performed.

Asthma

Asthma is a condition whereby the bronchi or tubes of the lungs are hyperreactive and constrict, causing a reduction of air flow, a tightness of the chest, and wheezing and coughing. Asthma may begin in childhood or adulthood. Some people may only have symptoms when they have a respiratory infection, when they exercise, when they are under emotional stress, when they are exposed to pollutants, or when they are near something to which they are allergic (cat dander, mold). Symptoms can be mild (cough) or severe, requiring high-flow oxygen and even intubation (placement of a tube in the throat to breathe). Drug treatment includes steroids (taken orally, intravenously, or inhaled), bronchodilators (taken orally or inhaled) and other agents.

Lung Cancer

Lung cancer is the leading cause of cancer deaths in our country in both men and women. The death rate for lung cancer is more than double among men because they are more likely to smoke cigarettes. However, as more women indulge in cigarette smoking, their rate of lung cancer is increasing. The lung cancer rate increases with age: the average age for those diagnosed with lung cancer is sixty.

Ninety percent of all lung cancer is attributed to cigarette smoking. The more one smokes, the greater the risk of contracting the disease. Those who smoke two or more packs a day have death rates fifteen to twenty-five times greater than non-smokers. Those who smoke filtered, low-tar cigarettes have lower lung cancer risks, but still have death rates much higher than nonsmokers. While it is true that not all smokers develop lung cancer, lung cancer is very seldom found among those who do not smoke. Other environmental contaminants correlated with lung cancer are asbestos, radon, X-ray exposure, second-hand smoke, and air pollution. A genetic factor, Alpha 1 antitrypsin deficiency, is responsible for a small proportion of lung cancer cases.

Warning symptoms for lung cancer include chronic cough, blood in the sputum, or shortness of breath. Some of these symptoms are similar to those of COPD; however, their onset is more rapid. Lung cancer may be localized to the lung or may metastasize to the lymph nodes, bones, and brain. When it has spread, lung cancer can also cause systemic symptoms such as weight loss, bone pain, or hormonal problems. Lung cancers are generally deadly. Although some patients live for months to years, many die within months of diagnosis. Less than 10 percent of those with lung cancer survive five years.[41]

There are two types of lung cancer, defined by cell type. Nonsmall cell lung cancer is the most common type and is sometimes treatable with surgery (lung transplant), radiation, or chemotherapy. Small cell lung cancer is even more strongly associated with smoking, is rapid-growing, and is more deadly. If cancer is advanced, chemotherapy may be offered, but it may only extend life for months.

Encouraging the public to not start to smoke and to stop smoking are the best ways to stem the tide of lung cancer deaths. Although chest X-rays may detect the disease, lung cancer is often advanced by the time it is diagnosed.

Sensory Disorders

Disorders of the sensory system, primarily hearing and vision, increase with advancing age. These disorders can have profound effects on the ability to perform daily activities and can cause withdrawal or depression. Chapter 3 discussed three age-associated

Cigarette Smoking: A Deadly Addiction

Cigarette smoking is the singlemost important cause of preventable illness and death in the United States. Each year, cigarette smoking causes one of every five deaths in the country—over 400,000 people. Despite the documented dangers of smoking cigarettes, one of four adults smokes cigarettes. For those over 65, the figure is lower (almost 12 percent of women and 14 percent of men),[42] likely because many of those who smoke have already died by that age. Cigarette smoking decreases life expectancy by five to eight years. By age 75, two-thirds of those who smoke are dead compared to only one-third of nonsmokers.

There is overwhelming evidence that cigarette smoking is harmful to every body system. Most importantly, it is a known cause of cancer, heart disease, stroke, and chronic obstructive pulmonary disease. Smoking doubles or triples the risk of stroke and heart disease. Smoking increases the risk of many cancers: lung, cervix, head and neck, esophagus, bladder, pancreas, and kidney. It is now known that cigarette smoking is associated with reduced bone density, skin wrinkling, increased cataract risk, and gum disease. Finally, nicotine is addictive; it may relax an anxious person, but it causes increased blood pressure, increased blood clotting, and irregular heartbeat.

The most well-known effect of cigarette smoking is that it causes lung cancer. Its negative impact on lung tissue also causes emphysema, chronic bronchitis, and other respiratory problems. Even in very young smokers, lung tests detect evidence of disease and reduced function. The lungs have a tremendous reserve capacity, so symptoms are not noticed until widespread irreversible damage has been done. Those who smoke have more frequent and severe respiratory infections, chronic cough, and phlegm production. The dangers of passive smoking (being around those who smoke) are an increased risk of lung cancer, respiratory disease, and cardiovascular problems.

Most people who smoke would like to quit, and many try several times before succeeding as nicotine is an addictive drug. Smoking cessation that includes skills-training (coping with the desire for a cigarette), supportive counseling, and long-term relapse prevention counseling have been reported to be effective. The more intense and varied the counseling and support, the higher the success rate. It is recommended that prescription nicotine delivery systems (patches, gum, inhalers) be offered to those who want to quit as they are also helpful.[43]

Quitting smoking pays. Within a year after quitting, a person's risk of heart disease is cut in half and the risk of lung cancer, stroke, and respiratory conditions declines. Even older smokers who quit lessen their risk of death or heart attack.

---

decrements believed to be part of the aging process: presbyopia, cataracts, and presbycusis. The following section will address three other sensory disorders that occur with increasing frequency in old age: glaucoma, macular degeneration, and tinnitus.

Glaucoma

Glaucoma is a disease characterized by an increased pressure within the eyeball due to a build-up of fluids. Because the drainage system for optical fluids is blocked, or because excessive fluid is produced, pressure builds up and progressively deteriorates the receptor cells in the retina and the optic nerve.

Ultimately, untreated glaucoma results in vision loss. It is a leading cause of blindness among older people. When glaucoma comes on suddenly, nausea, vomiting, and eye pain occurs, which should be treated immediately. More commonly, however, glaucoma comes on gradually, affecting peripheral vision first. Glaucoma is often called the "sneak thief of sight" because the vision loss is so subtle that significant damage may occur before it is diagnosed. Warning signs are headache, nausea, blurred vision, and the appearance of halos or rainbows around lights. Those who are at increased risk for glaucoma are African Americans, people who have a family history of glaucoma, or people who are diabetic, hypertensive, or anemic.

There is no cure for glaucoma, but various types of drugs either eliminate the build-up of excess fluid or encourage drainage to reduce pressure in the eye and subsequent nerve damage. These medications are recommended to be continued for life, although many elders have difficulty complying. One study reported that, in a group of almost 2,500 patients over sixty-five, one-fourth never even filled the prescription, and the average number of days a year without prescribed glaucoma therapy was 112.[44] This evidence underscores the need for patient education before the elder leaves the physician's office.

Other treatments include laser therapy to enlarge the drainage channel and ultrasound to create small holes that reduce pressure build-up. The elderly should be regularly screened for glaucoma.

Macular Degeneration

Among elder Americans, macular degeneration is the leading cause of legal blindness. One in four people over age sixty-five, and one in three over age eighty, is affected. Women are more likely affected than men, and individuals with brown eyes are less affected than those with blue eyes. Macular degeneration is a deterioration of the outer layers of the retina's center, called the macular area, which is needed to see fine detail. Elders may complain that the shape of objects seems distorted, or they may have difficulty driving or reading. However, this disease does not affect peripheral vision and generally affects only one eye, so compensation is possible. Elders with macular degeneration are recommended to install bright lights and increase light-dark contrast in their homes (e.g., dark furniture and white walls).

Researchers are unsure what causes macular degeneration, but heredity, hypertension, sunlight exposure, low estrogen levels, and diet may play a role in its development. To prevent macular degeneration, researchers recommend wearing sunglasses to protect against UV radiation, stopping smoking, and eating a low-fat diet rich in fruits and vegetables. There is no medication for the disease, but special low-vision aids such as magnifying eyeglasses help elders with macular degeneration. Laser therapy, which seals off leaky blood vessels, is a treatment method that can only be used in the early stages of the disease. However, many cannot undergo the procedure, and only about a third of those who do are permanently cured.

Tinnitus

Tinnitus is described as a high-pitched ringing in the ears when no external physical sound is present. Most people experience tinnitus occasionally, but some experience an incessant ringing or buzzing. For some, tinnitus is only a nuisance, but it can also be so severe that it can cause insomnia, loss of concentration, and psychological distress. Tinnitus is often associated with hearing loss. Tinnitus increases with advancing age and may affect more than one in three elders.

The most common cause of tinnitus is exposure to excessively loud noise, however, there are multiple other causes including medical conditions (hypertension, ear infection, nutritional deficiency), and obstruction of the ear canal with wax, tumors, or medications (e.g., aspirin). Tinnitus can worsen with loud noises, caffeine, nicotine, excessive alcohol, and stress.

Treatment involves improving the underlying medical condition, if possible. Other treatments include medications, stress-reduction techniques, or masking units, which create neutral noise to block out the tinnitus. Antidepressants, anticonvulsants, antianxiety agents, and/or antihistamines can be helpful. Masking units, which create neutral noise to block out the tinnitus, may be tried. Techniques to control stress, such as biofeedback and relaxation exercises, may also help. Support groups are available in many areas to help sufferers cope with their symptoms.

Neurological Disorders

Elders commonly complain of confusion, dizziness, shakiness, or disorientation. Some of these neurological symptoms are secondary to other disorders.

For instance, AIDS or depression can cause dementia, or strokes can cause confusion, memory loss, hallucinations, or seizures. Elders may also exhibit neurological symptoms when they have an acute infection such as pneumonia or a urinary tract infection. Further, many medications that elders are prescribed have the side effects of confusion, dizziness, or disorientation. Neurologic disorders such as Parkinson's disease and Alzheimer's disease are also more common among elders. This section will discuss Parkinson's disease, tardive dyskinesia, essential tremor, and Ménière's disease. Those neurological diseases that predominantly affect mental function, including Alzheimer's disease, were discussed in chapter 7.

Parkinson's Disease

Parkinson's disease is a slow, progressive, disorder that affects the part of the brain that controls movement. Approximately 3 percent of the population over age sixty-five has this disorder. Symptoms may include involuntary shaking of the extremities (tremors) that occur at rest, slowness in movement, body rigidity, masklike facial expression, and speech and gait disturbances. Most people with the disease have difficulty starting and stopping movements, have tremors at rest, but not with movement, and, in the later stages, exhibit a pill-rolling movement of the fingers and an uncontrollable shaking of the head. Individuals with advanced Parkinson's disease stand in a bent posture, walk with a shuffling gait, have very soft voices, and write in a small script. Muscle weakness in the arms, face, and tongue are preliminary symptoms of the disorder, followed by uncontrollable movements of the face, arms, and hands. Parkinson's disease may be associated with depression. As the disease progresses to affect the ability to walk, there is an increased rate of death.[45]

Parkinson's disease is caused by a shortage in the brain of a neurotransmitter chemical called dopamine. The disease is treated with levodopa (L-dopa), which increases the level of dopamine in the brain. This drug produces dramatic effects at first, but its effects become less predictable with prolonged use. Other medications are often prescribed that affect the balance of neurotransmitters in the body and enhance the action of levodopa. Selegiline (deprenyl) has been shown to delay the onset of disability in early Parkinson's disease. Surgery on the brain and other newer treatments are occasionally used. The latest technique for advanced Parkinson's disease is electrical stimulation of the brain by an implanted device that is connected to a battery-operated generator placed under the collarbone. It is believed that the stimulator disrupts excessive electric activity in the brain.[46]

Theories abound over what causes the dopamine shortage in the brain. Men are more likely to be afflicted than women, although the age of onset is similar. In addition, African Americans are seldom affected. In families where parkinsonism is common, sufferers experience its symptoms earlier in life. However, there is no correlation in incidence among identical twins. It is generally agreed that environmental factors such as pesticides, illicit drugs, carbon monoxide, and metal poisoning, play a role. One research project looked at the demographic features of a group of patients with Parkinson's disease and reported that exposure to pesticides was the strongest predictor of the disease.[47] Antipsychotic medications, which decrease dopamine in the brain, can induce a Parkinson-like syndrome, called tardive dyskinesia.

Tardive Dyskinesia

Tardive dyskinesia is a common movement disorder primarily caused by long-standing treatment with antipsychotic drugs. The disorder resembles Parkinson's disease in that the patient exhibits abnormal, involuntary facial and arm movements. Most commonly, the facial muscles contort into tics and grimaces, eye blinking, lateral chewing movements, and abnormal tongue and lip motions. Leg crossing, foot tapping, and rocking back and forth while standing are also evident in many cases. It is believed that these features are caused by chronic depletion of neurotransmitters. One study reported that one of three elders who took antipsychotic medication had tardive dyskinesia within less than a year.[48] It is estimated that up to one-half of those taking the drug on a long-term basis has tardive dyskinesia. Older people and women are at higher risk of developing dyskinesia. The condition may appear when the patient begins antipsychotic drug therapy or not until the drug treatment has been in place for years. It may even appear for the first time when the antipsychotic drugs are withdrawn, or persist for years after treatment is discontinued.

There is no satisfactory treatment for tardive dyskinesia. Ironically, some of the drugs that caused the disorder in the first place may be helpful in reducing some symptoms in low dosages. The best way to prevent tardive dyskinesia is to avoid long-term, high dosages of antispychotic drugs. The person with the disorder is often mentally ill and may be depressed or suicidal, so counseling should be an important part of therapy.

Essential Tremor

When hands tremble with movement, but not at rest, the culprit is generally not Parkinson's disease, but essential tremor. Essential tremor is a benign condition that becomes more common in advanced age. In general, the hands tremble about six to ten times a minute. It may start in the dominant hand (the one used for writing) then spread to the other hand, the head, or the voice. Tremor of the head (in a yes-yes or no-no motion) is also common. At times, the symptoms are mild and not bothersome; however, they can become so severe as to interfere with activities of daily living. This tremor runs in families and decreases following alcohol ingestion. Beta blockers (e.g., propranolol) are used to control the symptoms, as is the anticonvulsant primidone. In rare cases, surgery is needed.

Ménière's Disease

When vertigo, tinnitus, and hearing loss occur together, the diagnosis may be Ménière's disease. Ménière's disease is characterized by a build-up of fluid in the inner ear labyrinths, although why this occurs is not known. In general, this condition occurs in middle age and continues into old age, causing irreversible and progressive hearing loss. Violent attacks of dizziness are less common in elders, but a vague constant sense of disequilibrium is common. Balance tests, hearing tests, and brain scans help in the diagnosis. Treatment

involves diuretics, motion-sickness drugs, anti-anxiety drugs, niacin (B vitamin), and steroids. Surgery or other invasive treatments may be necessary. Other treatments that show promise are dietary changes; particularly salt reduction; eating small meals; avoiding caffeine, nicotine, and alcohol; and treating allergies, if present.

Digestive Disorders

Digestive disorders are a common complaint in the middle and later years. Although many symptoms are caused by dietary practices, sometimes they are associated with pathologic conditions, such as cancer. Thus, all digestive complaints should be thoroughly investigated. Gastrointestinal conditions are more common now than in the early part of this century. Many digestive disorders are associated with diet. Although diet is not the only variable affecting gastrointestinal complaints, a diet high in fiber and complex carbohydrates and low in animal fat is likely to reduce the number and severity of these problems.

Periodontal Disease

Great improvements have been made in oral health over the past few decades, and more elders are entering their golden years with a mouth full of natural teeth. However, it is estimated that approximately one of six elders has lost all natural teeth. The amount of tooth loss is likely to decrease in the future due to water fluoridation, increased focus on dental education in the early years, and the greater tendency for today's adults to visit the dentist.

The most important contributor to tooth loss among elders is periodontal or gum disease. This is a chronic bacterial infection of the gums (gingivitis) that may eventually destroy tooth roots and even erode the jaw bone. Gum disease in elders is aggravated by medications that dry the mouth. Periodontal disease begins as bacteria collect at the union of the tooth and gum and form plaque, a sticky substance composed of food debris and bacteria. If not removed daily, the plaque hardens into calculus, which must be removed by a dental professional. Symptoms include swollen, red, or bleeding gums,

gums that bleed during brushing or eating, gums that are separating from the teeth, bad breath, and loose teeth. If during routine dental exams, pockets are found that are 4 to 5 mm deep or more, then that individual has periodontal disease.

Periodontal disease is effectively treated with antibiotics, deep cleaning, antibacterial mouthwashes, and surgery. Surgery entails making cuts at the gum line to improve access to affected roots. One study showed that in a sample of people with severe gum disease, a two-week treatment with antibiotics was an effective alternative to tooth extraction and gum surgery.[49] Tooth loss and periodontal disease can be reduced with regular brushing and flossing, dental checkups, and smoking cessation. A soft-bristled toothbrush and fluoride toothpaste should be used twice daily. Elders with coordination decrements may use aids such as floss-on-a-stick, sponge-on-a-stick (toothettes), or electric toothbrushes to assist in dental hygiene.

Many elders do not have access to dentists and have the lowest rates of dental visits of all age groups. Visits are especially low among minorities, the oldest-old, and those in institutions. One barrier to dental services is financial; Medicare does not cover dental care, and elders are responsible for the majority of their own dental expenses. Institutionalized elders are seldom able to care for their own teeth, staff often does not have time for it, and dentists rarely visit nursing homes. An excellent paper on the need for dental services among elders is Dolan and Atchinson.[50]

Heartburn and Gastroesophageal Reflux Disease

Heartburn is a common disorder among adults, especially women. Ten to twenty percent of Americans suffer regular bouts of heartburn. The most common symptom is a burning sensation behind the breastbone that occurs one or two hours after eating or while sleeping. Sharp pain under the breastbone may also occur. Gastric juice, the strong acid in the stomach that breaks down food, leaks back into the esophagus because the muscle between the esophagus and the stomach does not close properly. Although the stomach lining secretes

a protective layer of mucus, the esophagus does not. Because the lining of the esophagus cannot tolerate the acid, it becomes irritated and inflamed, causing pain. Sometimes gastric juices and small amounts of food are brought all the way back to the mouth or respiratory tract. Heartburn symptoms occur in almost everyone at some time or another but are most common among those who are elderly, overweight, or pregnant. Heartburn can be caused by some foods (garlic, onions, and fatty foods). A side effect of some medications may also cause heartburn. Heartburn is also more likely to occur when the waist is constricted by tight clothing. Heartburn may be relieved temporarily by sitting upright, taking antacids, belching, eating smaller meals, and avoiding tight clothing. More permanent solutions are to quit smoking; lose weight; reduce or avoid alcohol, coffee, and fatty foods; and increase physical activity.

Many times heartburn can be diagnosed by symptoms alone. Sometimes X-rays are taken after a person swallows a radiopaque drink, or an endoscope is passed into the esophagus and stomach to take a direct look. Fortunately, heartburn can nearly always be managed, and even cured with medication. A variety of types of medications are used, including nonprescription antacid salts (calcium carbonate, for example) and drugs that reduce stomach acid production. Even chewing gum after meals has been found to reduce symptoms by diluting the stomach acid. If heartburn is not treated, or when these over-the-counter medications do not work, gastroesophageal reflux disease may be present. In the long term, those with continuous bouts of heartburn are at higher risk for cancer of the esophagus. Prescription medications are available (called proton pump inhibitors) that block stomach acid more effectively than over-the-counter blockers. Fortunately gastroesophageal reflux disease can nearly always be managed with proper drug therapy. Surgery should only be considered as a last resort.

Hiatal Hernia

A hiatal hernia occurs when part of the stomach protrudes into the chest cavity through the opening where the esophagus passes through the diaphragm.

Experts believe it is caused by a weakness in the diaphragm. The disorder causes inflammation of the esophagus as stomach acid is regurgitated into the lower part of the esophagus. Hiatal hernia is common in elders in developed countries; some degree of hiatal hernia occurs in many elders and seems to be more common in women.

Most hiatal hernias are asymptomatic. When symptoms do appear, the most common complaint is heartburn. Pain may occur when the esophagus becomes inflamed from stomach acid secretion. Overeating, lying flat, or coughing increases the discomfort. The condition is also aggravated by obesity, straining when defecating, and wearing clothes too tight at the waist. The most common drug treatment for this condition is antacids. Physicians usually recommend weight loss for the obese. Elevating the head and shoulders when sleeping and eating small, frequent meals will reduce the symptoms. If the condition is severe, surgery may be considered. Such an operation returns the stomach to its proper place, repairs the diaphragm, and constructs a valve around the esophagus to prevent back-flow of stomach acid. However, this surgery does not have a high record of success and should only be tried when other methods have failed.

Diverticulosis

Diverticular disease, rare in the early part of the century, is now the most common disorder of the colon in the United States. A diverticulum is formed when the mucous membrane lining the colon is pushed out through the muscular layer of the bowel wall, forming a pouch. These small distended sacs increase in size and number after a person turns fifty and are present in many of those over seventy (figure 8.1). Experts believe that a low-fiber diet contributes to the development of the disease. Constipation, obesity, and emotional tension also play a role.

The disorder is often asymptomatic. When symptoms are present, pain in the left abdominal region is the most common, and rectal bleeding sometimes occurs. The problem is generally not severe unless the pouches become inflamed (diver-

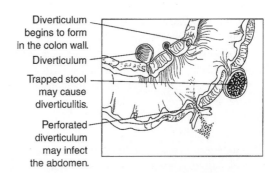

Figure 8.1   How Diverticula Develop.
Illustration reproduced by permission from *Drug Therapy* 1987; 6:57.

ticulitis). If the sacs rupture into the abdominal cavity, hospitalization and antibiotic treatment are required to reduce the chance of peritonitis, an inflammation of the abdominal lining. For those who have chronic attacks, or whose condition worsens despite treatment, part of the colon is removed. In most cases, a high-fiber diet and increased fluid intake will both prevent and treat this condition. Certain foods, such as small seeds, should be avoided.

Colorectal Cancer

Colorectal cancer is a significant cause of death, and its incidence and death rate rise sharply after age fifty. The incidence of colon cancer is two and one-half times more common than rectal cancer. Colon cancer is not always deadly. When cancer is localized to the bowel, five-year survival rates are 80 to 90 percent. However, when cancer has spread (for example to the liver or lymph nodes), the five-year survival rate drops to 30 to 40 percent.

The most common early symptom of colorectal cancer is rectal bleeding. However, constipation or diarrhea, the passage of stools of increasingly narrow diameter (pencil-thin), or systemic symptoms such as weight loss may also occur.

Many factors have been correlated with the development of colon cancer. The presence of outgrowths in the colon (polyps), many years of colon inflammation, or a family history of colon polyps or colon cancer put individuals at increased colon cancer risk.[51,52] Additionally, there is something about the American lifestyle that predisposes its residents to develop more colon cancer than people from Japan, China, or less-developed countries. A diet high in animal fat and low in fruits, vegetables, and fiber has been implicated, as has alcohol and cigarette use. Drinking water with a high level of chlorine has also been associated with colon cancer.[53]

Some factors may reduce colon cancer risk. Studies suggest that the B vitamin folate,[54] calcium,[55] and aspirin play a protective role against colon cancer.[56] Colorectal cancer may be detected through a rectal examination, testing of stool for occult (invisible) blood or through direct visualization of the colon through a sigmoidoscope or colonoscope. For these examinations, a tube is passed a varying distance into the rectum, and a physician visually examines the inside of the colon for signs of cancer. Any polyps, where cancers are thought to originate, are removed. It is estimated that one-third of all people over age fifty have one or more polyps. Experts recommend annual testing of stool for occult blood and rectal exams for all over the age of fifty, as well as sigmoidoscopic or colonoscopic exams every few years. (See chapter 11).

Colon cancer, unless it is has spread, is almost always treated with surgery. The cancerous bowel is removed and the intestine is either reconnected, or a colostomy is performed. A colostomy is a surgical procedure in which the end of the intestine is routed through the abdominal wall, creating an artificial opening in the abdomen called a stoma. The feces are then collected in a disposable plastic bag and regularly emptied. Because cancer recurs in over 50 percent of the cases, radiation and chemotherapy are commonly used after surgery.

Hemorrhoids

Hemorrhoids are the most common problem of the anal area, and Americans spend over $110 million annually on over-the-counter medications to relieve their symptoms of anal burning, pain, and itching. Hemorrhoids are enlarged and swollen hemorrhoidal blood vessels located where the network of anal and rectal blood vessels meets. Hemorrhoids

may be internal or external. Sometimes the internal hemorrhoids become so enlarged that they protrude through the anal opening. Hemorrhoids may occasionally bleed, causing streaks of bright red blood on the stool after straining.

Hemorrhoids have many possible causes. Heredity seems to play a role, and there is a relationship with occupation, posture, and diet. Those who must sit or stand for long periods are at increased risk. Physical straining during a bowel movement may also have an effect. Women who have had many children are at higher risk. A high-fiber diet may decrease hemorrhoidal irritation by decreasing constipation. Meticulous anal hygiene with gentle cleansing and blotting rather than rubbing is also helpful. Sitz baths, donut pillows, bedrest, or pushing the hemorrhoids back into the anal opening may reduce discomfort. Over-the-counter hemorrhoidal medications such as petroleum jelly, zinc oxide, calamine lotion, local anesthetics, and witch hazel are useful.

Physicians most commonly treat internal hemorrhoids by either tying them off at their base with elastic bands so they eventually fall off, or, less often by filling them with a chemical that shrinks them (sclerotherapy). Photocoagulation, the use of light to burn them off, is a relatively new therapy that is rapid, painless, and effective. Other treatments not commonly used are the laser and electrocoagulation (cauterizing tissue with electric current). As a last resort, surgical removal, or hemorrhoidectomy, may be necessary.

Constipation

Constipation is the most common digestive complaint in our country and is most common in individuals over sixty-five.[57] Although constipation seldom results in death, for some, it can be debilitating. Older people commonly report that it interferes with their quality of life and feeling of well-being. One study of home-bound elders found that 45 percent complained of constipation, and half of these described it as a major health problem.[58]

There is some disagreement about the definition of constipation. Some define it by low fre-

Constipation: Daily Hassle Causing Misery

This patient said constipation had always been a problem for him but since being treated for prostate cancer, it had gotten steadily worse. He told his physician this, but the physician simply nodded his head. The patient was irritated by this, and said he "couldn't interpret head nods." When one particular episode of constipation lasted five days, he called the physician, whose response was that constipation was a common side effect of a prescribed medication and recommended a bulk agent, a stool softener, and a laxative, which helped relieve the problem. The patient, however, was angry that his physician had not warned him that constipation might develop and apparently did not think through this issue beforehand. The physician did nothing to prevent the problem; rather, he attended to the problem only after repeated complaints.

The difference between lay and medical interpretations of constipation is analogous to the difference between daily hassles and traumatic life events. Constipation is like a nagging hassle that is capable of making the daily life of frail elders absolutely miserable. Physicians usually leave the management of hassles to others and focus on the equivalent of traumatic life events—emphasizing the medical treatment of disorders that are most likely to cause death and disability (e.g., heart disease, cancer, stroke, or infectious diseases). Physicians often respond to only one part of the patient's distress, which frequently results in a dissatisfied patient in continued distress.[58]

quency of bowel movements, while others believe that constipation implies hard stools with increased difficulties in passing. Medically, it is defined as fewer than three bowel movements per week.[59] Differences in perception of constipation makes it difficult to accurately assess the prevalence of constipation because the medical definition differs so radically from the layperson's view. Only 4 percent of men and 6 percent of women age seventy to seventy-nine and 6 percent of men and 11 percent of women over age eighty meet the medical definition of constipation. However, more than one-fifth of men and women seventy to seventy-nine and almost one-third of those over age eighty report use of laxatives at least once a month.[60] One study found that the self-reported prevalence of constipation increases with age (tripling from age forty-five to sixty-four to age sixty-five and older), and women are affected three times as much as men.[61] It is clear that many more elders consider themselves constipated than meet the medical definition.

The five most common complaints linked to constipation are straining to pass feces, hard

stools, inability to defecate when desired, infrequent bowel movements, and abdominal discomfort associated with defecation. Those who are constipated often complain of nausea, malaise, abdominal pain, and diminished appetite. There is tremendous variability in frequency of stool passage, with the range of normality being between three times daily to once every three days. It is not necessary to have a daily bowel movement for ideal health. However, elders often place undue concern over the regularity of their bowel habits and prefer to have daily movements, even if they must rely on laxatives. One-third to one-half the elder population uses laxatives, most saying they use them to reduce straining. The majority of nursing home residents use laxatives.

Although complaints of constipation increase with age, constipation is not part of the aging process. Constipation in elders may have multiple causes, ranging from inactivity, low-fiber diet, medication effects, or chronic illness. A low level of mobility or immobility is one of the most significant causes of constipation because it reduces intestinal motility. Some drugs (e.g., antidepressants, painkillers) and dietary supplements (e.g., calcium and iron) have a constipating effect. Long-term laxative use, particularly stimulant laxatives, may damage the nerve cells in the colon wall, promoting further constipation and dependence on laxative therapy. Many chronic illnesses are associated with increased risk of constipation, including cancer, depression, spinal cord lesions, Parkinson's disease, and hypothyroidism.

Constipation may be a transient event due to travel, change in activity level or diet, medication use, or emotional stress. On the other hand, constipation may be a sign of a serious physical problem, such as bowel blockage, fecal impaction, urinary incontinence, or colon cancer. When one suffers from constipation alternating with diarrhea or the passage of stools of increasingly narrower diameter, colon cancer or inflammatory bowel disease may be the cause, and a physician should be contacted.

Evaluation of the cause of constipation should include a detailed medical history, a physical examination, and selected laboratory tests. Management of constipation needs to be individualized and depends on other physical illnesses present and the cognitive status of the individual. It may include as simple a regimen as increased physical activity or adding fiber to the diet.[62] Medication and food supplement usage needs to be part of the medical history. Modifying diet and participating in daily physical activity are the two simplest and most effective ways to treat constipation. Constipated elders should be encouraged to increase their intake of fluids, especially fruit juices, and foods containing fiber such as bran or prunes. Ten to twenty grams of fiber daily are recommended, as well as at least 6 cups of water daily. If elders are not able to consume enough fluids, then fiber supplementation can aggravate constipation, and alternatives need to be explored.

Sometimes changes in daily routine may also be effective. Importantly, elders need to respond to the natural urge to have a bowel movement rather than ignoring it. Elders should set aside time each day to have a bowel movement, preferably after a meal to take advantage of the physiological reflex to empty the bowels after a meal. The use of a footrest while on the toilet can be helpful. If laxatives are necessary, natural laxatives (e.g., senna tea or mixtures of dried fruits such as prunes, raisins, figs, dates, prune juice, or currants) in paste or liquid form, may be useful. Chronic laxative use can cause the bowel to become less functional and is not recommended. For occasional use, bulk laxatives are helpful. See chapter 10 for an overview on laxative types.

Fecal Incontinence

Few symptoms are more distressing to elders and their families than fecal incontinence, the involuntary loss of stool. In many cases, incontinence leads to institutionalization. It has been estimated that five of every 1,000 men and thirteen of every 1,000 women over age sixty-five suffer from fecal incontinence. The frequency of this condition in elders in the community is unknown; however, its prevalence among hospitalized elderly patients and nursing home residents is high. Elders may suffer from minor incontinence (partial soiling), incontinence of flatus or liquid stool, or major incontinence when the elder is unable to control the passage of normally formed stool.

For some, fecal incontinence is secondary to another disease process (e.g., Alzheimer's dementia) and is generally irreversible. However, many causes of fecal incontinence are treatable, including fecal impaction/constipation, rectal prolapse, stroke, inflammatory bowel syndrome, trauma, diabetes mellitus, or tumors. A thorough work-up is warranted to determine whether the problem is reversible, although elders may be too embarrassed to broach the subject with their physician.

Urgency of stool commonly occurs when the stool is liquid; an elder has the sense of having to defecate, but cannot make it to the bathroom facilities. Urgency is best treated with agents to firm up stools, such as bulk laxatives or over-the-counter antidiarrheals. The best treatments for stool incontinence are directed toward its specific causes. However, using the toilet at a regularly scheduled time each day and/or regular use of rectal suppositories to initiate bowel movements can be helpful. Kegel exercises to strengthen the pelvic floor have been recommended. Biofeedback has had some success in improving fecal incontinence. Those with fecal incontinence are recommended to carry a tote bag containing supplies and a change of clothes. Avoiding odor- or gas-producing foods (broccoli, cabbage, fish, beans, eggs, and carbonated beverages) can help. In rare cases, surgery may be needed.

Skeletal Disorders

Arthritis and osteoporosis are the most common skeletal disorders affecting elders. Arthritis is the number one crippler of all ages in the United States. It is estimated that over 40 million Americans are affected, and this number is expected to rise to 60 million by 2020. Arthritis affects both men and women and all ethnic/racial groups, although Asians are less affected. However, the extent of these disorders varies: some afflicted elders are severely disabled, while others have little to no limitations of their daily routine. Skeletal disorders are by far elders' most frequent complaint because the diseases are painful and restrict movement, making it especially difficult to conduct activities that require strength or stamina. These disorders usually appear

in midlife and progress slowly with age. Because most skeletal disorders cause similar symptoms (aches, pains, limited movement, and stiffness), they are often grouped together, dubbed "rheumatism," and left untreated. However, all symptoms should be investigated because skeletal pain or disability in older people may be the only sign of a serious condition, such as bone cancer or a fracture. Further, treatment varies, dependent on the diagnosis.

For most arthritic conditions and osteoporosis, treatment consists of preventing further degeneration, controlling pain, and encouraging as much independence as possible. Additionally, prevention of accidents is an important goal of therapy.

Osteoarthritis

Osteoarthritis is the most common type of arthritis in the world, the most reported chronic illness in the United States, and a major cause of disability. Osteoarthritis is the process of degeneration of the joints caused by the bone wearing down the cartilage (figure 8.2). The resultant inflammation, swelling, and pain in the joints are common symptoms. Increasing knowledge about the disease is leading scientists to suppose that osteoarthritis is not one single disease, but rather a group of similar conditions, affecting many joints in the body though a process of joint destruction and repair.[63] Risk factors

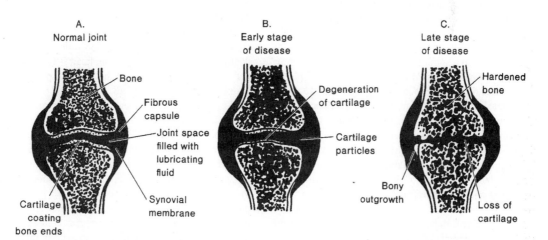

Figure 8.2   Osteoarthritis.
Reprinted with permission from the Arthritis Foundation's brochure, *Osteoarthritis*.

Chronic Illness: Joan Gehrman's Story

Excerpted from an interview by her son, Roger Strong, a nurse practitioner.

Joan Gehrman is a diminuitive little woman, 4'9" tall and about 80 pounds. Her small size belies her strong will, independence, and spunkiness. She lives in a small senior apartment that consists of a tiny bedroom, living room, bathroom, and kitchen. Small enough so she can get around, but filled with enough furniture, photos, and memorabilia to make it "home." Her caretaker, whom she has known for eight months, sits in the living room, reading the paper while Joan rests in her bed. The caregiver is paid minimum wage by the state to provide care that allows Joan to stay at home. Joan is lucky; the caregiver is gentle, knowledgeable, and a good cook (after Joan taught her to make all her specialties).

Joan is an educated woman. She graduated from Smith College and has held various jobs including substitute teaching and volunteer work. She went back to school in her sixties at a local community college, making the Dean's list for four semesters in general education. She is divorced and has lived alone for more than thirty years.

Joan tells me of her life with chronic illnesses. These past twenty to thirty years she characterizes as the "tarnished years" rather than the "golden years." She first developed arthritis in her forties, and her arthritis still pains her greatly. "It's one pain all over, but I have been able to control it. Just thinking about it [the pain] can kill you sometimes." She has undergone two total hip replacement operations and two total knee replacements in the past, and recently she has suffered a spiral fracture of her left femur (thigh bone), which required an operation and the placement of metal plates and wires to allow her to walk. After the fracture, she spent a week in rehab, but she thought it was too much like a nursing home and didn't like the way they were managing her constipation, so she went home. She gradually increased in strength so that she was able to ambulate a block or two, but then began to weaken again, and the fracture is not healing properly.

In describing her multiple medical problems, she states: "I feel quite surprised and angry. I can't do things like I used to do and see my ability decreasing; I can't live this way." However, as often as she describes the negatives of living with chronic illness, she refuses to give up hope. "I am not going to let my body run me because my mind refuses to accept it conditionally. If my mind can stay in control, then I won't give up. I did not give up. I had the power to fight it. The power within me allowed me to continue. Surgeons have been able to patch me, to keep me going."

Joan also has a long history of sluggish bowels or constipation and takes laxatives on a daily basis to stay "regular." In addition to her arthritis and constipation. Joan has significant heart disease, which initially started out as coronary artery disease and has progressed to congestive heart failure.

In her sixties, she underwent three coronary artery bypass operations (CABG) in a single year. "The first two didn't work, so I went for a third," she says, and bears the scar down her chest and the long, serepentine scars down her legs to prove it. After the surgery, she made big changes in her diet—low fat, low cholesterol, and low salt—and has stayed slim for the past twenty years. She takes quite a few medications for her heart failure, including nitrates and ACE inhibitors, and has recently begun to require oxygen at home.

Her chest pain has been getting worse, although she does not call it pain, merely pressure. When she gets chest pressure, she takes nitroglycerine under her tongue and some ativan (a benzodiazepine) and falls asleep, and when she awakens the chest pain is gone. She has recently had episodes where she has chest pain and then blacks out and falls down. Her doctors tell her this is because her heart is failing and not enough blood is going to the brain, or perhaps it is due to little strokes. In any case, she is too weak for further surgery and doesn't want any more tests, so she lives with it. She looks on the bright side, "It could be worse." The falls are worrisome, because she takes a blood thinner (Coumadin), and there is always a chance she will suffer internal bleeding. She takes the Coumadin because she had blood clots in her legs in the past that went up into her lung and damaged it. When it has been suggested that she stay in bed or in a chair unless her caregiver is there, she may agree, but invariably she gets up to do things for herself. She now needs help bathing and cooking and sometimes with getting dressed.

Chronic Illness: Joan Gehrman's Story (*continued*)

She has three children, but only keeps in close contact with one, a nurse practitioner who works full-time. She pages him during the day to ask him questions about her condition or medications, and he visits her daily to make sure she is OK. He does the shopping, takes her to the doctor, manages her caregiver, and helps with her finances. She knows as she becomes weaker that it may be necessary for him to stay at her house overnight, but for now she desires her privacy. He has promised never to put her in a nursing home.

As she has weakened, she is beginning to talk more about the end of her life. "I have been active all my life, and it is time for a rest now. I am listening to my mind, it will tell me when it is time to call this 'all over.' In my mind, when I became eighty, I knew I would not have much time left, and I will be ready to go. I am eighty years old, I don't expect it to keep beating forever. I have had a long, interesting life. The party has to come to an end sometime."

include advancing age, repetitive motion, family history, obesity, or previous joint injury or surgery. Elders with osteoarthritis have a decreased range of motion, cracking joints, and pain in the finger joints, knees, and hips. In general, pain is mild to moderate and gradual in onset, worse when the joint is moved, and improved with rest. Diagnosis can be made through examination or X-ray.

Treatment of osteoarthritis focuses on reducing symptoms because there is no cure for this disease. In general, treatment involves analgesics (low doses of aspirin, acetaminophen, or other nonsteroidal anti-inflammatory agents), heat/cold, walking aids, and weight loss. Steroid medications injected into the joint can provide weeks or months of relief. Capscaisin, an extract of hot pepper, can be applied to the affected joint and affords some relief. A new agent, Hyalgan, derived from the combs of roosters, increases joint lubrication when injected into the joint weekly for three to five weeks, lasting several months. Studies report improvement in osteoarthritis symptoms among those who consumed vitamin C (at least 150 mg) and vitamin D.[64] Hormone replacement therapy may be helpful. Glucosamine, a dietary supplement available over the counter, and orthoses (splints or braces) that are properly fitted to help align joints may reduce pain and disability associated with arthritis. Aerobic exercise, muscle strengthening, and range-of-motion exercises may also help. When pain or disability is severe, surgeons

often operate to correct deformities or replace joints. The most common operations are total hip replacements or total knee replacements.

Rheumatoid Arthritis

Although not nearly as widespread as osteoarthritis, rheumatoid arthritis is more likely to cause pain, crippling, and disfigurement and not only affects the joints, but also other body systems. The disease may occur between ages twenty and fifty so that many people enter old age with a history of the disease. Rheumatoid arthritis is two to three times more common in women than men.

Rheumatoid arthritis is caused by persistent inflammation in the tissue lining the joints. The joints in the small bones of the hand and foot are most often affected; however, it can also spread to the larger joints. Without treatment, the joint and ligaments are destroyed, producing permanent stiffness, joint dislocation, and deformity. What causes the inflammation is not completely understood, but many believe it is due to the "rheumatoid factor," an antibody that binds to existing antibodies in the blood. When the antibody binds other substances, these complexes settle into the joint where the body mounts an immune response. Rheumatoid arthritis may also affect the eye, the lung, the heart, or the nerves, causing peripheral sensory deficits.

Those with rheumatoid arthritis experience joint swelling, inflammation, and morning stiffness that last from one to five hours. In some cases, weight loss, weakness, and fatigue occur. The disease is characterized by flare-ups and remissions. Just as the pain leaves one joint, it may reappear in another. In some cases, the disease is inactive, and the individual has no symptoms. Older adults may already have deforming nodules on the joints and permanent joint damage because of lack of treatment in earlier years. Today, early treatment can prevent severe crippling in most cases.

Rheumatoid arthritis may be affected by estrogen. Women who take oral contraceptives or have been pregnant have a significantly reduced rate of rheumatoid arthritis.[65] Similarly, those who take postmenopausal estrogens experience lower rates of rheumatoid arthritis than those who do not.[66]

Rheumatoid arthritis can be treated in a variety of ways. High-dose aspirin therapy over months or years reduces pain and joint inflammation, but stomach ulcers or tinnitus are common side effects. Other nonsteroidal anti-inflammatory drugs (e.g., ibuprofen) are also used. If these do not provide significant relief, more potent drugs, such as antimalarial drugs, anticancer drugs, or steroids are helpful.

In the past, treatment consisted of high-dose aspirin therapy until the later stages of rheumatoid arthritis, but most physicians are prescribing a more aggressive treatment in the earlier stages to reduce the crippling and pain. Drugs used are methotrexate, an anticancer drug, and low-dose steroids.

In addition to medication, experts recommend a balance of rest during flare-ups and exercise several times a day during remission to achieve the fullest possible range of motion in each joint. Applying moist heat to afflicted joints temporarily reduces pain, swelling, and stiffness, and makes exercise easier.

When immobility and constant pain occur, various types of surgery to repair joints and tendons and to correct deformities may be performed. Psychological support for the affected individual is important because the pain, disability, and consequent dependence cause stress that further aggravates the disease. An important component of care for the patient with rheumatoid arthritis is to receive help from a physical or occupational therapist for assessment, splints, devices to assist in tasks of daily living, and training in how to protect the joints from further destruction.

Gout

Gout is an arthritic disorder caused by a malfunction in either the production or elimination of uric acid. Uric acid is a waste product of the breakdown of proteins. It accumulates in the bloodstream if too much is produced or if elimination is inefficient. Excessive levels of uric acid in the bloodstream may form uric acid crystals, which deposit in the fluid of particular joints. The problem often appears in only one joint, commonly the big toe, periodically causing a gouty attack that usually lasts from a few days to two weeks. Symptoms of a gouty attack are excruciating joint pain and inflammation. Attacks generally recur with increasing intensity and frequency but may not reappear for months or years. Between attacks, the individual has no symptoms. For those who have suffered severe gouty attacks for years, disfiguring tophi deposits composed of chalky uric acid crystals form around the ears and joints. These deposits are large and evident through the skin.

Primary gout is caused by a hereditary metabolic disorder and is usually detected between age fifty and sixty. The great majority of primary gout cases occur in men, although some women may get gout after menopause. Secondary gout, which is much more common, can be caused by multiple factors and occurs in both men and women. It commonly occurs as a side effect of thiazide diuretic use because the drug partially blocks urate excretion by the kidneys. Secondary gout may also occur with obesity, alcohol intake, kidney disease, joint injury, stress, or dehydration.

Gout is diagnosed by extracting fluid from an affected joint and finding uric acid crystals. Some drugs help reduce the overproduction of uric acid, while others help victims excrete more uric acid in the urine. These medications may have to be continued for life. For those who do not have attacks often, instead of taking medications to prevent an attack, they may choose to deal with the symptoms when an attack occurs. Nonsteroidal anti-inflammatory drugs (e.g., ibuprofen), but not aspirin, can be highly effective for an attack, as are corticosteroids either taken orally or injected into the joint. Those rare individuals with primary gout should reduce intake of shellfish and organ meats during an acute attack because these foods are high in purines, a chemical that aggravates the condition.

Osteoporosis

Osteoporosis is an age-related disorder characterized by a reduction in bone mass and an increased susceptibility to fractures. Gradual bone loss occurs in everyone with advancing age, however, osteoporosis is more severe than an age-related loss. Bones in the back, hips, and forearm are most likely to be affected. Osteoporosis is the major cause of fractures in the later years. It can also cause collapsed vertebrae leading to spinal deformities such as dowager's hump, loss of height, and chronic back pain. Oftentimes osteoporosis is not discovered until

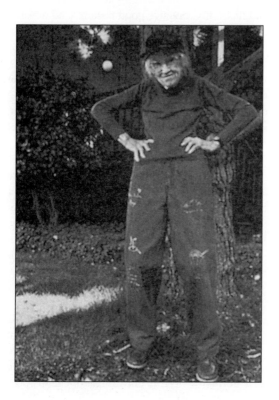

the patient has suffered a fracture and the disease is very advanced. Those with advanced osteoporosis are so fragile that even a minor fall might result in a severe fracture and subsequent disability and dependence.

Although osteoporosis frequently affects the spine, the most serious consequence is hip fracture, which has a much greater impact on a person's life. Experts believe that osteoporosis plays a role in hip fracture in one-third of all women and one-sixth of all men. Those with osteoporotic hip fractures take longer to heal, and the accompanying immobilization causes further bone loss. Twelve to 20 percent of elders who fracture a hip die within the year. Of those who survive, only about one-third are able to regain their previous independence, and half of those who survive the fracture must have long-term nursing home care.[67] Other consequences of osteoporosis include poor posture and associated back pain, and diminished lung function due to spinal deformities.

Those at increased risk for osteoporosis are older people, whites, smokers, people who consume excessive alcohol, and people who lead a sedentary lifestyle. Women are four times more likely to have osteoporosis than men. Those who are underweight or have a slight build are at increased risk, while those with heavier bones boast reduced risk. Individuals with a family history of fractures or osteoporosis are at increased risk. High caffeine or carbonated soda intake increases the risk of osteoporosis, while consumption of milk products reduces risk. Women with thyroid disease who are treated with thyroxine are also at increased risk.[68]

Research shows that estrogens play a role in osteoporosis, although the exact mechanism is not known. It is clear that osteoporosis worsens after menopause, and that estrogen-replacement therapy reduces bone loss and incidence of fractures. Women who had menopause before age forty-five, who had their ovaries removed without estrogen replacement, and who have diets low in calcium are at high risk of osteoporosis and consequent fractures.

Although bone loss is progressive throughout life, it often has no symptoms. Standard X-rays are poor at quantifying bone loss, but newer radiological techniques that measure bone density are able to diagnose osteoporosis more accurately. The tests are used for individuals at high risk for osteoporosis and those who have suffered a fracture. Bone density measurements are also undertaken to evaluate whether therapy is effective at reducing or reversing osteoporosis. The most common means used is the dual X-ray absorptiometry (DXA, known as a "DEXA scan"), although other methods are used. DEXA scans are covered by Medicare for women at risk. A new device uses ultrasound to measure bone density. It can be used during a routine examination, and it is faster and less expensive than a DEXA scan.

The first line of treatment of osteoporosis involves increasing dietary calcium and physical activity. Most physicians also presribe hormonal replacement therapy. A person with osteoporosis should begin a gradual physical activity program of weight-bearing exercises to increase muscle and bone strength. Calcium and vitamin D are important in both the prevention and treatment of osteoporosis because high calcium intake, through diet or supplementation, is associated with reduced rates of bone loss and fractures. In general, doses of about 1,000 to 1,500 mg of calcium and 600 IU of vitamin D are recommended.

Other drugs used to reduce fracture risk include bisphosphonates and calcitonin, a calcium-retaining hormone taken by injection or nasal spray. Fluoride may also be prescribed to stimulate bone reformation. A newer treatment, raloxifene, impacts with the estrogen receptor in the bones to reduce osteoporosis while also lowering cholesterol levels.[69]

Experts debate who should be screened and who should be prescribed drugs for osteoporosis because many women with osteoporosis never suffer any adverse effects, and bone density is not the only predictor of fracture risk. Even though these treatments are often prescribed for years, there are few studies that look at their long-term effectiveness. Finally, all drug treatments have side effects. The safest way to prevent osteoporisis is to increase calcium intake with diet or supplements and regularly engage in weight-bearing exercise.

Back Pain

Almost every individual has experienced back pain. Although back pain can be a symptom of another illness, the vast majority of back pain among middle-age and older adults is related to a strain on the muscles of the spine and on the supporting ligaments. Back pain caused by strain often occurs suddenly while lifting or bending. The person will complain of pain and be unable to move the back easily. In contrast, the pain from a herniated disk shoots down one leg past the knee. This pain is accompanied by tingling, weakness, and loss of reflexes in that leg. A collapsed vertebra (often caused by osteoporosis) may cause sudden onset of severe pain that radiates around the trunk. And, back pain of gradual onset may be a symptom of bone cancer, small fractures in the bone related to osteoporosis, or rheumatoid arthritis.

Doctors can generally identify the cause of the pain by examination, and an X-ray is not always needed. The best way to prevent back pain is to participate in exercises to enhance strength and flexibility, practice good posture, and develop correct technique in lifting and bending. Once a back has been injured, it is more susceptible to future back problems.

Among elders, spinal stenosis is a common cause of back pain. Spinal stenosis is a narrowing of the central canal of the spine, generally from osteoarthritis, that pinches nerves branching out from the cord. In addition, bone spurs may develop, further impinging on the spinal canal and squeezing nerves. Stenosis may occur anywhere along the spine but most often affects the lower back, causing pain in the legs or shoulders. The symptoms of spinal stenosis may begin gradually. People complain of pain along the spine, which sometimes radiates down the leg (sciatic pain) or the neck and shoulder. As the disease progresses, weakness and numbness of the extremities may appear. Diagnosis of spinal stenosis generally requires a CT (computed tomography) or MRI (magnetic resonance imagery) scan. It is important to realize that many people without pain have abnormal back X-rays, and many people with pain have normal X-rays. In one sample of healthy people, nearly three-fourths had at least one abnormality on the MRI.[70]

Treatment for back problems involves light aerobic exercise, such as swimming or walking, floor exercises to strengthen back muscles and improve posture, and if needed, weight loss. Back supports that restrict some spinal motion and support lax abdominal muscles may provide some relief with short-term use. However, they can reduce muscle strength and tone. Anti-inflammatory medications or steroid injections into the joints can help reduce pain. Heat, ice, ultrasound, acupuncture, stress management, and biofeedback may also be recommended. Physical therapy, chiropractic, and massage are also helpful in many cases. Modified activity and exercises have shown to be more effective in recovery than bedrest. In severe cases, surgery may be indicated, although not everyone has relief after surgery.

Endocrine Disorders

Endocrine disorders generally occur in early or middle adulthood, and none increase in incidence after age sixty-five. Diabetes and thyroid problems are the most significant endocrine problems affecting elders.

Diabetes

Diabetes is a metabolic disorder characterized by a deficiency in either the production or utilization of insulin, which is a hormone produced by the pancreas that allows body cells to take up sugar (glucose) from the bloodstream for energy. When there is a lack of insulin, the body cells cannot use the glucose in the bloodstream, so they continually send messages that sugar is needed. The liver responds to the cell's messages and dumps even more glucose into the blood. Thus, people with diabetes manifest high blood sugar but it is unusable unless insulin can assist it to get into the cells where it is needed. High blood sugar can damage the kidney, peripheral nerves, and the eyes. Diabetics often suffer increased blood cholesterol and hypertension: three out of four diabetics die of diseases related to the heart and blood vessels.

There are two types of diabetes, type I and type II. Type I (also called juvenile-onset) diabetes generally occurs in children or young adults. It is rapid in onset and characterized by the inability of the pancreas to produce insulin. Because of its early onset, Type I diabetics suffer complications from this disease for decades, including increased risk of heart disease, eye and kidney problems, and potentially early death. Additionally, they are susceptible to diabetic emergencies whereby their blood sugar goes out of control, and they suffer thirst, excessive urination, confusion, and even coma. These individuals require insulin daily for the rest of their lives. The etiology of this type of diabetes is unknown. Type I diabetes accounts for only about 5 percent of the total number of diabetes cases in our country.

Of the older people who have diabetes, the majority have type II. Type II diabetes is variously known as adult-onset or noninsulin-dependent diabetes mellitus (NIDDM). The term NIDDM can be confusing because some of these individuals are taking insulin. In adult-onset diabetes, the pancreas still produces insulin, but the body cells become less responsive to it. These diabetics actually have increased levels of insulin in their blood, but also manifest increased blood sugar levels. Unlike juvenile-onset diabetes, this type progresses gradually, is modifiable by diet and exercise, and runs in families. These individuals rarely manifest diabetic emergencies like those with juvenile-onset. However, they are subject to the same complications in other organs such as the heart, nerves, eyes, and kidneys. Treatment focuses on diet and lifestyle changes and strict regulation of blood sugar with oral medications or insulin, if needed.

Sixteen million people in the United States are estimated to have diabetes, but only half of them are aware of it. The prevalence of diabetes increases with age. Overall, about 20 percent of the older population have diabetes. African Americans, Hispanic Americans, and Native Americans have a greatly increased risk of diabetes. Adult-onset diabetes is associated with female sex, obesity, overeating, a propensity to store fat on the abdomen, and family history of the disease.

Symptoms of type II diabetes may be subtle. Usually elders complain of weight loss, fatigue, and frequent urination. Diagnosis of tingling in the legs, vascular disease, and cataracts may trigger a search for diabetes. It is recommended that elders who are obese, who have a family history of diabetes, who have hypertension or elevated cholesterol, and who are African American, Hispanic, or Native American undergo diabetic screening. The most common screening for diabetes involves a blood test to measure the amount of sugar in the blood, called the fasting plasma glucose test. To detect more cases of diabetes early, before complications set in, the American Diabetes Association has recommended that all adults forty-five and over be screened for diabetes, and if results are normal, every three years thereafter. For those who have known risk factors for the disease, such as obesity or family history, they should be screened before forty-five.

Once a person is diagnosed with diabetes, ongoing monitoring of diet, blood glucose, and medication dosages is required. The first line of treatment for type II diabetes is weight loss and a diet high in complex carbohydrates and fiber and low in refined sugar and fat.[71] More specifically, a diabetic may consume less than 10 percent of calories from saturated fat and between 10 to 20 percent of calories from protein. The remaining calories are to be derived from unsaturated fats and complex carbohydrates. This diet decreases the body's insulin requirements and helps lower blood cholesterol. Exercise is another important component of treatment because it increases the body's sensitivity to insulin and also facilitates weight loss. For about 70 percent of adult-onset diabetics, dietary changes, weight loss, and physical activity can control symptoms. However, getting elders to comply with an exercise program and dietary change is not always easy.

In general, if blood sugars are still elevated, treatment includes one or more prescription drugs. Some oral medications increase the release of insulin by the pancreas. These effectively lower blood glucose but may lower it too much (hypoglycemia) or cause weight gain. Some fear that the elevated insulin levels in the blood contribute to cardiovascular disease. Newer agents act to block glucose production in the liver and have less risk of hypoglycemia. Another new agent makes the tissues more sensitive to insulin. If oral agents fail (as they do in one-third of all type II diabetics), insulin injections may be added. The goal of treatment is to keep the blood sugar in a narrow, near-normal range to reduce the complications of diabetes.

In general, individuals with abnormal blood sugar should measure their own blood glucose many times a day to better understand their response to food and exercise and to maintain optimal tight control. Just as it is difficult to get elders to comply with diet and exercise recommendations, so it may be difficult to get them to frequently monitor their blood sugar and diabetic regimen. In addition, tight control can result in weight gain and higher risk of hypoglycemia. Despite these risks, tight control is a lifesaver. When blood sugar is kept in a tight, near-normal range, there is a marked reduction in diabetic complications for both those with type I and type II diabetes.[72] Maintaining control of cholesterol and hypertension associated with diabetes are also important to prevent complications.[73]

Diabetes is associated with complications in almost every body system, but can be minimized if the diabetic maintains tight control of blood sugar. Diabetics have an increased rate of atherosclerosis, strokes, and heart disease. Coronary artery disease is twice as common in diabetic men and five times as likely in diabetic women than in those without the disease. In addition, diabetics often have high blood cholesterol levels and high blood pressure. Because of poor circulation and peripheral nerve damage, elders are highly susceptible to infections, especially in the foot, and too often require amputation. In addition, diabetics suffer neuropathy (nerve damage) in their legs, which can be extremely painful. Diabetics often suffer visual decrements, sometimes losing vision completely, resulting from eye inflammation. Kidney failure (requiring dialysis) and kidney infections are also much more common among diabetics. Women with diabetes are more susceptible to vaginal and urinary infections. Men who have had diabetes for a long period of time may exhibit erectile dysfunction, and women may become anorgasmic. The high rate of insulin production in adult-onset diabetes can promote artherosclerosis and cardiac disease. Diabetics should be monitored carefully for early diagnosis of complications. To decrease damage to other organs, it is imperative that other medical problems are adequately treated.

Thyroid Problems

Elders can suffer from either a deficiency (hypothyroid) or excess (hyperthyroid) of thyroid hormone, although a deficiency is more common. Whites, women, the middle-aged, and those over seventy-five are at a higher risk for thyroid problems. Because of its high prevalence, many groups recommend routine testing of all elders for thyroid disease.[74]

Hypothyroidism can be subtle among elders and appears as slowed thought processes, decreased ability to respond to stress, constipation, weight gain, decreased cold tolerance, depression, or hallucinations. These symptoms are so common that it is difficult to determine whether they are due to medications, disease, or old age.[75] If untreated, hypothyroidism is lethal. Hypothyroidism is also associated with abnormalities in cholesterol levels.[76] Regular administration of thyroid hormone reverses the condition, and the dose can be carefully monitored by blood tests.

Hyperthyroidism is an excess of thyroid hormone and causes the opposite symptoms of hypothyroidism: increased heart rate, increased sensitivity to heat, sweating, diarrhea, weight loss, irritability, and tremors. This condition can also be dangerous in elders because they may have a myocardial infarction (heart attack) due to the excessive strain on the heart. Elders may not show typical symptoms, but may manifest rapid heart rate, fatigue and weight loss.[77] Because hyperthyroidism can be caused by a number of mechanisms, the treatment varies.

Breast Cancer and Genitourinary Disorders

Elders are at high risk for a number of chronic problems of the genital and urinary systems, and breast and prostate cancers become more common with advanced age. As in other chronic illnesses, treatment of genital and urinary disorders is more successful when the problem is diagnosed before the disease is advanced. Unfortunately, many older people are reluctant to bring these problems to the attention of the physician until the medical problem has become serious. The following section will discuss breast cancer, benign prostatic hyperplasia, prostate cancer, and urinary incontinence.

Breast Cancer

Breast cancer is the second leading cause of cancer death among women in the United States. It occurs infrequently in men. The incidence of breast cancer among women increases with age. While women age sixty-five and older are only 14 percent of the female population in our country, they account for 43 percent of the cases diagnosed with invasive breast cancer. Almost three-fourths of breast cancer cases occur in women over age fifty.

The causes of breast cancer are unknown, although studies give us information on risk factors. Breast cancer is associated with a high dietary fat intake, obesity, alcohol intake, and inactivity. Those with a family history of breast cancer are at increased risk of developing breast cancer early in life, but the importance of this risk factor diminishes with age. Environmental toxins, particularly pesticides, may also affect risk.[78] Another risk factor may be the length of time estrogen circulates in the body. For instance, women who menstruate early, have a late menopause, or have no children have had more estrogen cycles than those who do not. Although those with risk factors mentioned above are at increased risk of developing cancer, every woman is considered at risk since many women get breast cancer who have none of these risks.

Prevention of breast cancer may be possible in the future, but currently the best way to decrease morbidity and mortality from the disease is through early detection. Clinical breast exams (by physicians) and self-breast exams are widely recommended, although there is little evidence that they reduce death rates. Mammography is the single most effective means to detect breast cancer early for those fifty and over. Randomized controlled trials in the United States and abroad have shown clear reductions in breast cancer mortality among women receiving regular mammograms. Mammography uses extremely low doses of radiation to detect abnormalities in breast tissue that are too small to be noticed with self-examination. If a mammogram or breast exam is abnormal, the lump in the breast is biopsied. Recommendations vary regarding the frequency with which elder women should receive mammograms, however, most organizations advocate mam- mography every one to three years for women over age sixty-five, continuing throughout old age.

Unfortunately, older women who would most benefit from mammography are the least likely to utilize the service. Only about one-third of women over sixty-five have ever had a mammogram, and the proportion decreases with advancing age. Additionally, low-income and minority women are less likely to receive mammograms. A major reason why women might not have had a mammogram in the past was that Medicare did not cover the cost. Medicare now pays for periodic mammograms. The low participation currently is more likely because physicians are not informing their elderly women patients of its value.

Treatment for breast cancer differs, depending on the type of cancer, whether it has spread into the lymph nodes, and whether it is a cancer recurrence. For tumors localized to the breast, surgery or radiation is the first-line treatment. Surgeons may remove only the lump (lumpectomy), the breast (simple mastectomy), or the entire breast, lymph nodes in the arm pits, and adjacent muscle tissue (radical mastectomy). Radical mastectomy is no longer regarded as the treatment of choice for localized disease since lumpectomy followed by radiation therapy boasts the same survival rate as more drastic operations without the disfigurement. Often radiation or chemotherapy is used before surgery to shrink the tumor. The success rate of treatment for breast cancer is high: over three-fourths of those with breast cancer live five years after surgery, and about 60 percent are alive ten years later. However, for black women, the five-year survival rate is lower.

Unfortunately, many women do not see a physician until the cancer has already spread. Even after treatment, many of these women have a recurrence of cancer in the breast, or the disease metastasizes to other parts of the body. Recurrences are treated with combinations of surgery, chemotherapy, and hormonal therapy. Hormonal therapy involves medications, primarily tamoxifen, that decrease the effect of estrogens.

Evidence shows that older women are less likely than younger women to be treated vigorously for breast cancer, even when their condition is the same.[79] Furthermore, older women are less likely to be offered breast reconstruction.[80] Dealing with breast cancer and the loss of a breast may be emotionally traumatizing. The local Reach to Recovery support group, sponsored by the American Cancer Society, may be helpful.

Research on prevention of breast cancer is progressing. There is some evidence that reduction of alcohol use, a diet low in fat and high in fruits and vegetables, and consumption of monounsaturated oils or soy products may protect against breast cancer. Tamoxifen, a drug originally used for breast cancer chemotherapy, is now being used in high-risk women to prevent breast cancer. Although it reduces the incidence of breast cancer, it increases the chances of developing uterine cancer and blood clots in the lungs and major veins.

Benign Prostatic Hyperplasia

With age, almost all men experience a gradual enlargement of the prostate gland, called *benign prostatic hyperplasia (BPH)*. By age sixty, more than half of all men have BPH, and by age eighty-five, about 90 percent of men have some evidence of BPH with about one-fourth of these having symptoms. Because the prostate surrounds the urethra, its growth often compresses the urethra, leading to a host of urinary symptoms. The most common symptoms of BPH (also called prostatism) are hesitancy upon starting urination, reduced force of the urinary stream, increased urinary frequency, dribbling of urine after urination, and an inability to fully empty the bladder despite increased urge to urinate. Because of urine remaining in the bladder, there is an increased risk of urinary tract infection. Those affected may awaken frequently during the night to pass a small amount of urine. Symptoms develop gradually and although bothersome, are not life-threatening.

BPH can be diagnosed by a medical history, a rectal examination, lab tests of kidney function and urine, and testing of the flow of urine. Sometimes a catheter is inserted into the bladder after voiding to determine whether there is urine remaining in the bladder.

An enlarged prostate requires treatment only if the patient is suffering urinary blockage, urinary tract infections, or damage to the urinary system from the prostate. Most men with BPH do not need to be treated at all. In most cases, symptoms stabilize and do not worsen. Unless the symptoms are severe and causing significant inconvenience, patient education and watchful waiting may be the best answer. To reduce urinary symptoms, those with BPH should avoid over-the-counter cold med-

ications, diuretics, antidepressants, or other drugs that may cause urinary retention. Alcohol, caffeine, or carbonated beverages should also be avoided.

Surgical treatment is offered to men whose symptoms disrupt their lifestyle. The most common treatment for an enlarged prostate is a simple operation, called a *transurethral resection of the prostate (TURP)*. A small loop is inserted through the penis, and the part of the prostate causing the obstruction is scraped, widening the urethra. This procedure can be done on an outpatient basis, is relatively low risk, and has few side effects. However, not all men have relief after surgery and most have "retrograde ejaculation" where their semen pass into the bladder upon ejaculation. Further, the prostatic tissue may regrow, and up to 20 percent of the operations must be repeated. It is the second most common surgical procedure (after cataract surgery) covered by Medicare. A more radical surgery that is less commonly used for an enlarged prostate is a prostatectomy, in which the entire prostate is removed

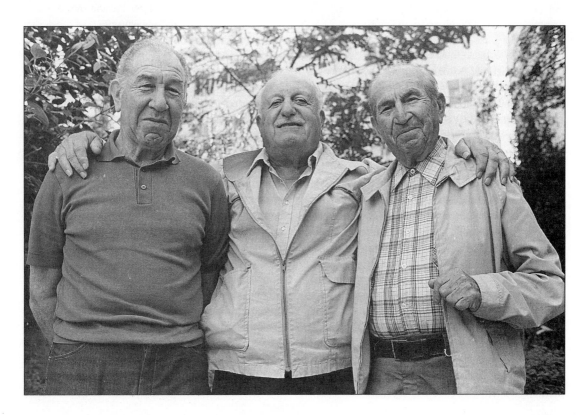

through the abdomen. This operation has more side effects and requires a longer convalescence. The effects of prostatic surgery on erectile function are discussed in chapter 6.

Alternatives to surgery include dilation of the urethra with a balloon catheter, similar to that used to widen blood vessels. Although symptoms may recur faster than with surgery, this procedure is simple and seems to have lasting beneficial effects. Within the last few years, a drug, called Proscar, was developed to shrink the prostate. Although it reduces the size of the prostate, it does not reduce the bothersome urinary symptoms for everyone. One controlled trial reported that after four years of drug treatment, the men had reduced urinary symptoms, increased urinary flow, and reduced probability of surgery.[81] Further, it is expensive, and the prostate grows again when the drug is discontinued. Another class of drugs may hold some promise. Studies are underway to determine their short- and long-term effects. See chapter 10 for details on drugs to shrink the prostate. An indwelling urinary catheter or intermittent self-catheterization is recommended in some cases.

Prostate Cancer

Prostate cancer is the most commonly diagnosed cancer in the United States (excluding skin cancers) and is second only to lung cancer as a contributor to cancer deaths in American men. In 1999, an estimated 179,300 new cases will be diagnosed, and 37,000 men will die of prostate cancer.[82] Eighty percent of the cases are diagnosed among men over age sixty-five. One in every five men in the United States will develop invasive prostate cancer before their death. The incidence of prostate cancer is increasing, probably because more men are receiving screening tests and being diagnosed with this cancer.

Prostate cancer is one of the more complicated cancers. On the one hand, it is a leading cause of cancer death in American men. On the other, it is a common part of aging, and many cases are not deadly. Unlike many other cancers, prostate cancer can be relatively slow growing, and some cancers may be insignificant. Autopsy studies reveal that up to one-half of all elderly men autopsied had prostate cancer. Some experts estimate that only a

very small proportion of men with prostate cancer will die from the disease. In fact, many men die with prostate cancer rather than from it. When prostate cancer is localized to the prostate, it is easily curable; however, it is more difficult to treat and more deadly if it has metastasized. For those with metastasis, the chance of living five years is only about 30 percent. Prostate cancer can affect a man for one to two decades, remaining quiescent for years, only to recur and spread.

The search for the cause of prostate cancer remains elusive. It is clear that incidence increases with advancing age, and the majority of men over age ninety have prostate cancer. African American men or men who have a family history of prostate cancer are at higher risk. Some studies suggest dietary factors may be protective (e.g., tomatoes, low fat, vitamin E, selenium). Environmental toxins have been implicated as a cause, but as yet, there is no explanation for the relationship.[83]

The principal screening tests for detection of asymptomatic prostate cancer are the digital rectal examination (DRE) and measurement of the serum tumor marker prostate specific antigen (PSA). A PSA greater than 4.0 ng/ml is the accepted threshold for further diagnostic evaluation. An elevated PSA will prompt more diagnostic work-up, which may include a needle biopsy of the prostate gland. There is a lot of controversy surrounding screening for prostate cancer; some organizations recommend screening for all men, and others assert that there is insufficient evidence to screen (see chapter 11).

Before choosing a treatment strategy, the disease progression, the aggressiveness of the cancer, survival rate, the dangers of each treatment, patient's preference, and health status should be taken into account. Cancer confined to the prostate can be treated by removal of the prostate (prostatectomy), which is usually curative. However, surgery may have serious side effects of impotence and incontinence. It is clear that men with a life expectancy of less than ten years rarely benefit from prostatectomy. If an elder is unable to tolerate surgery, radiation therapy is useful, however, this may also result in incontinence, diarrhea, or erectile dysfunction. Radiation may be directed at the entire pelvis or radioactive seeds implanted in the prostate may target therapy at the tumor. Some studies suggest that men with prostate cancer that has not spread and that appears to be growing slowly may elect no treatment at all and instead may engage in "watchful waiting," treating the cancer only when it begins to spread. This is justified because many of these cancers take many years to spread, and the death rate associated with untreated local cancer is low.[84,85] Other researchers assert that any man with a life expectancy of more than ten years should undergo surgery as an effective, curative treatment.[86]

Cancer that has spread outside the prostate is more deadly and is managed by hormonal therapy or removal of the testes (castration, also known as orchiectomy). Both procedures stop the production of testosterone and reduce bone pain. Hormonal therapy is a pharmacological castration in which a wide variety of estrogenlike substances may be used to block testosterone production. These treatments cause side effects such as erectile dysfunction, osteoporosis, weight gain, and hot flashes. Much more research needs to be done on how to determine which treatments are effective and how those who may benefit from treatment may be differentiated from those who may not.

Urinary Incontinence

Urinary incontinence ranges from the occasional passing of a few drops of urine while sneezing to the inability to control the voiding of urine at all times. Incontinence becomes more prevalent with age and is more common in women. Some experts estimate as many as 13 million people suffer from urinary incontinence. The prevalence of urinary incontinence among older people varies, depending on the setting. One study found that 19 percent of older men and 38 percent of older women living at home had incidences of urinary incontinence.[87] As expected, rates in hospitals and nursing homes are higher: half of all nursing home residents have some degree of incontinence.

Contrary to popular myth, incontinence is not an inevitable consequence of aging, but is a symptom of an underlying disorder. Causes include neu-

rological problems that affect central nervous system, medication side effects, infection of the genital or urinary system, and weakening of the pelvic muscles from childbirth. Almost all cases of incontinence can be eliminated or improved. However, too few people are evaluated. This is partly due to shame about incontinence or the physician's reluctance to bring up the topic, especially among the demented or institutionalized. Because many patients are embarrassed to discuss the issue, physicians need to broach the subject to their patients. Furthermore, physicians should evaluate and treat all patients with incontinence because its physiological and psychosocial effects are serious.

There are four types of incontinence, each with different causes and treatments. *Stress incontinence* occurs when abdominal pressure, caused by coughing, sneezing, laughing, or jumping, triggers leakage of urine. It is commonly due to weakness of the muscles supporting the bladder and urethra. This predominantly occurs in women and is caused by childbirth, estrogen deficiency, or previous pelvic surgery. *Urge incontinence* occurs when an individual suddenly feels the urge to urinate but cannot hold it long enough to reach the toilet. Local irritation or infection, or neurological problems, commonly occurring in dementia and stroke, can trigger such involuntary bladder contractions and cause leakage. *Overflow incontinence* occurs when an individual does not feel an urge to urinate, so the bladder fills to capacity and a small amount of urine flows out. The most common cause of overflow incontinence is prostate enlargement. Other causes include local nerve injury and medication use. *Functional incontinence* occurs when a continent elderly person is unable or unwilling to urinate normally. Causes might be mobility impairment, use of sedative medication, or psychological disturbances. Many elders have mixed incontinence, particularly a combination of urge and stress incontinence.

A variety of treatments can eliminate or decrease incontinence: the treatment of choice depends on the type. Behavioral changes can reduce or eliminate incontinence. Females with stress incontinence may benefit by exercises that strengthen the muscles of the pelvic floor, developed

Exercises for Urinary Control

If urine leakage is leaving you on the sidelines of the physical activities you enjoy, you've already taken the most important step toward recovery by seeing your doctor. But solving the problem often depends on teamwork between you and your doctor to settle on a solution that works for you.

Years ago, A. H. Kegel, MD, developed exercises to help his patients preserve and regain bladder control. Since then, these exercises have helped many patients by strengthening the pelvic floor muscles that control the flow of urine.

The two exercises below may help you if you perform them faithfully for three to four months. Many people with incontinence have avoided more aggressive forms of treatment by performing these exercises. If you do not improve your control of urine in this period, call your doctor, and he or she may suggest another solution. To maintain control, it is important for you to continue to do these exercises regularly.

Before you perform the exercises, you'll need to familiarize yourself with the muscles of your pelvic floor. To identify the back part of your pelvic floor muscles, imagine you are trying to hold back a bowel movement by tightening the ring of muscles around your anus, but don't tense the muscles of your legs, buttocks, or stomach. To identify the front part of your pelvic floor muscles, which control the flow of urine through the urethra, try to stop and restart the flow when you are urinating. When you've identified these muscles, you're ready to start the exercises.

Exercise 1. Working from the back (anus) to the front (urethra), tighten your muscles while counting to four slowly, then release. You can do this exercise anywhere—while sitting or standing, watching television, or waiting for a bus. There is no need to interrupt your normal daily activity.

When performing this exercise, do not tighten your stomach, thigh, or buttock muscles or cross your legs. This will help you feel only the pelvic muscles. When learning the exercises at home, women can check if they're exercising the right muscles by placing one finger inside the vagina and feeling the contraction. Men can check if they're exercising the right muscles by placing a finger between the scrotum and anus and feeling the contraction. Do this exercise for two minutes at least three times a day or for a total of 100 repetitions a day.

Exercise 2. Every time you urinate, start and stop your urine stream five times. (You should avoid this exercise if you have a urinary tract infection as it can result in discomfort.)

Excerpted from Baum, N., Appel, R.A., Moss, H. 1994. Helping incontinent patients resume activity. *The Physician and Sports Medicine* 22:79. Reproduced with permission of McGraw-Hill Inc.

by A. H. Kegel.[88] These exercises are very effective, but must be done daily and continued for three or four months.[89,90] Voiding at regular intervals (every two to three hours) and avoiding alcohol, caffeine, or carbonated beverages may also help. Other supportive measures may include having accessible toilets or substitutes and avoiding excessive sedation. Even a simple intervention, like crossing your legs when sneezing or coughing, can have a significant impact on stress incontinence.[91] Hormone replacement therapy in women may relieve incontinence; other medications may decrease bladder spasms or increase the strength of the urethral sphincter. Another technique to reduce incontinence is biofeedback, in which patients are trained to use internal muscles to control urine expulsion. Specialized physical therapy may also be helpful. For elders with impaired cognitive function, habit retraining may be effective. This technique puts elders with functional, urge, or stress incontinence on a strict toileting schedule.[92] This does not cure incontinence, but it can reduce embarrassing episodes. Although time-consuming for staff, it is very successful.

Devices are available that delay urine flow or collect the urine after it leaves the bladder. The Reliance urinary control insert is a tiny rod, about one-fifth the size of a tampon, that is inserted into the urethra, and a balloon inflates to block urinary flow. This device is removed when it is time to urinate and is discarded. An Impress Softpatch is a small triangular pad with gel adhesive that is placed over the urethra and acts like a seal; it is also disposable. An Introl Bladder Neck Support Prosthesis, inserted into the urethra, can help support a droopy bladder. Interestingly, a super-sized tampon inserted prior to exercise also reduces incontinence; to reduce vaginal irritation, it should be wetted slightly.[93] Newer treatments, such as the injection of collagen around the urethra to narrow the urethra[94] or nerve implants (Interstim Continence Control Therapy) to signal the bladder to fill or empty may play an important role in the future. Surgery to repair the pelvic floor is often successful for those with stress incontinence.

For patients who never regain continence, catheters are the major means of management. Catheters are tubes inserted through the urethra and into the neck of the bladder allowing the urine in the bladder to be drained. Elders can learn to catheterize themselves every few hours rather than have a permanent catheter that drains into a bag. Occasionally catheters are placed through the abdomen. However, catheters provide a direct route for bacteria to get into the bladder, and those using catheters have higher rates of urinary tract infections. Patients may also wear absorbent adult diapers, or men can wear a condom catheter where a drainage tube is attached to a condomlike penile covering. However, these aids should only be used as a last resort.

Urinary incontinence has widespread implications for elders and those around them. In our culture, the act of urination is considered a private activity. Any loss of continence in public is considered socially unacceptable and may be cause for embarrassment, chastisement, or ostracism by others. Because of its social importance, even partial incontinence is greatly feared, and those who have it often withdraw from social activities. Because

urinary incontinence is difficult to manage at home, it is often the major factor in deciding to place an elder in a nursing home. Even some nursing homes refuse incontinent applicants because of the increased workload they generate. The costs of labor, laundry, and supplies used to manage incontinence and its complications contribute significantly to the growing costs of nursing home care. Because of its wide-range of physical, psychological, and social effects, every effort should be made to treat this disorder.

Skin Disorders

Older people are susceptible to the same skin diseases as younger groups. However, some disorders are more common in the later years: psoriasis, senile pruritis, stasis dermatitis, decubitus ulcers, and skin cancer. Several studies indicate that approximately half of those over age sixty have a pathological skin condition, and those in institutions display a significantly higher percentage. This section will address psoriasis, pruritis, and skin cancers. Pressure sores will be discussed in chapter 9.

Psoriasis

Psoriasis is a noncontagious, chronic scaly skin disorder that affects 1 to 2 percent of the U.S. population. Psoriasis appears as reddened, dry, often itchy patches with a silvery surface scale located especially on the scalp, elbows, trunk, and legs. These patches demarcate areas of excessive cell turnover in the skin. Skin cells that normally take four weeks to develop now develop in only four days. Generally the disease causes only disfigurement and itching, however, more serious complications may result if body involvement is extensive. Psoriasis is characterized by exacerbations and remissions. It may be worsened by psychological stress, infection, or physical damage to skin.

Psoriasis runs in families, although no clear pattern of inheritance has been identified. Men and women are equally affected, and psoriasis most often appears for the first time between ages fifteen and thirty-five. Whites and East Africans have the highest prevalence of this disorder.

Treatment is directed at slowing cell turnover and moistening dried skin. First-line treatment is topical steroids, coal tar-based preparations, or a combination of oatmeal baths and emollients. Sunlight, warm water, weight loss, humidifiers, or vitamin D derivatives may also help. Ultraviolet light, in combination with topical treatment, is also effective. Occlusion therapy, whereby topical agents are applied and then the affected area is swathed in plastic overnight, may be useful as well. In severe cases, oral steroids or oral chemotherapy drugs may be used.

Senile Pruritis

Senile pruritis or itching is the most common skin condition of older people. Pruritis may be caused by a great number of factors and varies widely in severity; the disorder may cause mild discomfort or may drive one to acute mental distress.

The most common reason for itching is skin dryness. With age, the natural emollients of the skin decrease, and this tendency toward dryness is aggravated by cold and dry weather, sun and wind exposure, frequent bathing, or wearing rough fabrics, especially wool. Aside from itching, the skin looks abnormally dry and may be cracked in a block fashion, often with skin scaling. Frequent bathing or use of hot water is not recommended. Treatment involves tepid baths with minimal soaping followed by application of a heavy oil-based moisturizer while the skin is still wet. Aloe vera gel may be very effective. Oral medications are also available both over the counter and by prescription to treat itching.

In as many as half of all elders, an underlying cause for the itching is present. Pruritis may be caused by lice or mite infestation; fungus; an allergic reaction; emotional upset and tension; drug reaction; or a chronic disease such as diabetes, kidney disease, liver disease, or cancer. Because itching may be a symptom of other medical conditions besides simple dry skin, a medical evaluation should be conducted to rule out other possibilities.

Many elders who are diabetic, have chronic leg edema due to heart failure, or who have poor veins in the lower extremity suffer from *stasis der-matitis*. This appears as darkly pigmented (often purplish or reddened) skin, generally on the ankles and shins, that appears shiny and scaly. Edema is often present, and hair growth is reduced. This area may itch and is more susceptible to injury and poor healing. Treatment consists of applying topical emollients, reducing the edema through diuretics, raising the legs, using support stockings, or applying steroid creams.

Skin Cancer

Skin cancer is the most common type of cancer in the United States. There are multiple types of skin cancers with variable incidence, severity, risk factors, and treatment. Usually, only melanoma is deadly, and even it can be easily cured if identified and treated early. In general, the incidence of skin cancers increases with advancing age and is related to total lifetime sun exposure. Ultraviolet light damages the skin's genetic material and increases the likelihood of skin tumors. Risk factors include leisure-time and occupational sun exposure, age, and fair complexion (blue eyes and light skin). Skin cancers are on the rise in the United States and are appearing at younger ages. This increase is blamed on increased sun exposure through tanning and depletion of the protective ozone layer that filters ultraviolet light.

Basal and squamous skin cancers are the most common types of cancer in the United States among both sexes. Most commonly, squamous cancer is diagnosed in those aged sixty-five to seventy, and basal cell cancer is diagnosed in the ages of sixty to sixty-four. These skin cancers are almost always curable by simple procedures, they grow slowly, and rarely metastasize. Basal and squamous skin cancers are most common among whites and are generally located on the face, eyelid, top of head, forearms, or shoulders. Forty percent of these cancers start on or inside the ears. The most common are basal cell carcinomas, which are limited to hair-bearing areas (e.g., face, back) and generally appear as a smooth, pale, pearly nodule that may ulcerate or bleed.

Squamous cell cancers are common in sun-exposed areas, but may occur anywhere on the skin, including the mucous membranes. They appear as nodules on scaly, reddened patches with irregular borders that have a tendency to bleed. When they arise from a "precancerous" reddened or scaly patch, called actinic keratosis, they are less likely to metastasize than when they arise on their own. Tumors that develop on the lip or on sites of old scars are also more likely to be malignant. Squamous cancers are twelve times more lethal than basal cell cancers.

Precancerous actinic keratoses can be easily treated with liquid nitrogen. Older people who have many of these may be treated with applications of Retin-A or chemotherapeutic agents. Basal and squamous cancers generally are removed by simple excision, either by burning and scraping, by freezing, or with a laser. People with skin cancer or precancerous lesions are advised to protect their skin from further sun damage and to use broad-spectrum sunscreens.

The most serious and generally the only skin cancer that metastasizes and may be fatal is malignant melanoma. This skin cancer is becoming increasingly common with the incidence rising dramatically over the last few decades. In 1930, the lifetime risk of an American developing melanoma was 1 in 1,500; today, it is one in eighty-seven and continues to rise.[95] The lesions usually start as small, dark molelike growths that increase in size, change color, become ulcerated, and bleed with slight injury. A molelike lesion that changes size,

has irregular borders, is multicolored, is surrounded by reddened skin, becomes softer or harder, or is associated with pain or itchiness should be checked by a physician. The mnemonic ABCD is used: **A**symmetry, irregular **B**order, uneven **C**olor, and **D**iameter greater than 6 mm. They appear most often on lower legs and feet in women and the trunk in men, although they may occur on the face, on the nails, or in the mouth as well.

People at highest risk for melanoma have a large number of brown moles (fifty or more); have fair skin, freckles, and blond or red hair; have a history of severe sunburn in the childhood or teen years; and have lived or vacationed in sunny areas. Melanoma must be removed early to be cured. Even when the tumor is removed completely, it may already have spread, although the metastasis may not be detected until years later. When the tumor begins to spread to other body organs, systemic chemotherapy or radiation may be recommended; however, metastatic melanoma is usually fatal. Those who have any risk factors should thoroughly and regularly check their skin for suspicious moles. There is controversy regarding whether sunscreens are effective at preventing melanoma. Sunscreens may incompletely protect against damage and provide a sense of false security; however, newer broad-spectrum sunscreens may be helpful. Experts recommend sun-protective clothing such as a broad-brimmed hat and long sleeves.

SUMMARY

Old age is often accompanied by chronic illnesses. Chronic conditions are progressive, generally irreversible, and long-term. Although chronic illnesses are widespread in elders, most cause only minor limitation of daily routine. Some chronic illnesses (heart disease, cancer, and stroke) are the three leading causes of death among elders. Rather than a cure, medical management of chronic conditions involves treating symptoms and preventing further deterioration. The social, financial, and emotional considerations of chronic illnesses are a critical part of coping with disease. Health care workers and the family and friends of those with health problems need to be attentive to such variables when dealing with the chronically ill.

Lifestyle factors are increasingly recognized as having an important role in the development and treatment of many chronic illnesses. The most effective way to prevent these diseases or reduce their progression is to modify negative health behaviors, such as stopping smoking or increasing exercise. Prevention of chronic illness involves a personal, lifelong effort to improve health habits. For many, both young and old, the benefits are too distant and the short-term costs too great.

This chapter provides an overview of the common chronic illnesses among elders. Rarely does anyone get through old age without at least one of these illnesses; many elders have several of them. Each illness discussed includes a description of the disease, its risk factors, and ways to diagnose and treat its symptoms. When available, prevention strategies are also included. The discussion of diseases is intended to assist those who work with elders to understand the diseases that their client or patient might have in order to serve them more effectively. Even more importantly, this information may motivate those with poor health habits to improve them before a chronic illness develops.

ACTIVITIES

1. Create a brief case study of an older individual with a chronic health problem or problems. Include the impact of the disease on the overall quality of life of that person. Be sure to include psychological, social, and economic aspects. Assuming the individual in the case has a spouse, describe the impact upon that family member.

2. After studying the common chronic health problems of elders, which diseases will you be likely to suffer in your later years, due either to heredity or current health behaviors? Be complete. Remember that many are extremely common. What might you do to prevent or reduce the impact of one or more of these problems? Are you working on modifying any of these habits now? If, so, which ones? If not, discuss the factors keeping you from doing so.

3. Visit the campus library and peruse the recent medical journals. Choose an article that presents new information on some aspect of a common disease of elders. Write a brief summary of the findings and discuss the implications of this new information on the outcome of the disease and its effect upon the individual.

4. You have been asked to coordinate a health fair for elders in your community. You have twenty booths to fill with either agencies, screening facilities, or health education materials. Considering the information on chronic disease gathered in this chapter, list information or screening you would provide in each booth that would be most helpful to this age group.

5. Talk to the director of smoking cessation classes available in your area. What is the percentage of elders attending? In the director's experience, what is the success rate with elders? How does it compare to other age groups?

6. Visit a public place (shopping mall, drug store, or supermarket) and tally how many individuals have visible health problems, as well as their approximate ages. What health problem seems to be the most common? Can you detect any difference in types and numbers of problems with age?

BIBLIOGRAPHY

1. Hoffman, C., Rice, D., and Sung, H-Y. 1996. Persons with chronic conditions: Their prevalence and costs. *Journal of the American Medical Association* 276:1473–79.

2. Strauss, A.L. 1975. *Chronic illness and the quality of life.* St. Louis: C. V. Mosby Co.

3. Parsons, T. 1958. Definition of health and illness in the light of American values and social structure. In *Patients, physicians, and illness.* E. G. Jaco, ed. Glenco, IL: Free Press.

4. "Chronic illness and families: Too much help hurts." 1994. *Family Practice News* (April 15):14–15.

5. Gould, K.L., Ornish, D., and Scherwitz L., et al. 1995. Changes in myocardial perfusion abnormalities by positron emission tomography after long-term, intense risk factor modification. *Journal of the American Medical Association* 274:894–901.

6. Weverling-Rijnsburger, A.W., Blauw, G.J., and Lagaay, A.M., et al. 1997. Total cholesterol and risk of mortality in the oldest old. *Lancet* 350:1119–23.

7. Gillman, M.W., Cupples, L.A., and Millen, B.E., et al. 1997. Inverse association of dietary fat with development of ischemic stroke in men. *Journal of the American Medical Association* 278:2145–50.

8. Pearson, T.A. 1998. Lipid-lowering therapy in low-risk patients (Editorial). *Journal of the American Medical Association* 279:1659–60.

9. Launer, L.J., Masaki, K., and Petrovitch, H., et al. 1995. The association between midlife blood pres-

sure levels and late-life cognitive function. *Journal of the American Medical Association* 274:1846–51.

10. Pearce, K.A., Evans, G.W., and Summerson, J., et al. 1997. Comparisons of ambulatory blood pressure monitoring and repeated office measurements in primary care. *Journal of Family Practice* 45:426–33.

11. Whitcomb, B.L., Prochazca, A., LoVerde, M., and Byyny, R.L. 1995. Failure of the community based Vita-Stat automated blood pressure device to accurately measure blood pressure. *Archives of Family Medicine* 4:419–24.

12. Whelton, P.K., Appel, L.J., and Espeland, M.A., et al. 1998. Sodium reduction and weight loss in the treatment of hypertension in older persons. *Journal of the American Medical Association* 279:839–46.

13. Insua, J.T., Sacks, H.S., and Lau, T-S., et al. 1994. Drug treatment of hypertension in the elderly: A meta-analysis. *Annals of Internal Medicine* 121:355–62.

14. Rexrode, K.M., Carey, V.J., and Hennekens, C.H., et al. 1998. Abdominal adiposity and coronary heart disease in women. *Journal of the American Medical Association* 280:1843–48.

15. Wald, N.J., Watt, H.C., and Law, M.R., et al. 1998. Homocysteine and ischemic heart disease: Results of a prospective study with implications regarding prevention. *Archives of Internal Medicine* 158:862–67.

16. Graham, I.M., Daly, L.E., and Refsum, H.M. 1997. Plasma homocysteine as a risk factor for vascular disease. *Journal of the American Medical Association* 277:1775–81.

17. Stampfer, M.J., Colditz, G.A., and Willett, W.C., et al. 1991. Postmenopausal estrogen therapy and cardiovascular disease—ten year follow-up from the Nurse's Health Study. *New England Journal of Medicine* 325(11):756–62.

18. Gullette, E.C.D., Blumenthal, J.A., and Babyak, M., et al. 1997. Effects of mental stress on myocardial ischemia during daily life. *Journal of the American Medical Association* 277:1521–26.

19. Black, D.A. 1987. Mental state and presentation of myocardial infarction in the elderly. *Age and Ageing* 16:125–27.

20. Marrugat, J., Sala, J., and Masia, R., et al. 1998. Mortality differences between men and women following first myocardial infarction. *Journal of the American Medical Association* 280:405–9.

21. Hennekens, C.H., Dyken, M.L., and Fuster, V. 1997. Aspirin as a therapeutic agent in cardiovascular disease: A statement for healthcare professionals from the American Heart Association. *Circulation* 96:2751–53.

22. American Heart Association. 1998. *1999 Heart and Stroke Statistical Update.* Dallas: American Heart Association.

23. Kimura, T., Yokoi, H., and Nakagawa, Y., et al. 1996. Three-year follow-up after implantation of metallic coronary-artery stents. *New England Journal of Medicine* 334:561–66.

24. Every, N.R., Parsons, L.S., and Hlatky, M., et al. 1996. A comparison of thrombolytic therapy with primary coronary angioplasty for acute myocardial infarction. *New England Journal of Medicine* 335:1253–60.

25. Hlatky, M.A., Rogers, W.J., and Johnstone, I., et al. 1997. Medical costs and quality of life after randomization to coronary angioplasty or coronary bypass surgery. *New England Journal of Medicine* 336:92–99.

26. Selby, J.V., Fireman, B.H., and Lundstrom, R.J., et al. 1996. Variation among hospitals in coronary-angiography practices and outcomes after myocardial infarction in a large health maintenance organization. *New England Journal of Medicine* 335:1888–96.

27. Jollis, J.G., DeLong, E.R., and Peterson, E.D., et al. 1996. Outcome of acute myocardial infarction according to the specialty of the admitting physician. *New England Journal of Medicine* 335:1880–87.

28. Normand, S.L.T., Glickman, M.E., Sharma, R.G., and McNeil, B.J. 1996. Using admission characteristics to predict short-term mortality from myocardial infarction in elderly patients. *Journal of the American Medical Association* 275:1322–28.

29. Goldstein, R.E., Andrews, M., Hall, W.J., and Moss, A.J. 1996. Marked reduction in long-term cardiac deaths with aspirin after a coronary event. *Journal of the American College of Cardiology* 28:326–30.

30. Soumerai, S.B., McLaughlin, T.J., and Spiegelman, D., et al. 1997. Adverse outcomes of underuse of beta-blockers in elderly survivors of acute myocardial infarction. *Journal of the American Medical Association* 277:115–21.

31. Center for Disease Control. 1998. Changes in mortality from heart failure—United States,

1980–1995. *Morbidity and Mortality Weekly Report* 47:633–36.

32. Consensus Trial Study Group. 1987. Effects of enalapril on mortality in severe congestive heart failure: Results of the cooperative North Scandinavian enalapril survival study. *New England Journal of Medicine* 316:1429–35.

33. Dracup, K., Baker, D.W., and Dunbar, S.B., et al. 1994. Management of heart failure: II. Counseling, education, and lifestyle modifications. *Journal of the American Medical Association* 272:1442–46.

34. Stafford, R.S., and Singer, D.E. 1996. National patterns of warfarin use in atrial fibrillation. *Archives of Internal Medicine* 156:2537–41.

35. Alberts, M.A., Bertels, C., and Dawson, D. 1990. An analysis of time of presentation after stroke. *Journal of the American Medical Association* 263:65–68.

36. Pancioli, A.M., Broderick, J., and Kothari, R., et al. 1998. Public perception of stroke warning signs and knowledge of potential risk factors. *Journal of the American Medical Association* 279:1288–92.

37. Sivenius, J., Riekkinen, P.J., Sr., and Laakso, M. 1995. Antiplatelet treatment in elderly people with transient ischaemic attacks of ischaemic strokes. *British Medical Journal* 310:25–26.

38. Dutch TIA Trial Study Group. 1991. A comparison of two doses of aspirin (30 mg vs. 283 mg a day) in patients after a transient ischemic attack or minor ischemic stroke. *New England Journal of Medicine* 325(18):1261–67.

39. Bailar, J.C., and Gornik, H.L. 1997. Cancer undefeated. *New England Journal of Medicine* 336:1569–74.

40. Keintz, M.K., Rimer, B., Fleisher, L., and Engstron, P. 1988. Educating older adults about their increased cancer risk. *The Gerontologist* 28:487–90.

41. Lassen, U., Osterlind, K., and Hanson, M., et al. 1995. Long-term survival in small-cell lung cancer: Posttreatment characteristics in patients surviving 5 to 18+ years—An analysis of 1714 consecutive patients. *Journal of Clinical Oncology* 13:1215–20.

42. Centers for Disease Control. 1997. Cigarette smoking among adults—United States, 1995. *Morbidity and Mortality Weekly Report* 46:1217–20.

43. Fiore, M.C., Bailey, W.C., Cohen, S.J., et al. 1996. *Smoking Cessation: Information for Specialists.*

Clinical Practice Guidelines for Smoking Cessation Specialists. No. 18. Rockville, MD: U.S. Department of Health and Human Services, Public Health Service, Agency for Health Care Policy and Research and Centers for Disease Control and Prevention, AHCPR Pub. No. 96-0694.

44. Gurwitz, J.H., Glynn, R.J., and Monane, M., et al. 1993. Treatment for glaucoma: Adherence by the elderly. *American Journal of Public Health* 83:711–16.

45. Bennett, D.A., Beckett, L.A., and Murray, A.M., et al. 1996. Prevalance of Parkinsonian signs and associated mortality in a community population of older people. *New England Journal of Medicine* 334:71–76.

46. Limousin, P., Krack, P., and Pollak, P. et al. 1998. Electrical stimulation of the subthalamic nucleus in advanced Parkinson's disease. *New England Journal of Medicine* 339:1105–11.

47. Hubble, J.P., Cao, T., and Hassanein, R.E., et al. 1993. Risk factors for Parkinson's disease. *Neurology* 43(September):1693–97.

48. Saltz, B.L., Woerner, M.G., and Kane, J.M., et al. 1991. Prospective study of tardive dyskinesia incidence in the elderly. *Journal of the American Medical Association* 266:2402–6.

49. Loesche, W.J., Giordano, J., Soehren, S., et al. 1996. Non-surgical treatment of patients with periodontal disease. *Journal of Oral Surgery, Oral Medicine, Oral Pathology, Oral Radiology, and Endodontics* 81:533–543.

50. Dolan, T.A., and Atchison, K.A. 1993. Implications of access, utilization and need for oral health care by the non-institutionalized and institutionalized elderly on the dental delivery system. *Journal of Dental Education* 57:876–87.

51. Winawer, S.J., Zauber, A.G., and Gerdes, H., et al. 1996. Risk of colorectal cancer in the families of patients with adenomatous polyps. *New England Journal of Medicine* 334:82–87.

52. Giovannucci, E.L., and Colditz, G.A., et al. 1994. A prospective study of family history and the risk of colorectal cancer. *New England Journal of Medicine* 331:1669–74.

53. Doyle, T.J., Zheng, W., and Cerhan, J.R., et al. 1997. The association of drinking water source and chlorination by-products with cancer incidence among postmenopausal women in Iowa: A

prospective cohort study. *American Journal of Public Health* 87:1168–76.

54. Giovannucci, E.L., Stampfer, M.J., and Colditz, G.A., et al. 1998. Multivitamin use, folate, and colon cancer in women in the Nurses' Health Study. *Annals of Internal Medicine* 129:517–24.

55. Rozen, P., Fireman, Z., and Fine, N., et al. 1989. Oral calcium suppresses increased rectal epithelial proliferation of persons at risk for colorectal cancer. *Gut* 30:650–55.

56. Giovannucci, E., Egan K.M., and Hunter, D.J., et al. 1995. Aspirin and the risk of colorectal cancer in women. *New England Journal of Medicine* 333:609–14.

57. Sonnenberg, A., and Koch, T.R. 1989. Physician visits in the United States for constipation. 1958–1986. *Digestive Disease Science* 334:606–11.

58. Wolfsen, C.R., Barker, J.C., and Mitteness, L.S. 1993. Constipation in the daily lives of frail elderly people. *Archives of Family Medicine* 2:853–58.

59. Towers, A.L., Burgio, K.L., and Locher, J.L., et al. 1994. Constipation in the elderly: Influence of dietary, psychological and physiological factors. *Journal of the American Geriatrics Society* 42:701–6.

60. Harari, D., Gurwitz, J.H., Avorn, J., Bohn, R., and Minaker, K.L. 1996. Bowel habit in relation to age and gender. Findings from the National Health Interview Survey and clinical implications. *Archives of Internal Medicine* 156:315–20.

61. Johanson, J.F., Sonnenberg, A., and Koch, T.R. 1989. Clinical epidemiology of chronic constipation. *Journal of Clinical Gastroenterology* 11:525–36.

62. Romero, Y., Evans, J.M., Fleming, K.C., and Philips, S.F. 1996. Constipation and fecal incontinence in the elderly population. *Mayo Clinic Proceedings* 71:81–92.

63. Creamer, P., and Hochberg, M.C. 1997. Osteoarthritis. *Lancet* 350:503–9.

64. McAlindon, T.E., Felson, D.T., and Zhang, Y., et al. 1996. Relation of dietary intake and serum levels of vitamin D to progression of osteoarthritis of the knee among participants in the Framingham Study. *Annals of Internal Medicine* 125:353–59.

65. Spector, T.D., Roman, E., and Silman, A.J. 1990. The pill, parity, and rheumatoid arthritis. *Arthritis and Rheumatism* 33:782–89.

66. Vandenbroucke, J.P., Witteman, J.C., and Valkenberg, H.A. 1986. Non-contraceptive hormone and rheumatoid arthritis in perimenopausal and post-menopausal women. *Journal of the American Medical Association*. 255(10):1299–1303.

67. Cummings, S.R., Kelsey, J.L., Nevitt, M.C., and O'Dowd, K.J. 1985. Epidemiology of osteoporosis and osteoporotic fractures. *Epidemiologic Review* 7:178–208.

68. Stall, G.M., Harris, S., Sokoll, L.J., and Dawson-Hughes, B. 1990. Accelerated bone loss in hypothyroid patients overtreated with L-thyroxine. *Annals of Internal Medicine* 113(4):265–69.

69. Delmas, P.D., Bjarnason, N.H., and Mitlak, B.H., et al. 1997. Effects of raloxifene on bone mineral density, serum cholesterol concentrations, and uterine endometrium in postmenopausal women. *New England Journal of Medicine* 337:1641–47.

70. Wood, K.B., Garvey, T.A., Gundry, C., and Heithoff, K.B. 1995. Magnetic resonance imaging of the thoracic spine. Evaluation of asymptomatic individuals. *Journal of Joint and Bone Surgery* 77:1631–38.

71. American Diabetes Association. 1999. Position statement: Nutrition recommendations and principles for people with diabetes mellitus. *Diabetes Care* 22(suppl).

72. Wahl, P.W., and Savage, P.J., et al. 1998. Diabetes in older adults: Comparison of 1997 American Diabetes Association classification of diabetes mellitus with 1985 WHO classification. *Lancet* 352:1012–16.

73. Brown, D.F., and Jackson, T.W. 1994. Diabetes: 'Tight control' in a comprehensive treatment plan. *Geriatrics* 49:24–36.

74. Helfand, M., and Redfern, C.C. 1998. Screening for thyroid disease: An update. *Annals of Internal Medicine* 129:144–59.

75. Bemben, D.A., Hamm, R.M., and Morgan, L., et al. 1994. Thyroid disease in the elderly. Part 2. Predictability of subclinical hypothyroidism. *Journal of Family Practice* 38:583–88.

76. Bauer, D.E., Ettinger, B., and Browner, W.S. 1998. Thyroid functions and serum lipids in older women: A population-based study. *American Journal of Medicine* 104:546–51.

77. Trivalle, C., Doucet, J., and Chassagne, P., et al. 1996. Differences in the signs and symptoms of

hyperthyroidism in older and younger patients. *Journal of the American Geriatrics Society* 44:50–53.

78. Hoyer, A.P., Grandjean, P., and Jorgensen, T., et al. 1998. Organochlorine exposure and risk of breast cancer. *Lancet* 1816–20.

79. Hillner, B.E., Penberthy, L., and Desch, C.E., et al. 1996. Variation in staging and treatment of local and regional breast cancer in the elderly. *Breast Cancer Research and Treatment* 40:75–86.

80. Hynes, D.M. 1994. The quality of breast cancer care in local communities: Implications for health care reform. *Medical Care* 32:328–40.

81. McConnell, J.D., Bruskewitz, R., and Walsh, P., et al. 1998. The effect of finasteride on the risk of acute urinary retention and the need for surgical treatment among men with benign prostatic hyperplasia. *New England Journal of Medicine* 338:557–63.

82. American Cancer Society. 1999. Cancer facts and figures-1999, Atlanta, GA.

83. Haas, B.E., and Sakr, W.A. 1997. Epidemiology of prostate cancer. *CA—A Cancer Journal for Clinicians* 47:273–87.

84. Lu-Yao, G.I., and Yao, S.L. 1997. Population-based study of long-term survival in patients with clinically localized prostate cancer. *Lancet* 349:906–10.

85. Johansson, J.E., Holmberg, L., and Johansson, S., et al. 1997. Fifteen-year survival in prostate cancer: A prospective population-based trial in Sweden. *Journal of the American Medical Association* 277:467–71.

86. Lange, P.H. 1997. New information about prostate-specific antigen and the paradoxes of prostate cancer (Editorial). *Journal of the American Medical Association* 273:336–37.

87. Herzog, A.R., Diokno, A.C., and Brown, M.B., et al. 1990. Two-year incidence, remission and change patterns of urinary incontinence in non-institutionalized older adults. *Journal of Gerontology* 45:M67–74.

88. Kegel, A.H. 1948. Progressive resistance exercises in the functional restoration of the perineal muscles. *American Journal of Obstetrics and Gynecology* 56:238–48.

89. Hahn, I., Milson, I., and Fall, M., et al. 1993. Long-term results of pelvic floor training in female stress urinary incontinence. *British Journal of Urology* 72:421–27.

90. Fonda, D., Woodward, M., D'Asstoli, M., and Chin, W. 1995. Sustained improvement of subjective quality of life in older community-dwelling people after treatment of urinary incontinence. *Age and Ageing* 24:283–86.

91. Norton, P.A., and Baker, J.E. 1994. Postural changes can reduce leakage in women with stress urinary incontinence. *Obstetrics and Gynecology* 84:770–74.

92. Ouslander, J.G., and Schnelle, J.R. 1995. Incontinence in the nursing home. *Annals of Internal Medicine* 122:438–49.

93. Nygaard, I. 1995. Prevention of exercise incontinence with mechanical devices. *Journal of Reproductive Medicine* 40:89–94.

94. Herschorn, S., Steele, D.J., and Radomski, S.B. 1996. Followup of intraurethral collagen for female stress urinary incontinence. *Journal of Urology* 156:1305–9.

95. Rigel, D.S. 1996. Malignant melanoma: Perspectives on incidence and its effects on awareness, diagnosis, and treatment (Editorial). *CA—A Cancer Journal for Clinicians* 46:195–98.

ACUTE ILLNESSES AND ACCIDENTS

Old age is no place for sissies.

Bette Davis

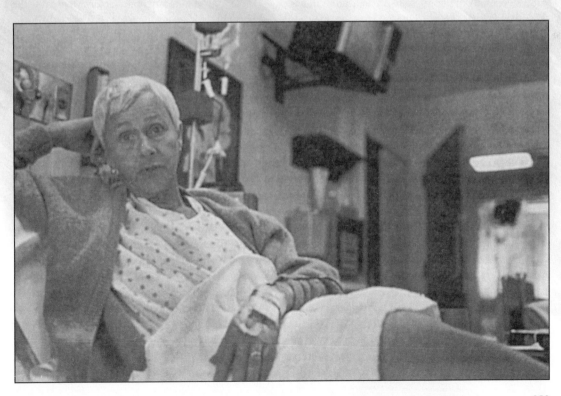

Long-standing chronic illnesses account for the largest proportion of death and disability of elders. However, acute illnesses (primarily influenza and pneumonia) and accidents are also important. For a number of reasons, elders are more likely to suffer severe consequences from infections and accidents than other age groups. Acute illnesses and accidents are also major causes of admissions to hospitals and consequently comprise a high proportion of the health care expenditures for those over sixty-five.

This chapter will look at acute illnesses common among older adults, both those caused by infection and those environmentally induced (hypothermia and hyperthermia). Common types of accidents among elders, factors that increase accident susceptibility, and accident prevention will also be addressed.

COMMON ACUTE ILLNESSES AMONG ELDERS

Elders generally are no more likely to acquire infections than younger people, but when they do, they are at higher risk for complications or death from them. Mortality from pneumonia and influenza is particularly high in the older population and, when considered together, the two are the fifth-leading cause of death among elders. Furthermore, elders are at much greater risk of nosocomial (hospital-acquired) infection as compared to the general population.

A number of factors, including age-associated physiological changes, the prevalence of chronic illnesses, and environmental influences, play a role in placing older people at a higher risk of illness or death from common infections. Susceptibility to viral or bacterial infections increases when immunity is reduced. Diminished pulmonary function, especially the ability of the lungs to clear foreign matter, increases the risk of pneumonia or other respiratory tract infections. In addition, age changes in the skin, such as reduced blood supply and subcutaneous fat, and thinning of the outer layer of skin increase susceptibility to skin and wound infections.

The high prevalence of chronic illness among elders plays a role in their high rate of acute illnesses. Many chronic diseases predispose elders to infections. For example, chronic bronchitis increases susceptibility to pneumonia and other respiratory infections. Elders with diabetes are more likely to develop urinary tract infections or foot ulcers.

Chronic disease may also indirectly promote infection. Some instruments used to treat chronic illnesses (e.g., catheters and intravenous equipment) predispose the user to infections. Malnutrition, common among cancer patients, is also thought to lower resistance to illness. Many drugs used to treat a chronic disease, (e.g., corticosteroids used to treat asthma and lung diseases), lower resistance to infection. In addition, the immobility caused by some chronic illnesses can predispose individuals to pneumonia, urinary tract infections, and decubitus ulcers. Finally, those who have a chronic disease are more likely to become sicker and to take longer to get well when faced with an acute illness than others without such diseases.

Certain environmental factors increase the opportunity for acute illnesses. Extremes of environmental temperatures may cause hypothermia or hyperthermia, especially among those who are frail. A hospital or nursing home setting encourages infection because confining many ill people in a small area increases their chances of contracting an infection. It is estimated that up to 20 percent of nursing home residents acquire an infection, most commonly, urinary tract infections and decubitus ulcers.

Elders have a higher rate of latent infections than younger groups. Some types of bacteria or viruses, which have been residing in the body in a latent state for years, can suddenly reappear. Tuberculosis and herpes zoster (shingles) are the most common among those over age fifty.

Diagnosis of acute illnesses is more difficult in elders than other age groups because important warning signs of infection, such as fever and elevated white blood cell count, may be atypical or absent. Those with congestive heart failure and those who take drugs, such as aspirin, corticosteroids, or other anti-inflammatory agents, are even less likely to develop a fever. In older people, nonspecific symptoms often accompany an infection: confusion, psychosis, fatigue, appetite loss, a decline in performance, or lack of interest in their environment. A physician or family member may ignore these vague symptoms, attributing them to age-related decline, a drug side effect, or a pre-existing chronic illness. Finally, elders themselves are less likely to report such symptoms to their physician.

Respiratory Infections

Acute respiratory illnesses are a significant problem for the elderly: they face a higher risk of complications and death from pulmonary infections than younger people. In 1996, influenza and pneumonia were the fifth-leading cause of death among persons sixty-five and older in the United States.[1] The risk increases among those who

smoke, inhale second-hand smoke, have chronic lung diseases, or are immobilized or have just undergone surgery.

The Common Cold

Although generally not disabling, the common cold is by far the most prevalent acute infection in the United States, costing billions of dollars in cold remedy purchases and immeasurable losses in productivity each year. It is a small consolation that each individual is susceptible only once to a particular cold virus because more than 200 types of viruses have been identified. The incidence of colds among elders is reduced because they have already been exposed to many of the cold viruses. The sheer number of different viruses makes the development of a vaccine very unlikely.

The common cold is a viral infection of the cells that line the nose and throat. In response to

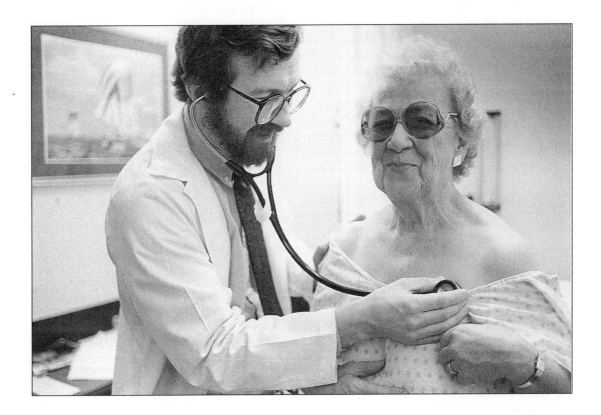

the virus, the mucous membranes lining the respiratory passages secrete large amounts of fluids. These fluids contain virus particles that are infectious. Viruses that cause colds are more likely to be spread by contaminated hands than through the air. For example, a person with a cold touches his eyes or nose, then touches the doorknob. The next victim touches the doorknob, then touches his eyes or nose. The best way to prevent a cold is by frequent hand washing with warm water and soap, avoiding touching the eyes and nose, and avoiding people with colds.

Symptoms of a cold appear one to three days after infection. Stress, poor general health, lack of sleep, and smoking predispose one to a cold. The most common symptoms include nasal congestion, runny nose, scratchy or sore throat, sneezing, and coughing. The treatment is simple: let it run its course without drugs, drink plenty of liquids, and rest. For those who must have symptom relief for nasal congestion, sore throat, and aches, several over-the-counter drugs are available. Some studies indicate that regular intake of vitamin C reduces both the duration and symptoms of the common cold. Zinc gluconate lozenges, taken every two hours at the first sign of a cold, have also been reported to significantly reduce the duration of the common cold.[2] Because the cold is caused by a virus, antibiotics (drugs that fight bacteria) are ineffective. The excessive prescribing of antibiotics for viral infections is a significant problem in the United States as it has contributed to the emergence of antibiotic-resistant bacteria strains. Despite this, antibiotic prescriptions for the common cold account for a significant proportion of the total antibiotic use in the United States.[3]

In the adult years, the likelihood of contracting a cold is reduced, and cold symptoms become milder in nature. However, among older people, a cold is more likely to lead to complications, such as sinusitis, ear infections, acute bronchitis, and pneumonia. Signs of an infection that require medical care are an extended fever, a bloody discharge from the nose or mouth, recurring chest pains, greenish or thickened nasal discharge or phlegm, persistent cough, earache, sinus pain, or severe sore throat.

Influenza

Influenza, commonly called the flu, is a viral infection that affects the respiratory tract and skeletal muscles. The flu differs from a cold in that the symptoms are more severe: sudden onset of high fever, headache, severe muscle aches, chills, loss of appetite, and total prostration for several days. Three types of influenza have been identified: A, B, and C. Type A influenza, generally the most severe and debilitating, has been responsible for five worldwide epidemics. Type A influenza occurs during the winter and spring and is marked by high absenteeism from work and school. Type B causes symptoms similar to type A, but is usually less severe and is associated with localized outbreaks. Type C is very similar in symptoms and treatment to the common cold.

Although elders are less likely to contract influenza than younger people, the mortality among those over age sixty-five is much higher, accounting for more than 80 percent of those who die from influenza. This increased mortality is attributed to the fact that the flu lowers elders' resistance to more serious infections, usually pneumonia. In 1918, the flu epidemic killed about 65,000 people (mostly the very old and very young), primarily from secondary infections. Elders are more likely to have heart disease, emphysema, bronchitis, kidney disease, and diabetes than younger groups, so they are at high risk of developing secondary infections after a bout with influenza.

Symptomatic treatment is similar to that for the common cold. In addition, the antiviral medication, Symmetrel (amantadine hydrochloride), is effective in preventing influenza A infections if taken daily during flu season. Amantadine has also been shown to reduce the duration and intensity of the flu if taken after contracting the virus. However, this medication has a high rate of side effects among the elderly, including hallucinations, abnormal gait, and heart failure.

Because of the high death rate of type A influenza, older people, the chronically ill, the institutionalized, and those who have significant contact with elders are advised to be vaccinated annually during autumn; the vaccine reduces the chance of getting the flu by more than half.[4] Many studies confirm that a yearly flu vaccine reduces the risk for pneumonia, hospitalization, and death in elders during a flu epidemic. It is considered an indispensible part of the medical care of those over sixty-five.[5]

The flu virus chosen for the vaccine changes each year. The Centers for Disease Control develops the vaccines by using the type of flu virus that predominated the previous year. A yearly vaccination is required because the immunity protects only against one type of virus and lasts only a few months. The most common side effect of the vaccine is muscle soreness at the injection site. There is some evidence that yearly flu shots can boost the immune system in a more general way as well.[6]

Many individuals mistakenly believe they can contact the flu from the flu shot, but this is impossible. What generally occurs is that individuals catch a cold in the days surrounding the date of their flu vaccine, and they attribute it to the injection. Use of the vaccine significantly reduces the rate of hospitalization, complications and death from influenza. Despite the proven success of the flu shot, only about 65 percent of the elder population in the United States received the vaccine in 1997, with even lower participation among Hispanic American elders and those of other racial/ethnic groups.[7] Medicare covers influenza immunizations. It is estimated that influenza vaccines save money that would otherwise be used in medical care—about $100 for each elder vaccinated.[8]

Acute Bronchitis

What begins as a cold or flu can develop into bronchitis, characterized by a productive cough that brings up a large amount of phlegm. Other symptoms that may occur are chest pains, wheezing, chest congestion, shortness of breath, and mild fever. If the infection is from a virus, antibiotics are not recommended. Even if it is bacterial, the infection may clear on its own. However, elders with pre-existing lung diseases might be prescribed antibiotics as they may have more difficulty clearing the phlegm due to lung damage. Antibiotics may also be prescribed to reduce the secretions. Generally, this infection runs its course in a week or two. If a cough persists, pneumonia or pertussis (whooping cough) needs to be ruled out by a health professional.

Many doctors feel that cough suppressants are unnecessary because coughing serves to clear the mucus; however, over-the-counter expectorants may be useful. Increased fluid intake, humidifiers, or steamy showers can also help. Some individuals require bronchodilators (inhalers) to reduce cough and shortness of breath.

Pneumonia

In general, pneumonia is caused when bacteria that normally inhabit the mouth get aspirated or sucked into the lungs, and the lungs cannot effectively eliminate the pathogens. Although pneumonia can be caused by viruses, fungi, or protozoa, bacterial pneumonia is the most common among older people. Often the bacteria get a foothold after a viral infection (e.g., cold or flu). Individuals who smoke, have respiratory diseases, have heart failure, and are malnourished are at increased risk. People who are bed-bound or immobilized after surgery are likely to develop pneumonia in the lower lobes of their lungs unless they are encouraged to breathe deeply and cough. Those with lung cancer also commonly get pneumonia. Hospitalization itself places one at risk because of increased exposure to bacteria.

People with pneumonia generally exhibit a cough that produces sputum, chest pain with inhalation, shortness of breath, chills, or fever. Elders may not exhibit classic symptoms; instead, they may have mental confusion, weakness, or congestive heart failure. Blood tests to measure white blood cell count, cultures of the blood, microscopic examination of the sputum, and chest X-rays are commonly used diagnostic tests.

Both the incidence of and mortality from pneumonia increase with advancing age. Pneumonia is most common among residents of nursing homes and the critically ill. Elders are more likely to be ill, require hospitalization, have extended hospital stays, have more complications, and die more frequently from pneumonia than younger adults. The cost of care for treating older people with pneumonia is estimated to be more than $1 billion a year.

Before antibiotics were discovered, over half the deaths in the sixth decade of life and 65 percent in the seventh decade of life were due to pneumonia. In his medical text written over a century ago, Sir William Osler defined pneumonia as "a friend of the aged" because it produced a relatively quick and often painless death among the frail old.[9]

Antibiotic therapy has significantly reduced the numbers of people dying from pneumonia. Sometimes antibiotics are prescribed after determining the type of invading bacteria, usually diagnosed from the blood, lung fluid, or sputum. Because it may take days for bacteria to be cultured from these fluids, physicians generally have to guess what type of bacteria is causing the pneumonia and begin treatment with broad-spectrum antibiotics that can kill many types of bacteria. Antibiotics can be provided orally, intravenously, or by injection.

A vaccine to protect against a common type of pneumonia is available, called the pneumococcal vaccine. Although not 100 percent effective, the vaccine significantly reduces the chances of dying from pneumococcal pneumonia. The vaccine is recommended for those over sixty-five years, and earlier if chronic illnesses are present. This vaccine has been widely studied in diverse populations; however some studies report a reduced risk of pneumonia, others find no effect. It appears that the vaccine works better in adults who are healthier and able to mount an adequate immune response. However, those most at risk of dying from pneumococcal pneumonia are those with chronic illnesses and the very old. The general consensus among experts is to immunize both healthy and debilitated elders and possibly revaccinate at age seventy-five. The vaccine lasts about six years, and it is hoped that immunizing elders while they are healthy will protect them later when

they are less able to fight off infection. In a national survey, fewer than half the elders questioned had ever received the vaccine, with the numbers even lower for Hispanic Americans and persons of other ethnic/racial groups.[7] Just as with the influenza vaccine, the cost of the pneumococcal vaccine is covered by Medicare.

Aspiration Pneumonia

A particular threat to elders is aspiration pneumonia, developing when sputum, stomach contents, or food are sucked into the lungs. The stomach acid causes damage to the lung tissues, and the bacteria introduced into the lungs can cause infection. Elders at particular risk are frail elders who have trouble swallowing, are bedridden, confused, semiconscious or sedated, and are fed with a nasogastric tube. Victims of stroke, Parkinson's disease, or Alzheimer's disease fit into this risk category. As a preventive measure, bedridden patients should have their heads and shoulders raised when eating or drinking and should not be prescribed drugs that depress respiration or produce sedation.

Tuberculosis

For many years, tuberculosis was not a significant health problem in our country. However, in the 1980s, the number of cases increased for two reasons: the high numbers of people with AIDS becoming infected because of their reduced immunity, and the emergence of a drug-resistant strain of tuberculosis. The number of tuberculosis cases in our country reached its peak in 1992, and since then, the cases have steadily declined. In 1997, less than 20,000 cases were diagnosed. The incidence of tuberculosis is highest among the elderly: almost one-fourth of the tuberculosis cases in the United States occur among those age sixty-five and older. Also, immigrants who reside in the United States are four to five times more likely to have tuberculosis than the rest of the population. That group accounted for about 40 percent of the total cases of tuberculosis in 1997.[10] It is most likely that they initially became infected in their country of origin. The decrease in the number of cases of tuberculosis over the last few years has been attributed to aggressive control programs.

Tuberculosis is a communicable disease caused by tubercule bacteria. The bacteria are found in the sputum of infected persons and are spread when they become airborne by coughing and sneezing. However, only about one in four persons exposed to the bacteria is infected; of those who do get infected, only one in ten develops symptoms.[11]

In most infected persons, the tubercule bacteria remain dormant in the body for decades. The bacteria can reactivate in those who are frail or have reduced immunity, causing a full-blown infection. In those over sixty-five, tuberculosis infections are a recurrence of the primary disease acquired many years earlier. About 5 to 15 percent of those with latent tuberculosis will develop an active disease during their lifetimes. Corticosteroid drugs that depress immunity, diabetes, and nutritional deficiencies may cause the tuberculosis bacteria to reactivate. Even if older people never had tuberculosis, they may acquire it in a nursing home when one resident reactivates a latent infection, infecting others.

In elders, the symptoms of tuberculosis are generally not dramatic: a chronic cough, loss of appetite or weight, or night sweats. The bacteria can infect virtually every organ system (lungs, kidneys, and bones), and the symptoms depend on which organs are affected. Because tuberculosis can mimic many other diseases, physicians often make the diagnosis by excluding other diseases. However, many physicians neglect to think of tuberculosis, delaying treatment.

The tuberculin skin test determines if an individual has ever been exposed to tuberculosis. If the test is positive, the individual is at risk of reactivating the latent infection later in life. However, when an individual is actually ill with tuberculosis, has another serious illness, or is taking some medications (like corticosteroids), the test may erroneously be negative because their immune system is suppressed. Active infection is proven only when a bacterial culture grows the tuberculosis bacteria. However, it may take six weeks or more to grow, so if tuberculosis is suspected,

appropriate medication should be started immediately. If the culture later shows that no tuberculosis is present, the medication is discontinued. Some physicians recommend that any elder who develops tuberculosis also be tested for the human immunodeficiency virus (HIV).

Tuberculosis must be treated with a combination of several antibiotics over a long period of time (nine to thirty-six months). In some cases (especially in the foreign-born), a highly dangerous form of tuberculosis (multidrug resistant) may be present. It is very difficult to treat and has a high mortality rate. Infected individuals must continue the prescribed drug regimen and have periodic medical evaluations so they can be monitored for treatment effectiveness, drug toxicity, and development of drug-resistant bacteria. Elders can be treated at home. In some areas of the country, those undergoing treatment for tuberculosis are observed taking their medication (directly observed therapy) because, if drug treatment is not taken as directed, the bacteria are more likely to become resistant and highly dangerous. Because the disease is highly infectious, the health of family members also must be under surveillance.

Gastrointestinal Illnesses

Gastrointestinal symptoms such as indigestion, abdominal pain, heartburn, diarrhea, and gas are very common complaints among older people. Some problems related to the gastrointestinal tract are serious and need immediate attention; others are bothersome at times, but not life-threatening. It is extraordinarily difficult for elders and their physicians to identify the cause of many abdominal complaints. This section will discuss the most common gastrointestinal illnesses among older people.

Cavities

Dental caries, more commonly called cavities, are localized areas of tooth destruction that are treated by drilling out the cavity and filling it with a metallic substance. Only 5 percent of Americans never get dental caries, or cavities. Among the

young, most cavities develop on the biting surfaces of teeth. With advancing age and gum reces-
sion, cavities are more likely to develop along the
roots because they are less protected by enamel.
Up to 70 percent of elders with natural teeth
develop root cavities. Elders are also susceptible
to cavities around old fillings. Good oral hygiene
and regular dental care reduces the risk.

Ulcer Disease

Ulcer disease occurs when stomach acid produces small holes in the lining of the stomach or
duodenum (first part of the intestine). Ulcer disease affects up to one in ten Americans. The most
common complaint is abdominal pain that often
occurs in the middle of the night, and may be
relieved by food or antacids. Duodendal ulcers are
more common than peptic ulcers (also known as
gastric ulcers or stomach ulcers). Ulcers can be
self-limiting, or may erode through the stomach or
intestinal wall and cause a surgical emergency.
Occasionally an ulcer signifies a malignancy.

In the past, ulcers were assumed to be caused
by stress. New evidence confirms that the vast
majority of ulcers of the stomach (peptic or gastric) and first part of the intestine (duodenal) are
associated with a bacterium, *Helicobacter pylori*
(*H. pylori*). By age sixty, more than half of elders
carry the bacteria and may have chronic inflammation of the stomach lining. *H. pylori* doesn't
always cause ulcers, and many people carry this
bacteria without any symptoms or signs of ulcer
disease. The infection is generally acquired during
youth, although researchers are not certain exactly
how it is transmitted. The bacteria is most easily
detected by breathing into a bag and analyzing its
contents, or through an endoscopy (a lighted flexible scope guided from the mouth into the stomach
and small intestine), and culture and biopsy of the
intestinal or stomach lining. Treatment can eradi-
cate the bacterium and reduce symptoms. These
various regimens involve taking antibiotics with
medications that block acid secretion. Some regimens require only a few days of treatment, others
require three weeks, and treatments vary in side
effects and cost. The cure rate with the medication

is as high as 90 percent.[12] When the bacteria are
eliminated, the infection rarely recurs.

The second most common cause of peptic ulcer
disease is the use of nonsteroidal anti-inflammatory
drugs (e.g., aspirin, ibuprofen, or naprosyn) that
inhibit prostaglandin production and destroy
the stomach's ability to protect itself from the damaging effects of stomach acid. People with ulcer disease should avoid nonsteroidal anti-inflammatory
drugs, smoking, alcohol, and caffeine. Medications
that reduce acid secretion promote healing (see
chapter 10).

Gallbladder Disease

The incidence of gallbladder problems and gallstones increases with age. Gallbladder operations
are one of the most common surgeries performed in
the United States. Three times as many women suffer from gallstones as men: Native American women
are particularly susceptible. Other identified risk factors for elders are a diet high in cholesterol and fat,
inactivity, hypertension, diabetes, and smoking.

Gallstones are calcium or cholesterol deposits
in the gallbladder that can become as large as an
egg. Most people never even know they have gallstones, only experiencing indigestion, belching,
bloating, nausea, vomiting, and episodes of pain
when fats are ingested. However, if a gallstone
blocks a duct entering or exiting the gallbladder, it
can cause an abrupt onset of severe crampy pain
below the rib cage or in the right shoulder, called a
gallbladder attack. Sometimes nausea and vomiting accompany the pain. The problem usually
resolves on its own if the gallstone successfully
passes through the duct. If recurring bouts are
common, the best diagnostic tool to determine if
surgery is needed is an ultrasound.

Physicians differ in their opinions regarding
the best treatment for gallstones. Some advocate a
cholecystectomy (laparoscopic surgery) to remove
the gallbladder before an acute attack to prevent
complications. The gallbladder is removed with the
help of a viewing tube and special surgical instruments inserted through small abdominal punctures.
In many cases, the surgery can be done on an outpatient basis, and the individual can go home the

same day of surgery. The procedure causes minimal discomfort, decreases recovery time, reduces complications and scarring, and is less expensive than traditional surgery. The procedure is so successful that the number of laparoscopic surgeries on the gallbladder is on the rise, and there is concern that many are unnecessary.

Some physicians advocate a more conservative approach for older people; they suggest not removing the gallbladder until the patient develops a gallbladder attack that does not resolve. However, those older people who have to have an emergency gallbladder removal have a much greater risk of death than those who have elective surgery. More conservative treatments include losing weight, taking antacids, and avoiding fatty foods.

Two nonsurgical treatments are available in some places for those at high risk for surgery, but their success is not yet well-documented. One is a drug that dissolves gallstones when it is placed directly into the patient's gallbladder through a catheter. In the second treatment, the patient is placed in water, and shock waves are focused upon the gallstones to break them into smaller pieces, eliminating the need for surgical removal.

Diverticulitis

Diverticulitis is characterized by an inflammation of the diverticula, which are numerous tiny pouches that protrude from the colon wall. The formation of diverticula increases with advancing age. It is estimated that about 10 percent of people in their forties and 80 percent of people in their eighties have diverticula.[13] Most people do not even realize they have diverticulosis unless a pouch becomes inflamed or ruptures, causing abdominal pain, bloody stools, and change in bowel habits. Diverticulitis is the acute stage of the chronic illness, diverticulosis. These acute complications occur only in about 20 percent of those who have diverticulosis.

It is hypothesized that the cause of diverticulosis is reduced stool bulk due to insufficient dietary fiber intake. Consequently, it takes longer for the stool to pass through the lower gastrointestinal tract. Pressure in the colon is created by increased straining and more forceful contractions of the colon. This elevated pressure eventually weakens the muscle wall of the colon, allowing the inner mucosal lining to slip through. Diverticulitis occurs when a piece of digested food, such as a seed, is trapped in the pouch because feces block the pouch, preventing it from emptying properly. As a result, a bacteria-laden mass forms in the pouch, blocking the blood supply and causing the pouch to become infected and swollen. If it ruptures, an abscess (collection of pus) or a fistula (the colon mistakenly hooks up to another structure such as the bladder, vagina, or another part of the intestine) may form.[14]

Symptoms of diverticulitis include abdominal pain or tenderness in the left side of the abdomen, constipation, and possibly a low-grade fever. The usual treatment for mild cases is a liquid diet, stool softeners, and antibiotic therapy. If symptoms do not improve, hospitalization with intravenous feeding and broad-spectrum antibiotic treatment are necessary. About one in five cases will require surgery to remove the portion of the colon with the affected diverticula. When inflammation is controlled, fiber is added to the diet to prevent further recurrence.

Appendicitis

Appendicitis is caused by a bacterial infection within the appendix, a small pouch located at the juncture between the large and small intestine. The disease usually progresses rapidly. If surgery is not accomplished promptly, the appendix may rupture, causing life-threatening complications. Appendicitis is most common in the teen years, and most cases are reported in those under thirty. Although patients over age sixty account for only 5 to 10 percent of all cases of appendicitis, they comprise more than half of all deaths from the disease.[15] They also have a higher complication rate. A perforated appendix may occur in as many as 70 percent of appendicitis cases among older people. Other complications are postoperative wound infections and increased incidence of blood clots, pneumonia, and heart attacks.

Appendicitis is more risky in the elder population. They may have a reduced immune function and several coexisting chronic diseases that make diagnosis, surgery, and recovery more difficult. Because of fear of hospitals, they may not seek care until the infection is advanced. Also because elders may not have the classic symptoms of appendicitis (fever, nausea, pain in the central abdomen that moves to the right side), they may not be diagnosed properly, increasing the chances of an abscess or a ruptured appendix.

It is often difficult to diagnose appendicitis among elders: up to 50 percent of the time a healthy appendix is removed, and about 20 percent of the time a case of appendicitis is missed, leading to a burst appendix and other complications.[16] Instead of relying on symptoms, it is recommended that a patient get a computed tomography (CT) scan. One study reported that the CT scan results were accurate 98 percent of the time. Since it takes only fifteen minutes to perform, the CT scan will likely become the prime tool to diagnose appendicitis. In addition to benefiting the patient, the cost savings for hospitals is about $500 per patient, and the number of unnecessary appendectomies will be reduced.[17]

Fecal Impaction

Fecal impaction is a consequence of untreated constipation, resulting in hard, dry stools that cannot be passed. This condition is more common than one might think. One year-long study reported that over 40 percent of the patients admitted to geriatric wards had a fecal impaction.[18] The most common symptoms of impaction are lack of appetite, abdominal pain, nausea, and vomiting. The diagnosis may be difficult because patients sometimes have watery diarrhea. This is actually liquid stool passing around the central solid impaction and should *not* be treated with antidiarrheal medications. A rectal examination is critical for accurate diagnosis. Ways to prevent fecal impaction are listed in the previous section on constipation. Treatment for fecal impaction is manual extraction of the fecal mass or an enema. Once an individual has suffered from impaction, bowel abnormalities persist. For example, a larger stool volume is required to stimulate contractions of the colon before an urge to defecate is felt.

Diarrhea

There is no evidence that age itself is a risk factor for diarrhea, but elders are more likely to have conditions that increase its likelihood. Most cases of diarrhea are caused by a nonspecific infection (bacteria, virus, or parasite) that resolves itself in a day or two. The most important risk factor for diarrhea is living in a nursing home because staff, visitors, and new admissions increase the opportunity for new infections to be brought into nursing homes. Further, nursing homes have a high proportion of residents who are demented and incontinent, increasing the likelihood that infection will be spread by the oral-anal route. Frail elders are more likely to become ill when exposed to infectious agents, probably due to lowered immune response. Finally, institutionalized elders are likely to be inactive, even immobile, lengthening the time it takes for waste to go through the intestines, consequently increasing the chance of infections in the intestinal tract.[19] Because the residents are frail and are less able to tolerate dehydrating illnesses, outbreaks of infectious diarrhea cause excess illness and deaths. Health care providers in institutions should learn to initiate early treatment of diarrhea with oral rehydration therapy to prevent dehydration.

Diarrhea can also be a side effect of medication or a symptom of a variety of medical problems. Antibiotic therapy commonly causes a side effect of diarrhea. Medical problems with diarrhea as a symptom are many: cancer, fecal impaction, emotional stress, food intolerance, food poisoning, acute intestinal infection, and abdominal disease. Generally, the treatment is to increase fluid intake in order to reduce dehydration, and to introduce simple constipating foods such as those in the BRAT diet—bananas, rice, apple juice, and toast. Available oral rehydration solutions containing sugar, salt, and water can be given by mouth or through an external feeding tube. It is important not to give antimotility drugs (Lomotil) because they worsen the inflammation. Mild drugs, such as

Pepto-Bismol, may be effective. A medical history and a physical examination are necessary if diarrhea is not resolved in a day or two.

Urinary Tract Infections

Urinary tract infections are the most common type of infections in the elderly, afflicting from 5 to 15 percent of elder men and 10 to 30 percent of elder women. Unlike urinary tract infections in the young that are associated with sexual activity, infections in the elderly are more often associated with debility resulting from chronic illness.

Elders often have health conditions that predispose them to urinary infections, such as incomplete emptying of the bladder, contamination from fecal matter, enlarged prostate, and diabetes. Urinary tract infections are the most common hospital-acquired infections. It is estimated that more than half the population of institutionalized elders has a urinary infection at any one time, often without symptoms. Those who are immobile, are diabetic, and use urinary catheters are at significantly greater risk, which partially accounts for the high incidence of urinary infections among the institutionalized. All patients with permanent urethral catheters acquire a urinary tract infection eventually.[20]

Cystitis and Pyelonephritis

Bladder infections are referred to as cystitis and are less dangerous than kidney infections (pyelonephritis). In the young, urinary infections are more likely to affect the bladder than the kidney. In elders, the opposite is true. The most common infecting organisms are *Escherichia coli* (*E. coli*) bacteria, which normally reside in the intestinal tract. If the infection is limited to the bladder, increased frequency of urination, burning, lower abdominal pain, or fever may be noticed. When the infection spreads to the kidneys and bloodstream, possible symptoms include confusion or bizarre behavior, lower back pain, fever, or general malaise. Many times, elders experience no symptoms with a urinary tract infection.

Treatment varies with the type and location of the infection. Sometimes urinary tract infections resolve on their own without drug treatment. For elders, recommendations are to perform a urine culture to determine the type of bacteria present, then choose a broad-spectrum antibiotic and prescribe it for ten days to two weeks.[21] If the infection spreads to the blood (septicemia), higher strength or intravenous antibiotics and hospitalization are often necessary.

Sexual activity, especially if it is frequent or prolonged, increases the risk of cystitis. Many people call it "honeymoon cystitis." An interesting consequence of the Viagra craze is the increase of cystitis among older women whose husbands were prescribed Viagra. In one medical practice, out of 100 men prescribed the drug, fifteen of their sexual partners (between ages fifty-five and seventy-five) developed cystitis.[22] The easiest strategy to reduce the risk of urinary infections is to drink plenty of fluids and to urinate after sexual activity to cleanse the urethra of bacteria that might have invaded the urinary tract from the anus. For those who get recurrent cystitis from sexual intercourse, taking antibiotics immediately afterwards has been shown to reduce the risk of future infections. It is recommended that sexual activity be avoided when symptoms of cystitis are present.[23]

Other strategies may reduce the number of urinary tract infections. A high fluid intake makes it more difficult for bacteria to get a foothold and is a good general health practice for many other reasons as well. Elder women have a less acidic vaginal pH because of the estrogen decline in menopause. This results in different types of bacteria normally residing in the vagina than when younger. Several researchers have reported that estrogen cream inserted into the vagina acidifies the vagina, significantly reducing the frequency of urinary tract infections in elder women.[24] Another study documented that drinking cranberry juice reduced the frequency of recurrent urinary tract infections among older women.[25] Cranberry juice contains a compound that reduces the ability of bacteria to adhere to walls of the bladder. Women need to be reminded to wipe from "front to back" after a bowel movement to reduce the opportunity that the bacteria normally residing in the colon will not move to the urethra.

Prostatitis

Bacterial prostatitis is rare in younger men, but it is the most common type of urinary infection among men age sixty and over. Its incidence among older men is primarily related to increased prostate size and the use of urinary catheters. The most common type, acute prostatitis, has a rapid onset characterized by fever, chills, and weakness. Local symptoms include increased urinary frequency and pain when urinating. The bacterial cause, usually *E. coli,* can usually be found in a simple urinalysis. When appropriate antibiotics are initiated, the response is dramatic, but these infections often disappear on their own without treatment.

Kidney Stones

About 12 percent of men and 5 percent of women will suffer from kidney stones at some time in their life. These are mineral deposits, mainly calcium oxalate, that form in the kidney. Generally, if they remain in the kidney, they do not cause much pain, but if they move into the ureter, a thin tube connecting the kidney with the bladder, they can cause severe crampy pain, nausea, vomiting, blood in the urine, and urinary frequency. Small stones (a little smaller than the width of a pencil eraser) can often pass on their own in days to months. When this occurs, the individual is advised to drink lots of fluids and take painkillers when needed. However, larger stones require more treatment. Lithotripsy uses shock waves, which are a type of sound waves, to break up the stone. The person is lightly sedated, then immersed in a water bath or asked to lie on a water mattress. The stone is pinpointed and the waves travel through the body until they arrive at the stone, breaking it apart. Lithotripsy has a 70 to 90 percent success rate, and individuals often recover in one to two days. Alternatively, uretoscopy, where a tiny instrument is inserted up through the urethra and the stone is extracted or fragmented, has a higher success rate (over 90 percent) and a slightly longer

recovery period (3 to 4 days). In extreme cases, surgery may be required.

Some people are more prone to developing kidney stones than others; this increased risk is probably related to genetic differences in calcium excretion. A high fluid intake can help prevent stones. It used to be believed that too much calcium intake increased the risk for kidney stones. However, calcium-rich foods and calcium supplements are increasingly recommended to prevent osteoporosis. One large-scale study in women found that those with a higher dietary calcium intake had 35 percent less risk of developing kidney stones.[26]

Vaginal Infections

Thinning and drying of the vaginal walls (atrophic vaginitis) predisposes some elderly women to vaginal infections. Although most postmenopausal women with vaginitis experience no symptoms, a few experience increased vaginal discharge, soreness, burning, or occasional spotting of blood. These symptoms are usually relieved with estrogen cream applied inside the vagina.

Like younger women, elder women can develop other types of vaginal infections, such as bacterial vaginosis or candidiasis (yeast). Bacterial vaginosis is the most common vaginal infection and is characterized by a milky discharge that smells fishy. It is best treated with oral antibiotics or antibiotic creams placed into the vagina. Candidiasis is characterized by itching, redness, and a whitish discharge. This is often a side effect of antibiotic therapy. Women who take broad-spectrum antibiotics often develop yeast infections during or following treatment because the bacteria normally found in the vagina are destroyed, allowing the yeast to grow. Women who take corticosteroids and who are diabetic are also at high risk for yeast infections. Elder women are far less likely to be affected by such sexually transmitted vaginal infections as trichomonas, chlamydia, or gonorrhea than young women, likely because of fewer sexual partners.

Several treatments are available for those with vaginal infections. Eating a cup of yogurt a day that contains live acidophilis bacteria reduces the risk of yeast infections. Over-the-counter antifungal creams or suppositories are also effective. For those who do not want to take strong drugs, an alternative remedy is to place a boric acid capsule into the vagina every night for a week. In both fungal (yeast) and bacterial infections, women may not experience any symptoms, and infections may regress spontaneously without treatment.

Pressure Ulcers

Decubitus ulcers, also called bedsores, pressure ulcers, or pressure sores, are localized areas of tissue death that develop when soft tissue is compressed between a bony prominence and an external surface for a prolonged period of time. The skin tissue is progressively destroyed by unrelieved pressure that does not permit an adequate blood supply to the skin. If left untreated, pressure ulcers rapidly spread into underlying tissues, eventually invading the bone. Pressure ulcers occur predominantly among those who are immobilized in bed or a wheelchair and are common among disabled, hospitalized, or institutionalized elders. Estimates vary widely, but about one in four nursing home residents and one in ten hospital patients has pressure ulcers. If ulcers are left untreated, they can result in severe disability and death. Experts estimate that nearly 2 million patients in hospitals and nursing homes in our country develop pressure ulcers, and 60,000 people die each year from them.

The amount of pressure and time needed to produce an ulcer depends on the condition of the individual. Changes in the skin can occur with as little as two hours of pressure on an area. A sore may begin with a reddened area of the skin, and, if not attended, can progress to a deep cavity of dead tissue that is highly susceptible to infection and, ultimately, gangrene. Once the skin ulcerates, it takes an average of one year to heal.[27]

Pressure ulcers are common among those with spinal injuries, the frail, and the immobile, even with good nursing care. Those who are obese, underweight, malnourished, incontinent,

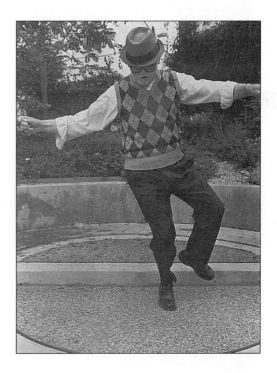

diabetic, confused, or highly sedated are also at high risk for pressure sores. In the obese, fat tissue does not have many blood vessels, which makes the skin more susceptible to blood loss. On the other hand, those who are very underweight do not have sufficient fat or muscle to cushion bony protuberances. The localization of bedsores depends on whether the person is sitting or lying. The most likely locations for bedsores are on the heel, lower back, knee, pelvis, hip, or buttocks. Refer to figure 9.1 for common sites of pressure ulcers.

A pressure ulcer must be regularly cleaned and protected so it does not worsen. Special mattresses, frequent turning and skin substitutes (known as tegaderm, tegasorb) can be used to prevent further breakdown and aid healing. Antibiotics are sometimes needed if the ulcers are infected. Patients recovering from pressure ulcers need a high protein diet to supply the body with nutrients to build antibodies and repair tissues. Serious pressure ulcers are treated with laser therapy or tissue grafts.[29]

Pressure ulcers form where bone causes the greatest force on the skin and tissue and squeezes them against an outside surface. This may be where bony parts of the body press against other body parts, a mattress, or a chair. In persons who must stay in bed, most pressure ulcers form on the lower back below the waist (sacrum), the hip bone (trochanter), and on the heels. In people in chairs or wheelchairs, the exact spot where pressure ulcers form depends on the sitting position. Pressure ulcers can also form on the knees, ankles, shoulder blades, back of the head, and spine.

Nerves normally "tell" the body when to move to relieve pressure on the skin. Persons in bed who are unable to move may get pressure ulcers after as little as one to two hours. Persons who sit in chairs and who cannot move can get pressure ulcers in even less time because the force on the skin is greater.

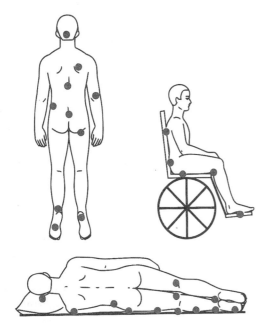

Figure 9.1
Common Sites for Pressure Ulcers.[29]
From Agency for Health Care Policy Research. Preventing pressure ulcers: a patient's guide. 1992. Rockville, MD: Author. No. 92-0048.

The best prevention for pressure ulcers is attentive nursing care. Ideally, institutions should determine which patients are at high risk for pressure ulcers upon admission and give them special attention throughout their stay. Daily skin inspection for those at special risk (chair and bedbound) is important. Their diet should be high in proteins, calories, and fluids, and they should be kept active, if possible. Because the biggest factor in pressure sore development is pressure of bone against an external surface, moving the chair-bound or bedbound patient every two hours is imperative. Some experts believe some patients need to be turned every half-hour, using specific lifting and turning techniques. Incontinent patients must be kept clean and dry because urine can lead to skin breakdown. Dynamic devices circulate air or fluid in a mattress and are useful for high-risk patients. Static devices to relieve pressure, such as sheepskin pads, waterbeds, and foam padding, are sometimes helpful for patient comfort. Good skin care, including body oils and massages, increases blood flow to the skin.[29]

Since pressure ulcers are a common and serious problem in nursing homes, it is imperative that education be directed to all levels of health care providers, patients, family, and caregivers. A program for prevention of pressure ulcers should be developed with an understanding of the abilities and needs of the groups receiving the education. The program should include seven core topics: cause and risk factors for pressure ulcers, methods to assess risks, how to assess skin, selection and proper use of support surfaces, how to develop and implement an individualized skin care program, how to position and move to decrease risk of tissue breakdown, and how to document important information about the patient.[29] Implementation of such programs in the nursing home setting would significantly reduce the suffering and excess deaths caused by lack of attention to pressure sores.

Shingles

Herpes zoster, also called varicella zoster virus, but most commonly called shingles, is an extremely painful latent infection. It invades the body when a person is young in the form of chicken pox. Since the body does not destroy all the viruses, those that remain find refuge in the nerve tissue near the spinal cord, where they remain dormant for years. Disease, stress, or weakened immunity may trigger an attack although the majority of affected persons are apparently healthy. Even though most adults carry the latent virus, only about 20 percent ever get shingles. Although shingles may occur among all age groups, it is more commonly reactivated in those aged fifty and older.

Upon reactivation, the zoster virus travels from the spinal nerves to the skin, causing a very painful rash of pea-sized blisters, usually on a band clustered on one side of the trunk or face. Some people experience only mild discomfort: others experience excruciating pain, especially where clothing touches the skin. The rash and pain usually last from two to three weeks. In up to one-half of those elders with shingles, nerve pain persists for months or years after the rash disappears (called postherpetic neuralgia). The biggest challenge in treating shingles is how to deal with the chronic pain still present long after the blisters heal. For some, the extended period of severe pain may be so demoralizing that it leads to prolonged depression.

Treatment depends on the severity of the infection. For those with mild shingles, talcum powder, cornstarch, calamine lotion, wet compresses, and analgesics are helpful. A cream made with hot peppers (capsaicin) reduces nerve sensitivity and pain in many cases. For more serious infections, physicians used to prescribe cortisone to prevent the complication of long-lasting pain after the shingles attack. However, cortisone depresses the immune system and may cause the shingles to spread to other parts of the body. An antiviral drug designed for herpes zoster, called famciclovir, is now prescribed because it has been shown to heal the rash quicker, slow the replication of the virus, and reduce the duration of postherpetic neuralgia by half.[30] Treatment should be started as soon as possible for the maximum effect of the drug. Shingles is highly contagious;

however, individuals who have had varicella (chicken pox) or who have received the varicella vaccine do not have to worry about acquiring a second infection.

Acquired Immune Deficiency Syndrome (AIDS)

AIDS is caused by the human immunodeficiency virus (HIV) that is transmitted from person to person in blood and semen. Over time, the virus disables the immune system by attacking specific types of lymphocytes, the T-helper cells. Once the virus infects the body, the person may have no symptoms for years, then may manifest only vague symptoms such as fatigue, loss of appetite, night sweats, diarrhea, or increased susceptibility to colds. Later, the person becomes more disabled, loses weight, and becomes very susceptible to opportunistic infections (that is, infections that usually do not affect those with normal immunity). Examples of opportunistic infections include tuberculosis, widespread herpes, cytomegalovirus, pneumocystic pneumonia, or fungal meningitis. When individuals with HIV antibodies in their blood (HIV positive) develop a major opportunistic infection or manifest other severe signs of infection, they have AIDS. The three major mechanisms to contract AIDS for any age group are intercourse (anal and vaginal), sharing needles among intravenous drug abusers, and blood transfusions.

AIDS is epidemic in the United States. In 1996, almost 70,000 individuals over twelve years old had AIDS. Eleven percent of that total were individuals fifty years and older. This proportion has remained stable since 1991. Of those fifty and over, about three-fourths were between fifty and sixty, 14 percent were between sixty and sixty-four, and 12 percent were sixty-five and older. For the over-fifty group, males accounted for 84 percent of the cases, and African Americans accounted for 43 percent of the total. In both the thirteen to forty-nine and the fifty and above age groups, the highest exposure category was men having sex with men.[31]

AIDS Education: Seniors Need It, Too

Tampa, Florida—Sue Saunders is 65 and has AIDS. As far as she's concerned, the more people who know it the better.

Saunders pioneered a project in her hometown of Fort Lauderdale to educate Floridians over age 50 about the risk of developing acquired immune deficiency syndrome.

Her first challenge was getting the attention of an age group largely ignored when it comes to AIDS education.

"Yes, there is sex after 50. After 60. After 70. People think after 50 we die from the neck down," Saunders said. "People look at you like you're crazy. What? You mean Grandma and Grandpa are still having sex?"

Ten percent of all AIDS cases in the country are people over age 50, according to the Florida Department of Elder Affairs. In Florida, the figure is higher—ranging between 12 and 14 percent.

One in eight Floridians living with AIDS is 50 or older, state health officials said. Yet when groups are addressed that are considered at risk of contracting the virus that causes AIDS, older Americans are often left out.

Eighteen months ago, Saunders began inviting herself to small South Florida groups to discuss prevention, promote education and warn seniors to abstain from sex or use condoms.

"You're telling people 50 to 90 years old: 'You are at risk for a fatal disease. You just went to bed with a guy and you don't know where he's been.'"

Saunders was healthy and active. She was divorced, in love, and in a longtime relationship. Her Bahamian boyfriend was the spark of her life. They spent lazy days on the water, fishing. Life was good. That was in 1990.

Suddenly her boyfriend was diagnosed HIV positive. Nine months later, he was dead. She feared the same thing would happen to her and began saying goodbye to her four grown children.

A son took her to an HIV-infected doctor in Laguna Beach, Calif. That visit helped change her life.

She dropped the self-pity and went to the Broward County Health Department but found little information. After six months doing research, she went to Bently Lipscomg, elder affairs secretary, who found $170,000 to fund SHIP, the Senior HIV Intervention Project.

Saunders worked long and hard getting into the crowded retirement condominiums along Florida's Gold Coast to give her message. In these building complexes, women outnumber men seven-to-one, she said.

The women are starved for affection. The men are having a ball. They can have all the women they want.

"Everybody says, 'It can't happen to me. I'm not a prostitute. I don't fool around,'" she said. "You're never too old. And all it takes is one partner—if he or she is infected."

Older people are rarely targeted for prevention. The health care system, including doctors, often is reluctant or uneasy about discussing AIDS and sex with them, said Dave Bruns, elder affairs spokesman.

"Not only is it an insult, it's rampant ageism," Bruns said. "Just who do they think is buying all this Viagra?"

There are 67,282 cases of AIDS state-wide and 8,400 of those infected are age 50 or older, according to the Florida Department of Health.

When Saunders left the SHIP program recently, the demand for lectures was enormous. "Everybody wanted us to come talk to them," she said. They were scheduling 20 to 30 presentations a month.

The project was so successful, a second program was launched in the Tampa Bay area under Edith Ellerson in June. She encountered similar apprehension as she started talking at senior centers, assisted-living residences, senior nutritional programs.

Gradually, the audiences became more receptive and willing to listen. She brings condoms, urges listeners to be tested and find out first about themselves, then question their partners.

"You're not only sleeping with your partner, but with whomever your partner slept with for the past five years, and whoever they slept with—like a pyramid or domino effect," she said.

By Pat Leisner, Associate Press Writer
Copyright Associated Press

In 1996, 13 percent of those age fifty and over diagnosed with AIDS died within a month of their diagnosis, more than twice the percentage of those thirteen to forty-nine. One possibility for the short interval from diagnosis to death are age-associated changes in the immune system that may make elders become sicker and die sooner than younger persons. Or, elders may not respond as well to antiviral medications as the young. However, it is more likely that older persons are not promptly tested for HIV following the onset of HIV-related illness, and when they are diagnosed, it is later in the course of the disease than the young. There are several reasons for this. Physicians often neglect to conduct sexual histories and to consider HIV infection in their elder patients, possibly because of discomfort or disbelief of elder sexuality. Further, elder gay men may be less open to talking to the physician about their sexual practices than younger men. Finally, AIDS is difficult to identify among older people because the symptoms are vague and mimic many age changes and chronic illnesses common to elders. Many elders with AIDS may have a dementia that is easily misdiagnosed as Alzheimer's disease. For whatever reason, later diagnosis means a delay in initiating therapy to prevent the progression of the disease.

Older persons may not be tested for HIV because they do not believe they are at high risk for HIV infection, or they may be unwilling to admit their risky sexual behaviors. Two large national surveys found that older people were one-sixth as likely to use condoms and one-fifth as likely to have been tested for HIV as people in their twenties.[32] Another study found that older women with heterosexually acquired AIDS were less likely than younger women to have used a condom before their HIV diagnosis, and were less likely to have been tested for HIV before being hospitalized with an infection due to AIDS than a comparison group without AIDS.[33] Finally, heterosexual elders are less informed about AIDS, AIDS risk factors, and safe sex practices than younger persons, although homosexual elders are better informed.[32]

Health professionals must educate older persons about AIDS because the lack of education allows them to believe they are not at risk. Schools of medicine and nursing also need to prepare health professionals to confront the reality of AIDS in older people because it will likely become even more prevalent in that age group in the years to come.

Current protocols for treating people with AIDS are changing rapidly as new treatments are developed. Most people infected with HIV can be treated with antiviral medications including AZT and newer protease inhibitors that are quite costly but that slow disease progression. Individual opportunistic infections are treated with antibiotics and other medications. Managing AIDS cases in older patients is particularly difficult; physicians must manage the opportunistic infections, chronic diseases, and polypharmacy in the face of their patients' diminishing physical reserves, as well as the multiple problems inherent in treating persons with AIDS. However, AIDS is fatal: treatment only prolongs the course of the disease because there is no cure.

The proportion of older people with AIDS will increase in the future as the young who are currently infected with HIV grow older and the progression of AIDS is slowed with antiviral medications. In time, AIDS may become another chronic disease, like diabetes, that requires a lifetime of medical management. The increase of AIDS among elders brings many new dilemmas. For one, the medications used to forestall the illness are very costly, from $20,000 to $40,000 annually. Little is known about the interaction of HIV medications with other chronic illnesses, or about HIV medication regimens commonly prescribed to elders. There is still a stigma attached to AIDS that may affect the care that elder AIDS patients receive.

Although most AIDS patients are cared for in the home by informal caregivers, many also rely on home health services and hospice care. Nursing homes are often used in the latter stages of the disease. A program in New York called SAGE (Senior Action in a Gay Environment) provides social support and education services to older gay men and lesbian women who are dealing with HIV/AIDS—either to those infected or their caregivers, friends, or relatives. For more information, contact SAGE at 202-741-2247.

Dehydration

Dehydration, defined as the rapid loss of greater than 3 percent of body weight, is a common condition among the elderly. Two factors place them at high risk for dehydration: insufficient fluid intake and excessive fluid loss. Older people are less likely to be thirsty and, when they do drink, they may not drink a sufficient quantity of water. Insufficient fluid intake becomes more significant when the need for fluid increases, such as infection, diarrhea, and fever, and some medications. The traditional symptoms of dehydration are not as obvious among elders, making early diagnosis difficult. If left untreated, the death rate may exceed 50 percent.[34]

Dehydration is often due to an infection, and the dehydration can become serious enough to require hospitalization. One regional survey of hospital discharges reported that the average age of patients admitted with dehydration as one of the main diagnoses was eighty years, and the average length of stay was almost two weeks.[35] Hospital care of patients with dehydration is expensive, costing more than $1 billion a year.[34]

Evaluation of dehydration involves a thorough assessment of medication use (especially diuretics), medical illnesses, and bowel and bladder function. Once identified, adequate oral hydration is generally sufficient when the underlying cause is treated. In some cases, fluids must be given intravenously.

Dizziness

Dizziness is a common complaint of elders and can mean different things to different people. Dizziness is not a disease, but a symptom of many diseases or disorders. Serious illnesses, medication reaction, dehydration, infections, or other conditions may cause dizziness. Those with persistent dizziness should visit a physician because a thorough exam will often reveal its cause.

There are two major types of dizziness: vertigo and disequilibrium. *Vertigo* refers to a particular type of dizziness characterized by the sensation of movement felt in the head (room is spinning). A common cause is a viral infection that has disturbed the balance mechanism of the inner ear. Vertigo may occur as a side effect of medication or injury to the head. In contrast, *disequilibrium* causes unsteadiness in the body, not the head. The individual may feel he or she is about to faint. This could be caused by low blood pressure or a medication side effect.

One type of vertigo is *benign positional vertigo*. Some people develop short episodes of vertigo, lasting less than a minute after changing the position of the head. This is thought to be caused by tiny granules of calcium that build up in the semicircular canals of the inner ear. Treatment involves moving the head to a position to bring on the vertigo, and holding it there for a few minutes. Then the head is moved 90 degrees and held again for a few minutes. Over the next few days, the head is to be kept upright. These simple maneuvers can reposition the granules and provide permanent relief.

Orthostatic hypotension is a temporary condition of low blood pressure that occurs with position change. In this condition, the heart does not move the blood with enough force to supply the brain adequately. Symptoms include sudden feelings of faintness, light headedness, or dizziness when standing up quickly. Because the muscles of the aging blood vessels are weak and the arteries are inadequate in helping convey blood to the head, older people are particularly susceptible to this condition. Older persons who do not sit or lie down at the first sensation of dizziness may lose their balance.

Light-headedness might occur during stressful circumstances, sometimes accompanied by heart palpitations and panic. Many people can induce this state by breathing deeply and rapidly for a few minutes (hyperventilating). Hyperventilation triggered by anxiety or depression may be the underlying cause of many patients' complaints of dizziness.

Environmentally Induced Acute Illnesses

Because humans are warm-blooded animals, body temperature remains fairly constant whether the environmental temperature is hot or cold. When the body is cold, metabolic rate increases to warm the blood, capillaries in the extremities constrict to preserve warm blood in the core, and the body shivers and develops goose bumps to reduce the loss of body heat from the skin surface. When the body is too warm, the metabolic rate slows, the capillaries in the extremities widen to release heat, and perspiration is produced to cool the body surface by evaporation.

The normal body temperature fluctuates about 2 or 3°F within a twenty-four-hour period, generally decreasing at night and increasing during the day. This section will discuss hyperthermia (raised body temperature) and hypothermia (lowered body temperature), two emergencies that result when the body temperature lies outside the normal range. Both hyperthermia and hypothermia are more common and more serious in older people. Elders need to be educated concerning the symptoms of temperature-related conditions and their consequences since they may be fatal.

At highest risk of hyperthermia and hypothermia are the frail, chronically ill, users of certain prescription drugs, the poor, and those who live alone. Many medicines can impair the physiological response to heat and cold: diuretics, many heart medications, antidiabetes drugs, psychoactive drugs, and antihistamines. Elders taking these medications should be aware of their increased vulnerability to heat and cold.

Hyperthermia

Hyperthermia occurs when the body temperature is 100°F or more because of infection or high environmental temperatures. Hyperthermia can result in illness, injury, even death. Except for children fourteen years and below, the incidence of hyperthermia increases with age, especially for those over fifty-five. Major risk factors for heat-related illnesses and death are use of medications that impair heat loss, poor physical condition, chronic heart and respiratory conditions, recent fever, diarrhea, or dehydration, and obesity. Several

---

A Case of Heatstroke[39]

A 63-year-old man who worked as a messenger collapsed on a city sidewalk on the first warm day of spring. In the emergency department, he was in a deep coma. His skin was hot, dry, and mottled. Blood pressure was low, heart rate was 170 beats per minute, breathing was slowed, and rectal temperature was 112°F. His pupils were unreactive.

The patient was covered with ice and wet sheets, and fans were directed across his body. Shivering noted at the onset of cooling was suppressed by giving him a shot of a particular drug with an intravenous diazepam. He was given sugar water and electrolytes intravenously. One hour after arrival in the emergency department, his temperature was 101°F, and he was dried and covered with a light sheet. He continued to get intravenous solutions; within two hours, he had an adequate output of urine, and blood pressure increased. Rapid pulse decreased slowly over the next 8 hours.

On the next day, the patient was disoriented but able to follow simple commands. All abnormal lab findings began to resolve by the third day. On the sixth day, results of a neurological examination were normal except for mild cognitive impairment.

factors may impair the normal physiological response to extended heat exposure. In general, elders require a higher core body temperature to initiate sweating, and less sweat is produced per gland.

Increased hospital admission rates of older people have been recorded during heat waves.[36] About 80 percent of all deaths from heat occur in those over age fifty. Heat-related deaths due to weather conditions are underreported because hot weather conditions also increase mortality from respiratory and cardiovascular diseases. Thus, even if the death was caused by hyperthermia, it would likely be reported as respiratory or cardiovascular disease on the death certificate.[37] A particularly deadly heat wave occurred in Chicago in 1995, claiming over 700 lives. Those at highest risk for death were frail elders confined to bed, the socially isolated, and elders without access to air conditioning.[38]

The most common heat-related illnesses among elders, especially the frail, are heatstroke and heat exhaustion. *Heatstroke,* a life-threatening emergency, is characterized by a high internal body temperature (at or above 105°F) caused by lack of sweating, and altered mental status (delirium and disorientation). Heatstroke may be caused by exertion among healthy persons who work in hot environments or by medical problems or medications that impair thirst and sweat mechanisms during hot weather. Most episodes of heatstroke occur in temperatures over 90°F with humidity over 50 percent. To treat heatstroke, the body temperature must be reduced rapidly by ice water washes or baths. Medical personnel should be contacted as soon as possible.[39] Despite medical care, heatstroke is often fatal.

Heat exhaustion is slower in onset and is not life-threatening. This condition results from excessive loss of water and salts and often occurs in elders who use diuretics. Weakness, light-headedness, and fatigue are common symptoms. Treatment for heat exhaustion is to reduce the body temperature if it is elevated and to give liquids to replace depleted fluids and electrolytes.

To prevent heat-related conditions in hot weather, elders should keep cool, avoid heavy exertion, and drink adequate fluids. The hottest hours of the day should be spent indoors, preferably with air conditioning. If their homes have no cooling system, elders should go to the mall or the library in the hottest part of the day. Elders should drink more water than is necessary to satisfy their thirst. Alcoholic drinks and salt tablets should be avoided. Cool baths or showers, increased ventilation, forgoing vigorous exercise, and dressing in lightweight clothing will reduce the effects of the heat. Because problems with heat regulation are most extreme among frail elders, it is important that they be under surveillance of family members, neighbors, or health professionals during hot weather.

Hypothermia

While a cold environment can be harmful at any age, it is especially hazardous for the old; nearly half the victims of hypothermia are elderly. With advancing age, elders tend to lose muscle mass, and their blood vessels at the skin surface are less able to constrict in response to cold. Hypothermia occurs when the body temperature drops below 95°F because of exposure to a cold environment without sufficient protection. The combination of frailty, immobility, and the inability to regulate body temperature can result in hypothermia. Hypothermia may even occur after exposure to mildly cool temperatures. For example, a frail person might get hypothermia after spending an extended period of time indoors at temperatures between 60 and 65°F without adequate warm clothing.

People with hypothermia have a high risk of death, but elders are more likely to die of hypothermia than younger people. Experts believe the incidence of hypothermia is underreported. Because its symptoms mimic those of other disorders, elders who die of hypothermia often manifest a number of other chronic conditions that are more likely to be listed as the cause of death.

Hypothermia may take a few days to develop. When body temperature is reduced, the following occur: metabolic rate decreases, heart rate slows, pulse weakens, blood flow decreases to the brain, reflexes are slowed, and the victim may become confused, feel drowsy, or fall into a coma. A person with hypothermia often shivers uncontrollably, has a slow, irregular heartbeat, slurred speech, slow shallow breathing, feels sluggish, and lacks coordination. The victim may not complain about feeling cold. The signs of hypothermia may be confused with those of a stroke, diabetic coma, heart attack, or other conditions.

Treating victims of accidental hypothermia involves warming their core body temperature with hot water bottles, electric blankets, or another's body heat. If conscious, the victim should be administered warm fluids. If unconscious, the victim's head should be lowered and feet raised to prevent shock. Upon hospitalization, the victim sometimes is administered transfusions of warm blood. The most serious problem during hypothermia and rewarming of the body is ventricular fibrillation, a form of irregular heartbeat that can lead to death. The odds of recovery depend on the severity, length of exposure, and previous general health. Hypothermia can worsen pre-existing chronic conditions such as heart disease and diabetes. Serious hypothermia can damage the kidney, liver, or pancreas.

Hypothermia can be prevented by keeping the house warm in cold weather, wearing warm clothing, using an electric blanket, maintaining fluid and calorie intake, refraining from alcohol consumption, and keeping active. Elders should be encouraged to dress warmly in cold weather, even if they don't feel cold, and to wear a hat outdoors. For the poor, subsidizing fuel costs and financial support for home weatherization programs reduce the incidence of hypothermia. Prevention of hypothermia is similar to prevention of hyperthermia: frail older people living alone should be monitored by family, neighbors, or social service workers.

A newly discovered cause of hypothermia that may significantly affect the older population occurs in the hospital environment. Surgical procedures usually are accomplished in cold operating rooms with lightly clad patients. Further, almost all anaesthetics impair the body's natural response to cold: patients can no longer shiver to generate warmth, and their blood vessels cannot constrict to retain heat. When this effect is combined with below–body temperature intravenous fluid and blood administration, the reduced body temperature may affect recovery after surgery. Once the patient is wheeled into the recovery room and the anaesthetic wears off, the body temperature may be 4°F below normal. In this situation, the brain produces high concentrations of stress hormones to quickly increase body temperature. These chemicals can adversely affect the heart.

Two Cases of Hypothermia[44]

Case 1: In December 1996, an 80-year-old woman was found lying dead in a ditch near the nursing home in which she resided. The decedent had Alzheimer's disease, Parkinson's disease, and congestive heart failure, and had been reported missing from the nursing home approximately 12 hours earlier. She was fully clothed, and an autopsy indicated no evidence of life-threatening trauma, pre-existing infection, or new intracranial hemorrhage. The outside temperature during the period she was presumed to be outside was approximately 40°F. There was no detectable blood alcohol. The cause of death was listed as hypothermia attributed to environmental exposure.

Case 2: In February 1997, an 83-year-old man was found dead in his home. He had no known history of medical problems. He was partially dressed, and there were no signs of traumatic injury. The temperatures during the preceding days had been below freezing, and there was no heat in the house. The cause of death was listed as exposure to cold.

Frank and his colleagues compared two groups of people who went in for surgery,[40] other than on the heart, but were at high risk of cardiac problems. One group was covered only with thin cotton blankets during and after surgery, and the other group had their temperatures kept normal with blankets with tiny jets that bathed the patient in warm air. The group kept warm had half as many heart complications within twenty-four hours after surgery as those who were not, showing that hypothermia induced by surgical procedures may have significant consequences.[41]

ACCIDENTS

Unintentional injuries are the seventh-leading cause of death among elders. Even though elders constitute less than 13 percent of the total population, they comprised 30 percent of all accidental deaths in 1994.[42]

Not only are elders as a group more than twice as likely to suffer accidents than younger people, but also their rates of illness and death are higher following an accident. Elders are more apt to become injured during an accident, their injuries are more often serious, they are more likely to be hospitalized, they take longer to heal, and they are more likely to die than younger groups. Older accident victims also remain in the hospital significantly longer than their younger counterparts.

Accidents are responsible for a significant proportion of hospital care expenses. The average length of hospital stay for accident victims over age sixty-five is longer than for most diseases. Aside from the cost, the consequences of accidents may be increased dependence, permanent physical damage, institutionalization, and death. In some cases, there may be no lingering physical effect, but self-confidence is reduced, causing excessive cautiousness because of the fear of a future accident.

Even though the risk of injury or death due to accidents increases with advanced age, chronological age itself is not the cause. Individual susceptibility is very important. Age-associated physiological deficits in vision, hearing, muscular strength, and coordination play a role, as do drug side effects, symptoms of some chronic health problems, and psychological factors. The following section will explore the multiple factors that make some elders more susceptible to accidents than others. Also, the most common types of accidents among this age group will be discussed: falls, driver and pedestrian accidents, burns, and choking. Finally, the importance of medical assessment after the accident and accident prevention strategies will be addressed.

Factors Increasing Accident Susceptibility

Contrary to popular opinion, an accident is not due to fate, chance, or luck; instead, it is a combination of individual susceptibility and environmental hazards. Elders are particularly susceptible to accidents due to age-associated physiological decrements. Also, numerous chronic and acute illnesses can increase the risk of accidents, as can the side effects from medications. Nutritional status, psychological state, and environmental hazards are other factors that predispose elders to accidents. The following paragraphs will describe the multiplicity of factors that promote accidents in elders.

Although the effects of aging vary considerably among elders, there is a general decline in the neurosensory system that reduces awareness of and reaction to environmental hazards. Decreased visual acuity is a significant factor in falls among elders.[43] Hearing deficits, commonly experienced among elders, may result in a failure to hear signs of an impending accident. Additionally, temperature and pain receptors in the skin are not as efficient in many elders, increasing the possibility of scalding and hypothermia.

Multiple chronic diseases among elders increase their susceptibility to accidents. Circulatory disorders causing transient light-headedness can temporarily impair blood flow to the brain. Orthostatic hypotension results from a temporary loss of blood flow to the brain as the blood pools in the lower extremities when one gets up rapidly after lying down or sitting. It is believed that orthostatic hypotension occurs in up to 30 percent of elders living at home and more than 50 percent of those in nursing homes.[44] Many elders also report intermittent dizziness that impairs their ability to maintain balance. Small strokes and cardiac arrhythmias temporarily reduce blood to the brain and can cause falls. Because diabetics have reduced blood flow to their legs, they have reduced pain and pressure sensation in their feet, increasing their susceptibility to falls.

Diseases of the central nervous system also increase accident risk. For instance, people with organic brain disorders may experience disorientation, memory loss, poor judgment, poor comprehension, or emotional imbalances that affect awareness and appropriate response to the environment.

Musculoskeletal disorders often increase accident susceptibility. Arthritis can reduce joint flexibility so that when balance is lost, it is difficult to recover quickly enough to avert a fall. A significant number of falls may be due to "drop attacks," a condition in which an elder experiences a sudden weakness of the legs, loses control, and falls. The elder does not lose consciousness, but needs assistance in rising. Drop attacks are thought to be due to arthritic changes in the neck that impair blood flow to the brain, especially when the head is tilted backwards.

Individuals with gait disturbances are more susceptible to accidents, especially falls and pedestrian accidents. The stooped posture and shuffling walk of some older people make them more susceptible to tripping and decreases their ability to catch themselves when they begin to fall. Many elders have increased body sway, further increasing the tendency to fall. Not surprisingly, these postural limitations are most common in the very old and frail. Many musculoskeletal diseases cause gait disturbances that increase the likelihood of accidents (e.g., arthritis and Parkinson's disease). Elders relying on walking aids, such as canes and walkers, are even more susceptible to accidents.

Other problems in walking may be due to foot conditions, such as sore or deformed feet. The American Podiatry Association estimates that 80 percent of those over age fifty have at least one foot condition. Elders with such conditions are more likely to wear loose-fitting shoes or floppy slippers, or to go barefoot, causing further gait disturbances and increased risk of falls or other injuries.

The side effects of many medications increase the likelihood of accidents. Psychoactive drugs such as antipsychotics, antidepressants, or antianxiety medications can produce drowsiness and reduce awareness of environmental hazards. Both barbiturates and alcohol are an important cause of falls at night and during a hangover because they commonly produce drowsiness, distort judgment, and impair motor response. A large number of drugs may induce postural hypotension with consequent dizziness and possible falls; these include diuretics, sedatives, antidepressants, and diabetic medications.

Psychological status also affects accident susceptibility. Any illness, regardless of symptoms, tends to cause a detachment from the environment. Preoccupation with illness reduces alertness and decreases self-care, which increases susceptibility to accidents. Depressed people have slower psychomotor function, and they are unable to react quickly enough to the environment to avoid danger. Some mental illnesses make an individual oblivious to his or her surroundings, resulting in poor judgment.

Accidents are more likely to occur during or after periods of transient emotional stress. When individuals are temporarily tense, angry, anxious, or frightened, they are preoccupied with emotions and less alert to danger. Furthermore, in an intense emotional state, the ability to respond to danger is temporarily impaired. An elder who is usually cautious may become accident-prone under the stress of loss and grief. Conversely, an older person who suffers repeated falls, scalds, or other accidents may be under psychological distress.

Some older people are at higher risk of accidents because of denial or anger at their physical limitations. Some may deny their physical limitations because the limitations are a concrete reminder of growing old. They may insist that they are as capable as ever and can do the same activities with the same intensity as when they were young. This denial can place older persons at risk of falling because they may refuse to ask for or accept assistance, may insist on living alone when it is no longer safe for them to do so, or may engage in activities that put them in danger.

My Children Are Coming Today

My children are coming today. They mean well. But they worry.

They think I should have a railing in the hall. A telephone in the kitchen. They want someone to come in when I take a bath.

They really don't like my living alone.

Help me to be grateful for their concern. And help them to understand that I have to do what I can as long as I can.

They're right when they say there are risks. I might fall. I might leave the stove on. But there is no challenge, no possibility of triumph, no real aliveness without risk.

When they were young and climbed trees and rode bicycles and went away to camp, I was terrified. But I let them go.

Because to hold them would have hurt them.

Now our roles are reversed. Help them see.

Keep me from being grim or stubborn about it. But don't let me let them smother me.

From E. Maclay. 1977. *Green Winter.* New York: Reader's Digest Press.

Although it is healthy to try to be as independent as possible, sometimes the desire for independence outstrips an individual's physical capacity. In this situation, the person needs assistance in developing alternative ways to perform daily tasks that maintain dignity. The sense of helplessness in those who are dependent can produce unconscious feelings of rage and fear. These individuals may take risks because they no longer have goals or a strong will to live. However, despite family support and counseling, some older people refuse to alter an unsafe living situation. If they are competent to make that decision for themselves (e.g., they understand the possible consequences of their behavior), there is nothing to be done except to encourage the elder to accept support in the home.

Some contributors to accident susceptibility can be reduced or eliminated. For instance, the types of drugs or their dosage can be changed, vision and hearing impairments can be lessened, and symptoms of some chronic illnesses can be reduced. However, some health problems cannot be corrected, and the individual must learn to adjust to them.

Some experts estimate that the number of accidents could be reduced significantly if environmental hazards were eliminated. Unlike individual factors that increase susceptibility to accidents, environmental hazards are simple to find and remove. Several types of home checklists are available for that purpose. These lists are valuable for everyone to assess their living space to prevent future accidents. More importantly, a list should be used when a human service worker does a home visit, and deficiencies should be remedied. This type of accident prevention may even save the life of a frail elder.

Common Types of Accidents

The majority of accidental deaths among elders are from falls and vehicular and pedestrian accidents. From ages sixty-five to seventy-four, accidental deaths from motor vehicles are the most common, but among those seventy-five and older, falls are the most common. When both elder groups are combined, falls are the most common cause of accidental deaths, causing one-third of all accidental deaths. The second most common cause of accidental deaths are those relating to motor vehicles. Deaths due to choking, surgical and medical complications, fires, and burns are responsible for most of the remainder of the accidental deaths among those sixty-five and over.[42] Figure 9.2 compares the accidental injury death rates by age. This section will discuss the five most common types of accidents resulting in death that occur among elders: falls, motor vehicle and pedestrian accidents, fires and burns, and choking.

Falls

Falls commonly occur among elders, both at home and in institutions. The number of falls experienced and the number of injuries and deaths by falls increase with advanced age. Despite the high inci-

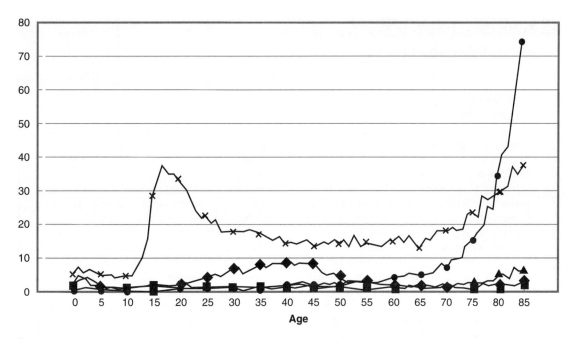

● Falls

◆ Poisoning
(solids, liquids)

■ Drowning

▲ Fires

✕ Motor vehicle

Figure 9.2
Unintentional-Injury Death Rates by Age: 1994.

dence of falls among elders, most falls are not serious. Researchers estimate that even though about one-third of people aged sixty-five and over fall every year, only 10 to 15 percent result in injury.[45,46] About half the injuries are bone fractures. Experts estimate that fall-related fractures cost the nation $10 billion a year in acute care costs.[47] Fractures in the elderly are serious and are often followed by declining health, decreased mobility, reduced independence, and premature death. Falls are a strong predictor of nursing home placement.[48]

Many factors are associated with an increased risk of falls. A fall can be a sign of illness, such as pneumonia, stroke, or dehydration. Mood-altering drugs, such as tranquilizers, antidepressants, sleep medication and antianxiety agents, are consistently shown to be related to increased falls and hip fractures. It is not known whether the side effects of particular drugs are responsible for the falls, or whether the types of illnesses for which the drugs are prescribed are to blame. One study found an association between incidence of hip fracture and the recent filling of prescriptions for certain tranquilizers and sleep medications, such as Valium, Librium, and Dalmane, which take a long time for the body to eliminate. The rate of hip fracture increased with dosage, but when the drug was discontinued, the risk of falling reverted to that of a

Falls, Their Consequences, and Prevention

- A 90-year-old woman has lived independently since her husband died fifteen years ago. Although her daughter helps her with her shopping and she no longer drives, she is able to do everything for herself and is fiercely independent. After suffering a stomach flu, she becomes dehydrated and dizzy and falls in her apartment. The first time, she is bruised; the second time, she catches the side of her leg on the table and develops a laceration. The third time, she fractures her hip and is unable to get to the phone to summon help. She is discovered about 8 hours later after her daughter notes she does not answer the phone. She is taken to a local hospital where the hip is repaired surgically. She recovers somewhat, but requires a stay in a nursing home because she has become weaker. She dies of pneumonia three months later.

- A 76-year-old woman is nearly blind, but can get around her tiny apartment by feel. When she develops an episode of heart failure, she is hospitalized. The medication she is given for sleep causes confusion, and when she awakens at night to go to the bathroom, she forgets she is not at home. She stumbles to the bathroom and falls, with the IV pole on top of her. Her confusion worsens, and she cannot remember to stay in bed. She is given drugs to sedate her, which worsen the confusion and delirium until she is agitated and is restrained in the bed. Her recovery is delayed, and she loses the ability to ambulate because of bedrest.

- An 86-year-old man lives with his elderly wife in a tiny house that is so full of furniture and memorabilia that it is difficult to walk through. He has Alzheimer's disease and tends to wander at night. A home visit by a nurse uncovers safety hazards in the home. The home has steep steps covered with a slippery shag carpet. The man frequently walks through the house in crocheted slippers his wife has made for him. The light is poor, there are no grab rails, and some parts of the home have only narrow pathways to walk through the clutter. The wife is assisted in reducing the clutter by giving furniture to her children and neighbors, she purchases a baby monitor to better monitor her husband's activities, attaches a gate to the bottom of the steps, and moves her husband's bed downstairs. He is dressed in no-slick shoes, and light bulb wattage is increased to improve visibility.

nonuser.[49] Another study reported that those elders using antidepressants, even the newer medications, had a risk two to three times those not on medication.[50] In a study of nursing home residents, antidepressant use was strongly related to falls among women, but there was no relationship between falls and antidepressants among the men.[51]

Although the frequency of falling is highest among the frail, when vigorous older people fall, they are more likely to have serious injuries. Those older people who are strong and mobile may be in more danger because they can get into situations where significant damage might occur (e.g., participating in sports, carrying heavy items, or climbing a ladder), while the frail elder usually cannot.[52] Men over sixty-five have a higher rate of deaths from falls than do women, possibly reflecting a higher likelihood of risk-taking activities.

Almost half the falls in the home among elders involve floors, rugs, and stairs. Tripping over the edge of a rug, slipping on scatter rugs and highly waxed floors, and moving from one flooring type to another are common causes of accidents. Staircases, especially those that are poorly lighted without handrails, can be hazardous. Elders often miss the first or last step. However, environmental dangers seldom cause accidents among healthy and active elders. Those who are physically or psychologically vulnerable are at much greater risk. Pets may cause falls among elders. Examples are tripping over a dog underfoot and loss of balance from unexpected pulls by a leashed dog.

The Public Health Service estimates that two-thirds of all deaths due to falls are preventable. Many risk factors for falls can be modified. Use of a home safety checklist by the elder or caregiver is helpful in reducing environmental hazards. Review of medications and dosages, avoidance of alcohol or sedatives, and frequent evaluations of vision and hearing can reduce the propensity for accidents. Falls can be reduced by physical conditioning programs to increase strength, balance, and mobility among elders. One study with community elders was successful in reducing the incidence of falls by modifying medications after review and instituting an exercise program.[53] Another study was able to increase balance among elders through tai chi.[54] Appropriate footwear helps balance and stability. Loose-fitting slippers or stocking feet should not be worn. There is evidence that hard, thin-soled shoes provide more stability and "foot awareness" than thick-soled walking or running shoes.[55]

Orthostatic hypotension, a rapid fall in blood pressure upon rising, causes dizziness that can lead to a fall. One study of nursing home residents reported that more than half the subjects had a significant blood pressure drop upon rising. Those on antipsychotic or antiparkinsonian drugs were more likely to experience the effect. And it didn't matter whether the blood pressure was initially high or low, the degree of change was most important. The phenomenon occurred most often before breakfast.[44] Gradual position changes upon rising, allowing the body to acclimate, can also serve to prevent falls.

Institutionalization, even with its increased patient surveillance, does not decrease the risk of falling. In fact, severe falls are much more common among the institutionalized than those living at home. Institutionalized patients are at higher risk of falling because they are more likely to have many underlying illnesses, be confused and disoriented, have problems moving about, and take medications that affect brain function. Furthermore, patients with a history of falling and those with visual problems were more apt to fall. Although those who fall in institutions have a low death and injury rate, there is often significant immobility after a fall, resulting in extended stays at the institution, and demoralizing the patient and family.

There is a widely held belief that physically restraining frail elder patients reduces the incidence of falls. Depending on the patient's condition and institutional protocol, a patient at high risk may be strapped to the bed or wheelchair. Side rails may be used, and in severe cases, even straitjackets. However, it is now well-documented that restraints are ineffective in preventing falls and, in fact, may increase falls and serious injury.[56–58] Physical restraints may agitate the patient, consequently increasing the accident risk as he or she attempts to become free. Another way to restrain is to use medication such as tranquilizers and sedatives. However, numerous studies document that such drugs place elders at higher risk of falling than those not taking them.

The number of accidents among institutionalized elders can be reduced by training all personnel in transferring patients and assessing the facility for hazards that might increase falls. Periodically assessing medication type and dosages, using night lights, and orienting the newly admitted patient to the hospital environment are also helpful. One randomized trial found that a comprehensive individualized assessment and interventions targeting environmental and personal safety, wheelchair use, psychotropic drug use, transfers, and ambulation resulted in significantly fewer falls.[59]

Only about 1 percent of all falls result in hip fractures; however, hip fractures account for most of the disability, death, and medical costs associated with falls. Hip fractures alone are responsible for two of five admissions to nursing homes.[60] Hip fractures occur about twice as frequently among older women than older men. Women with osteoporosis are most susceptible to hip fracture. The incidence of hip fractures increases exponentially with age: among those age ninety and older, one-third of women and one-sixth of men will suffer a hip fracture at some point before they die.[61]

The effects of hip fracture upon the individual are tremendous. Following hip fractures, elders are hospitalized, and approximately 5 percent suffer serious complications and death while there. Only about one-third of elders are able to go back home after hospitalization from a hip fracture: the majority must go to a nursing facility. Those elders who survive hospitalization suffer a mortality rate of over 40 percent in the first six months afterwards.[62] In one study of elderly women a year after a hip fracture, less than a third returned to former levels of functioning, only about one-fifth were able to walk independently, and one-fifth were still depressed at one year.[63]

Mortality increases during the first four to six months after a hip fracture. Rehabilitation must be implemented during this time frame. Because of the trend toward shortened length of stay in the hospital setting, it is important to advocate home and nursing home rehabilitation programs.

Falls may create psychological consequences among elders. One study describes "post-fall syndrome," the anxiety an individual has regarding the ability to walk after experiencing being on the floor for an hour or more before being found after a fall. Even if they had only minor injuries, after they have recovered, they will only attempt to walk if accompanied by another person or by holding on to furniture. Similarly, "fallaphobia," an abnormal fear of falling by a person who has fallen before, may include a panic attack (sudden anxiety, dizziness, heart palpitations) when attempting an activity that previously resulted in a fall. Fallaphobia may occur even when a fall is not serious. Up to a quarter of those who have fallen limit their daily activities because of fear of falling again.[46]

Paradoxically, the preoccupation with the fear of falling, although it might reduce a person's engagement in a fall-related activity, may also increase the risk of falling. The goal is to minimize the person's anxiety and maximize strength, balance, and safety. Such reassurance can be accomplished by education, therapy, and correction of physical and environmental hazards associated with that activity. Although some degree of fear of falling may be prudent, unnecessary restriction of activity leads to a downward spiral of dependency.

Motor Vehicle Accidents

"I can barely hear, barely see, and can barely walk. Things could be worse though. At least I can still drive."[71]

Motor vehicle accidents are the leading cause of accidental death among elders age sixty-five to seventy-four and the second leading cause of those seventy-five and over.[42] Overall, older drivers account for the fewest miles driven, the least number of crashes, and lowest crash rate of all age groups. They rarely drink and drive, speed, or drive without a license. Elder drivers are involved in a small percentage of all accidents compared to other age groups. However, when the data are analyzed on a per-mile basis, drivers aged seventy-five and over have the worst record: 11.5 crashes per 100 million miles. In contrast, the average number of crashes for all drivers is 3.0 per 100 million miles, and for the sixteen to nineteen age group, it is 9.2 crashes per 100 million miles. The rates are similar for injuries.[64] Further, elders are more likely to sustain serious injuries, hospitalization, and death from motor vehicle accidents than younger age groups.[65]

Although there is a clear association with increasing risk and advancing age, there is wide variability among elders in miles driven and driving skills. A number of physiological factors can predispose older people to motor vehicle accidents. Vision problems are significant because these commonly occur in older people, and their gradual onset may make the elder unaware of their level of disability. Furthermore, the motor vehicle licensure vision chart may not adequately screen for vision problems. Elders commonly have reduced peripheral vision, have diminished night vision, and are more susceptible to glare than younger groups. Elders are more likely to have chronic illnesses such as diabetes, heart disease, Parkinson's disease, and stroke, which are associated with increased risk of driving accidents. Mental impairments, related to Alzheimer's disease or strokes, may affect judgment

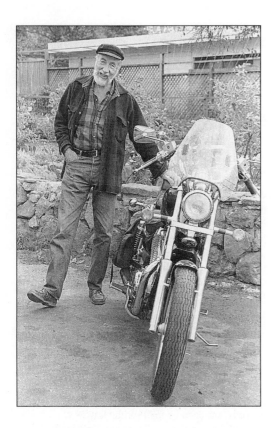

and increase the rate of driving errors. Arthritis and osteoporosis make it more difficult to turn the head in order to directly note traffic patterns. Feet problems or coordination difficulties, as well as diminished reaction times, can cause difficulties. Antihistamines, benzodiazepines, opioids, and many other prescription drugs may cause confusion, drowsiness, and impaired reflexes, consequently reducing driving skill.

Much research has been conducted to identify physical and cognitive factors that impact driving skills among elders. According to one report, important factors to consider are the person's past driving record, signs of alcohol abuse, lapses of attention or memory, diminished reaction time, use of medications that cause drowsiness or impair judgment, ability to follow directions, and the results of a vision test.[66] One study found that adverse driving events (crash, tickets) were more common in those individuals who could only walk a block a day, who had foot abnormalities, and those with slight mental impairments. Only 6 percent of those with none of these three problems had an adverse event, compared to 12 percent of those with one problem, 26 percent of those with two problems, and 47 percent with all three problems.[67] Another report tested driving ability, visual perception, and memory of older drivers and compared them with a group of young drivers. The older drivers without mental impaiments drove as well as the young. But those with mild mental impairment, no matter what their age, made serious driving errors. The authors suggest that mild mental impairment be used as a criterion for license restriction or revocation.[68]

There are certain driving patterns that are characteristic of elderly drivers. Older drivers are more likely to not yield the right of way, to not observe signs and signals, and to have turning violations. On the other hand, they are less likely to be cited for reckless driving or drinking while driving. In urban areas, elderly drivers are overrepresented in accidents involving turns, parking, or head-on crashes.[69] Elders often drive with a spouse or "copilot" in the car for assistance. Although two may see some hazards more easily than one, this is dangerous because two partially impaired individuals cannot react to an emergency situation with only one behind the wheel.

How can it be determined whether an individual is still safe to drive? Although standard procedures exist to diagnose almost every health problem of older people, there is no agreement about how to assess their driving ability. Over 2,500 physicians subscribing to a prominent medical journal in geriatrics responded to a survey assessing their reported behaviors and knowledge concerning driving in their older patients. Their procedures in dealing with older drivers were varied. There was also a lack of consensus on the criteria that physicians used to assess their patients' driving skills. Interestingly, three-fourths of the respondents did not keep records of their patient's driving status, and almost two-thirds never referred a patient to the state licensing agency.

What is Your Opinion? Elder Drivers

Dear Ann Landers: You printed a letter laying it on the line about the hazards of elderly drivers. My father, who is nearly 90, was having eye problems. One afternoon, his vehicle was not in his garage, so I went over later and asked where he'd been. His answer was, "My eyes were bothering me. I couldn't read and couldn't watch TV so I went for a drive." Scary, isn't it?

From Anchorage, Alaska: A 78-year-old man was driving the car that hit me. He refused to admit that he was in the wrong lane to make a turn. The police officer gave him a ticket. He contested it and won. I don't think he lied. I doubt that he knew what he was doing. So now this elderly, befuddled man has a clear record and will probably cause another accident. I hope he doesn't kill somebody.

Boca Raton, Florida: A friend of mine who is 87 years old received his new driver's license in the mail. It's good for six-and-a-half years. Another friend, who had a stroke and is paralyzed on his left side, drives over to see him every day. He also received his license in the mail without taking a test. Florida is a great state to live in with many benefits for seniors, but some of its laws need updating.

Fort Myers, Florida: I know an 85-year-old man from Ohio who received his driver's license by mail. This man ran over "three trash cans" and left the accident scene not knowing he had killed three little girls. He was not required to have a doctor's test or an eye test, and he thought he ran over three trash cans. What does it take to get the laws changed?

New Jersey: My grandfather should have stopped driving years ago, but no one wanted to deprive him of his independence. What happened? He hit a family standing on a corner and changed everyone's lives forever. Grandpa and his wife are now in a great deal of physical and emotional pain, not to mention the survivors of the family he hit. Please, Ann, print this message in large type: SENIORS: WHEN YOU FEEL YOURSELF SLIPPING, STOP DRIVING BEFORE YOU KILL YOURSELF AND SOME INNOCENT BYSTANDERS.

Desert Hot Springs, California: So you were shocked at the issuance of a driver's license to an 88-year-old Florida woman? I live in California and am 87. I received my renewal license in February. Issuance has been by mail for the last 24 years, each for a full four-year term. P.S.: I am totally deaf.

This Is Ann talking now. Mandatory retesting for drivers over the age of 70 should be a must in every state. Driving should not be a lifetime right.

Permission granted by Ann Landers and Syndicate (Creators).

Nevertheless, 87 percent agreed that they had a legal responsibility to assess a patient's driving ability but were uncertain about how to do it and what their responsibility was toward their older patients who drive.[70] Because physicians are aware of the physical and mental limitations of their patients, and because their views are respected, they are in a position to recommend driving limitations to protect the elder as well as other drivers and pedestrians. Limitations such as driving only in town during nonrush hours and only in daylight may be a reasonable compromise.

When family members of friends voice concern or when an elder accumulates traffic citations, reducing or eliminating driving should be considered. Referral to a doctor, the department of motor vehicles, or an occupational therapist may be helpful in this evaluation; although, as mentioned above, physicians are not certain how to assess an elder's ability to drive and tend to leave the decision up to the individual. This issue has to be handled very carefully because serious psychosocial consequences may result when an individual is no longer permitted to drive.

In our country, the ability to drive represents competence and independence and is a message to others that they are functional and capable adults. The problem is compounded by the lack of public transportation in many areas. Giving up driving often means a loss of social contact and status. They start to feel old and dependent. Families and medical personnel may be concerned about safety of the elder, but decisions must be made, taking into account both benefits and risks of the elder driver remaining behind the wheel.[71]

Elders, in general, are often aware of their decreasing abilities and adjust their driving accordingly. One study of older drivers reported that the majority stopped driving gradually, usually by eliminating night driving, driving in heavy or fast traffic, and reducing miles driven when they noticed a decline in their ability. Most in that group decided on their own when it was time to stop driving.[72] The second, but less common, pattern of discontinuing driving was a sudden disabling event, prohibiting driving ability.[71] However, more subtle visual or cognitive deficits may limit elders' ability to self-regulate driving practices.

Educating elders about those factors that increase their risk of car accidents can reduce their incidence. Older people must be cautioned about driving when they are using drugs that interfere with driving skill, such as those affecting perception and reaction time. Keeping elders updated on the current driving rules might also increase their confidence and reduce accidents. The American Association for Retired Persons (AARP) offers such a community education program for drivers over fifty-five. It is an eight-hour program, usually given in two days. The focus is to help older people understand physical changes that come with aging and their effect on driving skills. To find out if AARP's program is offered near you, write them at 1909 K Street, N.W., Washington, D.C. 20049. Elderly drivers who complete driver education courses have significantly fewer accidents and traffic violations, and attendance is often rewarded with insurance premium reductions.

Our country is experiencing a rapid growth in the number of older drivers, and in a few years, the baby boomers will be elders. Almost one of three drivers are over fifty-five, and the number of drivers over seventy-five is increasing the most rapidly. Although many elders escape physical and cognitive disorders, as a group they are more likely to exhibit such impairments that compromise driving safety. Because there are many areas in the country that do not have adequate public transportation, many elders continue to drive (either by necessity or desire) to preserve independence and social contacts, despite these limitations. The effect this will have on driving statistics in our country may be significant.

Driving license requirements set up by each state have the potential to directly affect the safety of the elder driver. Driving problems may be detected more quickly if frequent testing of elders is required. But measurements of driving abilities should be based on individual skills, not age alone. Who will test, what will be measured, and what instrument will be used to determine driving ability? As of yet, there is no unified approach to assessing the driving skill of the older driver. In 1991, thirty-eight states required vision tests, and four required a written test for all drivers wishing to renew their licenses. Those states requiring vision testing had fewer fatal crashes among drivers seventy and older than those states not mandating such tests.[73]

Pedestrian Accidents

Death rates for pedestrians struck by vehicles increase after middle age. Not only are elder pedestrians more likely to be hit by a motor vehicle, but they also are more likely to die from it. Their injuries are more serious because the bones of an elder are more likely to break, and their wounds take longer to heal than their younger counterparts. Death rates are highest among pedestrians living in downtown areas and progressively decrease in less populated living environments.[74]

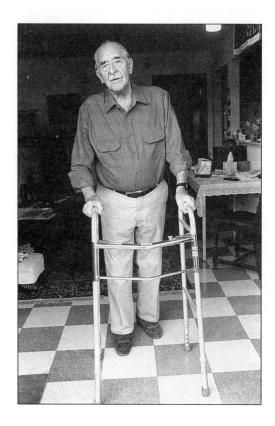

Reducing Your Risk of Pedestrian Accidents

- To guarantee plenty of crossing time, wait for a new green light before starting across the street.
- Whenever possible, wait to cross with other pedestrians.
- Look both ways before stepping into a crosswalk, even when the light indicates you may walk.
- Be alert for drivers who are turning. Before crossing the street, get their attention by making eye contact.
- Cross only at intersections. Do not jaywalk and do not walk between parked cars or in front of or behind a stopped bus or truck.
- Wear reflective or white clothing or reflector patches if out at night. Carry a flashlight.
- Stand on the curb, not on the street, while waiting to cross.
- Whenever possible, walk on sidewalks, not on the road. If you must walk on the road, use the left side facing the oncoming traffic.
- Concentrate on the traffic around you as well as what you are doing and where you are going.
- If you are on medication or have used alcohol, be wary of their side effects.
- Do not carry umbrellas or packages in a way that blocks your vision or hampers your ability to walk.

Although older pedestrians are generally more cautious than younger groups, hearing and vision impairments, problems in walking, and other disabilities increase their susceptibility to pedestrian accidents. The majority of elder pedestrian accidents occur at crosswalk intersections. There are many reasons that crosswalks are particularly hazardous. Older people are less able to judge the speed and distance of oncoming vehicles. Crosswalk green lights often do not last long enough for slow-moving elders to safely cross the street. One study found that less than 1 percent of people seventy-two and older had a normal walking speed sufficient to cross the street in the time typically allotted at average intersections. Even in neighborhoods with light adjusted for elders, only 7 percent could get across in time.[75] Providing for more realistic crossing time to reflect elder's range of abilities would not only decrease injuries, but also would give elder pedestrians a greater feeling of independence. Another way to help elders cross busy intersections is to use a wide median strip at signalized intersections. Difficulty in ascending and descending street curbs also increases pedestrian accident risk. In this case, ramps would make the crossing more accessible. Additionally, the lack of extra energy to run out of harm's way increases with age and disability.

Most fatal pedestrian accidents among older people occur in early evening. Whether it is because the driver is unable to see the older pedestrian or vice versa is not clear. However, a significant number of elder pedestrian deaths and injuries occur after the pedestrian has violated a traffic law or done something unsafe. One community reduced pedestrian accidents by 43 percent after initiating changes such as lengthening traffic signals, installing pedestrian signals on traffic islands, making signals and crosswalks more visible, increasing enforcement of speed limits, and making educational presentations to seniors.[76] A few communities have installed a built-in crosswalk warning system that consists of flashing lights embedded in the street on both sides of the crosswalk. When a pedestrian steps into the walkway, lights are either activated by a button pushed by the pedestrian, or a sensory device is activated when the person enters the crosswalk. In any case, the row of embedded lights are activated, warning motorists. This signal costs a lot less than a traffic light ($20,000 instead of up to $150,000 for a traffic light).[77]

Fires and Burns

Accidents due to fire and burns are not nearly as common as falls among elders, but when they occur, they are more likely to cause serious injury or death. About one-fourth of those killed each year from fires and burns are sixty-five and over.[42] Most deaths from fire are caused indirectly: about four-fifths are due to smoke and gas inhalation. Careless personal behaviors, especially leaving lighted cigarettes untended, are the primary causes of fire accidents in younger adults. Among older adults, faulty electrical products such as electric blankets or electric heaters more commonly cause fires. The second most common causes of fires and burns are cooking accidents. One type of preventable accident occurs among older women wearing bathrobes with dangling sleeves while they are making tea. Severe burn injuries are caused as the sleeve ignites when it drags across a lighted burner when reaching for the kettle on the back burner. Accessible fire extinguishers in the kitchen are important to reduce the consequences of cooking accidents.

When a fire occurs, elders are more susceptible to injury or death than the young. If they are frail, they are less able to respond quickly enough to prevent injury. Many times, fire-related injuries are due to cognitive impairments. Furthermore, many older people live alone and have nobody to alert them and get them to safety. Not uncommonly, elders trap themselves in their homes because they have installed multiple locks that are difficult to open when an emergency arises. The risk of accidents from fires and burns can be greatly reduced by installing smoke detectors and checking them periodically to be sure that they work. It is also helpful to devise a fire escape plan.

Although not as serious, burn injuries due to hot liquids, or scalding, are much more common than burns due to fire. Elders are particularly vulnerable to scalding because of their decreased pain and temperature sensation. Many elders, especially those with diabetes or other health problems, soak their feet in hot water then later realize they have severely burned themselves. Water temperature and duration of exposure affect the severity of the burn. Tap water at 140°F will cause a serious burn after only a few seconds, whereas water at 120°F will cause the same burn in ten minutes. Almost all scald injuries could be prevented by adjusting the temperature of the household water heater to 120°F or below.

Choking

Respiratory obstruction, or choking, is common among the very old and the very young. Elders, however, are more likely to die from choking than children: over 2,000 elders died by choking in 1994.[42] Choking occurs when an obstruction (food, vomited matter, mucus, or even water) enters the windpipe instead of the esophagus, blocking air passages. Choking is more likely among people who have difficulty swallowing, such as those with neurological problems (e.g., stroke, Alzheimer's and Parkinson's diseases). Other factors that contribute to unintentional aspiration of food or fluid into the lungs are overmedication, alcohol intoxication, poor eating position, poorly fitting dentures, missing teeth, and emotional excitement.

Home Safety Checklist

General Considerations
Can the person climb the stairs to enter and exit?
Is the neighborhood safe?
Is the house clean?
Is the house insulated and well-ventilated?
Are there signs of neglect (old food, dirty clothes, unwashed dishes)?
Is the food supply sufficient?

Exterior
Are step surfaces nonslip?
Are step edges visually marked to avoid tripping?
Are steps in good repair?
Are stairway handrails present? Are they securely fastened to fittings?
Are walkways slip- and trip-free?
Is there sufficient outdoor light available to provide safe walking at night?
Are the stairways and landings free of stored items?
Are garden hoses and tools out of the walkway?
Is the walkway free of leaves and snow?

Interior
Are lights bright enough to compensate for limited vision?
Are light switches accessible upon entering rooms?
Are night lights strategically placed throughout house, especially on stairs and route from bed to bath and bed to kitchen?
Are lights glare-free?
Are stairway carpets and molding edges securely fastened and in good condition?
Are throw rugs at the head or foot of the stairs?
Are throw rugs secured with non-slip backing?
Are handrails present and secure on both sides of staircases?
Are step edges outlined with colored adhesive tape and slip-resistant?
Are carpet edges taped or tacked down?
Is the floor material in good repair?
Are rooms uncluttered to permit unobstructed mobility?
Do low-lying objects (coffee tables, step stools, etc.) present a tripping hazard?
Are telephones accessible?
Are any phone or electrical cords located in walkways?
Is furniture secure enough and nontrippable to provide support if leaned upon for mobility assistance?

Are chairs of proper height and equipped with armrests to help in getting in and out?
Are wheelchairs and other walking aids in good working condition? Can they be safely used in all areas of house?
Are there any overloaded electrical outlets or frayed electrical wires?
Is the hot water heater set at 120°F or below?
Does the resident have an escape plan in case of fire?

Kitchen
Are storage areas easily reachable without having to stand on tiptoes or chairs?
Are the linoleum floors slippery?
Is there a nonslip mat by the sink area to soak up spilled water?
Are chairs wheel-free, equipped with arm rests, and of proper height to sit down and get up?
If the pilot light goes out on the gas stove, is the odor strong enough to alert the person?
Are step stools strong enough to provide support? Are their treads in good repair and slip-resistant?
Is a smoke alarm present and functional?

Bathroom
Are doors wide enough to provide unobstructed entering with or without a device?
Does door threshold present a tripping hazard?
Are floors slippery, especially when wet?
Are skid-proof strips or mats in place in the tub or shower?
Are tub or grab bars available? Are they securely fastened to the walls?
Are toilets low in height? Is an elevated toilet seat available to assist getting on and off the toilet?
If a throw rug is used, does it have a nonslip rubber backing?

Bedroom
Are night lights and/or bedside lighting available for getting up at night?
Is the path from the bed to the bath clear?
Are beds of appropriate height for ease in getting in and out of bed?
Are bed mattresses sag-resistant at the edges to provide good sitting support?
Are floors nonslip and trip-free? Can the person easily reach objects on closet shelves?
Is a smoke alarm present and functional outside the bedroom door?

The typical choking victim is unable to speak, makes high pitched sounds when gasping, grabs the throat, turns pale, and then blue. If the individual can speak or cough, the obstruction is likely partial, and you should not interfere with his or her own attempts to dislodge the object. Sometimes people who are choking may show no evidence of distress except they suddenly stop eating and talking, then collapse. The act may be misinterpreted as a heart attack. In any case, a choking person will sustain permanent brain damage from lack of oxygen unless the object is removed within minutes.

If it looks as if the individual is not able to cough up the object (cannot speak, cough, or breathe), get someone to call an ambulance, then work quickly to unblock the airway. The safest and easiest first aid procedure for removing a foreign object from the windpipe is to perform a series of quick thrusts to the victim's abdomen. The thrusts push in the abdomen which force air out of the lungs to push the object out of the airway. The rescuer stands behind the victim and wraps her arms around the victim's waist (above the navel and below the rib cage). A fist is made with one hand, then grabbed with the other hand. Subsequent quick inward and upward thrusts into the abdomen should be continued until the airway is cleared or the victim becomes unconscious. If the victim is too big to reach around and give effective abdominal thrusts, give chest thrusts. When alone, give yourself abdominal thrusts with your fists, or press your abdomen onto a firm object, such as the back of a chair. Continue using stronger thrusts until the object is expelled.[78]

Medical Assessment after an Accident

The first concern of medical personnel after an accident is to look for signs of treatable injury. As soon as the acute problems from the accident are stabilized, the circumstances surrounding the accident should be explored. A careful accident history includes the following questions: What was the person doing at the time? Were physical symptoms present before the accident? What symptoms occurred at the time of the accident? It is seldom easy to determine the circumstances leading up to an accident because elders may be very vague about how it happened, or they may not remember any physical symptoms preceding it. In falls, many are not willing to disclose how they fell because they may have been doing something dangerous or foolish. If witnesses were present during the episode, they should be questioned so the cause of the accident can be better determined. Questions regarding the presence of environmental hazards should also be asked.

A comprehensive physical assessment should be part of the evaluation after an accident. Unfortunately, physicians too often make the assumption that accidents are due to old age and merely examine and treat the injuries without ascertaining their cause. Accidents are often the result of disease, drug side effects (sleepiness, dizziness, weakness, and confusion), or other serious conditions. Disorders of vision, hearing, and balance are common correlates of accidents and should be checked. Many chronic and acute illnesses predispose one to falls, so both a physical examination and medical history are necessary. One study reported that, in a physical assessment of 160 nursing home patients who had recently fallen, more than two active medical problems were identified for each patient. Ninety-two percent of those problems were identified for the first time during the postfall exam.[79]

Health professionals can reduce accident susceptibility by correcting vision and hearing disorders, diagnosing acute illnesses and bringing them under control, reducing the symptoms of chronic illnesses, and altering drug dosages. Patients with balance problems may be directed to do exercises that increase balance and instill confidence. Those with gait problems may be prescribed a cane, walker, or wheelchair. Since elders who use mobility aids are more susceptible to falls, elders should be taught to use them properly. When a physical limitation cannot be reduced, it is important that health professionals explain the limitation and counsel elders on accepting their disabilities and learning to accommodate them. Rehabilitation therapists are especially helpful in this regard.

A home visit can clarify whether an environmental hazard contributed to the accident. A checklist will enable the assessor to determine the safety of the environment and suggest improvements that reduce accident risks. A home visit is especially important for those who are already frail. Family members should be instructed on safety practices and how to reduce environmental hazards, especially if the elder has a history of falls.

Accident Prevention

There is a great need for both health professionals and elders to learn how to prevent accidents. Not only do accidents cause unnecessary deaths, but also those who survive may have serious disabilities and be dependent upon others for the remainder of their lives. Estimates vary, but as many as two-thirds of the accidents occurring among elders may be prevented by treating underlying medical conditions and reducing environmental hazards.

As mentioned previously, safety programs for elders and their families and friends can significantly reduce the environmental hazards associated with many accidents. Education is also important for health and social service providers so they can recognize environmental hazards when they visit elders in their homes. The National Safety Council (444 N. Michigan Avenue, Chicago, IL 60611) provides materials to assist providers in educating elders regarding accident prevention, including a home-safety checklist.

It is reasonable that family and friends of frail elders, especially those living alone, are concerned about their safety. But overprotectiveness can undermine self-confidence, increase unnecessary cautiousness, and promote anxiety. There are many constructive ways that family and friends can assist the frail elder living at home. For instance, caregivers can help eliminate environmental hazards, make daily phone calls or visits, and monitor drug intake. To reduce elders' fear of falling and not being found for days, some communities have services that provide daily visits, phone calls, or monitoring devices.

SUMMARY

Although chronic conditions account for the majority of death and disability among elders, acute conditions and accidents remain an important cause of illness and death. For a number of reasons, older people are more likely to suffer from infections and accidents than other age groups.

Acute illnesses may be more difficult to diagnose in elders because symptoms may be vague, and warning symptoms may be absent. Common acute illnesses of elders include respiratory infections, gastrointestinal conditions, urinary tract infections, vaginal infections, and environmentally induced illnesses (hypothermia and hyperthermia).

Even though elders comprise only 13 percent of the population in the United States, they comprise 30 percent of all accidental deaths. Common accidents among elders include falls, vehicular and pedestrian accidents, burns, and choking. Because so many factors can contribute to an accident, health professionals should conduct a thorough assessment to prevent further accidents and to treat underlying conditions. Accident prevention programs are effective in reducing accident susceptibility among elders.

ACTIVITIES

1. Last year, what was the death rate from accidents among persons sixty-five and older in your state? What about specific accident types? How do death rates among elders differ from those between ages eighteen to sixty-four? Using statistics, draft an argument opposing any driving for those drivers over age seventy. Now, do the same for a proposal supporting reduced restrictions on elder drivers.

2. What programs in your community reduce accidents among elders (e.g., driver education for those over sixty-five, safety checks of homes)? Compile a list of ways your community could further decrease accidents among elders.

3. Interview a group of elders and a group of younger people about their fear of accidents and how they consciously prevent accidents. Do elders seem to be more preoccupied with avoiding activities that may cause accidents? In your estimation, are some too cautious?

4. Question elders on their knowledge of prevention and treatment of acute illnesses. How do they know whether their conditions are severe enough to see a doctor? What methods do they use to prevent or treat minor acute illnesses?

5. Attend a senior nutrition site, senior center, or other places where elders congregate, and look for environmental hazards that may cause falls. Write a letter to the director outlining the problems and suggestions to reduce them.

6. Using a checklist for home safety, assess the safety of your home or that of an older friend. (Be sure to ask permission first.) Discuss your findings with the occupant.

7. Consider an accident you were involved in within the past two years. What was the cause? How might it have been prevented? Discuss this accident in terms of individual susceptibility and environmental factors.

8. Simulating some of the age changes outlined in Chapter 5 (such as putting petroleum jelly over eyeglasses, or using a walker or wheelchair), attempt to cross the street, manipulate curbs, enter and leave the car, and go up or down stairs. Discuss how accidents may happen. When you do this, pair up with a friend to reduce your risk of accidents!

9. Find out how nursing homes cope with patients with colds, the flu, or other infectious diseases. How is disease contagion prevented?

10. Find data on severe climatic changes occurring in the United States. What age group suffered the most from these temperature extremes? Were all elders at risk or just those with pre-existing health problems?

11. Research the years of major influenza and tuberculosis epidemics. What age groups were affected most? What age groups of elders still living survived those epidemics?

12. With a partner, devise a list of errands (e.g., buying milk at the grocery, visiting the bank or post office, attempting to find a specific book at the library) that elders may need to do in the course of their daily life. You don't have access to a car, so you must walk or take public transportation. Make an effort to act as if you are a frail elder with reduced mobility, hearing, and vision. Make a list of the physical barriers and psychological concerns you may encounter, as well as ways in which merchants have reduced barriers. To simulate being in a wheelchair, you may consider bringing along a stroller—but remember, you can't go down curbs!

13. Discuss/debate various legislative proposals to reduce the risk of elder drivers (e.g., driving tests, regulations about distance/time of day, age restrictions). Debate proposals to raise the driving age for younger drivers and contrast the arguments "for and against" with those regarding older drivers. Would some legislative proposals be more difficult to enact? Why?

14. List considerations important in assessing whether an individual is a good driver. Devise a protocol, including various types of tests, that you think would accurately predict whether someone was able to drive safely.

BIBLIOGRAPHY

1. National Center for Health Statistics. Health, United States, 1998, with socioeconomic status and health chartbook. Hyattsville, MD: U.S. Department of Health and Human Services, Public Health Service, CDC, National Center for Health Statistics, 1998: 217.

2. Moosad, S.B., Macknin, M.L., Medendorp, S.V., and Mason, P. 1996. Zinc gluconate lozenges for treating the common cold. A randomized, double-blind, placebo-controlled study. *Annals of Internal Medicine* 125:81–88.

3. Gonzales, R., Steiner, J.F. and Sande, M.A. 1997. Antibiotic prescribing for adults with colds, upper respiratory tract infections, and bronchitis by ambulatory care physicians. *Journal of the American Medical Association* 278:901–4.

4. Govaert, T.M.E., Thijs, C.T., and Masurel, N., et al. 1994. The efficacy of influenza vaccination in elderly individuals. *Journal of the American Medical Association* 272:1661–65.

5. Gross, P.A., Hermogenes, A.W., and Sacks, H.S., et al. 1995. The efficacy of influenza vaccine in elderly persons: A meta-analysis and review of the literature. *Annals of Internal Medicine* 123:518–27.

6. McElhaney, J.E., Meneilly, G.S., and Beattie, B.L., et al. 1992. The effect of influenza vaccination on IL2 production in healthy elderly: Implications for current vaccination practices. *Journal of Gerontology* 47:M3–M8.

7. Centers for Disease Control. 1998. Influenza and pneumococcal vaccination levels among adults aged > 65 years—United States, 1997. *Morbidity and Mortality Weekly Report* 47:797–802.

8. Nichol, K.L. Margolis, K.L., Wourenma, J., and Sternberg, T.V. 1994. The efficacy and cost effectiveness of vaccination against influenza among elderly persons living in the community. *New England Journal of Medicine* 331:778–87.

9. Osler, W. 1892. *The principles and practice of medicine.* New York: Appleton and Co.

10. Centers for Disease Control. 1998. Tuberculosis morbidity—United States, 1997. *Morbidity and Mortality Weekly Report* 47:253–57.

11. Snider, D.E., Salinas, L., and Kelley, G.D. 1989. Tuberculosis: An increasing problem among minorities in the U.S. *Public Health Reports* 104:646–53.

12. Soll, A.H. 1996. Medical treatment of peptic ulcer disease: Practice guidelines. *Journal of the American Medical Association* 275:622–29.

13. Thompson, W.G., and Patel, D.G. 1986. Clinical picture of diverticular disease in the colon. *Clinical Gastroenterology* 15:903–16.

14. Ferzoco, L.B., Raptopoulos, V., and Silen, W. 1998. Acute diverticulitis. *New England Journal of Medicine* 338:1521–25.

15. Lau, W.Y., Fan, S.T., Yiu, T.F., et al., 1985. Acute appendicitis in the elderly. *Surgery, Gynecology, and Obstetrics* 161:157–60.

16. Rothrock, S.G., and Schneider, R.E. 1992. Overcoming limitations and pitfalls in the diagnosis of appendicitis. In *Updates in Gastroneurology II,* S.G. Rothrock, ed. Atlanta: American Health Consultants, pp. 19–31.

17. Rao, P.M., Rhea, J.T., and Novelline, R.A., et al. 1998. Effect of computed tomography of the appendix on treatment of patients and use of hospital resources. *New England Journal of Medicine* 338:141–46.

18. Read, N.W., Abouzekry, L., and Read, M.G., et al. 1985. Anorectal function in elderly patients with fecal impaction. *Gastroenterology* 89:959–66.

19. Bennett, R.G., and Greenough, W.B. 1993. Approach to acute diarrhea in the elderly. *Gastroenterology Clinics of North America* 22:517–33.

20. McCue, J.D. 1993. Urinary tract infections in the elderly. *Pharmacotherapy* 13:51S–53S.

21. Nygaard, I.E., and Johnson, M. 1996. Urinary tract infections in elderly women. *American Family Physician* 53:175–82.

22. Little, W.N., Park, G.T., and Patton, H.M. 1998. Sildenafil and cystitis (letter). *New England Journal of Medicine* 339:700.

23. Stamm, W.E., and Hooton, T.M. 1993. Management of urinary infections in adults. *New England Journal of Medicine* 329:1328–34.

24. Raz, R., and Stamm, W.E. 1993. A controlled trial of intravaginal estriol in postmenopausal

women with recurrent urinary tract infections. *New England Journal of Medicine* 329:753–56.

25. Avorn, J., Monane, M., and Gurwitz, J.H., et al. 1994. Reduction of bacteriuria and pyuria after ingestion of cranberry juice. *Journal of the American Medical Association* 271:751–54.

26. Curhan, G.C., Willett, W.W.C., Speizer, F.E., and Stampfer, M.J. 1998. Beverage use and risk for kidney stones in women. *Annals of Internal Medicine* 128:534–40.

27. Brandeis, G.H., Morris, J.N., Nash, D.J., and Lipsitz, L.A. 1990. The epidemiology and natural history of pressure ulcers in elderly nursing home residents. *Journal of the American Medical Association* 264:2905–10.

28. Granick, M.S., Eisner, A.N., and Solomon, M.P. 1994. Surgical management of decubitus ulcers. *Clinics in Dermatology* 12:71–79.

29. Panel for the Prediction and Prevention of Pressure Ulcers in Adults. 1992. *Pressure ulcers in adults: Prediction and prevention.* Clinical Practice Guideline, no. 3. AHCPR Publication No. 92-0047. Rockville, MD: Agency for Health Care Policy and Research, Public Health Service, U.S. Department of Health and Human Services, May.

30. Tyring, S., Barbarash, R.A., and Nahlik, J.E., et al. 1995. Famciclovir for the treatment of acute herpes zoster: Effects on acute disease and postherpetic neuralgia. *Annals of Internal Medicine* 123:89–96.

31. Centers for Disease Control. 1998. AIDS among persons aged >50 years—United States, 1991–1996. *Morbidity and Mortality Weekly Report* 47:21–27.

32. Stall, R., and Catania, J. 1994. AIDS risk behaviors among late middle-aged and elderly Americans. *Archives of Internal Medicine* 154:57–63.

33. Schable, B., Chu, S.Y., and Diaz, T. 1996. Characteristics of women 50 years of age or older with heterosexually acquired AIDS. *American Journal of Public Health* 86:1616–18.

34. Weinberg, A.D., and Minaker, K.L. 1995. Dehydration: Evaluation and management in older adults. *Journal of the American Medical Association* 274:1552–56.

35. Daly, J. 1993. *Medicare discharge data, 1984–1987.* Brockton, MA: Health Services

Research and Development, Brockton/West Roxbury Veterans Affairs Medical Center, July.

36. Fish, P.D., Bennett, G.C., and Millard, P.H. 1985. Heatwave morbidity and mortality in old age. *Age and Ageing* 14:243–45.

37. Centers for Disease Control. 1998. Heat-related mortality—United States, 1997. *Morbidity and Mortality Weekly Report* 47:473–76.

38. Semenza, J.C., Rubin, C.H., and Falter, K.H., et al. 1996. Heat-related deaths during the July 1995 heat wave in Chicago. *New England Journal of Medicine* 335:84–90.

39. Delaney, K. 1992. Heatstroke: Underlying processes and lifesaving management. *Postgraduate Medicine* 91:379–88.

40. Centers for Disease Control. 1997. Hypothermia-related deaths—Virginia, November 1996–April 1997. *Morbidity and Mortality Weekly Report* 46:1157–59.

41. Frank, S.M., Fleisher, L.A., and Breslow, M.J., et al. 1997. Perioperative maintenance of normothermia reduces the incidence of morbid cardiac events. *Journal of the American Medical Association* 277:1127–34.

42. National Safety Council. 1997. *Accident Facts.* Chicago: National Safety Council.

43. Lord, S.R., Clark, R.D., and Webster, I.W. 1991. Visual acuity and contrast sensitivity in relation to falls in an elderly population. *Age and Ageing* 20:175–81.

44. Ooi, W.L., Barrett, S., and Hossain, M., et al. 1997. Patterns of orthostatic blood pressure change and their clinical correlates in a frail, elderly population. *Journal of the American Medical Association* 277:1299–1304.

45. Hindmarsh, J.J., and Estes, E.H. 1989. Falls in older persons: Causes and interventions. *Archives of Internal Medicine* 149:2217–22.

46. Tinetti, M.E., Speechley, M., and Ginter, S.F. 1998. Risk factors for falls among elderly persons living in the community. *New England Journal of Medicine* 319:1701–7.

47. Sattin, R.W. 1992. Falls among older persons: A public health perspective. *Annual Review of Public Health* 13:489–508.

48. Tinetti, M.E., and Williams, C.S. 1997. Falls, injuries due to falls, and the risk of admission to a

nursing home. *New England Journal of Medicine* 337:1279–84.

49. Ray, W.A., Griffen, N.P., and Schaffner, W., et al. 1987. Psychotropic drug use and the risk of hip fracture. *New England Journal of Medicine* 316:363–69.

50. Thapa, P.B., Gideon, P., and Cosst, T.W., et al. 1998. Antidepressants and the risk of falls among nursing home residents. *New England Journal of Medicine* 339:875–82.

51. Ruthazer, R., and Lipsitz, L.A. 1993. Antidepressants and falls among elderly people in long-term care. *American Journal of Public Health* 83:746–49.

52. Speechley, M., and Tinetti, M. 1991. Falls and injuries in frail and vigorous community elderly persons. *Journal of the American Geriatrics Society* 39:46–52.

53. Tinetti, M.E., Baker, D.I., and McAvay, G., et al. 1994. A multifactorial intervention to reduce the risk of falling among elderly people living in the community. *New England Journal of Medicine* 331:821–27.

54. Wolfson, L., Whipple, R., Derby, C., and Judge, J., et al. 1996. Balance and strength training in older adults: Intervention gains and Tai Chi maintenance. *Journal of the American Geriatrics Society* 44:498–506.

55. Robbins, S., Waked, E., Allard, P., McClaran, J., and Krouglicof, N. 1997. Foot position awareness in younger and older men: The influence of footwear sole properties. *Journal of the American Geriatrics Society* 45:61–66.

56. Tinetti, M.E., Liu, W.L., and Ginter, S.F. 1992. Mechanical restraint use and fall-related injuries among residents of skilled nursing facilities. *Annals of Internal Medicine* 116:369–74.

57. Capezuti, E., Evans, L., Strumpf, N., and Maislin, G. 1996. Physical restraint use and falls in nursing home residents. *Journal of the American Geriatrics Society* 44:627–33.

58. Capezuti, E., Strumpf, N.E., and Evans, L.K., et al. 1998. The relationship between physical restraint removal and falls and injuries among nursing home residents. *Journal of Geriatrics* 53A:M47–52.

59. Ray, W.A., Taylor, J.A., and Meador, K.G., et al. 1997. A randomized trial of a consultation service to reduce falls in nursing homes. *Journal of the American Medical Association* 278:557–62.

60. Tobis, J.S., and Reinsch, S. 1990. Falls in the elderly. *Western Journal of Medicine* 153:433.

61. Riggs, B.L., and Melton, L.J. 1986. Involutional osteoporosis. *New England Journal of Medicine* 314:1676–84.

62. Magaziner, J., Simonsick, E.M., and Kashner, M. et al. 1989. Survival experiences of aged hip fracture patients. *American Journal of Public Health* 79:274–78.

63. Mossey, J.M., Mutran, E., Knott, K., and Craik, R. 1989. Determinants of recovery 12 months after hip fracture: The importance of psychosocial factors. *American Journal of Public Health* 79:279–85.

64. Massie, D., Campbell, K., and Williams, A. 1995. Traffic accident involvement rate by driver, age and gender. *Accident Analysis and Prevention* 27:73–87.

65. National Highway Traffic Safety Administration. 1994. *Traffic safety facts: Older drivers.* Washington, D.C.: U.S. Department of Transportation.

66. Wiseman, E.J., and Souder, E. 1996. The older driver: A handy tool to assess competence behind the wheel. *Geriatrics* 51:36-8, 41–2, 45.

67. Marotolli, R.A., Cooney, L.M., and Wagner, D.R., et al. 1994. Predictors of automobile crashes and moving violations among elderly drivers. *Annals of Internal Medicine* 121:842–46.

68. Fitten, L.J., Perryman, K.M., and Wilkinson, C.J., et al. 1995. Alzheimer and vascular dementias and driving. *Journal of the American Medical Association* 273:1360–65.

69. Transportation Research Board. 1988. *Transportation in an aging society.* Special Report 218. Washington, D.C.: National Research Council.

70. Miller, D.J., and Morley, J.E. 1993. Attitudes of physicians toward elderly drivers and driving policy. *Journal of the American Geriatrics Society* 41:722–24.

71. Perrson, D. 1993. The elderly driver: Deciding when to stop. *The Gerontologist* 33:88–91.

72. Marotolli, R.A., Ostfeld, A.M., and Merril, S.S., et al. 1993. Driving cessation and changes in mileage driven among the elderly. *Journal of Gerontology* 48:8255–60.

73. Levy, D.T., Vernick, J.S., Howard, K.A. 1995. Relationship between driver's license renewal policies and fatal crashes involving drivers 70 years or older. *Journal of the American Medical Association* 274:1026–30.

74. Allard, R. 1982. Excess mortality from traffic accidents among elderly pedestrians living in the inner city. *American Journal of Public Health* 72:853–54.

75. Langlois, J.A., Keyl, P.M., and Guralnik, J.M., et al.1997. Characteristics of older pedestrians who have difficulty crossing the street. *American Journal of Public Health* 87:393–97.

76. Centers for Disease Control. 1989. Queens Boulevard Pedestrian Safety Project—New York City. *Morbidity and Mortality Weekly Report* 38:61–64.

77. Hamberg, L. 1998. Pulsing lights warn drivers of pedestrians. *San Francisco Chronicle* (October):A11.

78. American National Red Cross, 1993. *Community First Aid and Safety.* Mosby-Yearbook: St. Louis, MO.

79. Rubenstein, L.A., Robbins, A.A., and Josephson, K.R., et al. 1990. The value of assessing falls in an elderly population: A randomized clinical trial. *Annals of Internal Medicine* 113:308–16.

10

Medication Use

The desire to take medicine is perhaps the greatest feature which distinguishes man from animals.

Sir William Osler

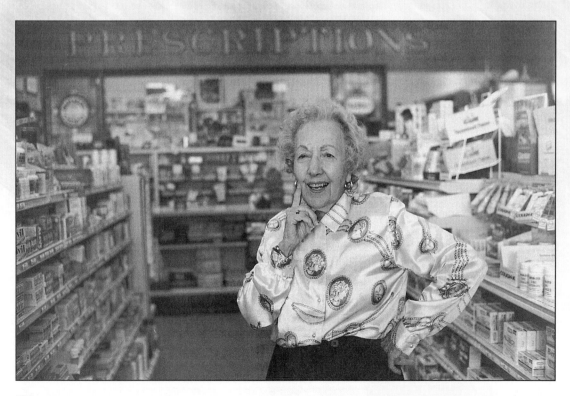

The development and use of medicines to prevent and treat a broad range of health problems is one of the many advances of modern medicine. Antibiotics to control bacterial infection, vaccines to prevent communicable disease, and drugs to treat the symptoms of chronic illnesses have improved the quality of life for many who would have suffered, even died without them. Drugs also rid us of small irritants, such as headaches, itching, minor aches and pains, and constipation. However, despite their many benefits, drugs may cause adverse effects, sometimes even causing death.

As a group, our nation's elders consume more medications than any other age group, mainly because they have the highest prevalence of chronic illness and age-related ailments. Drug therapy provides significant benefits in managing chronic symptoms and minor conditions that would otherwise impair the quality of life. However, drug use among elders comes with a high cost, not only economic, but also an increased risk of serious adverse drug effects. Elders are at a higher risk of adverse drug reactions than other groups because of age-related changes in physiology, decrements due to chronic diseases, and use of multiple drugs. In addition, adverse drug events among the older population reflect the inadequacy of health professionals in assessing drug need, prescribing appropriate drugs, supervising drug therapy, and educating elders to be active partners in their health care.

Because medication issues are of paramount importance to elders, their relatives, and those who work with them, details on the classes of drugs most commonly used among that group will be discussed. Both over-the-counter (OTC) and prescription medications will be described. Everyone, young and old, should be aware of the benefits and risks of the medications they purchase and use. Finally, alternatives to medications will be briefly addressed.

ELDER MEDICATION CONSUMPTION AND EXPENDITURES

Elders in the United States use a disproportionate amount of both prescription and nonprescription medications: they comprise 13 percent of the total population but account for more than 30 percent of the total drug expenditures. Many individuals take more than one drug. As expected, those who report depression, poor health, high hospitalization rate, and lower functional status are more likely to take medications. Use of prescription drugs increases with age, although use of nonprescription drugs does not. Surprisingly, some elders who report fair or poor health take no prescription medications, and a small group takes neither prescription nor over-the-counter medications.[1]

The prevalence of drug use is high among institutionalized elders: one study reported an average of eight prescriptions per resident, even though each resident takes only four to six medications daily. This figure is high because the institutionalized are often prescribed drugs that others purchase over-the-counter; thus, aspirin, laxatives, and antacids are often counted as part of the total and inflate the figure. Institutionalized elders are particularly high users of medications that affect the central nervous system, most likely because of the high prevalence of behavior problems and dementia in nursing home residents. Because of the concern with the high numbers of elders in nursing homes prescribed nervous system drugs, the Nursing Home Reform Act of 1987 was passed to restrict their use (see chapter 13).

Most physician visits result in a medication prescription, and physicians are more likely to add medications to a patient's list than to discontinue them. Approximately two-thirds of all physician visits for patients over 65 result in a new prescription, with the average number of drugs prescribed per visit estimated at 1.5. With advancing age, elders are more likely to receive prescriptions, and elder women are more likely to receive a prescription than men.[2]

Over half of the nation's elders do not have insurance coverage for prescribed drugs because Medicare does not cover drug therapy unless hospitalized. If elders join a managed care health maintenance organization, prescription medications may be covered. The alternative is to purchase supplementary insurance or be poor enough to qualify for

What Is Your Opinion? Pharmaceutical Companies' Profits

The pharmaceutical industry is the most profitable industry in the United States, earning $75 billion each year. This is good news for stockholders, but bad news for medication consumers. The pharmaceutical business has more than tripled the profit margin of the average Fortune 500 company. Prescription drug prices continue to increase faster than inflation. It is not uncommon for prices to increase 12 percent in one year. Profits are expected to increase even more in the future because of the introduction of new, high-priced drugs to the marketplace. Some medications can cost consumers thousands of dollars annually. Many experts believe pharmaceutical companies are guilty of price gouging and assert that a cap should be placed on the companies' profit margins. However, it is unlikely that Congress will cap profits since the pharmaceutical industry supports one of the strongest lobbying bodies.

In an international survey comparing the cost of eight common antidepressant and antipsychotic drugs, on the average, Americans paid twice as much as Europeans and Canadians for the same drug. One drug cost three times more.[4] In our country, pharmaceutical companies set the charges, but in other countries, nationalized health care plans negotiate prices with drug companies, thus getting "bulk" discounts. With the rise in managed care, health plans are negotiating with pharmaceutical companies for lower prices, even threatening to remove drugs from their formulary if prices are not reduced. If drugs are not in their formulary, they are not covered under that insurance plan, and clients who are prescribed these drugs must pay out-of-pocket or use a substitute.

What should be done? Continue to permit drug companies to charge what they want for all drugs? Put a cap on those drugs required by many people, but currently unaffordable because of their high prices? Put a cap on profit margin for all drugs? Should the government negotiate with the pharmaceutical companies for lower prices for Medicare beneficiaries? Should the government develop a national health care plan and negotiate price controls for all its citizens?

Drug mark-up is not limited to pharmaceutical companies; pharmacies also vary in how much they profit from prescription drugs. For some drugs, the difference among pharmacies is significant.

Medicaid (see chapter 12). On the average, about 3 percent of the elders' household income is spent on prescription drugs, but the figures vary greatly. Seven percent of all elder households spend at least 10 percent of their income on prescription drugs. For severely disabled elders, outpatient drug prescriptions are responsible for over half their out-of-pocket health care expenditures. When elders do have insurance, this decreases their out-of-pocket expenses by about 50 percent.[3] The lack of insurance for prescription drug costs may serve as a barrier to effective treatment for many elders because they may take lower dosages than needed or may do without the medication altogether.

FACTORS AFFECTING MEDICATION USE

Our country is afflicted with widespread chemophilia, a love of chemicals. Many people would rather be prescribed a pill to make them feel better than take personal responsibility to modify negative health behaviors to prevent disease. The overflowing medicine cabinets of most households exemplify our country's obsession with drug cure-alls. This "quick fix" attitude is encouraged by the pharmaceutical marketing practices to physicians, and now, directly to the consumer. Pharmaceutical companies promote the idea that there is a "pill for every ill," a chemical solution to every physical, emotional, or social problem. Also, they spend more money to market their products than they do on research and product development.

Since pharmaceutical companies must rely on physicians to sell their prescription products, their goal is to maximize their profits by encouraging physicians to write as many prescriptions as possible. This is accomplished in many ways. The companies advertise heavily in professional journals and send salespeople to inform physicians of their latest products, giving out free drug samples, prescription pads with the name of the drug product printed on them, and coffee mugs, pens, and refrigerator magnets with the newest drug logo. Drug companies commonly offer educational symposia at plush resorts for physicians and their spouses. After the American Medical Association adopted guidelines in 1990 to limit gifts to physicians to those of nominal value and those with direct educational benefit, the number of expensive gifts, vacations, and free meals has been reduced. However, other marketing practices of pharmaceutical companies have come under increased scrutiny as being unethical. They include offering pharmacists payments to encourage physicians to switch prescriptions, awarding doctors points toward airline travel if they prescribed a product, or setting up fraudulent payments for "research grants," which are really prescribing incentives.[5]

Although physicians profess not to be influenced by the claims of the drug company representatives, such interaction is often their only source of continuing education on pharmacology. One study found that 11 percent of the information presented to physicians from drug company representatives was inaccurate and favored the drug being promoted, and some statements were even dangerous.[6] Even print ads, which are regulated by the FDA, can contain inaccuracies. An analysis of 109 ads in major medical journals in 1990 found that a whopping 92 percent may have violated FDA regulations that require ads to fully disclose side effects and appropriate uses.[7] In that study, 32 percent of the headlines misled the reader about the drug's efficacy, 57 percent of the ads had little or no educational value, and 44 percent may cause a physician to prescribe the drug incorrectly. One study documented the influence that pharmaceutical company contacts have on physicians. It was reported that doctors who had accepted money to speak at a company symposium or to conduct research were 19 times more likely to request that a drug be added to the hospital pharmacy. Those who met with representatives of the company were thirteen times more likely

and those who had accepted a gift or free meal from the pharmaceutical company were five times more likely to request that their hospital pharmacy stock a particular medication.[8] Another study documented an increase in the use of an expensive antibiotic in one hospital immediately following a hospital dinner sponsored by a pharmaceutical company.[9]

For years, drug companies have advertised over-the-counter drugs on television and in magazines to tout their particular brand. More recently, drug companies are advertising prescription drugs with widespread appeal in magazines, billboards, and on television, providing the consumer with toll-free numbers for more information or referrals. Drugs most often advertised to the public are those for allergies, menopausal symptoms, baldness, and impotence. Consumers are being encouraged to discuss these newer (often more expensive) medications with their physician and, if the pharmaceutical company has its way, to leave the office with a prescription. Pharmaceutical companies are now spending more to advertise to the general public than to physicians. As a result, increasing numbers of consumers are going to their physicians with specific prescription requests.

Advertisements may be effective at encouraging individuals with treatable medical problems to see their physicians, but they are often confusing and misleading. Consumers rarely read the "small print," which details the medication's indications, uses, and side effects.

Physicians' drug-prescribing practices are influenced by many factors besides drug companies: where they trained, their past success in prescribing the medication, the medical journals they read, their perceptions of the severity of the problem, whether they believe the patient is likely to be noncompliant, their attitudes toward the elderly, and the pressure they receive from patients.

Ideally, physicians first explore nondrug alternatives before turning to medications. Then, if drugs are necessary, they choose the most effective and inexpensive drug at the lowest dose for the shortest time possible to minimize adverse effects. However, sometimes the easiest way to terminate an elder's office visit is to hand over a prescription for his or her vague complaints. On the other hand, many patients want to receive a prescription, because it is a sign that their pain is real and can be helped. Without a prescription, patients may feel the problem is untreatable or that the physician did not take their complaints seriously.

PHARMACOKINETICS

Pharmacokinetics is the study of what happens to a drug after it enters the body: how it is absorbed from the gut into the bloodstream, distributed throughout the body, metabolized (broken down), and finally excreted. An understanding of pharmacokinetics is necessary to determine why older people may respond differently to drugs than younger adults and to determine the drug dosage needed to maximize benefits and minimize side effects. For instance, how quickly a drug is absorbed and how long the active drug circulates in the blood before it is broken down determines how often the drug must be taken. For most medications, the effectiveness and toxicity are related to their concentration in the blood. In these cases, blood levels of the medicine can be measured to assure that the patient is receiving enough medication to be effective, but not so much as to be toxic.

The passage of a drug through the body is affected by many factors, such as kidney and liver function, amount of circulating blood, body weight, and body fat. Age-associated changes, chronic illnesses, dehydration, vitamin deficiencies, presence of other drugs in the bloodstream, and immobility can also affect drug response. Drug dosages and frequency must usually be altered to minimize toxic effects in affected elders.

In 1998, the Food and Drug Administration (FDA) began to phase in a requirement that all prescription drugs be labeled to include information pertinent to the use by those over age sixty-five, to be completed by 2003. The educational package inserts now contain a summary of the studies conducted on the use of the drug among elders, including special considerations in prescribing optimal dosages. However, the FDA does not require additional studies to be conducted on elders.

Changes in Drug Absorption

When taken by mouth, most drugs are absorbed into the bloodstream from the stomach or small intestine. Injected drugs enter the bloodstream directly. Although a number of changes in the digestive system may accompany aging, experts in pharmacokinetics do not believe these significantly affect drug absorption. Digestive diseases or food and other drugs taken at the same time are more likely to affect drug absorption than age changes alone.

Changes in Drug Distribution

After a medication is absorbed into the bloodstream, the blood carries it to all body tissues. Some drugs dissolve in the blood and are carried that way. However, the majority of drugs "hitch a ride," that is, they attach themselves to carrier proteins in the blood. Drugs may also be stored in fat or muscle to be released when the blood concentration of the drug declines. Drugs circulate throughout the body, even if the drug is only meant for one organ, such as the heart. Cells at the site of action have receptors on their surface that bind chemically with the drug, creating the intended effect. Medication side effects are often caused by the drug binding to targets that are similar to those at the intended site of action.

A number of age-related changes cause elders to distribute drugs differently. Elders generally weigh less than younger adults so dosages appropriate for younger adults may be excessive for elders. Because many medications are distributed in body fat or body water, changes in these constituents can significantly affect drug distribution. For instance, drugs distributed in body fluids are more concentrated in elders because they have less body fluid. Conversely, drugs stored in fatty tissues may last longer in elders because they have more fatty tissue. Underweight elderly patients often receive higher than necessary doses of medications because their weight is not taken into account in the prescribed dosage.

Another influence on the distribution of medication within the body is the degree to which the drug attaches itself to a carrier protein (often albumin) in the bloodstream. Most drugs can bind or unbind with this protein and thus can be carried throughout the body. When a drug is bound to albumin, it is inactive: only the unbound drug has a pharmacological effect. Since the percentage of the unbound drug is an important determinant of drug distribution, changes in the albumin levels will affect drug action. The amount of albumin in the body can be determined by a blood test.

Even though the albumin level in the blood does not decline with age, it is reduced significantly in elders who have advanced illness or malnutrition. Low albumin levels may result in a decreased proportion of bound (inactive) drug and an increased proportion of the unbound (active) drug. Consequently, more of the drug will be distributed to the site of action, increasing toxicity. A small decrease in albumin causes large increases in blood concentrations of active drug. Furthermore, with age, each albumin molecule becomes less efficient at binding drugs. Thus, if an elder is taking many drugs that bind to albumin in the bloodstream, the active drug concentrations will increase. Low albumin levels are directly related to a number of adverse drug reactions in elders.

Changes in Drug Metabolism

The liver metabolizes many medications before they are eliminated from the body. It is hypothesized that reduced liver function due to age-associated changes could cause medications to remain in the body longer. However, others assert that the liver has a great deal of reserve, and any age-related decrements in its function have little effect on drug metabolism.

Changes in Drug Excretion

Most drugs are eliminated from the body through either the kidneys or the liver. The liver breaks down some drugs; the remainder is either secreted into the intestine along with bile or released into the bloodstream to be excreted by the kidney. Other drugs leave the body unchanged. There is no appreciable change in liver excretion with age; however, elders with liver disease may need reduced dosages of some drugs.

The kidney continuously filters the blood, eliminating drugs in the urine. Although there is high variability among older people, kidney blood flow and filtration ability decrease significantly with age. The consequent decrease in kidney function allows a drug to circulate longer in the body, thus increasing its effect.

Before medications excreted by the kidney are prescribed to older people, their kidney function should be measured. Most dosages for elders are two-thirds to one-half the adult dose. The reduced dosage recommendations for many medications given to the elderly are based primarily on decreased kidney function.

Because of the great variability of age changes, disease states, and other drugs used concurrently by elders, physicians should carefully monitor blood levels of the drug, observe the patient's response, and adjust dosages to prevent adverse reactions. Textbooks, drug company testing information, and articles in professional journals can assist a physician in adapting dosages for elders. In addition, prescription drugs now require labels that detail the possible effects on elderly patients, which will serve to educate physicians.

POLYPHARMACY

Polypharmacy is the practice of using a number of medications at the same time. This behavior is common among elders because they often take a number of medications to treat multiple illnesses. A variety of medication behaviors are included in the definition of polypharmacy. Duplicate medications may be used simultaneously, creating excessive drug concentrations in the body. Also, several drugs taken in the same period might interact with one another, creating either a heightened or

Delerium Mistaken for Senility

When her regular physician was out of town, M. M., an 89-year-old African American woman developed weakness and fell, and her neighbors called an ambulance. She had a lot of tests done in the emergency room and was diagnosed with a urinary tract infection and dehydration. She was started on intravenous fluids and antibiotics and admitted to the hospital. When she was seen the next day, she was confused and agitated, trying to get out of bed, insisting she had to use the bathroom. An indwelling catheter was placed, but she still felt she had to urinate and kept trying to get to the bathroom. She slipped through the hospital bed rails and fell and bruised herself all along one side. She pulled out her intravenous line, and it had to be replaced. She was given a benzodiazepine to calm her and help reduce her agitation. This resulted in brief periods of sleep, but when she was awake, she remained confused. She could recall only her name, but she did not know where she was, what day it was, or the phone number of any friends or family members. For her safety, she was put into a chair with an attached tray that did not allow her to stand up, and she was given doses of various medications for sedation. It was thought she may be depressed, so she was started on an antidepressant.

When her bladder infection was cleared, a decision was made to transfer her to a nursing home. Her primary physician returned to town. He was contacted to help with the plan to send her to a nursing home. He telephoned the patient's elderly sister who lived in a nearby town, and they arrived to visit. They were shocked at the patient's appearance. They informed the medical team that she had been alert, highly functional, and able to care for her own needs at home where she had lived alone for many years. A review of her medical records revealed that she had been given at least six new medications; over the next week, her mental status cleared. She had little memory of the hospitalization and some weakness associated with being in bed, but was once again able to care for herself at home.

reduced drug effect. Furthermore, drugs are sometimes used to reduce the adverse effects of other drugs. Oftentimes, many drugs are prescribed because all are needed. For example, heart failure is treated with nitrates, beta blockers, an ACE inhibitor, and a diuretic. Polypharmacy places an individual at greater risk of adverse reactions, further health problems, increased expense of physician and hospital visits, and, in some cases, even death.

The practice of polypharmacy may be initiated by the physician or the consumer. Some consumers visit more than one physician without telling one about the drugs prescribed by the others. Or, they may use a number of OTC drugs in addition to their prescribed medication in order to deal with a severe health problem. Physicians do not regularly ask their patients the other drugs they are currently taking, and sometimes mistake a medication side effect for another illness.

Drug Interactions

Drug interactions are the unintended result of polypharmacy, caused by inappropriate drug dosages, taking two drugs at the same time that interfere with each other, or ingesting alcohol or OTC medications with prescription drugs. For example, the antiseizure medication, dilantin, causes the liver to break down other drugs more rapidly, thereby reducing their effects. In contrast, the anticoagulant warfarin (Coumadin) accentuates the blood-thinning action of aspirin. Herbs can also interact with medications. For example, Gingko biloba can cause excessive blood thinning when used with Coumadin. Elders are especially susceptible to drug interactions because they generally take many drugs. In addition, drug interactions may be more hazardous in elders because of their decreased reserves.

The intended drug action can be reduced or enhanced by particular foods. Perhaps the most hazardous and well-documented case involves a type of antidepressant called monoamine oxidase inhibitors. When foods high in the amino acid tyramine (aged cheeses or red wine) are consumed with this drug, the individual may suffer a very sudden rise in blood pressure. The presence of food in the stomach may impede or enhance the absorption of a drug into the bloodstream. For example, acetaminophen (e.g., Tylenol) is absorbed faster on an empty stomach. In contrast, the absorption of griseofulvin, an antifungal drug, is enhanced when one eats fatty foods before taking the drug. Some drugs, such as antibiotics or anti-inflammatory medications, are taken with food to minimize gastrointestinal upset. But tetracycline is inactivated when taken with foods containing calcium, such as dairy products.

Adverse Drug Effects

An adverse drug effect is an undesirable and unexpected response resulting from the administration of a drug. Gastrointestinal disturbances are the most common adverse drug effect. Others are confusion, depression, loss of appetite, weakness, urinary incontinence, falls, weight loss, postural hypotension, lethargy, unsteady gait, forgetfulness, tremor, or constipation. Note that many of these symptoms conform to the stereotypes of old age. As a result, many adverse drug effects that could be eliminated are ignored by old people, their families, and health professionals.

Although those over age sixty account for only 13 percent of the total population, they account for the highest percentage of hospitalizations and deaths from adverse drug effects than any other age group. There are many reasons for this. Elders generally have:

1. smaller bodies and different body composition. Elders generally weigh less, have less body water, and increased body fat.

2. decreased ability of the liver to process some drugs.
3. decreased ability of the kidneys to clear drugs out of the body.
4. increased sensitivity to many drugs, especially those that act on the central nervous system.
5. decreased ability to maintain blood pressure stability while on some drugs, predisposing elders to postural hypotension and dizziness upon rising too rapidly from sitting or reclining.
6. decreased temperature compensation. Many drugs reduce the ability to sweat or shiver, a dangerous condition in extreme heat or cold.
7. more diseases that alter response to some drugs. Elders with congestive heart failure, liver disease, or kidney disease have heightened drug effects.
8. more drugs to take, creating more adverse drug reactions and drug interactions.[10]

Adverse drug reactions may be due to human error—incorrect prescription, dosage, timing, and taking a drug that interacts with another already prescribed. These errors can occur when the drug is prescribed by a doctor, filled by a pharmacist, dispensed by others, or taken independently. It is believed that one in four adverse drug reactions is preventable. The bad news is their incidence is increasing, nearly tripling in the decade from 1983 to 1993.[10] Many experts assert that a majority of drugs commonly used by older people are not adequately tested in that population before approval.[10]

Medication Errors

New studies are uncovering the alarming frequency at which medication errors occur in hospitals, nursing homes, and physician's offices. One study at two hospitals affiliated with Harvard University noted that 247 adverse drug reactions (and 194 near misses) occurred in six months, or 6.5 percent of all hospital admissions. It was believed that one in four of those were preventable; most of the errors occurred in the prescribing stage. The most common cause was lack of knowledge about the drug itself; the second-leading cause was lack of knowledge of patient's history.[12] The researchers estimated that the number of deaths due to hospital errors in the United States exceeds the death rate from automobile crashes and all other accidents combined.[13] Adverse drug reactions cause an increased length of hospital stay, increased cost of treatment, and almost a three-fold increase in death rate.[14]

A report by the U.S. Government Accounting Office found that millions of elderly Americans are hospitalized and die from medication errors. They estimated that almost one out of five Medicare recipients who live at home are prescribed an unsafe medication (either the drug is not recommended for that age group, or it could be substituted for other, safer medications). They also estimated that the annual cost of hospitalizations associated with these prescriptions is $230 billion.[15] These include outdated prescribing practices by the physician, elders not telling pharmacists or physicians the other drugs they were using, and pharmacists not reviewing the medications taken by the patients.

What Is Your Opinion? Elder Drug Abuse

When we hear the words "drug abuse," the first thing that comes to mind is heroine, cocaine, smack, crack, or whatever drug is currently in the headlines. But what about drug abuse in older people? Well, older people do not use *those* kinds of drugs. *That* problem mainly has to do with younger people. But that is taking the narrow view that drug abuse means the drug-abusing person chooses to take drugs such as heroin, cocaine, etc. If, instead, we broaden the definition of "drug abuse" to include victims of the choices of others— such as patients of doctors—then the greatest epidemic of drug abuse in American society is among our older people.

Excerpted from Health Letter of the Public Citizens Health Research Group, April, 1993, p. 4.

Two studies in particular demonstrate the severity of medication errors among various elder populations. One study of older people in a community found that one-quarter to one-third of elders were receiving at least one medication that geriatricians believed was not appropriate for elders.[16] Another study of elderly residents in board and care facilities found between one-fifth and one-quarter of the residents were using possibly dangerous drugs.[17] Although each of these studies had some methodological flaws and may overestimate the danger, what emerges from these and other studies is the seriousness of adverse medication reactions among various elder populations and the need to understand their cause and to implement strategies to reduce such errors. One of the strategies should be to increase physicians' awareness of those drugs that should not be prescribed to older people.

COMPLIANCE

Compliance is defined as adherence to a prescribed medical regimen. Even if the physician accurately diagnoses a disease or disorder and prescribes the appropriate drug, the health problem cannot be cured or controlled unless the patient takes the medication as directed. Although elders differ little from other populations in compliance rates, compliance is especially important for elders because they are prescribed more drugs and are more susceptible to drug interactions and their adverse effects than other adult populations.

Noncompliant Behaviors

A number of behaviors can be classified as noncompliant. An individual may never begin a drug therapy, forget to take the drug, or take the drug improperly because of lack of education. It is easy to forget the physician's explanation about one's illness, and even easier to forget the detailed instructions on how to take the drug. As many as 90 percent of all noncompliance is due to taking less than the prescribed dose of medication, either through forgetfulness, intentional reduction to minimize adverse effects, or to save money.

TABLE 10.1	**Causes of Noncompliance Among Elders**

Patient Factors
1. Never start the drug therapy
2. Forgetfulness
3. Lack of knowledge
   a. Does not understand disease or importance of therapy
   b. Does not know how to take medication properly
   c. Visual or hearing decrements that preclude knowledge of medication use
4. Intentionally altering medication schedule
   a. Fear of dependence on medication
   b. Lack of trust in physician
   c. Dissatisfaction with results of medication

Nature of Disease and/or Therapy
1. High number of medications and dosage frequency
2. Long treatment time
3. Medication causes unacceptable side effects
4. High cost of medication
5. Disease has no symptoms
6. Unacceptable dosage forms (bad taste, can't swallow pills)
7. Low potential for therapy to cure disease or relieve symptoms

Physician Inadequacies
1. Lack of explicit written and oral instructions
2. Poor relationship with patient
3. Physician's lack of confidence in treatment
4. Complicated drug regimen prescribed
5. Lack of specific instructions on medication label

Noncompliance has a variety of causes: it may be caused by patient behavior, the nature of the disease or therapy, and the inadequacies of the physician. Noncompliance extends the recovery rate, consequently increasing the costs of drugs, physicians, and hospitalization. Table 10.1 describes the common causes of noncompliance among elders.

Education to Increase Compliance

Elderly patients often do not know the names, dosages, indications, or side effects of the medications they are taking. One survey of elder patients and their physicians found that the two groups agreed only about one-third of the time regarding what drugs the patient was taking. This agreement between the two parties decreased with the patient's advancing age, but was not explained by their cognitive deficits. Additionally, only about half the patients were able to identify why they were prescribed each of their drugs, but many did not know their potential side effects. Over one-third of the elders in that study wanted more information on their medications.[18]

Effective education increases the success of drug therapy. Although education does not guarantee compliance, it is a necessary prerequisite. Patient education should include an understandable description of the disease and its progression, treatment goals, and details about the drug therapy. Elders generally need more time to learn about the drugs they are prescribed. Many elders are hearing or vision impaired, and some are less educated or less fluent in English. One large-scale study of over 2,000 adult hospital patients found that 30 percent were not able to read medical material, and 50 to 80 percent of those were over age sixty. Of those tested, 41 percent were unable to read directions for taking medication on an empty stomach, 26 percent couldn't read information regarding the next appointment, and almost two-thirds could not understand a standard informed consent document.[19]

To compensate for these difficulties, the health professional should ensure that the patient not only understands the specifics of the drug therapy, but can also carry out the instructions. It is important to determine whether the client can administer the medication (e.g., swallow large pills, put drops in own eyes). The client should be quizzed about the regimen to assure understanding. Elders need time to ask questions about their health problem and treatment plan. Finally, if possible, someone close to the patient should also be involved in the drug education session, especially if she or he will monitor or administer the medication.

One of the most important, and neglected, means of patient education to increase compliance is clear instructions on drug labels and provision of supplemental educational materials. The more information put on the drug label, the better the client is able to understand the directions, and the higher the compliance rate. Whenever possible, verbal information regarding drugs or disease should be supplemented with large-print, readable, written materials that the client can refer to later. It is also important to assess whether the person's vision is adequate to take medication without supervision.

The following information should be discussed when any prescription is given:

Name of medication (both generic and brand name)

Amount of medication in each dose

Appearance of the medication

Why the drug is prescribed

Major benefits and risks of medication

Quantity to be taken

Dosage frequency

Method of administration

Duration of therapy

Precautions

Special instructions

What to do if dose is missed

Prescription refill information

Storage requirements

Adverse effects to report

Interactions with food, other medications, or alcohol

When effects of medication should be noticed

When to stop taking a drug

How long prescription should last

What to expect if medication is not taken

The Federal Poison Prevention Act requires childproof containers be used for both OTC and prescription medication. Medication is packaged in this way because it reduces the incidence of poisoning in children. However, many elders cannot open childproof containers because of impaired eyesight, manual dexterity, or strength. The most obvious consequence is that elders will not take the medication. Elders may break the container when trying to open it or injure themselves. Once the cap is off, elders may not recap the container or may transfer the medication to another vial without identification

or instructions for use. Uncapped medications may spoil or be ingested by grandchildren. The American Association of Poison Control Centers estimates that grandparents' medications account for almost one in five childhood poisonings.

Some new cap models, mainly squeeze-and-turn designs, are childproof, but many older adults are still able to open them. Elders should request this type of bottle, and if possible, they should try to open the bottle in the pharmacy. Medication without childproof caps should be stored away from children.

Memory Aids to Increase Compliance

Because elders often take multiple drugs, keeping track of which medications to take at what time can be a major impediment to compliance. There are many techniques to help people remember medication schedules. The time to take medication may be matched with another daily activity, such as breakfast or bedtime. Medication can be placed in an obvious place (beside the coffee, toothbrush, or razor) to jog the memory. Elders may also divide their week's medications into envelopes, pillboxes, or egg cartons labeled with the date and time of ingestion. The pharmacist may also consolidate medications into labeled bubble-packs. Elders may also use a medication calendar and check off boxes when drugs have been taken. The calendar may be brought to doctor's visits to allow the doctor to assess compliance. Finally, a timer may be set as a reminder. An electronic pill cap has been developed with a flashing red light and a loud bell that goes off a preset number of times a day.

The Issue of Noncompliance

The word *noncompliant* is used to describe a patient who does not conform to a physician's instructions. Noncompliance may be unintentional (lack of knowledge or forgetfulness) or intentional (a deliberate choice not to comply). Not taking prescribed medication as directed can result in a worsened condition, unnecessary hospitalization, even death. However, noncompliance does not always result in negative consequences. Some patients may make a necessary drug dosage adjustment to minimize adverse effects or discontinue unnecessary medication without the physician's consent.

Until the consumer health movement of the early 1970s, physicians and pharmacists withheld information on the medications prescribed. Now, the majority believe medical consumers have a right to know about their health status and all aspects of their medications—benefits, side effects, and alternatives. Furthermore, consumers have the right to decide whether or not to agree to a prescribed regimen. It is the physician's responsibility to give clients appropriate information to allow them to make these decisions rationally.

PROMOTING RATIONAL DRUG USE

A number of health professionals should be involved in effective drug therapy because each has the potential to minimize adverse drug effects and provide helpful drug information to elders. In a team approach, the physician, pharmacist, nurse, social worker, and the individual should cooperate to maximize benefits and minimize problems with drug therapy. The following paragraphs discuss the role of each team member in promoting rational drug use. The team approach, although effective, is rarely used in community settings.

The Physician's Responsibility

Physicians have the primary responsibility for drug therapy. They must accurately assess the health problem, prescribe the correct type and dosage of medication, and supervise drug therapy. It is estimated that two-thirds of the prescriptions filled by elders, almost 5 million a year, fall into one of the following categories:

1. The drug is not needed: that particular drug will not solve the health problem.
2. The drug is unnecessarily dangerous: another drug would give the same benefit with less risk.
3. The prescribed drug is correct, but the dose is unnecessarily high, increasing risk without extra benefits.[10]

In addition, the physician must be responsible for educating the patient about the disease and drug

therapy. Sometimes these responsibilities may be delegated to a nurse, health educator, or pharmacist. The following list outlines the many ways in which physicians may contribute to patient drug misuse, raising the risk of noncompliance.

Failure to obtain a complete drug history, including allergies to some medications,

Inaccurate diagnosis of the health problem,

Use wrong drug name, dose, or abbreviation,

Miscalculate dosage or frequency of dosage (e.g., due to reduced drug excretion and lower body weight)

Failure to consider food–drug and drug–drug interactions,

Failure to consider nondrug alternatives,

Inappropriate drug treatment (e.g., wrong drug, wrong dose),

Overmedication (prescribing unneeded or ineffective drugs or for an excessive length of time),

Failure to prescribe most inexpensive drug,

Failure to consider drug side effects,

Failure to consider decrease in kidney function with age,

Failure to consider effects of disease on liver function and change dose acordingly,

Failure to consider patient's lifestyle when recommending type of drug and dosage,

Failure to give clear instructions regarding medication,

Inadequate supervision of long-term medication, and

Failure to periodically review need for all medications.

Much of the physician's lack of knowledge of the special medication needs and concerns of older people can be attributed to a dearth of geriatric focus and pharmacology content in medical schools, as well as limited opportunities for continuing drug education for practicing physicians.

The Pharmacist's Responsibility

The traditional role of the pharmacist used to be to procure, store, prepare, and dispense drugs. Now, pharmacists in the hospital and community have

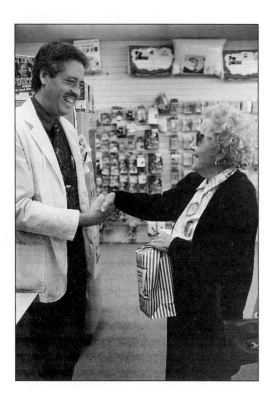

cies provide emergency service, delivery, and insurance billing service.

Many long-term care institutions and hospitals have instituted clinical pharmacy services to dispense and administer drugs, review drug utilization, and educate patients. When such services are implemented in an institutional setting, drug misuse drops significantly. New regulations from the Health Care Financing Administration have expanded the role of the pharmacist in long-term care institutions. Pharmacists now monitor drug regimens and dosages, eliminate unnecessary drugs, and assure that their patients understand and can administer their own medications when discharged.

The Responsibilities of the Nurse and Social Worker

The nurse's responsibility in drug therapy depends on the work setting. In a physician's office, nurses commonly provide drug education. In hospitals, nursing homes, or home health care, nurses carry out the plan of care devised by the physician; they administer medications, monitor drug reactions, and report problems to the physician. Nurses are in direct contact with the patient and are in a good position to determine if a new drug or change of dosage is needed. Nurses employed in nursing homes have a great deal of contact with patients over a long period of time, seeing patients much more frequently than do physicians. Thus, their responsibility for monitoring drug regimens and side effects is crucial.

Nurses are responsible for carrying out the Five Rights of Medication Administration: administering the right drug, in the right dose, through the right route, at the right time, to the right patient. Although this seems a straightforward task, data from a number of studies indicate a significant number of errors are made in medication administration both in hospitals and nursing homes.

Social workers should have a basic knowledge of medication-related problems and be able to refer clients with those problems to appropriate health care professionals. Social workers in community settings generally have close contact with elders so they are in a good position to monitor medication

expanded their role to prevent, recognize, and intervene in drug-associated problems.

Pharmacists serve as a resource for both clients and physicians, providing information on proper drug use and adverse effects of both prescription and OTC drugs. Further, pharmacists provide a confidential record-keeping service for their customers. This includes drug history, drug allergies, and medical history. They consult with the physician periodically to assure the client is using the drug properly and alert the physician of potential drug interactions, adverse drug effects, and the negative impact of prescriptions ordered by other physicians. They can identify symptoms of serious diseases in their clients and refer them to their physician when necessary. Pharmacists provide information on generic drugs and can assist the patient with medication scheduling and memory aids. In addition, they can instruct clients on the use of childproof containers and assess their need for easy-open containers. Finally, many pharma-

consumption and adverse effects. Social workers might also discuss problems with compliance or medication complications with their clients' physician. Unfortunately, few social workers are knowledgeable of common health concerns of elders and associated medication issues.

An important role of social workers who work with older people is to serve as their health advocate by recognizing medication-related problems, helping to resolve them, and encouraging health practices that could reduce drug use. Health advocates are in a position to inform elders about generic drugs and assist in developing memory aids to increase compliance. They can encourage elders to keep medication records and discuss all drugs with their pharmacist or physician. The social workers' advocacy role becomes more important for those elders living alone because they may be the only professional contact those older people have.

The Elder's Responsibility

Consumers must take responsibility for their medication use. They need to actively seek drug information from their physician and pharmacist, make decisions about the treatment plan, and monitor their own drug therapy program. Consumers can also decrease their chance of suffering adverse mediation events by familiarizing themselves with their medications, reading labels and directions carefully, asking questions about all new medications, and reminding health care professionals about their allergies.

Everyone needs to keep a record of all over-the-counter and prescription medications they are currently taking. This should include those taken daily and those taken only occasionally. The dosage, timing, and any adverse reactions should be noted. Further, the reason the medication is taken should also be listed. The medication record should be

---

Be a Savvy Drug Consumer

- Tell the physician all physical complaints; lack of complete data can lead to inappropriate drug use. It might help to bring a written list to the doctor's office.
- Be aware that a physical problem may be caused by adverse drug effects or drug–drug/drug–food interaction. Report them to the physician.
- Keep a personal medication record, including both prescription and OTC drugs. Share this record when you visit each physician.
- Tell the physician of any allergic reactions experienced previously with drugs.
- Question the physician about alternatives to drug therapy.
- Know when, how, and with what to take drugs, as well as which foods to avoid. Read all drug inserts and consult your pharmacist or physician with unanswered questions.
- Follow medication instructions exactly. If in doubt, contact your physician or pharmacist.

- Don't mix medications without permission from your physician.
- If the drug schedule interferes with your lifestyle, tell your doctor immediately.
- Do not share prescription medication with others.
- Do not mix similar-looking medications in a pill box.
- Do not take medications in the dark or when not fully awake.
- Do not drink alcohol when taking drugs.
- Keep medications away from children.
- Destroy all outdated medication.
- Ask that childproof containers not be used if they are a problem for you.
- Ask for a generic substitution, if available.
- Ask for large-print prescription labels if you have vision problems.

brought to every physician visit and to every pharmacy visit if it involves a new prescription.

It is best to use the same pharmacy so that the elder's complete medication history is on one record in one location. Elders should inform their pharmacists of their over-the-counter medications. Many physicians and pharmacists prefer that patients bring their medications to pharmacists and physician visits for review. If any adverse reactions are noted, the physician should be called immediately so that the drug or dosage may be modified.

The above responsibilities are very important to optimize medication use among older people. Realistically, however, some elders are frail and often need someone to be an advocate for them during their interactions with the medical profession. Elders are less apt to initiate discussion with their physician than other adults for many reasons. They may have difficulty understanding the nature of their illness because of sensory deficits, memory problems or lack of education. They may have difficulty asserting their needs. Any patient, elder or not, can benefit from assistance from family or friends when interacting with the medical profession.

If the older individual cannot be responsible for personal medication use, family and friends can reduce the risks of misuse by supervising or assisting with drug administration. A family member or friend can also monitor the elder's reaction to the drug, determine if symptom relief is sufficient, keep drug intake records, and serve as a health advocate. In addition, the helper should be alert to potential adverse drug reactions and should contact the physician when they occur.

Over-the-Counter Drugs Commonly Used by Elders

The FDA estimates that up to 300,000 different OTC products developed from 700 active ingredients are currently marketed in the United States. The drugs come in a variety of doses, forms, sizes, and strengths. The FDA regulates which drugs are sold by prescription and which can be sold over-the-counter. More than 600 over-the-counter drugs used to be sold by prescription; however, FDA

approval doesn't mean the drug is safe under all conditions for all people. It can cause side effects and can interact with other medications. Many OTC drugs have not been required to demonstrate their safety and effectiveness before becoming available to the public.[20] By law, all information needed to use the drugs appropriately must be on the label.

When consumers select and use OTC drugs, they take charge of reducing symptoms or curing a health problem themselves. The majority of all medical care in this country is self-care, especially among elders, and over-the-counter drugs play a major role. Almost everyone uses OTC drugs, either to supplement or substitute for medical care. Also, their use is growing; they are generally considered the first line of defense against common minor health problems.

Over-the-counter drugs should not be underrated. They are a quick and inexpensive drug therapy for temporary, minor conditions. Most OTCs are effective at reducing symptoms. In fact, some contain the same compounds as prescription drugs, differing only in dosage or packaging. Over-the-counter preparations save money and physician visits; many problems that are self-medicated are minor conditions that go away whether treated or not. These drugs can alleviate back pain, sore throat, gastrointestinal complaints, coughs, colds, constipation, and many other minor aches and pains.

On the negative side, some individuals are not able to accurately diagnose many of their own health problems and to choose an appropriate drug. Or, they may select a drug because of its packaging or advertising, not because of its suitability to treat the health problem. They may not read the labels, so drugs may be used improperly. As a result, the selected OTC drug may be ineffective, delaying needed care for a serious problem. For instance, what may be interpreted as heartburn may in fact be angina. Also, self-prescribed medications might confuse a physician's diagnosis. Furthermore, because OTC drugs are mistakenly believed to be less potent than prescription drugs, consumers may overmedicate. Some over-the-counter remedies contain a mixture of ingredients, including sodium, sugar, alcohol, potassium, and magnesium that can harm some individuals. Taking multiple remedies with combinations of ingredients can lead to a higher than recommended dose of some ingredients. Finally, there is a potential for drug interactions when some OTCs are taken with prescription drugs.

Despite the disadvantages, OTC drugs can contribute to good health if the right product is used for the right problem, and label directions are followed. The most common OTC drug families will be discussed in this section. When indicated, the brand names begin with capital letters, while the generic equivalents are in lowercase letters.

Pain Relievers

Analgesics, or pain relievers, are the most commonly used OTC drugs, and the most common symptom treated is headache pain. The umbrella term nonsteroidal anti-inflammatory drugs, NSAIDS (pronounced en-sayds), is used to describe a plethora of chemicals that work by inhibiting prostaglandin production. Prostaglandins are a specialized group of hormone-like compounds found in all body tissues. Prostaglandins have a variety of functions: they may regulate the flow of nerve impulses, protect the lining of the stomach, sensitize pain receptors, produce a fever, and inhibit blood clotting, to name a few. The main types of over-the-counter analgesics are aspirin (Anacin, Bayer, Bufferin), naproxen sodium (Aleve), ketoprofen (Orudis KT, Actron) or ibuprofen (Advil, Motrin IB, Nuprin). Acetaminophen (Tylenol, Pandol) is also used as an analgesic, although it works through a different pathway.

Aspirin is a widely used analgesic. Not only is it sold as a single product, but it is also an active ingredient in over 200 different OTC products. Aspirin effectively reduces pain, fever, and inflammation. It is inexpensive, generally safe, and the body does not build up tolerance for the drug. Aspirin is prescribed by physicians in high doses for arthritis and in low doses for prevention of blood clotting, heart attacks, and stroke. (In fact, if

an individual experiences symptoms of a heart attack, he or she should chew an aspirin immediately.) Aspirin is quite effective for joint, bone, or muscle pains that accompany arthritis, osteoporosis, fractures, even bone pain of advanced cancer. Aspirin use has also been associated with the reduced incidence of colon cancer, stomach cancer, rectal cancer, esophageal cancer, breast cancer, and Alzheimer's disease.[21] One study of almost 8,000 elders found that those who used aspirin regularly for at least three of the last five years had significantly less mental decline than those who did not use aspirin.[22]

Aspirin, although widely used, is not benign. Its most well-known side effect is the potential to damage the lining of the stomach, causing pain, bleeding, ulcers, and anemia. Although this side effect is more common in elders taking high dosages, it can occur with very low doses as well. Contrary to popular belief, buffered or coated aspirin products do not protect against stomach ulcers.[23] If gastric pain is experienced when aspirin or other NSAIDS are taken, they should be discontinued, and medical advice should be sought. In addition, high doses of aspirin may cause nausea, hearing and vision disturbances, abdominal pain, confusion, or dizziness. Elders with reduced kidney function have a higher risk of toxicity. Because aspirin reduces fever, it may interfere with one of the body's own mechanisms for healing. Further, aspirin also interacts with a number of prescription drugs and may affect the results of kidney function tests. Finally, because aspirin reduces the ability of the blood to clot, it can be detrimental if taken before surgery. It is important that more than one NSAID be taken at a time.

The other NSAIDS have similar uses and side effects. Some are now sold over-the-counter in lower doses than their earlier prescription products. These medications may be even more effective at reducing fever, pain, and inflammation than aspirin. However, they also irritate the stomach, causing bleeding or ulcers, and can cause kidney disease or confusion in elders. They cause about 80,000 deaths each year in Canada and the United States, most of whom are elderly. The use of NSAIDs by elders increases their risk of serious gastrointestinal side effects threefold. If they already have peptic ulcers, the risk is increased sixfold. There is evidence that if they are also given an antiulcer drug at the same time, such side effects are reduced.[24] In one study that monitored physician visits with elders, it was reported that of those visits that ended with a NSAID prescription, acetaminophen would have been sufficient in 40 percent of the cases. Unnecessary drugs were more likely to be prescribed when no personal histories were taken and the office visits were short.[25]

The most popular analgesic without aspirin is acetaminophen (Tylenol, Tempra, Panadol). It relieves minor pain and fever and, although it is not an anti-inflammatory, new evidence points to its utility in arthritis. It is less irritating to the stomach than aspirin and can be used by people allergic to aspirin. Unlike aspirin, it does not affect blood clotting or kidney function. However, an overdose of acetaminophen may cause permanent liver damage, especially in those who drink alcohol or are fasting; this effect occurs without any warning symptoms.[26]

NSAIDS and acetaminophen are ideal for short-term, intermittent therapy when the lowest possible dose is used. High doses or prolonged use of either acetaminophen or NSAIDS are associated with increased risk of side effects. If use is long-term, a physician should be consulted to monitor therapy.

Often, analgesics contain caffeine that can cause sleep problems in some people. One study of elders reported that those taking analgesic products containing caffeine had almost twice the difficulty falling asleep as those who did not.[27]

Antacids

Antacids relieve symptoms of upset stomach, heartburn, and indigestion by neutralizing excess stomach acid. There are over a hundred different antacid products on the market, and they come in many forms: pills, lozenges, gum, powder, and liquids. Some popular brand names are Alka-Seltzer, Tums, Milk of Magnesia, and Maalox. These antacids generally begin acting immediately and may be effective for up to forty minutes.

All antacids contain one or more of thirteen active ingredients, each with its own side effects. Aluminum hydroxide has a constipating effect, magnesium salts have a diarrheal effect, and antacids with high sodium content can cause fluid retention. Antacids may decrease the absorption of some drugs, aggravate symptoms of upset stomach, or mask symptoms of an ulcer. However, antacids are a very effective treatment for sporadic or daily symptoms of heartburn and are often prescribed by physicians. Tums, an antacid containing calcium carbonate, is recommended as a calcium supplement to reduce the risk of osteoporosis.

Newer antacids available over-the-counter are called H_2 blockers because they act on a histamine receptor in the stomach to prevent acid formation. Previously, these have been available only by prescription. They are widely advertised and include cimetidine (Tagamet HB), ranitidine (Zantac-75), nizatidine (AXID-IR), and famotidine (Pepcid AC).

Diarrhea Medications

These agents are available to treat transient bouts of mild diarrhea. Products containing bismuth (e.g., Pepto-Bismol) coat and protect the lining of the bowel and absorb some excess fluid. These may darken the tongue or stool. Kaopectate also serves to reduce the liquidity of the stool. Loperamide (Imodium) slows the activity of the gut, prolonging the time that fecal matter remains in the body. This drug may cause urinary retention and should not be used by men with an enlarged prostate. It has also been known to cause intestinal obstruction. If diarrhea persists, a physician should be consulted to rule out a parasitic infection or malignancy.

Antihistamines

Antihistamines block the effects of the allergy-producing substance, histamine, that is responsible for sneezing, watery eyes, runny nose, and itchy nose or throat in those with hay fever and other allergies. The most common nonprescription antihistamines are chlorpheniramine (ChlorTrimaton, Dristan, Contac) and diphenhydramine (Benadryl). The side effects are dry mouth, cognitive slowing, and drowsiness. People taking antihistamines should refrain from driving. Although many people with colds use antihistamines, these drugs do not relieve the sinus or nasal congestion of a cold and tend to thicken and dry bronchial secretions in the airway.

The antihistamines previously mentioned are also the active ingredients in most over-the-counter sleep medications. Interestingly, antihistimines are used, not because they block histamine production, but for their side effect of drowsiness.

An antihistamine nasal spray called Nasalcrom relieves allergy symptoms. The active drug, cromolyn sodium, prevents cells from releasing histimamines. However, it is primarily used for prevention, not for quick symptomatic relief. It takes weeks of regular use before any effect is noticed.

Laxatives

Laxatives, products that promote bowel movement or that soften the stools, are frequently used—some would say overused—by elders. Laxatives are helpful for occasional use in many elders and routine use in those with chronic health problems or who take medications with a side effect of constipation (such as codeine and morphine). However, many nondrug alternatives, including increasing dietary fiber, physical activity, and fluid intake, and taking natural laxatives, such as prunes, are better for chronic constipation. There are many types of laxatives, and each works differently.

Perhaps the safest of all laxatives are the fiber or *bulk laxatives* that increase volume and water content of stools. By increasing stool bulk, waste is moved through the colon more quickly. Common names are bran, psyllium (Metamucil), methylcellulose (Citrucel), and calcium polycarbophil (Fibercon). They are most useful for people with a low-fiber diet and should be taken with a lot of water to avoid intestinal obstruction. Common side effects include bloating and flatulence. Bulk laxatives are the least likely to be abused and do not

seem to interfere with intestinal absorption of essential nutrients. However, bulk-forming laxatives can reduce appetite because the individual feels full.

Stool softeners work within the intestinal wall to increase salts and water inside the intestines. They may be useful when stools are very hard to reduce straining. The most commonly used stool softener is docusate sodium (Colace).

Nonabsorbable sugar agents increase fluid in the gut by attracting fluid. Two examples are sorbitol lactulose (Chronulac) and polyethylene glycol (Golytely). Sorbitol is safe and inexpensive, and is a component in some sugar-free candies. These candies bear a warning label that high intake may result in diarrhea. Lactulose is also effective. Polyethylene glycol is used to clean out the intestines completely prior to diagnostic tests. These agents may be associated with some cramping and flatulence.

Saline laxatives (e.g., Milk of Magnesia) attract water to the intestinal tract where it is retained, stimulating movement in the intestines. Saline laxatives can cause dehydration and electrolyte abnormalities if not carefully monitored.

Lubricant laxatives, including mineral oil, though effective stool softeners, prevent absorption of fat-soluble vitamins and may cause fecal leaking or incontinence.

Stimulant laxatives increase intestinal motility by increasing fluid excretion into the gut and irritating the nerves supplying the intestines. These are some of the most commonly used and abused laxatives among the elderly. Examples include bisacodyl (Dulcolax), anthraquinones, senna (Sennakot), cascara (Peri-Colace), and phenolphthalein (e.g., Ex-Lax, Correctol, Feen-A-Mint). Prolonged use can lead to laxative dependency, fluid-salt imbalance, severe cramps, malabsorption, diarrhea, and dehydration. Phenolphthalein was recently removed from the market because of its newfound association with cancer.

Glycerine rectal *suppositories* stimulate the rectum to evacuate its contents. *Enemas* may be concocted from a variety of substances including mineral oil, tap water, phosphate (Fleet), or soapsuds. They soften and lubricate the stool in the rectum and assist evacuation by distending the rectum and cleaning it out.

Many experts assert that laxatives are the worst choice to treat constipation. They suggest that the source of the problem needs to be identified. Checking to see if prescriptions are causing constipation, increasing fluid and fiber intake, increasing physical activity, and going to the toilet after eating should be the first line of treatment. Laxatives should only be used temporarily as a last resort.[28]

Cold and Flu Medications

One of the most common self-limiting illnesses is the common cold, a viral infection of the upper respiratory tract. Influenza (flu) is also caused by a virus, and some strains affecting the respiratory tract have symptoms similar to a cold. Antibiotics are ineffective against viruses, so the only therapy is to reduce the symptoms while the cold or flu runs its course.

There are thousands of remedies on the market to temporarily relieve one or more cold and flu symptoms. While some remedies contain only one ingredient, the majority contains a combination of ingredients. It is for this very reason that they are not recommended or needed because the products likely contain ingredients to reduce symptoms that are not even present. Also, the more drugs ingested, the greater risk of drug interactions and side effects. Selecting simple medicines to treat the bothersome symptoms at the dose needed is more effective. An understanding of the medications used to treat the symptoms of a cold or flu can help the consumer best select the ingredients to treat their symptoms. The following drugs reduce many of the symptoms of the common cold.

Cough suppressants are useful to control coughs that cause chest pain or interfere with sleep or breathing. Dextromethorphan (Drixoral, Robitussin DM, Benylin) is the safest and most effective suppressant for dry coughs. Since coughing due to colds is usually caused by postnasal drip, a nasal decongestant, in addition to relieving nasal congestion, will ease the coughing. Although products with codeine work well, they cause constipation and can be habit-forming.

Expectorants thin and loosen the excessive phlegm common in the airways of a cold sufferer. An example is guaifenesin (Robitussin). Although these results are desirable, most OTC expectorants are ineffective because the dosage is insufficient.

Decongestants unclog blocked nasal passages and sinuses (stuffy nose) and prevent postnasal drip in the throat by constricting blood vessels in the nasal passages. They may be taken by pill, most commonly pseudoephedrine (Sudafed, Actifed), or by nasal drops or sprays, for example oxymetazoline (Afrin) or phenylephrine (Neo-Synephrine). Nasal drops or sprays are safer, work faster, and are more effective than pills. However, their use is restricted to only a few days because rebound congestion may occur, requiring higher and more frequent dosages for the same effect. Decongestants may cause nervousness, dizziness, urinary retention, dry eyes, or insomnia.

Analgesics ibuprofen (Motrin IB, Nuprin), aspirin (Bayer), acetaminophen (Tylenol), and others reduce the aching feeling that may accompany a cold or flu and reduce a fever.

Medicated lozenges and sprays ease the minor pain of a sore throat that accompanies a cold. Since a sore throat is caused by postnasal drip, a decongestant can reduce the soreness. The most effective and long-lasting ingredient in sore throat remedies is dyclonine (Sucrets Maximum Strength, Sucrets throat spray).

Topical Medications

Medications are available over-the-counter to treat skin irritations and minor bacterial and fungal infections. Redness, itching, eczema, or rashes may be treated with 1% hydrocortisone cream, a low-strength corticosteroid. Minor bacterial infections may be treated with topical creams such as neosporin or polysporin ointments. Vaginal yeast infections can be treated with a wide variety of OTC products, previously available only by prescription, including miconazone (Monistat), ticonazole (Vagistat 1), and clotrimazole (Gyne-lotrimin) available in creams and suppositories. Yeast infections of the genitals (jock itch) and feet (athlete's foot) may also be managed with over-the-counter remedies.

Another topical remedy is the nicotine patch (Nicotrol, Nicoderm CQ) to assist adults in smoking cessation. These patches contain nicotine that is absorbed through the skin into the bloodstream. These patches are expensive. Ideally, they are used in combination with a comprehensive behavioral smoking cessation program. Nicotine gum (Nicorette) is also available.

PRESCRIPTION DRUGS COMMONLY USED BY ELDERS

Prescription medications can only be procured under the direction of a physician and dispensed by a pharmacist. They are usually used to treat more serious disease conditions and are more likely to cause unexpected and adverse side effects. Over 5,000 prescription drugs are available and are classified into major drug families or groups that share important chemical characteristics and intended effects. Each family has several medications marketed under different brand names, but all contain the same or similar basic drug ingredients. This section provides an overview of the medications commonly prescribed to elders.

Analgesics

Although some analgesics can be purchased over-the-counter, others are available only by prescription. In most cases, pain can be relieved with over-the-counter analgesics. If pain is not managed, the next step is often a prescription combination drug that includes either acetaminophen or NSAID and low-dose opioid medications (derived from opium). Examples include acetaminophen and codeine (Tylenol #3), acetaminophen and oxycodone (Percocet, Tylox), and acetaminophen and hydrocodone (Vicodin, Lortab). For severe pain (e.g., back strain, migraine headache, kidney

stone, and postoperative or cancer pain), higher potency opioids should be prescribed. These include drugs naturally derived from opium (morphine and codeine) or synthetic drugs such as oxycodone (Roxicodone), hydromorphone (Dilaudid), methadone (Dolophine), fentanyl (Duragesic patches), and meperidine (Demerol). Opioids are available as pills, rectal suppositories, transdermal patches, nasal sprays, or lozenges, which are placed under the tongue for those who have difficulty swallowing. Opioids can be injected into the veins, muscles, skin, or spine.

Opioid medications have been used for centuries and are more effective and safer than many other types of pain medications. Many believe them to be underused, especially in the treatment of cancer pain, because the physician, patient, and family fear addiction. Many elders have chronic pain conditions that significantly impair their functional ability and quality of life and would be best treated with opioid medications.[29]

Opioid medications have multiple side effects (constipation, nausea, respiratory depression, confusion, sedation, and tolerance), especially among elders. However, NSAID medications, commonly used instead of opioids, also have high rates of adverse effects in older persons. Pain can also have significant adverse effects on functional status, physical activity levels, nutrition, psychological status, socialization, and quality of life. People in pain are generally willing to take these medications and to manage side effects with other pharmacological and nonpharmacological means. In addition, those with pain often maintain alertness and functional capacity while on opioid medications. Elders using the medications for cancer rarely become addicted; addiction rates are less than 1 percent in that group.

There are many other types of medications that can be used to manage pain, including corticosteroids, antidepressants, anticonvulsants, muscle relaxants, antiarrythmics, and local anesthetics. These medications are commonly prescribed for pain due to nerve damage that is less responsive to opioid medications (e.g., herpes zoster, diabetic neuropathy, sciatica).

Antibiotics and Antivirals

Antibiotics destroy or inhibit the multiplication of disease-producing bacteria that invade the body. There are a tremendous variety of antibiotics used alone or in combination to treat bacterial infections. Selecting an antibiotic depends on the infection location and the bacteria most likely causing that type of infection. Often body secretions such as urine, vaginal secretions, or sputum may be "cultured" to determine the type of bacteria causing the infection. This involves taking a sample of body fluids and growing it in the laboratory, then identifying the specific infecting bacteria.

The choice of antibiotic also depends on the way the drug is metabolized, how it is administered, and its toxic potential. Some antibiotics are metabolized by the kidney, others by the liver. Most antibiotics can be taken orally, others are only given intravenously or by injection. Their toxicities also vary widely—some can cause kidney problems, some cause increased sensitivity to sunlight, and others can affect hearing. People may suffer allergic reactions to antibiotics that range from a rash to respiratory collapse. Common side effects of antibiotics are gastrointestinal upset and vaginal yeast infections.

Antibiotics are sometimes prescribed incorrectly for conditions, like the common cold or influenza, where they are not useful. Additionally, some people discontinue antibiotics when symptoms subside rather than finishing the prescription. As a result, the infection returns, sometimes more virulently. Both practices contribute to the development of antibiotic-resistant bacteria.

A newer category of drugs is the antivirals. These medications are being developed to fight severe viral infections, and most work by not allowing the viruses to multiply. Amantadine is used both for prevention and treatment of influenza; however, it is very expensive and must be taken by inhalation. Another antiviral medication, AZT, is used daily by people with AIDS or AIDS-associated immunosuppression to decrease viral replication and slow the progression of the disease. Protease inhibitors are another type of antiviral used to interfere with the replication of HIV. In addition, acyclovir (Zovirax) is useful for attacks of herpes, both genital herpes as well as herpes zoster. Currently, researchers are developing many other antiviral drugs.

Antihistamines

The prescription antihistamines have the same effect as those purchased over-the-counter: both block the histamines released during an allergic reaction: sneezing, itching, watery eyes, and itchy nose and throat. Common brand names are Allegra and Claritin. However, the newer generation prescription antihistamines work differently than OTC drugs, and most do not have the side effect of drowsiness.

Anti-Inflammatory Drugs

Anti-inflammatory medications reduce joint swelling, stiffness, inflammation, and pain for people suffering from osteoarthritis or rheumatoid arthritis. The most widely used and effective drug for arthritis is aspirin, generally given in high dosages. In some cases, prescription anti-inflammatory agents are useful. The drugs in this category vary in effectiveness and side effects in different patients. However, there is increasing evidence that nonsteroidal anti-inflammatory drugs create a serious risk of peptic ulcer and death among the elderly who use them. Many physicians are now recommending acetaminophen to their arthritic patients to minimize this risk.

During severe exacerbations of arthritis, other drugs such as corticosteroids (prednisone, cortisone), methotrexate, gold salts, and higher-strength painkillers are sometimes used. Cortisone can be injected or taken orally to reduce inflammation. However, steroids have many serious side effects and should be used with caution in elders. They will be discussed later in this section. Methotrexate was originally used as chemotherapy for cancer patients. It is now being used for rheumatoid arthritis as well. Although this drug may cause gastrointestinal side effects, it is used for long-term treatment of severe cases. Gold salts are sometimes injected or taken orally to treat rheumatoid arthritis; however, it may be several months before improvement is noted, and their effectiveness has been questioned. Gold salts also have many adverse effects on the skin, blood, and kidneys.

Osteoporosis Drugs

The goal of drug treatment in postmenopausal women with osteoporosis is to reduce fracture risk by increasing bone mass. The most commonly prescribed drug is hormone replacement therapy (see below). However, for those who do not want or cannot tolerate estrogen, other drugs have demonstrated some effectiveness. Sodium flouride used to be the mainstay of treatment for osteoporosis because it increased bone density. However, it has become less popular because it is not clear that it decreases fracture risk. A new slow-release pill seems to be more effective if combined with a calcium supplement. Calcitriol (Rocaltrol) is a potent form of vitamin D and regulates calcium metabolism. The drug increases calcium absorption and increases bone mass in some bones.

Daily treatment with alendronate (Fosamax) has been reported to increase bone mass, reduce fractures, and reduce the progression of vertebral deformities. Although the drug was designed to treat bone cancer, alendronate is also used to treat postmenopausal osteoporosis, although it does not yet have FDA approval for that purpose. There have been many reports of severe damage to the esophagus. To counteract that problem, the drug should be taken with a full glass of water, and the patient should not lie down for at least thirty minutes afterwards. A related drug in the same group can be injected, and another is available in pill form to treat osteoporosisis of the spine.

Bronchodilators and Antiasthmatics

Drugs in this category act by enlarging constricted airways, improving the ability to breathe. They are used to treat asthma, chronic obstructive pulmonary disease (COPD), and acute respiratory infections accompanied by wheezing. These medications are most commonly dispensed as inhalants, but can also be taken in pill form. Inhalers have fewer side effects because the drug is absorbed where needed with less of it circulated through the body. Common inhalant drugs are Proventil (albuterol), Alupent (metaproterenol), corticosteroids, beclomethasone (Vanceril, Beclovent), and triamcinolone acetate (Azmacort). Proventil and Alupent can cause nervousness and increased heart rate and should be used cautiously in patients with heart conditions. Studies show the inhalant drugs to be highly effective, but many adults use them incorrectly because coordination is needed to correctly inhale the medication. This difficulty can be minimized with the use of an aerochamber or spacer that reduces the need to coordinate breathing with medication delivery.

Theophylline is a widely used drug that relaxes and expands the bronchial tubes, and stimulates the diaphragm for better breathing. This medication is often prescribed for people with asthma or emphysema when inhalers are not sufficient. Some evidence suggests that this medication adds a high degree of risk for small benefit, but many physicians and patients disagree. Theophylline can cause jitteriness, increased heart rate, nausea, or insomnia. Blood levels of this medication should be closely monitored in elders.

Corticosteroids

The steroids publicized in the news for their ability to increase muscle mass are anabolic steroids, a type of male sex hormone. In contrast, the type of steroids most often prescribed by physicians are corticosteroids, which act to decrease inflammation, suppress immune reactions, and promote healing. These drugs are used as creams for skin conditions, inhaled to treat the lungs and sinuses, and ingested for treatment of COPD, autoimmune diseases, cancer, or steroid-deficiency conditions. During acute stages of lung disease, corticosteroids are used to reduce inflammation in the lungs. In end-stage lung disease, patients need the corticosteroids continuously.

Corticosteroids are very effective; however, they have a number of side effects that limit their use. They suppress immune function, consequently decreasing healing time and increasing infection risk. They also cause thinning of the skin and bones, aggravate cataracts and diabetes, cause weight gain (particularly in the face and abdomen), increase fluid retention, and alter psychological and cognitive function. They can cause a sense of elation in some individuals, and psychosis in others. When these drugs are withdrawn, the dosage must be gradually tapered to prevent symptoms of withdrawal. To prevent steroid-associated osteoporosis, individuals should be prescribed supplemental doses of calcium and vitamin D while on long-term steroid therapy.[30] For these reasons, they should be used at the lowest dose and for the shortest possible time.

Drugs for Skin Problems

The steroid preparations previously discussed comprise the main drug treatment for skin problems of elders. These are applied to the skin directly or taken orally to treat a wide range of conditions including eczema, psoriasis, and pruritus. There are many different strengths and types of corticosteroids.

For those with multiple actinic keratosis (precancerous lesions), skin treatment with either 5-fluorouracil (5-FU) or Retin-A is generally prescribed. These agents irritate the skin, but prevent precancerous skin lesions from progressing to more invasive skin cancer. Fluorouracil inhibits cell division. When applied to the face, the skin becomes reddened, itchy, and irritated; complete healing sometimes takes months after the preparation is stopped. Retin-A is a topical vitamin A derivative used to treat acne, facial wrinkling, and precancerous skin lesions. People who use these preparations should avoid direct sunlight exposure.

Hormone Replacement

Sex steroids are widely used as hormonal replacement therapy to reduce symptoms of menopause and to reduce the risk of several chronic diseases and disorders. Several types of estrogen and progesterone have been developed for this purpose. Unless

women have had a hysterectomy, estrogen and progesterone are used in combination because estrogen prescribed alone increases endometrial (lining of the uterus) cancer risk. Hormone replacement therapy varies in type of estrogen and progesterone, method of administration, dosage prescribed, and timing. When the hormones are administered cyclically, women experience periodic bleeding, similar to a menstrual period. In other cases, smaller doses of one or both drugs are given continuously, and bleeding does not occur. Estrogen creams, prescribed to reduce the thinning and drying of the vaginal walls, and a transdermal estrogen patch, worn on the abdomen, are other ways to deliver estrogen.

Hormonal replacement therapy (HRT) instituted at menopause reduces menopause-associated symptoms such as hot flashes and vaginal dryness. Many studies report that HRT offers other important benefits for postmenopausal women. Multiple large observational and cohort studies and a few randomized controlled trials have shown that HRT significantly decreases overall death rates, particularly deaths from cardiovascular disease. Because cardiovascular disease is the number one cause of death among elder women, the benefits are clear, and are particularly relevant for women at high risk of cardiovascular disease. HRT alters the cholesterol profile of the blood, increasing levels of HDL ("good" cholesterol) and decreasing levels of LDL ("bad" cholesterol).

Estrogen replacement therapy also slows menopausal bone loss and consequent fracture risk. However, this benefit rapidly reverses when HRT is discontinued. HRT has also been associated with reduced risk of urinary incontinence, colon cancer, and urinary tract infections. Use of hormones is associated with improved mood, better cognitive function, and reduced risk of Alzheimer's dementia. Studies are ongoing to confirm these associations because many of the studies have methodological problems that limit firm conclusions.

Hormone replacement therapy has its drawbacks. For example, estrogen increases the risk of endometrial cancer. To counter this risk, all women with an intact uterus are prescribed progesterone because it has been shown to counteract that nega-

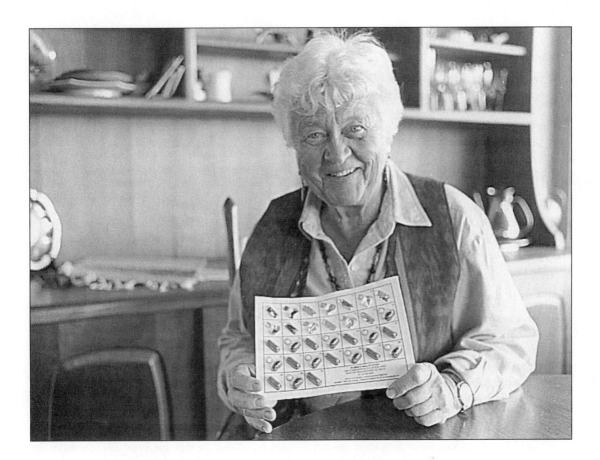

tive effect. Thus far, no clear relationship has been found between breast cancer incidence and hormonal replacement therapy. Although women are more afraid of breast cancer than cardiovascular disease, the risk of dying of heart disease is far greater than dying of breast cancer because heart disease is the number one killer of middle-aged and older women.

Currently, fewer than one-third of postmenopausal women use HRT in the United States. Because of the accumulating evidence, more physicians are becoming convinced of its benefits and are recommending HRT to many of their middle-aged and elder women patients. However, HRT is not for all women. Personal risk factors, family history, and motivation should be taken into account when making the decision.

Medications (including estrogens) that suppress the manufacture of testosterone may be prescribed to men with widespread prostate cancer to slow disease progression. Also, men may be prescribed testosterone to counteract a deficiency that is reflected by impotence, lack of energy, abnormal body fat distribution, and/or reduced sexual desire. Postmenopausal women may also be prescribed testosterone to increase sexual desire and energy; however, the dose needs to be carefully monitored to control masculinizing side effects, such as facial hair and deepened voice.

A variety of other hormonal medications are available. The most widely prescribed is thyroid replacement, used by people with an underactive thyroid gland. Megesterol (Megace) is a progesteronal agent used to increase appetite. Tamoxifen

(Nolvadex) is an antiestrogenic agent prescribed to women with breast cancer to slow the rate of growth of the tumor. Studies are ongoing to determine whether tamoxifen is useful in preventing breast cancer as well. Raloxifine (Evista) is another newer drug that, although not an estrogen, acts like one in the body. It appears to have positive effects on bone density and cholesterol. However, the effects on the uterus are not yet known, and it does not reduce uncomfortable menopausal symptoms. Studies need to be conducted to compare it with the benefits of estrogen. The drug might be useful for those menopausal women who cannot take estrogen who want to decrease their risk of cardiovascular disease, osteoporosis, and breast cancer.

Drugs to Reduce Cholesterol

Many drugs are now on the market to reduce cholesterol, with varying modes of action, and their use is on the rise. However, there is continuing debate about who should use cholesterol-lowering drugs. Some assert that these medications should be reserved for people with elevated cholesterol who are at high risk of developing fatal heart attacks—individuals with high cholesterol and who have had a previous heart attack. However, others assert that these medications should be prescribed to all individuals with elevated cholesterol, even without a history of heart disease.

Because the findings about who should take cholesterol-lowering drugs are often contradictory and confusing, meta-analyses (combining results from multiple studies) attempt to make sense of these data. These studies report that cholesterol-lowering drugs reduce cholesterol and cardiovascular disease among those with high or low risk for a heart attack (mainly white, middle-aged men). Those who have already had a heart attack seem to reap the most benefits in reduced deaths from a second heart attack. In addition, some studies reveal an alarming increase in noncardiac mortality (such as cancer and accidents) among low-risk participants taking cholesterol-lowering drugs.[31] It has been hypothesized that these negative effects are due to the dangerous side effects of these medications,

What Is Cholesterol?

Cholesterol, a waxy substance made in the liver, plays a crucial role in maintaining the cell membranes and building certain hormones. Cholesterol travels from the liver through the blood to its various destinations as a component of certain large particles, known as lipoproteins. Low-density lipoprotein (LDL), known as the "bad" cholesterol, dumps some of its cholesterol into the walls of the arteries. High-density lipoprotein (HDL), the "good" cholesterol, sweeps up the cholesterol from the arteries and carries it back to the liver. If the liver makes too much LDL or too little HDL—mainly due to a fatty diet, lack of exercise, and genetic factors—cholesterol can build up in the blood and form artery-clogging plaque deposits.

such as reducing reaction time. However, many of these trials studied older drugs, which may be more dangerous and less effective than newer ones. It is generally agreed that men with high levels of LDL and other risk factors for heart disease have the most to gain from these drugs.

Medications that lower cholesterol vary by type and mechanism of action. Cholestyramine (Questran) binds bile acids in the gut and prevents the absorption of cholesterol. Side effects include flushing, constipation, rashes, and blurred vision. This drug interacts poorly with other drugs and can alter absorption of fat-soluble vitamins. Gemfibrozil (Lopid) steps up the activity of an enzyme that breaks down LDL. It is recommend only for patients without previous cardiac disease, with high levels of triyglycerides and LDL, and with low levels of HDL.

Probably the most effective and most widely used class of drugs now on the market to reduce cholesterol levels are the "-statins." Statins work by inhibiting the production of cholesterol in the liver. Less production means less need for its carrier, LDL, so the liver pulls LDL out from the blood and destroys it. Thus, statins reduce LDL more than any other type of drug. Pravastatin (Pravachol) or simvastatin (Zocor) are two new statin drugs that have been shown to be associated with reduced risk of heart attack and stroke in people who have either heart disease or elevated cholesterol levels.[32, 33] Another study used another statin drug (lovastatin [Mevacor]) that reportedly cut cardiovascular risk in healthy people with only moderately elevated cholesterol levels.[34] Other statin drugs probably have similar effects, showing that they are valuable drugs for protecting the heart.

Although not technically a drug, niacin, a B-vitamin, also decreases LDL cholesterol production and prevents body fats from breaking down to release triglycerides into the bloodstream. Recent research documents it to be as effective in reducing cholesterol as many cholesterol-reducing drugs. In addition, it increases the proportion of good cholesterol (HDL) in the bloodstream. Its greatest side effect is skin flushing. The advantage of niacin is its cost, about $70 per year for the generic version.

Despite their potential benefits, cholesterol-lowering therapy remains controversial. Even though these medications are widely used by women, ethnic minorities, and the elderly, insufficient research has been conducted on these groups to demonstrate any benefit to lowering cholesterol. Further, these drugs are prescribed indefinitely, sometimes for life, when little data exist on their impact on other organ systems, especially the liver. Real-world use of these medications is often accompanied by high drop-out rates due to unacceptable side effects. Finally, except for niacin, the medications are expensive, with costs ranging from $500 to $1,300 per year.

Even though pills may reduce the risk of having a heart attack and dying from one, the first line of treatment to reduce cholesterol and other risk factors for heart disease is to develop healthy behaviors. Sidney Smith, M.D., the former head of the American Heart Association, stated, "I am continually amazed that patients are willing to take pills, have tubes snaked into their heart, even have their chest sawed open—but aren't willing to change their diet, get some exercise, or stop smoking."[35]

Gout Drugs

Allopurinol is the drug most commonly prescribed for the long-term management of gout. The drug maintains normal uric acid blood levels, thus preventing acute episodes of gout. It may cause anemia or skin rashes, and interacts with many other medications, including alcohol, antibiotics, or oral medications to treat diabetes.

If an individual chooses not to take continuous medication to prevent an acute gouty attack, drugs can be taken at the onset of an acute gout attack (e.g., an NSAID, such as indomethacin). Although colchicine is sometimes used as a preventive drug, it is more commonly used in larger doses to reduce the pain, swelling, and inflammation of an acute attack. It can cause severe anemia and is often associated with severe gastrointestinal upset.

Diabetic Drugs

Two major drug types help the body maintain blood sugar at a nearly normal level: oral hypoglycemics for those with diabetes who still produce insulin, and insulin for those who cannot produce it. Oral medications, called sulfonylureas (Orinase, Dymelor, Tolinase, Diabinese), stimulate the pancreas to release more insulin and also increase the receptivity of body cells to available insulin. These drugs are taken daily, generally in combination with a diabetic diet, to normalize blood sugar. Their major side effect is low blood sugar or hypoglycemia, which can result in confusion, abnormal behavior, and if persistent, brain damage. Newer oral medications, such as metformin hydrochloride (Glucophage), increase the sensitivity of the body's cells to insulin without the risk of hypoglycemia and are quite effective, allowing many individuals to forego the use of insulin. Glucophage medication can be combined with other oral medications to increase effectiveness.

For diabetics who do not produce insulin, daily insulin injections are necessary. Insulin injections may also be used for adult-onset diabetics who do not respond to diet change, weight loss programs, or oral hypoglycemic drugs. Appropriate dosage and careful monitoring are necessary: too much or too little insulin can be harmful.

A new method of administering insulin is the electronic insulin pump that is implanted in the abdominal cavity. It dispenses insulin in constant steady pulses through the day. Before each meal, the patient holds a transmitter device over the pump to tell it to deliver extra insulin. The surgery and the pump cost between $5,000 and $8,000. When the pump is compared with insulin injections, those who had the implanted pump had fewer episodes of low blood sugar and controlled their weight better. However, a significant number of pumps have malfunctioned.[36]

Gastric Acid Blockers

Gastric acid blockers are widely used to reduce the secretion of acid in the stomach. These drugs are useful for people who have stomach ulcers, chronic heartburn, stress, or who have been hospitalized because these conditions increase gastric acid secretion. They can be taken by mouth or intravenously, and may be used in conjunction with OTC antacids. The most widely used prescription antacids are the H_2 blockers, many of which are now available over-the-counter, including Tagamet (cimetidine) and Zantac (ranitidine). These drugs may cause confusion in elderly patients. The newer drugs, omeprazole (Prilosec) and lansoprazpole (Pravacid), completely block the mechanism that secretes acid into the stomach. Although they have fewer side effects, they are expensive. These newer drugs also can be effective for severe gastroesophageal reflux.

Psychoactive Drugs

Elders are prescribed a wide variety of drugs for many different disorders of the central nervous system. On the average, they are prescribed more psychoactive drugs than any other age group. Psychoactive drugs are used to treat migraine headaches, Parkinson's disease, seizures, depression, anxiety, psychotic behavior, and sleep problems. Some of these medications, including anticonvulsants and antidepressants, are often used in reduced dosages to treat nerve pain after a shingles outbreak, and for diabetic neuropathy, low back pain, or cancer pain. When used appropriately, these medications can be quite effective in reducing agitation and depression, improving functional status and improving sleep among elders.

Elders are more sensitive to central nervous system medications than other adults, and many physicians fear these medications are overprescribed, particularly among those in nursing homes. Because of these concerns, advocates pressed for tougher regulations on the use of psychoactive drugs in nursing homes. Subsequently, the Nursing Home Reform Act of 1987 mandated that these medications be closely monitored to prevent unnecessary use. This section discusses the many classes of psychoactive medications.

Drugs for Siezures

Some elders may have had seizure disorders since birth, but many develop seizures secondary to other illnesses such as strokes, brain tumors, alcoholism, head injury, or metabolic problems. Dilantin (phenytoin), Tegretol, Neurontin, and Depakote are some of the drugs used to prevent seizures. Dilantin is most often used, but it has many side effects (e.g., unsteady gait), and blood levels must be carefully monitored. Anticonvulsant medications are sometimes used to treat nerve pain conditions or to stabilize mood.

Drugs for Parkinson's Disease

Drug therapy for patients with Parkinson's disease increases dopamine in the brain, thus reducing the symptoms. Levodopa (Carbidopa) is the drug most often prescribed. Other drugs, such as antihistamines, cogentin, or the antiviral drug, amantadine, are used in combination to enhance the effect of levodopa. Pramipexole (Mirapex) is a new drug that has been shown to improve motor skills in the early stages of Parkinson's disease for those who are not yet receiving levodopa.

Sedatives

As a group, elders are high users of sleeping pills, responsible for 30 percent of all sedative prescriptions. Sleeping pills are useful in the hospital setting when elders have difficulty falling asleep or for short-term use during an acutely stressful event. It is recommended that they be taken for no more than seven to ten days. Despite their long-term use by many, they have never been shown to be effective sleep-inducers for any age group for more than two weeks. Benzodiazepines, barbiturates, and chloral hydrate can all induce sleep.

Benzodiazepines are a class of prescription drugs that have a wide variety of uses. The intermediate and longer-acting benzodiazepines are used to reduce depression and anxiety and help to relax muscle tension (see "Antidepressants" below). Those with shorter half-lives, such as temazepam (Restoril) and triazolam (Halcion), are used to induce sleep. Although the shorter-acting forms have less of a hangover effect, ingesting high doses or continuing for an extended period of time can cause memory loss, daytime sedation, and confusion. Benzodiazepines can worsen psychological symptoms in some individuals by causing agitation, impaired judgment, depression, and psychosis. Further, they are known to disrupt normal sleep patterns, and they are habit-forming.

Barbiturates are an older type of drug used to induce sleep. Common barbiturates are pentobarbital (Nembutol) and phenobarbital (Luminal). Barbiturates should not be used among elders, except in special, well-supervised conditions. These medications cause a hangover effect with excessive sedation during the day and can cause confusion, gait disturbance, falls, and drug dependence. It is common to have impaired memory the day after taking the drug.

Chloral hydrate (Noctel) is a drug that has been used since the 1800s to induce sleep. At low dosages, it relieves mild to moderate anxiety, and higher dosages relieve insomnia when taken at bedtime. It produces less of a hangover effect and is often prescribed to elders. A newer drug, Ambien, is also prescribed to elders.

Antipsychotic Drugs

Antipsychotics, or strong tranquilizers, are a diverse group of medications used to treat schizophrenia or reduce agitated, disruptive behavior. Elders likely to receive psychotropic drugs include those who are mobile, incontinent, cognitively impaired, or behaviorally disruptive. Elders who take antipsychotics fall into two groups: those with long-term mental illness who have taken these medications for years, and those who develop the organic diseases associated with old age, such as Alzheimer's disease, acute confusion (e.g., following surgery or a stroke), or those demented patients who have "sundown syndrome" (increased confusion and agitation in the evenings). These elders may be prescribed low doses of antipsychotics to calm them. However, there is increasing concern that these medications are used as a chemical restraint, especially in skilled nursing facilities. Federal regulations specify particular criteria under which these drugs can be used in nursing homes.

Elders who receive antipsychotics for the first time in their later years are highly sensitive to them and should be given very low doses and be carefully monitored. Side effects include rigidity, restlessness, drowsiness, dry mouth, blurred vision, constipation, urinary retention, and unsteadiness. Often other drugs must be given to counteract these side effects.

Perhaps the most severe side effect of antipsychotic drug use is tardive dyskinesia. These individuals exhibit tics and involuntary muscle movements thought to be caused by chronic depletion of neurotransmitters. Women and those on long-term antipsychotic therapy are most susceptible. Since these drugs are generally very effective, the best way to minimize the onset of tardive dyskinesia is to prescribe the lowest possible dose that controls the psychotic symptoms.

There are a wide variety of antipsychotic medications with differing uses and side effects. Those with schizophrenia are generally prescribed the high-potency medications, consequently placing them at a higher risk of acquiring tardive dyskinesia. The low-potency antipsychotic medications are less likely to cause tardive dyskinesia, but they are more sedating and more likely to cause dry mouth and urinary retention. If troubles occur on one medication, they can likely be ameliorated with a change in medications.

Antianxiety Drugs

Antianxiety drugs, benzodiazepines, also called mild tranquilizers, are prescribed to reduce anxiety and tension, relax skeletal muscles, and facilitate alcohol withdrawal. These drugs are useful for treating people with panic disorder and agoraphobia as well as those in pain. The short-acting antianxiety drugs were discussed under "Sedatives." The benzodiazepines commonly prescribed for anxiety are Librium and Valium. Other agents are lorazapam (Ativan) and alprazolam (Xanax), and newer agents such as busipirone (BuSpar).

Benzodiazepines should be prescribed only for temporary episodes of anxiety or panic disorder because tolerance and dependence occur with prolonged use. In addition, elders are more likely to manifest side effects than younger groups, such as daytime sedation, confusion, or dizziness. The newer antianxiety agents such as busipirone are not habit-forming, but may take up to six weeks to be effective. Busipirone is increasingly being prescribed to reduce the agitation common in elders with dementia.

Although problems with benzodiazepines have been known for years, these drugs may still be widely prescribed to elders. Multiple studies report that about one-fifth of elders are prescribed benzodiazepines each year, many using them daily. However, these drugs have never been shown to be effective for long-term use. Since it has been documented that elders suffer a disproportionate number of adverse effects, including an increased risk of falling, driving accidents, and impaired memory and thought processes, continuing assessment is crucial. Before antianxiety drugs are prescribed, other alternatives should be explored, including stress reduction, meditation, counseling, and physical activity.

Antidepressants

Antidepressants are prescribed to relieve depression and its associated symptoms of anxiety, insomnia, lack of appetite, and suicidal thoughts. They are also used to treat obsessive-compulsive disorder, insomnia, and nerve pain syndromes.

In the last several years, the use of antidepressants in the United States has increased tremendously. There are more than twenty antidepressant medication types on the market. Newer medications on the market are called serotonin-specific reuptake inhibitors (SSRIs), including fluoxetine (Prozac), paroxetine (Paxil), and sertraline (Zoloft). Antidepressants may also be classified as tricyclic, including amitriptyline (Elavil), desipramine (Norpramin), and imipramine (Tofranil) and as MAO inhibitors, including phenelzine (Nardil) and tranylcypromine (Parnate). Other types may work through other mechanisms: buproprion (Wellbutrin), trazodone (Desyrel), or vantafaxine (Effexor). Still other types of drugs for depression and bipolar disorder include mood stabilizers such as lithium carbonate (Eskalith, Lithobid) and some of the anticonvulsant medications.

All antidepressants work by increasing levels of neurotransmitters, including dopamine, norepinephrine, and seratonin, that transfer signals from one nerve to another within the brain. Because different drugs target different transmitters, and because transmitter imbalance varies among individuals, some drugs are more effective than others for a given individual. At times, these drugs are used in combination. The dosage must be started low and gradually increased to minimize side effects. Although some individuals have rapid responses, most note gradual onset of improvement in mood over four to six weeks. In general, these drugs are continued for months to years to prevent recurrent bouts of depression. Those with obsessive-compulsive disorder respond well to Prozac and Zoloft.

Some antidepressants (e.g. Elavil) cause sedation and should be taken before bedtime to help the insomnia associated with depression, while others (e.g., Prozac) are more activating and should be taken in the day. A wide variety of side effects have been reported, including constipation, anxiety, excessive sedation, sexual difficulties, and alterations in weight or appetite.

The tricyclic antidepressants can be lethal if taken in overdose; therefore, the quantity of pills dispensed to suicidal patients should be small.

Although the MAO inhibitor antidepressants are often effective, they are particularly hazardous to older people because of the risk of dangerously high blood pressure when foods containing tyramine (an amino acid) are eaten (smoked meat, aged cheese, pickled fish, red wine, and yogurt with active cultures). MAO inhibitors should not be used unless other treatments have failed.

All medications have side effects, but the newer class of antidepressants, the SSRIs, has fewer of them. Consequently, many physicians are less hesitant to prescribe antidepressants to elders or those with mild depression. Doctors should prescribe lower doses of antidepressants to elders to compensate for physiological changes accompanying old age and to reduce side effects. However, it is important that the patient be continually assessed to ensure the dose is high enough to be therapeutic. Also, SSRIs are more expensive.

Drugs for Alzheimer's Disease

Many drugs have been tested to reduce the effects of cognitive decline in Alzheimer's disease. Some have survived the test of time, others have not. One drug, tacrine (Cognex), is the first drug to be approved for Alzheimer's disease. Studies show improvements in cognitive function, quality of life, and postponed nursing home placement among those taking the drug. However, tacrine is only a temporary stopgap because it delays the cognitive decline only for a short time (about six months) and works only for one out of four who take the medication. Further, it has many side effects and is toxic to the liver.[37]

Donazepit (Aricept) is a drug that acts similarly to tacrine. It has also been reported to slow the decline common in Alzheimer's disease. Hydergine, an older drug, has also shown promise in reducing symptoms associated with dementia, including depression and indifference.

Cardiovascular Drugs

Drugs in this category include those used to treat hypertension, congestive heart failure, angina, and cardiac arrhythmias. Often older people have more than one cardiovascular problem and are prescribed more than one drug in this category. All drugs in this category require frequent monitoring by a physician.

Drugs for High Blood Pressure

There are a plethora of medications available to treat high blood pressure (hypertension) with a wide variety of side effects. The mainstays of hypertension treatment are two older classes of medications, the diuretics and beta blockers. However, the newer classes of medications often have fewer side effects, leading many physicians to prescribe them. The National High Blood Pressure Education Program, representing a consensus of a number of health care experts, emphasizes the importance of first prescribing diuretics and/or beta blockers because they are the only drugs shown in long-term studies to reduce death rate. Further, diuretics and beta blockers are the least expensive antihypertensive agents on the market.

Diuretics are the first-line treatment for hypertension and congestive heart failure. These drugs reduce the amount of salts and water in the body, consequently reducing water retention and blood pressure. Two types of diuretics are commonly used: potassium-depleting (thiazide diuretics) and potassium-sparing. When used excessively, diuretics can cause dehydration, salt imbalances, and postural hypotension (a drop in blood pressure when rising, resulting in dizziness and fainting).

Thiazide diuretics are widely used to lower blood pressure and are used by those with congestive heart failure to decrease edema (swelling caused by an accumulation of fluid). Adverse effects of thiazides are an excessive loss of potassium and an increased uric acid level that may cause gout, disturbed glucose metabolism, and increased cholesterol. Potassium supplements are usually prescribed to reduce potassium depletion. Elders on thiazides should frequently have blood tests to monitor their potassium, uric acid, cholesterol, and glucose levels to keep adverse effects to a minimum. A beneficial side effect of thiazide diuretics is that they help the body to conserve calcium: elders on thiazides have a reduced incidence of hip fracture and kidney stones.

Potassium-sparing diuretics rid the body of water without eliminating potassium. In addition, they do not seem to disturb glucose or uric acid metabolism like the potassium-depleting diuretics. However, in elders, the drugs may cause too much potassium to be retained, especially in those with decreased kidney function, and may result in cardiac problems. Patients on potassium-sparing diuretics should avoid foods high in potassium (e.g., bananas).

Beta blockers are effective at reducing heart rate, thus reducing its oxygen requirement: Metoprolol (Lopressor), atenolol (Tenormin), and propranolol (Inderal) are the most commonly prescribed. These medications are the drug of choice after a heart attack because randomized controlled trials have demonstrated significant benefits in reducing further heart attacks and improving survival rates. However, these drugs are markedly underprescribed in the elderly. Instead, elders are often prescribed the newer calcium channel blockers (see below), which do not have a good record of lowering death rate.[38]

If beta blockers and/or diuretics are ineffective or not tolerated, newer cardiac drugs may be added, called ACE inhibitors because they reduce the production of *a*ngiotensin *c*onverting *e*nzyme that constricts blood vessels. Commonly used ACE inhibitors are enalapril (Vasotec), captopril (Capoten), and lisinopril (Zestril, Prinivil). These agents are particularly effective for congestive heart failure (see below).

Calcium channel blockers are another newer family of drugs. They block calcium from entering cardiac and smooth muscles, inhibiting contraction of the coronary arteries and other blood vessels. This allows blood vessels to widen, reducing blood pressure. These drugs include diltiazem (Cadiazem, Dilacor), amiodipine (Norvasc), niphedipine (Procardia, Adalat), and verapamil (Isoptin, Calan). Some come in longer-acting forms that need to be used only once or twice a day. Channel blockers are very widely used, which concerns many cardiovascular experts. Even though calcium channel blockers have been shown to reduce blood pressure, there is no evidence of their long-term effects in reducing death rates from cardiovascular disease. Further, several studies document that channel blockers are associated with an increased risk of heart attack, gastrointestinal bleeding, and cancer among elders.[39]

For those with severe hypertension, even more medications may be added, including methyldopa (Aldomet), clonidine (Catapress), and prazosin (Minipress). These medications act in the brain to reduce hypertension or act directly on the blood vessels to dilate them.

Antihypertensive medications have a host of side effects that may decrease quality of life, including erectile dysfunction, chronic cough, and fatigue. Because hypertension usually has no symptoms and the medications used to treat it may cause distressing symptoms, medication compliance is often difficult. Health professionals treating hypertension need to thoroughly educate the patient about the disease and the consequences of uncontrolled hypertension upon the eyes, heart, and kidneys. In addition, if one drug causes a side effect, another drug may be prescribed to reduce those side effects, increasing compliance.

Drugs for Congestive Heart Failure

Diuretics are also used to treat congestive heart failure. In congestive heart failure, there is too much fluid in the system, which overloads the heart. Diuretics decrease the body fluids, while medications such as digoxin (Lanoxin) stimulate the heart to pump more efficiently. Digoxin can be extremely toxic, and drug levels should be monitored frequently. However, this drug is very effective at increasing the pumping of the heart in congestive heart failure and normalizing irregular heart rates. Some studies find this drug overprescribed among the elderly. Beta blockers, ACE inhibitors, and occasionally calcium channel blockers are important to effectively manage heart failure.

Drugs for Angina

Three major types of drugs are used to treat the pain and coronary arterial constriction of angina: vasodilators (nitroglycerine), calcium channel blockers, and betablockers. Vasodilators increase circulation to the working heart muscle by enlarging the arteries. Elders with angina can take vasodilators when the pain occurs, for example, by placing a nitroglycerine tablet under the tongue. Some types of nitroglycerine tablets are prescribed for daily use to reduce the frequency and severity of anginal attacks. To provide a constant level of vasodilation, elders with angina can also wear a transdermal patch that releases nitroglycerine through the skin.

Anticoagulants

Blood thinners, or anticoagulants, reduce blood clotting by blocking the action of vitamin K in the liver, which is essential in the blood clotting process. There are three drugs commonly prescribed for anticoagulation: aspirin, warfarin, and heparin. Aspirin, and other drugs that decrease the clumping of platelets, are frequently used as blood thinners, especially in the prevention of heart attack and stroke. Heparin is an anticoagulant that must be given by injection under the skin. It is sometimes prescribed on an outpatient basis, but is the most frequently used anticoagulant in hospitalized patients to prevent the formation of blood clots in the legs during the immobilization that follows surgery.

A widely used anticoagulant is warfarin (Coumadin). Those with a history of blood clots, chronic heart arrhythmias, and artificial heart valves must use warfarin to prevent the formation of clots. This is a very strong and dangerous drug, and dosage and blood clotting time must be carefully monitored. The most dangerous side effect of warfarin is excessive bleeding. Those on warfarin should not take vitamin K because it reduces the blood-thinning effect. In contrast, aspirin increases the action of warfarin. Further, warfarin interferes with many other medications.

A new generation of drugs has been developed to break down blood clots after a heart attack or stroke. Tissue-plasminogen activator (TPA) and streptokinase are therapies given intravenously, generally in the emergency room, if a heart attack or stroke is suspected. If given within three hours of the event, these drugs reduce the extent of disability. These cannot be used in every case of stroke, only those caused by blockages of the arteries.

Drugs to Shrink the Prostate

The prostate is composed of two main types of tissue: glandular tissue that produces some of the substances found in the semen, and smooth muscle that surrounds the urethra and periodically contracts, propelling certain prostate secretions into the urethra where they mix with sperm. In the aging process, the glandular tissue expands, causing the prostate to enlarge, while smooth muscle tissue surrounding the urethra contracts. Both changes can affect the urethra that tunnels through the prostate gland.

Within the last few years, a drug has been developed to shrink the size of the prostate gland. Finisteride (Proscar) works by blocking the production of testosterone into another form that prompts glandular tissue to develop. Although Proscar is relatively effective at reducing the size of the prostate gland, it is only somewhat effective in reducing urinary symptoms for most men. And, for those who do have reduced symptoms, the effects reverse quickly once the medication is discontinued. Proscar costs over $1,000 annually. The most frequently reported side effect is excessive development of the male breast.

Another class of drug, alpha blockers, do not shrink the glandular tissue; instead, they relax the smooth muscles in the gland lying close to the urethra, the neck of the bladder, and the urethra. Three medications within this class have been approved: terazosin (Hytrin), doxazosin (Cardura), and tamsulosin HCl (Flomax). Which medication is used is determined by which change is causing the symptoms—the enlarging of the glandular tissue or the contracting of the smooth muscle tissue. Studies are underway to determine the short- and long-term benefits of each drug.

GENERIC VERSUS BRAND-NAME DRUGS

When a drug company develops a new drug, it is patented and sold only by that company under a single brand name. After seventeen years, the patent runs out, and any drug company can manufacture the drug using another brand name or its generic name. A generic drug has the same ingredients as the original patent and must meet the same Federal Drug Administration (FDA) standards for quality. The generic drug must be shown to be chemically identical and have the same reaction in the body. About three-quarters of all generic drugs are manufactured by the same company that makes the parent drug. The name of a generic drug is a simplified version of its chemical name.

It is estimated that if physicians prescribed the generic form of a drug rather than the brand name, drugs costs would be reduced by more than $1 billion each year. A generic drug costs from 30 to 80 percent of the brand-name price. For example, doxycycline hyclate (a generic antibiotic) costs the pharmacy $0.31 per pill, compared to $3.15 for Vibramycin Hyclate (its brand name). The brand-name diuretic, Lasix, costs $0.19 per pill, compared to its generic equivalent, furosemide, at $0.07/pill.[40]

Thus far, of more than 5,000 approved prescription drugs on the market, one-third are still under patent and cannot be sold generically. However, there are currently about 2,400 prescription brand-name drugs that have tested and approved generic equivalents. Many people erroneously believe brand-name drugs to be better than generic drugs. A number of pharmaceutical companies encourage this belief by directing misleading advertising toward physicians and consumers that portray generic drugs as ineffective and unsafe. Pharmaceutical companies were also alleged to prevent the publication of a study comparing brand-name to generic thyroid replacement therapy for years. The study was finally published in 1997.[41]

Even though the generic prescribing rates have increased in the last three decades, most physicians still prescribe brand names. Physicians may prescribe the brand-name medication because they are familiar with it through the influence of pharmaceutical company representatives. Furthermore, generic drugs are not advertised or otherwise promoted by the drug companies. Physicians may also have more confidence in the brand name. Finally, a number of brand-name drugs do not yet have generic equivalents, so the physician must prescribe a brand name in some cases.

The patient is influential in whether a brand name or generic equivalent is prescribed or filled at the pharmacy. The patient may not trust a generic drug, believing it to be inferior because it is less expensive. Many elders have the attitude, "I want the best possible medication, and I'm willing to pay the price." Generic drugs may arouse suspicion because they differ in shape and color from the brand elders may have previously taken. Educating elders that generic drugs are safe, effective, and significantly less expensive than brand names would counteract negative attitudes towards generic drugs. Consumers need to learn to ask the pharmacist or physician to prescribe the generic equivalent, if available. Most states have passed legislation that permits the pharmacist to substitute a generic equivalent unless the physician specifically expresses that the substitution would not be in the patient's best interest. In addition, some HMOs and hospitals require generic substitution unless the physician specifically orders the brand-name drug.

ALTERNATIVES TO DRUGS

Although the focus of this chapter is on OTC and prescribed medications, there are many other alternatives to improve health and reduce suffering.

Herbal remedies are the primary medical treatments for over three-fourths of the world's population. Even in industrialized nations, about one-quarter of all prescription medications contain ingredients derived from herbs. Herbs are inexpensive, and many can be grown in the backyard. They do not require interaction with a health care provider. The movement in consumer advocacy towards being responsible for one's health and the high cost of prescription drugs make herbal therapy very appealing. However, it is important to realize that, just as with

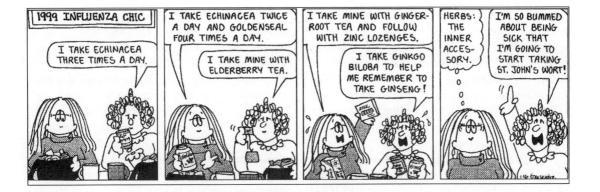

prescription and over-the-counter medications, herbs have benefits, risks, and side effects. They can interact with other medications or foods, and their metabolism is affected by advancing age. However, in comparison, there are very few deaths and injuries from herbs when compared with the adverse effects of drugs. Unlike drugs, the Food and Drug Administration does not regulate herbs because they are considered food supplements. This means that their manufacturers cannot make health claims (e.g., suggesting that garlic may lower cholesterol) or place warnings about potential risks on the label.

There is a tremendous need for rigorous controlled clinical trials to document the health claims of herbal healing proponents. Research is beginning to appear in medical journals, although certainly not in proportion to their use. Drug companies seldom fund studies on herbs that are already available without a prescription because, even if these natural products are found to be effective, they will not realize a financial gain. Further, the dosages of herbs are very difficult to measure because the ingredients are not controlled by the FDA. To complicate matters even further, some herbal preparations use different parts of the plant (leaves, buds, roots), different forms of the herb, and different methods of extraction, and dosages are not standardized. When clinical studies are conducted, the size of the study and the research methodology make it very difficult to interpret the results.

A brief description of some of the more widely used herbal remedies is included below. A few have documented benefits.

- *Aloe vera gel,* derived directly from the thick, fleshy leaves of the aloe vera plant, can be used on burns or dry skin conditions for improved healing.
- *Cascara sagrada* is used in many prescription and over-the-counter stimulant laxatives.
- *Echinacea* is thought to boost the immune system and fight infection and is used to treat colds and flu.
- *Garlic* has anti-infective and natural antibiotic properties, reduces blood pressure and blood clotting, may reduce blood cholesterol, and has been implicated in prevention of stomach cancer. Controlled studies have had mixed results.
- *Ginkgo biloba* is used to improve circulation, particularly to the brain, and improve memory and cognitive function. In a randomized controlled trial, it significantly improved memory and cognitive function.
- *Psyllium* seeds are used in the popular laxative Metamucil and also have cholesterol-lowering actions.
- *Red pepper* is the basis for the topical capsaicin which is effective for severe pain related to shingles, diabetes, and arthritis.
- *Saw palmetto* is used to reduce symptoms of an enlarged prostate and seems to interfere with testosterone production.
- *St. John's-wort* is gaining popularity as an antidepressant because it works like an MAO inhibitor. It is also helpful topically in wound healing. There is some hope that it stimulates the immune system.
- *Valerian* root has been used as a sleep aid or tranquilizer. Valium is a derivative of this plant.

Paralleling the increase in interest and consumption of herbal remedies is the increase and consumption of vitamin and mineral supplements to enhance health, prevent disease, and even to reduce the symptoms of common health problems. It is estimated that one of three individuals in our country takes at least one vitamin supplement. Evidence is accumulating of the benefits of vitamins and minerals (see chapter 5).

The traditional healing practices of a majority of the world do not include most of the medicines of which we have become so accustomed. They depend on other theories of healing that do not lend themselves to the scientific method. A sampling of the most popular practices will be discussed in chapter 12.

Many of the trips to the physician or the drug store can be managed, even eliminated, with lifestyle modifications. Health behavior change should be the first consideration in managing most chronic illnesses: in many cases, drug use may not be needed. For instance, weight loss, dietary change, and exercise can control adult-onset diabetes, and increased fiber intake, fluid, and daily exercise almost always help those who are constipated. However, for some diseases and disorders, drug therapy may be the most effective means to control symptoms and prevent the disease from worsening.

In addition to their benefits, almost every medication on the market is accompanied by unwanted side effects. The health professional and the consumer must be aware of the long-term and short-term benefits of the medication and how it compares with nondrug alternatives. A cautionary note: symptoms are a signal to the body that something is wrong. If self-care does not relieve the symptoms, seek a physician's advice.

The good news is that our bodies have extraordinary healing powers, and many of our health problems do not need a physician, a prescription, or a trip to the drug counter. As Dr. Lewis Thomas said, "The biggest secret of doctors is that most things get better by themselves; most things, in fact, are better in the morning."

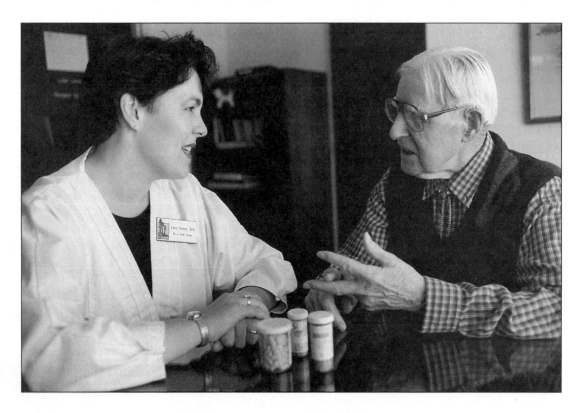

Summary

Elders use more medications than any other age group because of their high prevalence of chronic conditions. Advances in drug technology have revolutionized the management of symptoms of chronic illnesses in elders. However, with drug benefits come several risks. Elders are especially susceptible to adverse drug effects and drug interactions because of the high number of OTC and prescription drugs they take. Additionally, some age- and disease-related physiological states affect the drug dosages needed in elders. Adverse effects are more common among elders than any other patient group and can cause illness, hospitalization, or death.

Noncompliance with medication regimens is a prevalent, multifaceted problem. Effective patient education can increase compliance with drug regimens and reduce the risk of adverse drug effects. Nurses, pharmacists, physicians, social workers, and the consumer can work together to maximize rational drug use. Finally, other alternatives besides drugs should be attempted before drug therapy is initiated since no drug is risk-free. And, when drugs are used, the lowest possible dose for the shortest possible time is recommended.

Activities

1. Ask an older relative or friend to show you what OTC and prescription drugs he or she has at home. Find out how much this person understands about the medications' use, side effects, directions for administration, and shelf life. Ask which drugs are currently being used. Remember to ask specifically about OTC medications such as laxatives, which are commonly used, but infrequently reported. From your reading, do you note any drug misuse?

2. Go to the drug store and examine the multitude of medications available for purchase. Note the most common symptoms being treated. Note the differences between package labeling of brand-name versus generic drugs and price differences. Note how medications are clustered on the shelf and the varying dosage forms available. Observe individuals buying OTC drugs at the drug store for a half-hour period. How do they decide? Compare the purchases of elder and younger people. Keep a record and compare your results with those of other students in the class.

3. Collect as many types of childproof containers as you can from pharmacists and other class members. Have a container-opening session in class and assess which would be most difficult to open for elders with decreased visual and touch sensitivity and reduced physical strength. Interview five elders regarding their opinion of childproof caps. Are they aware they can request a regular container?

4. Ask ten people (any age) if they know what generic drugs are and if they request them. Be prepared to educate them on the difference between generic and brand-name drugs. Ascertain information regarding generic prescribing from a local pharmacy. What laws in your state encourage the use of generic drugs?

5. Collect all the OTC and prescription drugs in your home. Are the name and label clear on the prescription drugs? Do you know why it was purchased? Is the medicine still usable (look at the expiration date)? Is it being properly stored? Do you have unfinished prescriptions that you are no longer taking? Why? Concerning the OTCs, are they really needed? Have you tried nondrug alternatives for headache, insomnia, constipation, acid indigestion? How do you decide when you are ready to treat your symptoms with an OTC remedy?

6. Collect and analyze drug advertisements in medical journals and popular magazine publications. What type of medications are advertised in what type of publication? How many advertisements are geared to older people? How many purport to give scientific information in the advertisement? How do advertisements marketed directly to consumers suggest that consumers obtain their product? Attempt to read all of the small print associated with the advertisement. What new information have you garnered? If a toll-free number is available, call for more information.

7. Bring an OTC medication to class (every student in class should do so). Without reading the label information, see what the rest of the class believes the

medication is used for and how they know about the product. Then read the label. Any surprises? Discuss nondrug alternatives to each product.

8. Go to a health food store (or section) and examine the herbal remedies available. What does store personnel tell you about each remedy? Are written materials available to guide you? Compare prices with other medications.

9. Design an educational pamphlet that provides education to patients and assists them in deciding whether to use hormone replacement therapy. Review the pros and cons and discuss how to individualize the decision-making process.

10. Interview adults regarding their compliance with prescribed medications. Do most people take all medication as prescribed, or is it more common to stop taking medication after a time? Do your subjects report taking medications exactly as instructed? Does compliance depend on particular factors you can identify (for example, whether they can feel the medication effects, whether they are knowledgeable about the reason it was prescribed, whether the medication is for an acute or chronic problem, or whether their physician explained the importance of finishing the prescription)? Are any of them intelligent noncompliers?

11. Make a list of nondrug alternatives to common medical problems. For example, insomnia: use bed only for sleeping, eliminate daytime naps, drink warm milk before bed, go to sleep at same time nightly, increase physical activity.

Bibliography

1. Chrischilles, E.A., Foley, D.J., and Wallace, R.B., et al. 1992. Use of medications by persons 65 and over: Data from the established populations for epidemiologic studies of the elderly. *Journal of Gerontology* 47: M137–M144.

2. Nelson, C.R. and Knapp, D.E. 1997. Medication therapy in ambulatory medical care: National Ambulatory Medical Care Survey and National Hospital Ambulatory Care Survey, 1992. *Advance data from vital and health statistics,* no 290. Hyattsville, MD: National Center for Health Statistics.

3. Rogowski, J., Lillard, L.A., and Kington, R. 1997. The financial burden of prescription drug use among elderly persons. *The Gerontologist* 37:475–82.

4. Sasich, L., and Torrey, E.F. 1998. *International comparisons of drug prices for antidepressant and antipsychotic drugs.* Washington DC.: Public Citizen Research Group.

5. "Kickbacks." 1994. *Health Letter of the Public Citizens Health Research Group* (October):2.

6. Ziegler, M.G., Lew, P., and Singer, B.C. 1995. The accuracy of drug information from pharmaceutical sales representatives. *Journal of the American Medical Association* 273:1296–98.

7. Wilkes, M.S., Doblin, B.H., and Shapiro, M.F. 1992. Pharmaceutical advertisements in leading medical journals: experts' assessments. *Annals of Internal Medicine* 116:912–19.

8. Chren, M.-M., and Landenfeld, S. 1994. Physicians' behavior and their interactions with drug companies. *Journal of the American Medical Association* 271:684–89.

9. Shorr, R.D., and Green, W.L. 1995. A food-borne outbreak of expensive antibiotic use in a community teaching hospital (letter). *Journal of the American Medical Association* 273:1908.

10. Wolfe, S. 1993. *Worst pills, best pills II.* Washington D.C.:Public Citizens Health Research Group.

11. Phillips, D.P., Christenfeld, N., and Glynn, L.M. 1998. Increase in US medication-error deaths between 1983 and 1993. *Lancet* 351:643–44.

12. Bates D.W., Cullen, D., and Laird, N., et al. 1995. Incidence of adverse drug events: Implications for prevention. *Journal of the American Medical Association* 274:29–34.

13. Bates, D.W., Spell, N., and Cullen, D.J., et al. 1997. The costs of adverse drug events in hospitalized patients. *Journal of the American Medical Association* 277:307–11.

14. Classen, D.C., Pestotnik, S.L., and Evans, S., et al. 1997. Adverse drug events in hospitalized patients. Excess length of stay, extra costs, and attributable

mortality. *Journal of the American Medical Association* 277:301–06.

15. General Accounting Office. 1995. Prescription drugs and the elderly: many still receive potentially harmful drugs despite recent improvements. Washington D.C.: GAO/HEHS 95–152.

16. Wilcox, S.M., Himmelstein, D.U., and Woolhandler, S. 1994. Inappropriate drug prescribing for the community-dwelling elderly. 1994. *Journal of the American Medical Association* 272:292–96.

17. Spore, D.L., Mor, V., and Larrat, P., et al. 1997. Inappropriate drug prescriptions for elderly residents of board and care facilities. *American Journal of Public Health* 87:404–9.

18. Burns, E., Austin, C.A., and Bax, N.D. 1990. Elderly patients' understanding of their drug therapy: the effect of cognitive function. *Age and Ageing* 19:236–40.

19. Williams, M.V., Parker, R.M., and Baker, D.W., et al. 1995. Inadequate functional health literacy among patients at two public hospitals. *Journal of the American Medical Association* 274:1677–82.

20. General Accounting Office. 1992. *Non-prescription drugs.* Washington D.C.: GAO/PEMD 92–9.

21. Thun, M.J., Namboodiri, M.M., and Calle, E.E., et al. 1993. Aspirin use and risk of fatal cancer. *Cancer Research* 53:1322–27.

22. Rozzini, R., Ferrucci, L., and Losonczy, K., et al. 1996. Protective effect of chronic NSAID use on cognitive decline in older persons. *Journal of the American Geriatrics Society* 44:1025–29.

23. Kelly, J.P., Kaufman, D.W., and Jurgelon, J.M., et al. 1996. Risk of aspirin-associated major upper-gastrointestinal bleeding with enteric-coated or buffered product. *Lancet* 348:1413–16.

24. Silverstein, F.E., Graham, D.Y., and Senior, J.R., et al. 1995. Misoprostol reduces serious gastrointestinal complications in patients with rheumatoid arthritis receiving nonsteroidal anti-inflammatory drugs *Annals of Internal Medicine* 123:241–349.

25. Tamblyn, R., Berkson, L., and Dauphinee, W.D., et al. 1997. Unnecessary prescribing of NSAIDS and the management of NSAID-related gastropathy in medical practice. *Annals of Internal Medicine* 127:429–38.

26. Whitcomb D.C., and Block, G.D. 1994. Association of acetaminophen hepatotoxicity with fasting and ethanol use. *Journal of the American Medical Association* 272:1845–50.

27. Brown, S.L., Salive, M.E., and Pahor, M., et al. 1995. Occult caffeine as a source of sleep problems in an older popuation. *Journal of the American Geriatrics Society* 43:860–64.

28. Wolfsen, C.R, Parker, J.C., and Mitteness, L.S. 1993. Constipation in the daily lives of frail elderly people. *Archives of Family Medicine* 2:853–58.

29. AGS Panel on Chronic Pain in Older Persons. 1998. The management of chronic pain in older persons. *Journal of the American Geriatrics Society* 46:635–51.

30. Buckley, L.M., Leib, E.S., and Cartularo, K.S., et al. 1996. Calcium and vitamin D3 supplementation prevents bone loss in the spine secondary to low-dose corticosteroids in patients with rheumatoid arthritis. *Annals of Internal Medicine* 125:961–68.

31. General Accounting Office. 1996. Cholesterol treatment: Review of the clinical trials evidence. Washington D.C.: GAO/PEMD 96–7.

32. Shepherd, J., Cobbe, S.M., and Ford, I., et al. 1995. Prevention of coronary heart disease with pravastatin in men with hypercholesterolemia. *New England Journal of Medicine* 333:1301–7.

33. Sacks, F.M., Pfeffer, M.A., and Moye, L.A., et al. 1996. The effect of pravastatin on coronary events after myocardial infarction in patients with average cholesterol levels. Cholesterol and Recurrent Events Trial investigators. *New England Journal of Medicine* 335:1001–9.

34. Downs, J.R., Clearfield, M., and Weis, S., et al. 1998. Primary prevention of acute coronary events with lovastatin in men and women with average cholesterol level. *Journal of the American Medical Association* 279:1615–22.

35. "Should you be taking one of the new cholesterol drugs?" 1998. *Consumer Reports* (October):54–56.

36. Saudek, C.D., Duckworth, W.C., and Giobbie-Hurder, A., et al. 1996. Implantable insulin pump vs multiple-dose insulin for non-insulin-dependent diabetes mellitus. *Journal of the American Medical Association* 276:1322–27.

37. Knapp, M.J., Knopman, D.S., and Solomon, P.R., et al. 1994. A three-week randomized controlled trail of high-dose tacrine in patients with

Alzheimer's disease. *Journal of the American Medical Association* 271:985–91.

38. Soumerai, S.B., McLaughlin, T.J., and Spiegelman, D., et al. 1997. Adverse outcomes of underuse of beta-blockers in elderly survivors of acute myocardial infarction. *Journal of the American Medical Association* 277:115–21.

39. Psaty, B.M., Heckbert, S.R., and Koepsell, T.D., et al. 1995. The risk of myocardial infarction associated with antihypertensive drug therapies. *Journal of the American Medical Association* 274:620–25.

40. "The price of brand names." 1992. *People's Medical Society Newsletter* (October):8.

41. Dong, B.J., Hauck, W.W., and Gambertoglio, J.G., et al. 1997. Bioequivalence of generic and brand name levothyroxine products in the treatment of hypothyroidism. *Journal of the American Medical Association* 277:1205–13.

Prevention and Health Promotion

Our fascination with the more glamorous 'pound of cure' has tended to dazzle us into ignoring the more effective 'ounce of prevention.'

Jimmy Carter

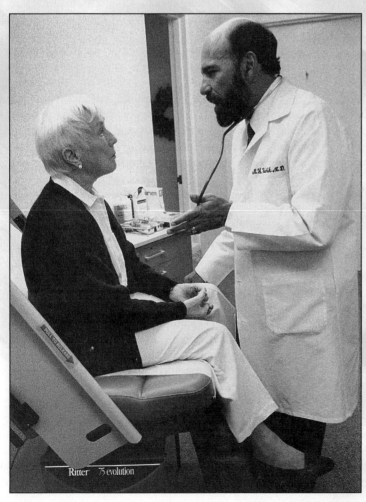

As evidence accumulates on the role that lifestyle plays in many chronic illnesses, the public is more knowledgeable and motivated to make positive lifestyle choices. The aging baby boomers, a generation known for its focus on health issues, is expected to be one of the healthiest cohorts of elders. Although preventive efforts are ideally instituted in childhood or early adulthood, it is not too late in the middle or later years to make positive lifestyle changes. For example, even quitting smoking in later life has substantial benefits on mortality and morbidity from lung disease, stroke, and multiple types of cancer.

Prevention includes many different activities with the goal of reducing premature death and disability. Making health behavior changes, such as eating more fruits and vegetables or stopping smoking, undergoing tests to find illness earlier, or having a nurse visit a home to assess it for accident risks are all types of prevention. Prevention may occur in a physician's office, in the community, or through individual efforts. This chapter will explore the various types of prevention activities and their applicability to elders. In addition, this chapter will define what is meant by "risk factors" and "screening tests" and will discuss our nation's commitment to prevention: *Healthy People.*

PREVENTION: AN OVERVIEW

Prevention includes any activity that reduces the incidence and severity of disease. Health promotion efforts involve education, community advocacy, or legislation to improve the health of an individual or a population. In general, health promotion activities focus on changing health behaviors to reduce the incidence of death and disability.

Preventive medicine, a relatively new medical specialty, has the goal of reducing the occurrence of illness, disability, and premature death through prevention. Most elders do not seek out a specialist to administer preventive services. Preventive care and health education are accomplished most often through a primary care physician, nurse, or other health care provider. These interventions may occur during special meetings set aside regularly (e.g., annual physical examinations) or interspersed during regular office visits.

Some prevention efforts go beyond the provider's response to individuals and are accomplished by health educators or by political advocacy groups. These may include legislative efforts to improve health (e.g., seat belt laws), community education (community forums, health fairs, billboards, television advertisements), or nationwide campaigns (e.g., the Great American Smokeout or the Five-a-Day campaign to increase consumption of fruits and vegetables).

There are three major types of prevention activities: primary, secondary, and tertiary. *Primary prevention* is what most people classically think of as "prevention"—administering a procedure to prevent illness or disability from occurring in the first place. The most common example is immunizations administered to children or adults for diphtheria, hepatitis B, pneumonia, influenza, or chicken pox. *Secondary prevention* includes the use of screening tests, which are medical tests administered to healthy individuals or populations who have no sign of disease in order to detect illnesses in an earlier, more treatable stage. *Tertiary prevention* includes the many types of treatments for those with existing illnesses. It is usually accomplished to prevent further disability, complications, or death. An example of tertiary prevention is reducing cholesterol levels in people with heart disease or carefully monitoring insulin therapy in people with diabetes. Tertiary prevention will not be discussed in this chapter because treatment for a variety of physical and mental illnesses was included in chapters 7, 8, and 9.

Health promotion includes education or counseling to improve health that might occur in a physician's office or a visit to a nutritionist. Health promotion also encompasses large-scale educational or legislative interventions designed to improve the health of both individuals and populations. Being told by a health care provider to quit smoking, receiving smoking cessation education in a physician's office, reading a billboard with an antismoking message, or seeing the Surgeon General's warning on a pack of cigarettes are all examples of health promotion activities. In general, health promotion efforts help people to change unhealthy habits to reduce the frequency or severity of disease.

WHAT IS A RISK FACTOR?

Risk factors are personal characteristics, physiological parameters, environmental conditions, symptoms, or preclinical disease states that increase an individual's likelihood of having or developing a disease. These factors might include behaviors, such as smoking; physiological parameters, such as elevated cholesterol levels; environmental conditions, such as pollution; or preclinical disease states, such as impaired glucose tolerance, which increases the risk for diabetes. Some of these risk factors are subject to personal control (e.g., smoking patterns, use of seat belts); others are not (e.g., family history of breast cancer, gender).

A risk factor is a statistical concept. Having a risk factor for a particular disease does not mean you will get the disease but it does make it more likely. Not having a risk factor may reduce your likelihood of getting a disease, but it does not protect you altogether. Risk factors are more applicable to populations or groups than to individuals. For example, it is true that the majority of those who smoke will develop smoking-related illnesses, but this does not mean that every smoker will become ill. Likewise, most people who develop lung cancer are smokers, but this does not mean that an individual who neither smoked nor was exposed to secondhand smoke cannot get lung cancer. It is important to note that individual variation does not change the strong association between smoking and lung cancer and other illnesses. Thus, just because your grandfather smoked three cigars a day for thirty years and never got cancer does not affect the strong association of multiple studies over many years linking cigarette smoking and lung cancer.

Some risk factors are more important than others. For instance, smoking is an extraordinarily strong risk factor for lung cancer, increasing risk 25 to 50 times of that of a nonsmoker. In contrast, a family history of breast cancer in one relative increases the risk of developing breast cancer only 2 to 3 times. Magnitude of risk factors is important,

but it is not the only factor that should be considered. If a disorder is very rare (say one in a million) and a certain risk factor doubles the risk of developing that disease, the absolute risk for an individual with a certain risk factor is now two in a million. Thus, the risk is increased, but chances are quite high that the individuals will not suffer that disease. On the other hand, some risk factors of relatively small magnitude (e.g., the increased risk of heart disease among those with a sedentary lifestyle) become far more important when you consider how common cardiovascular disease is in the general population. These concepts of risk are often muddied in news accounts of the relationship between risk factors and disease. Often, when risk factors are known for a disease, the public begins to believe the cause of the disease is known and may worry unnecessarily about getting that illness. It is more productive to reduce more important risk factors for the more common diseases (such as reducing dietary fat to prevent heart disease).

Attempting to modify the risks associated with diseases is difficult: individuals must make daily efforts to change long-standing habits or lifestyles for a long period of time, often without experiencing short-term benefits. Often individuals have no symptoms of a disease and a gain of a few "statistical" extra years of life is an intangible goal. In contrast, most medical procedures provide quick, noticeable results. For example, eating a low-fat, high-fiber diet for twenty years to reduce the incidence of cardiovascular disease may seem tedious and boring compared to a single coronary artery bypass operation after years of eating what you want. Lifestyle modifications are more likely to be followed if their benefits are observable. For example, people consuming a low-fat diet often report more energy and weight reduction in addition to the benefits they may note later in reduced cardiovascular disease incidence.

PREVENTION AND HEALTH PROMOTION EFFORTS TOWARDS ELDERS

Preventive efforts are most effective if aimed at the youngest members of our population and if they are continued over a lifetime. With age and increasing rates of disability and illness among adults, there is a new focus on health promotion and preventive efforts directed toward that group to maximize the length and quality of life in the middle and later years. Since elders visit physicians more than any other adult groups, they are a prime target for health promotion efforts.

This section will focus on particular prevention efforts for the elder population. Primary prevention activities encompass adult immunizations and the use of medications to reduce the onset of illness. Secondary prevention involves disease screening and health promotion activities conducted in a variety of settings to improve health and delay or eliminate the development of disease and disability.

Primary Prevention: Shots and Pills

Influenza Vaccination

Influenza is a debilitating, but generally self-limiting, viral infection causing incapacitating weakness, fevers, chills, and body aches. In elders, particularly the chronically ill, an influenza infection may be life-threatening. In fact, the vast majority of deaths attributed to influenza occur among those over age sixty-five. In addition, those with influenza are at high risk of developing secondary pneumonia infections.

The influenza vaccine is created annually based on scientists' assumptions regarding which virus strains may cause illness in that year. Although studies show this vaccine to be effective in reducing the incidence and severity of influenza, studies on the elderly are less conclusive. The vaccine is likely more effective at preventing illness and death among healthier elders (who may recover without the vaccine) than among the very old or frail (who are at higher risk of death from influenza). Despite its limitations, most experts recommend an annual influenza vaccination for all adults age sixty-five and older. Under development is a vaccination that would be inhaled, eliminating the flu shot.

Pneumococcal Vaccination

Pneumococcal pneumonia is a significant cause of illness, hospitalization, and death, especially among those over age sixty-five. The pneumococcal vaccine is made from several strains of the bacteria. Determining of the effectiveness of the vaccine has been difficult for a number of reasons. It seems that the vaccine is least effective for the sickest elders (those with immune system problems, alcoholism, renal failure, or cancer) who are those most likely to benefit from it. However, the vaccine is more effective in healthier elders. Ideally, the vaccine is administered while the person is in good health so that protection will be assured when health wanes. A pneumococcal vaccine is recommended for all elders over age sixty-five with normal immune systems. Even though frail elders are less likely to respond, most experts recommend they be vaccinated. Some experts recommend a single vaccination; others recommend that reinnoculation occur every five to ten years.

Tetanus Immunization

Tetanus is rare in the United States, but most cases occur among adults over age fifty. Many older people do not have up-to-date tetanus immunizations. The vaccine is effective at inducing immunity and should be given as a primary series in childhood with boosters every ten to twenty years.

Postmenopausal Hormone Replacement Therapy

Many diseases, including cardiovascular disease, osteoporosis and cancer, are influenced by female hormones. Hormone replacement therapy (HRT) has many positive effects, including improving cholesterol and reducing osteoporosis and fracture risk, and is associated with improved sexual functioning, increased quality of life, decreased urinary incontinence, decreased risk of urinary tract infections, better cognitive function, and reduced risk of Alzheimer's disease. On the negative side, HRT may increase the risk of breast cancer, can cause irregular bleeding, and requires long-term daily administration of medication. The decision to take hormones for prevention is controversial.

Multiple large observational and cohort studies and a few randomized controlled trials have shown that hormone replacement therapy significantly decreases overall death rates, particularly deaths from cardiovascular disease. Because cardiovascular disease is so common, many experts recommend that all women initiate hormone replacement therapy at menopause. Unfortunately, to date, few studies have examined the risks and benefits of long-term hormone replacement therapy. Further, few women prescribed hormone replacement therapy continue it, especially for a long term.

Despite many areas of uncertainty, a growing number of women are electing to undergo hormone replacement therapies. It is widely recommended that health care professionals discuss the benefits and risks of hormone replacement therapy with all menopausal and elder women patients, particularly those with elevated cholesterol, heart disease, or osteoporosis (or risk factors for those diseases). These women should be counseled about the availability of various estrogen and progesterone medication forms. The minimum amount of estrogen should be 0.625 mg of conjugated estrogen or its equivalent. All women with a uterus who are prescribed estrogen should also be prescribed progesterone (either continuously or a few days a month) to prevent uterine cancer. There are many types and dosages of estrogens and progesterones and many regimens for hormonal replacement.

Aspirin to Prevent Cardiovascular Disease

As a result of a large randomized controlled trial of U.S. male physicians, there has been increased interest in the role of aspirin in the prevention of heart attacks in middle aged and older men.[1] In this study of healthy male physicians age forty to eighty-four, those taking a low dose of aspirin every other day had a decreased risk of heart attack that was so significant that the study was terminated so that the group taking the placebo might start on the therapy also. A prospective, nonrandomized study of female nurses reported similar findings.[2] Aspirin therapy also was found to be beneficial for those with pre-existing heart disease or stroke to prevent further heart attacks or strokes.

Aspirin therapy has some undesirable side effects, including stomach upset, bleeding, or ulcers. In addition, all studies have not supported the protective role of aspirin: the physician's study showed a disturbing increased rate of sudden death in those receiving aspirin therapy. Because of its side effects, most groups do not recommend aspirin therapy for all patients. However, health professionals should discuss aspirin therapy with elders and consider it for those individuals at high risk of cardiovascular disease or stroke. Very low doses of aspirin, taken every other day, are just as effective and are associated with fewer side effects than higher doses.

Secondary Prevention: Screening

Screening tests are preventive services in which a special test or examination identifies patients who need further intervention. In general, screening tests are offered to a large group of people who have no signs of a particular disease with the goal of finding the disease at an early, treatable stage.

In some cases, screening tests are offered only to individuals at high risk. For example, only diabetics would require screening for problems that affect diabetics, such as diabetic kidney disease or blindness. This section will discuss tests that are recommended for everyone over age sixty-five.

There are certain characteristics to be met before screening is recommended on a wide scale.

1. The test must be able to detect the illness before any signs or symptoms of the disease are evident to the patient or the health care provider. Once symptoms are present, the individual should undergo any further diagnostic tests necessary, and treatment should proceed.

2. The test must be accurate with a minimum of false positives or false negatives. False positive results occur when the test is positive, but the individual does not have the illness, and false negative results occur when the test

is read as negative, but the individual does have the condition. Although no test is perfectly accurate, false positive results can cause mental distress and subject healthy people to unnecessary tests or procedures. For example, some of the screening tests for ovarian cancer have high rates of false positives, and women with these results may be subject to surgery to assure them they do not have cancer. In contrast, false negative results can delay treatment and provide a false sense of security. For example, mammography in younger women has a high rate of false negatives so a woman is told her mammogram is normal, when she is really harboring a cancer. Because of this reassurance, she may ignore other cancer warning signs or delay her next mammogram.

3. Screening and early treatment of disease should improve the health of the patient. Although it seems intuitive that early detection must be better, this is not always the case. For example, some illnesses are universally fatal, and discovering them earlier does not change the end result, but merely gives the individual more time to live with (and worry about) the diagnosis. For example, prostate cancer often grows slowly and may be present in many men who die of something else. Detecting it earlier and subjecting men to treatment (which may be harmful) may not make any difference in their life expectancy, especially if they die of heart disease before the prostate cancer becomes advanced.

4. The goal of screening and early detection is to reduce morbidity and mortality from particular diseases, helping people live longer, healthier lives. The best way to determine the value of a screening test is to compare a group of people who were offered screening with those who were not and compare how many people died in each group. If there were significantly fewer deaths in the group who was screened, the screening test is considered to be effective.

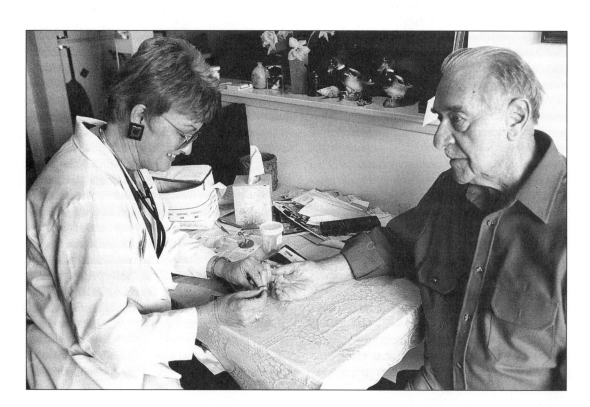

Screening can be accomplished as part of a health interview: the clinician questions the patient regarding behaviors that put them at risk for disease or injury, such as high-fat diet, smoking, inactivity, level of stress, alcohol intake, use of seat belts, and others. Some screening can be undertaken with standardized questionnaires, rather than relying on individual clinicians to ask certain questions. Standardized questionnaires exist for screening for alcoholism, depression, and dementia.

Screening practices are an integral part of the physical examination. Ascertaining information regarding the patient's health history and family history is a type of screening. Measurement of weight, blood pressure, vision, hearing, pulmonary function, and examination of body organs for cancer (oral cavity, breasts, abdomen, testicles, skin, pelvic exam, rectal/prostate exam) are also screening tests. Most people identify screening with laboratory tests, particularly measurement for anemia, diabetes, elevated cholesterol, HIV, electrocardiogram for heart abnormalities, tuberculosis patch test, the Pap smear for cervical cancer, prostate-specific antigen (PSA) test for prostate cancer, and the stool tests for microscopic blood. Finally, screening can entail more elaborate tests, such as X-rays (e.g., mammography), endoscopy of the intestines to detect cancer, and exercise treadmill tests. The same test can serve as a screening test or a diagnostic test. The difference is that diagnostic tests are performed on patients with symptoms of illness, while screening tests are performed on people who have no symptoms.

Although it may seem as if the best thing is for everyone to undergo every screening test, "just to be sure," in actuality this is poor preventive medicine for a number of reasons. First, as mentioned earlier, no test is perfect. Any test has a potential to indicate that you have a certain disease or condition when you really don't (false positive) or the test might indicate that you are free of a condition when you actually have it (false negative). The chance of a test being wrong increases if the condition is rare. For example, if the local health department decided to screen all school children for cancer using a blood test and the incidence of this cancer was one in a million. Even if the test were

99 percent accurate, of every 100 normal children who are screened, one would be told a wrong diagnosis. If you screen a million children, you might find the one who has cancer, but you must tell at least 100 children that they might have cancer when they don't. Obviously the false positives can cause a lot of unnecessary worry.

Aside from being inaccurate, screening tests may cause pain, embarrassment, and waste money that could be used to diagnose and treat more common health problems. Further, some tests may be very time-consuming.

So how do we know what screening tests are worth it? Many types of studies can help us answer this question, but the gold standard is the randomized controlled trial. This type of large-scale study randomly assigns its subjects into two groups— one group gets the intervention (for example, mammograms every year) and the other group does not. Then the study follows those subjects for many years to determine whether those who received the intervention are less likely to die (e.g., from breast cancer) than those who did not.

Other types of studies are used in evaluating screening tests, but these studies suffer from serious biases that are often not apparent. For example, a study might show that cancers detected by a screening test were smaller and less likely to have spread, and therefore, that this screening test should be recommended. However, this study does not tell us whether finding these smaller tumors helped these patients live longer, whether the people who consented to the tests were not as sick in the first place, or whether the screening had some toxic side effect that could cause more severe problems in the future.

Unfortunately, the majority of screening tests have not undergone randomized clinical trials. Even if a screening test has undergone a randomized clinical trial, it may not have clear-cut benefits. Even fewer studies address the efficacy of screening tests for elders, so most recommendations for that group are based on studies of middle-aged adults. Thus, in most cases, screening for the elderly is restricted to those who will live at least ten years longer. In general, screening tests are not recommended for elders with life-threatening chronic illnesses because they will not likely live long enough to benefit from the treatment. For example, an elder with end-stage heart disease who has had multiple heart attacks is likely to die of cardiovascular disease. Obtaining a mammogram and discovering the simultaneous presence of breast cancer would be counterproductive. First, the individual would likely not be healthy enough to undergo surgery, chemotherapy, and radiation treatments. Second, the diagnosis of cancer may be psychologically detrimental, reducing the quality of the few years of life that remain.

Various professional groups make recommendations regarding screening tests—who should undergo them, how frequently to be tested, and to what benefit. These groups include professional organizations by medical specialty (e.g., geriatrics, family practice, urology), patient or consumer groups (e.g., the American Cancer Society), expert panels, and government agencies. These groups vary in the method they use to make their decisions and their recommendations. Some groups convene councils of experts who use their expert medical opinion, experience, and review of the literature to determine recommendations. Others, such as the U.S. Preventive Services Task Force, use a highly structured, systematic review of the literature to determine recommendations that are later reviewed by experts. In general, the recommendations made by more structured reviews are more conservative and often do not recommend routine, population-based screening.

Professional groups differ in their bias, whether they state this or not. The American Cancer Society and oncologists (cancer specialists) see a lot of cancer patients and have seen first-hand the devastation that cancer can cause to the patient and family. Cancer specialists are more likely to recommend any screening that detects cancer early because they believe they have an ever-expanding arsenal for fighting cancer and a strong belief that any cancer that was "missed" could have been treated. Often the costs (both emotional and financial) of screening are not considered. In contrast, the U.S. Preventive Services Task Force is biased toward interventions that have been proven effective and adopts a more population-wide approach. For example, a screening test that offers significant risk to the patient and often misses a very rare but terrible disease may not be recommended by the U.S. Preventive Services Task Force, but may be recommended by those experts who commonly work with that disease.

Conflicting recommendations by different professional groups can cause confusion, both among the public and health care professionals, and can lead to the belief that "no one knows what to do." Over a year or two in the 1990s, for example, multiple groups came out with competing recommendations about mammography that were quite different and caused quite a public outcry from patients, physicians, the public, and politicians.

Sometimes there is a great deal of emotion wrapped up in recommendations, reflecting individual experience. For example, a woman who has survived breast cancer that was detected by a mammogram may advocate mammograms for everyone. Conversely, a woman whose cancer was missed by a mammogram and who is now dying may vehemently assert that mammograms are useless.

Ideally, screening recommendations are not made because of emotionality or personal experience but by following a scientific rationale. However, the science behind recommendations—particularly the review of studies and analysis of epidemiologic concepts—is quite complicated and not easily understood by the lay public.

The controversy surrounding the value of some screening tests should not obscure the fact that there are a core of recommendations for preventive services and screening tests that are widely agreed to have documented benefits. If everyone adhered to this core of recommendations, there would be dramatic improvements in health. Unfortunately, even when most professional groups agree on a screening recommendation, far too many professionals and laypersons do not comply. Professionals may not feel they have enough time to devote to screening measures, they may feel they are unskilled at recommending these tests, or they may be uncertain of their benefits.

Individuals also have varying values that affect their compliance with screening tests. By definition, screening tests are for those without symptoms. It is difficult to get those people who have no symptoms of illness to come to the doctor or hospital and pay for testing and counseling. It is also easy for physicians and their patients to focus on current complaints of existing chronic or acute illnesses rather than devote precious time to disease prevention and early detection.

Some individuals are quite frightened of illness and ask their physician for every test to prove they are not harboring something curable. Others adopt a more fatalistic attitude—"If I am going to get cancer, I am going to get it, and this test isn't going to help me at all." Some find screening tests stressful and develop anxiety or depressive states while waiting for the results. Often people's biases are surprising. A chronically ill patient with a limited life expectancy might insist on routine mammograms, while a healthy elder, who could benefit from such screening, might refuse. Although many people say they are in favor of

preventive efforts, few actually make appointments and follow-through on health professionals' recommendations for health promotion and disease prevention efforts.

The following screening recommendations for elders reflect the position of the U.S. Preventive Services Task Force because this organization provides guidance on all aspects of prevention, uses a highly structured, data-based methodology, and summarizes findings of other groups. They produced the *Guide to Clinical Preventive Services* that discusses each screening test for different age groups in a readable manner.[3] This is not to imply that these recommendations are the best, but they do provide a standardized list of the minimum screening tests elders should undergo.

Breast Cancer

Mammographic screening for breast cancer is relatively well-studied, and there are several large randomized controlled trials that suggest that

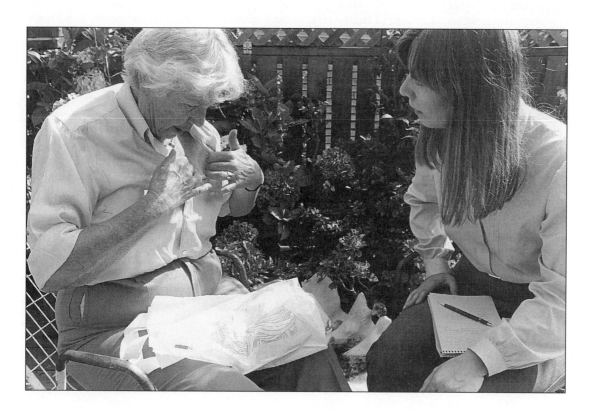

middle-aged women (age fifty to seventy) who underwent mammograms had a lower mortality rate than those who did not. Breast cancer risk continues to increase with advancing age, and the majority of breast cancers are diagnosed in women over age sixty-five years. However, few studies have assessed the benefit for women over age seventy. Mammograms are recommended every one to two years for women age fifty to sixty-nine by almost all professional groups, and most also support screening healthy women over age seventy. Medicare finances mammogram screening for elders. Although widely practiced, physical exams by the physician or breast self-exams have not been shown to reduce the risk of breast cancer death.

Prostate Cancer

Prostate cancer is the most common cancer in American men and is second only to lung cancer as a cause of cancer death. The principal screening tests for prostate cancer are the rectal exam and the prostate-specific antigen (PSA) blood test.

There is a tremendous amount of controversy regarding screening for prostate cancer in asymptomatic men. Prostate cancer differs from other cancers in that it is relatively slow-growing in many men and, even if left undetected, may not significantly impact life expectancy. Although tests such as PSA do detect prostate cancer earlier, it is unclear whether such earlier detection will increase either the quantity or quality of men's lives. The treatments for prostate cancer (surgery, radiation, hormones) have many undesirable side effects. Unfortunately, no randomized clinical trials have evaluated the benefits and risks of prostate cancer screening.

The American Cancer Society and other professional groups recommend annual screening with rectal exam and PSA blood tests, generally starting at age fifty, and earlier in African American men with a higher risk of cancer. In general, most organizations do not recommend screening for prostate cancer in men who have less than ten years to live. Some organizations recommend against prostate cancer screening; others have no recommendations but encourage patients to consult their physicians

to discuss the issue (e.g., U.S. Preventive Services Task Force). It is hoped that the results of randomized controlled trials will be available soon to help elders and their physicians decide what to do.

Colorectal Cancer

Cancers of the colon and rectum are common causes of death in the later years. Multiple types of tests have been recommended to detect asymptomatic colon cancer: the fecal occult blood test, rectal exam, barium enema, and colonoscopy or sigmoidoscopy. These tests vary widely in cost, ease of administration, and patient comfort. The fecal occult blood test involves taking stool samples and placing them on special cards that are later analyzed in a laboratory. The presence of blood in the stool that is not visible to the eye (occult) is a signal that there is increased risk of colon cancer, and more tests should be prescribed. A rectal exam involves a health practitioner placing a gloved finger in the rectum and feeling for abnormalities. For a barium enema, a radio-contrast material is placed in the rectum and X-rays are taken. Colonoscopy and sigmoidoscopy involve placing a tube into the rectum and actually looking at the lining of the bowel for possible cancers or precancerous lesions. Colonoscopy allows visualization of the entire large intestine, while sigmoidoscopy involves looking at the end portion of the large bowel.

In general, professional groups recommend annual rectal exams and fecal occult blood screening between ages forty to fifty. Starting at age fifty, individuals are also recommended to undergo more invasive tests (barium enema, sigmoidoscopy, colonoscopy) every three to ten years with discontinuation of screening after about age seventy. Compliance with these recommendations, particularly for the more invasive, uncomfortable, and embarrassing tests, is very low and expensive.

Cervical Cancer

The most common screening test for cancer of the cervix (the outlet of the uterus) is the Pap smear, named after its discover, George Papanicolaou. The

Pap smear is well known to reduce cervical cancer death rate. There is some debate about the frequency of Pap smears in younger women, with recommendations ranging from one to three years. Many groups recommend a discontinuation of regular Pap smears after age sixty-five in women with a lifetime of normal tests, although not all concur. Because many elder women, particularly the poor, ethnic minorities, and the oldest-old, have not received regular Pap smears in their younger years, it is sensible to initiate regular Pap smears to assure they reap the benefits of screening.

Cardiovascular Disease

Heart disease is the number one killer of older adults. In many adults, the onset of chest pain or angina signals a problem with the heart, but for some people, the first sign of heart disease may be a heart attack or sudden death. There are two major strategies for heart disease screening. One involves screening for the risk factors of cardiovascular disease (e.g., hypertension, sedentary lifestyle, elevated cholesterol, cigarette smoking) and helping people to modify those risks. Another is to try to determine which asymptomatic individuals have significant heart disease through medical tests.

Perhaps the most common test to detect the presence of heart disease is the electrocardiogram or EKG. This test involves placing electrodes on the skin and measuring the electrical activity of the heart. Unfortunately, resting EKGs are not a good screening test for heart disease—they are often abnormal in people without heart disease (high degree of false positives), and normal in people with significant disease (high degree of false negatives). An exercise EKG is somewhat better, but it is still too often normal in people who later die suddenly from heart disease. Some professional organizations recommend an exercise EKG for previously sedentary middle-aged and older adults prior to beginning an exercise program; however, the same difficulties are noted in this population. Namely, those with normal EKGs are often still at high risk of sudden death, and those with abnormal EKGs are often perfectly healthy.

Hypertension

Hypertension, a leading risk factor for heart disease, renal disease, stroke, and other illnesses, may be present in individuals of all age groups. Treatment to lower blood pressure is known to reduce mortality. Screening tests for hypertension are easily accomplished with the use of a blood pressure cuff (sphygmomanometer). Most professional groups assert that blood pressure should be measured every one to two years and, if pressure is elevated, at least three measurements should be accomplished. Some recommend a home monitor that records blood pressure at regular intervals over a period of time. If hypertension is discovered, individuals should receive counseling on other modifiable cardiovascular risk factors (e.g., diet, activity level, obesity, and elevated cholesterol).

Elevated Cholesterol

Elevation of blood cholesterol is one of the major risk factors for cardiovascular disease, even among elders.[4] This association is less strong among elder women and men over age seventy-five. Cholesterol levels and fractions (such as HDL and LDL) can be easily measured by a blood test. Many groups recommend screening middle-aged adults, but screening recommendations for elders are not as clear-cut because of lack of data and conflicting data regarding the benefits and risks. It is prudent to measure cholesterol levels in elders who have multiple risk factors for coronary artery disease. In healthy asymptomatic elders without chronic illnesses, cholesterol levels should probably be measured once or twice between ages sixty-five and seventy-five years. However, cholesterol levels seem to plateau at around age sixty-five (in women) and earlier (in men), so continued screening of those with previously normal levels may not be necessary.

Tuberculosis

The most widely accepted screening technique for tuberculosis is the Mantoux test (also known as PPD), in which a small amount of antigen (inactivated virus) is injected under the skin, then is "read" in forty-eight to seventy-two hours. The amount of swelling at the injection site is measured, and if it is greater than 10 mm, it is considered positive. Positive tests require a chest X-ray to look for active infection, which requires aggressive multidrug treatment. All residents and staff of skilled nursing facilities (nursing homes) should be screened for tuberculosis.

Vision Problems

Visual impairment is a common and potentially serious problem among the elderly. Because visual losses progress gradually, elders may be unaware of vision decrements that could affect their ability to drive safely and increase their risk of falls. Studies also document that elders wear corrective lenses that are not appropriate. Snellen eye charts use progressively smaller lines of type (generally letters) that are read with one eye covered to measure visual acuity. Regular screening with the Snellen test is widely recommended to detect vision loss among elders. Those with abnormal screening tests should be referred for further evaluation and treatment.

Glaucoma is a slowly progressive loss of vision that increases in incidence with age. The disease can be detected by various eye tests that assess the pressure in the eye or resultant damage to the optic nerve. These tests are usually conducted by optometrists and opthalmologists. Although the disease cannot be reversed, there is some evidence that if medication to reduce the pressure inside the eye is started early, the progress of the disease can be slowed or stopped. Treatment is life-long, and the medication has side effects. However, many people with increased ocular pressure never develop glaucoma, and there is no clear evidence that treatment prevents glaucoma or blindness, although large studies are underway to determine whether screening and early treatment reduces blindness from glaucoma. Although ophthalmology groups recommend regular screening, large task forces have not found sufficient evidence to recommend screening for all elders. Those at higher risk (diabetics, African Americans, or a family history of glaucoma) may be good candidates for screening.

Hearing Loss

Hearing loss is a substantial cause of disability among older adults and can be caused by multiple factors—including noise, illness and presbycusis (the loss of high-frequency hearing associated with aging). Although no studies have documented the effectiveness of routine screening for hearing loss, studies do show that if it is recognized and treated, hearing-impaired adults have an improved quality of life. Hearing loss can usually be detected by asking elders or family members questions about their hearing and providing information and referral when necessary. In addition, some experts recommend audiometric testing of all elders every ten years or so, while others recommend audiometric testing only in elders with suspected hearing loss.

Osteoporosis

Osteoporosis is a significant cause of pain and fractures among elders, particularly women. A number of screening tests are able to detect bone mineral density, osteoporosis, and fracture risk. The most commonly used tests are X-rays to estimate bone density, for instance, DXA (dual energy X-ray absorptionometry) scans to assess bone density on selected sites on the skeleton. A newer and less expensive technique measures bone density by using ultrasound on the heel of the foot.

Although a few groups propose universal screening for older women, most take no position or argue against routine screening on the basis of its high cost and questionable benefit. Many recommend screening for women at high risk of osteoporosis (e.g., white, thin, those whose ovaries were removed when younger). However, most groups suggest more general counseling and education to reduce osteoporosis and fracture risk. Elder women should receive counseling on measures to prevent fractures, including high intake of dietary calcium and vitamin D, calcium supplements, weight-bearing exercise, and smoking cessation. In addition, women should be informed about the potential benefits of hormone replacement therapy in reducing the risk of osteoporosis.

Problem Drinking

Alcoholism is a pervasive medical problem in the United States. However, even those who do not meet the criteria for alcoholism may have significant emotional, social, or medical problems related to drinking. Although the risk of alcoholism and problem drinking declines with age, elders who do drink excessively suffer detrimental effects (see chapter 7). Screening for problem drinking should involve careful questioning about alcohol consumption, including quantity, frequency, and degree of intoxication. Clinicians may want to use standardized questionnaires designed for this purpose. All people who drink should be provided with information of the dangers of excessive drinking, be referred to counseling when necessary, and be warned of the dangers of drinking and driving.

Health Promotion and Counseling

Alteration in health behaviors brought about by health promotion activities can greatly reduce the development and progression of many of the chronic illnesses that are common among older people. Based on their exhaustive review of the literature, members of the U.S. Preventive Services Task Force concluded that "clinicians are more likely to help their patients prevent future disease by asking, educating and counseling them about personal health behaviors than by performing physical examinations or tests. In other words, talking is more important than testing."[5]

Epidemiologists report that the greatest impact on chronic illness can be made through lifestyle changes rather than technological interventions, such as drugs or surgery. As many as 80 percent of the diseases that plague Americans, including heart disease, diabetes, and stroke, are related to lifestyle. It has been estimated that about half the deaths from cardiovascular disease and half the disabilities of diabetes could be prevented by changes in health behaviors alone. Over the last twenty years, there have been significant declines in cardiovascular disease, largely attributed to nationwide health promotion campaigns about risk factors that encourage citizens to decrease dietary fat, stop smoking, and increase physical activity.

Increasingly, evidence points to the importance of personal health behaviors in the cause and severity of many diseases and causes of death—from lung disease to heart disease, cancer, and strokes to accidents. The most obvious example is cigarette smoking, contributing to an estimated one in five deaths in the United States annually from heart disease, stroke, cancer, and pulmonary disease. Failing to use seatbelts and driving drunk account for the majority of automobile accidents. Poor diet and physical inactivity are major contributors to heart disease, cancer, diabetes, osteoporosis, and other common diseases. These factors are the major direction of health promotion efforts.

Health promotion includes a range of activities, from individual counseling and education to community or nationwide campaigns to improve health. In some cases, individual-based interventions are more effective. For example, a health care provider can provide education, support, and medication as needed to assist an individual to quit smoking. In other situations, community-based interventions are more optimal (e.g., lengthening the delay time on the street lights near a busy intersection frequented by frail elders). In some cases, legislative options are the most effective way to improve the health of a population; legislation requiring seat belts and automatic seat belt systems has been far more effective at increasing seat belt use than individual counseling.

Because of the many environmental variables that affect personal health, some health professionals consider health promotion to include mobilizing individuals to become active in political change to improve health care for a far greater number of people. For instance, elders may become active in efforts to change local laws regarding smoking or to advocate more stringent nursing home regulations or national health insurance. In this way, professionals involved in health promotion activities can work on two fronts—not only encouraging individual health behavior change, but also reducing political, social, and other environmental influences that ultimately impinge on health status.

Despite the evidence supporting the importance of counseling and education, most physicians continue to underuse health promotion activities. There are a number of reasons for this phenomenon. First, health promotion efforts take time, and many physicians are not trained to provide effective counseling and education. There is a tendency among both health care providers and their patients to emphasize the "here and now" of patient care. It often appears more pressing to deal with the patient's chronic disease management or acute complaint than switch the topic to discuss their cigarette smoking or use of seat belts.

There is a widespread misconception that screening tests and physical examinations are more effective than counseling. However, intervening in a disease state at the time of screening may be too late because the disease has already started to develop. It is far better to prevent the development of lung cancer, for example, than to discover it early. Also, many physicians are not convinced of the effectiveness of their counseling efforts. For example, if a physician encourages smoking cessation among smoking patients and only one of twenty-five smokers quits, he or she may feel like the effort was in vain. However on a population basis, this was an effective intervention.

Health promotion activities are a collaborative effort between the health care provider and the patient. Unlike many medical interventions that the clinician initiates and controls, the patient must initiate and sustain the health behavior change. To effectively integrate prevention into medical care, the physician cannot rely only on providing counseling during checkups but must incorporate this counseling into all visits. An excellent resource on integrating health promotion in medical care is *Health Promotion and Disease Prevention in Clinical Practice.*[5]

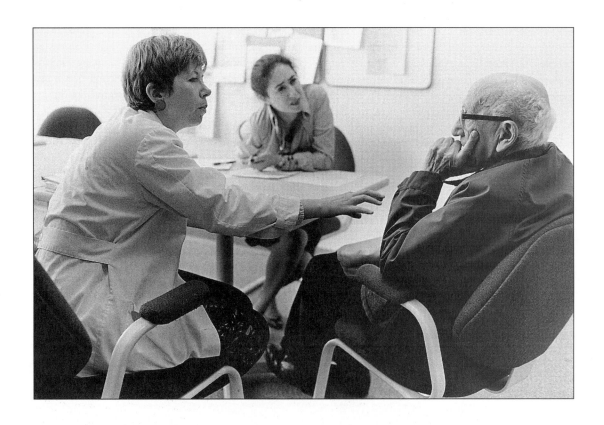

Changing Health Behaviors

Changing personal health behaviors is very difficult because it usually requires altering long-standing patterns that often involve physical discomfort or giving up valued comforts (e.g., reducing fat intake). When contemplating making life changes, it is hypothesized that several stages are involved. Understanding these stages helps the health professionals to tailor their prevention or health promo-

tion message to the individual.[6] The first and most difficult stage is acknowledging a problem: accepting that something is not right in our lives. We may decide we are eating too much, or are getting fat, or are not exercising enough. Those who admit they have a problem are not always willing to move to the next stage: deciding to make a change. Then, once a goal is set (e.g., I want to lose ten pounds), the options for achieving that plan are explored

---

Changing Personal Health Behavior

Generally, to make and sustain meaningful life-style changes requires the following:

1. Acknowledging the need for change.
2. Believing that there is more to gain than to lose. One must carefully balance the pleasures inherent in the old way of doing things (e.g., overeating, smoking, lounging) and the gains expected from the health behavioral change. If the positives outweigh the negatives, the change is more easily accomplished.
3. Feeling a sense of self worth and self-efficacy. A person needs to feel able to accomplish the desired changes to succeed.
4. Feeling a sense of ownership over the plan for change. It is important that the goals are set by the individual and not the practitioner. If an individual is not committed to the plan for change, it is unlikely that the change will be sustained.
5. Developing realistic goals and workable plans. Often in an overzealous attempt at self-improvement, an individual will set goals that are too lofty or unattainable. For instance, a previously sedentary person should not expect to be running a marathon in three months, or a two-pack-a-day smoker may find it difficult to stop "cold turkey" tomorrow. Incremental, achievable goals are preferable.
6. Finding positive reinforcement. Rewards are a well-documented way to change behaviors. Rewards can be extrinsic (I get a new wardrobe

when I lose twenty-five pounds) or intrinsic (sense of satisfaction).
7. Enlisting the support of others is key. Making health behavior changes as a family unit is often easier than making such changes on one's own. On the other hand, significant others may unwittingly sabotage health behavioral changes. For example, as one partner in a couple begins to lose weight and become more attractive, the other partner may have conflicting feelings of jealousy or a fear of abandonment and so may inadvertently encourage the changing partner to lose interest in the regimen.
8. Developing and implementing a strategy for monitoring progress. Individuals need to frequently and continually monitor their progress toward their goal, both on their own and with the support of someone else—either a health care professional or another significant person.
9. Initiating follow-up. Even after the goals are met, follow-up is important to prevent backsliding.
10. Maintaining patience and practice. It is hard to change ingrained patterns of behavior, and meaningful change takes time. Some backsliding is to be expected. It is important not to lose patience with the process and to practice new skills.

Adapted from Westberg, J., and Jason, H. 1996. Fostering healthy behavior: The process. In *Health promotion and disease prevention in clinical practice. S.H. Woolf, S. Jonas, and R.S. Laurence. Baltimore, MD: Williams and Wilkins*, pp. 145–62.

(e.g., cooking low-fat meals). Once a plan is selected and initiated, the next stage is to assess progress toward the goal (e.g., weighing ourselves), modifying the plan as needed (e.g., I can only exercise three times a week, so I will have to lose weight more slowly), and guarding against backsliding.

Stages of Behavior Change

Instead of targeting the same health promotion message to everyone, theorists have proposed that health promotion counseling be individualized. One way of doing this is to assess the openness of the client to behavior change. Five stages through which individuals progress when making behavioral change have been conceptualized: precontemplation, contemplation, preparation, action, and maintenance.

In the *precontemplation* stage, there is no intention to change behavior in the foreseeable future. Many individuals in this stage are unaware of their problems. *Contemplation* is the stage in which people are aware that a problem exists and are seriously thinking about overcoming it but have not yet made a commitment to take action. The *preparation* stage combines intention with previous failed attempts. Individuals in this stage are intending to take action in the next month and have unsuccessfully taken action in the past year. In the *action* stage, individuals modify their behavior, experiences, or environment in order to overcome their problems. Action involves the most overt behavioral changes and requires considerable commitment of time and energy. *Maintenance* is the stage in which people work to prevent relapse and consolidate the gains attained during action. For addictive behaviors, this stage extends from six months to an indeterminate period past the initial action.[7]

In this model, interventions by the health professional can be tailored toward the stage of change of the client. For example, in the precontemplation stage, the focus is to discuss the health hazards of a current behavior and to encourage the individual to change that behavior. For example, a smoker who does not even acknowledge that smoking is harmful to his health and that he should stop would not be likely to benefit by setting a quit date at that visit. Instead, the emphasis should be on convincing him of the harmful effects of smoking on his personal health and the benefits of quitting. In contrast, contemplators do not need to be told about the hazards of their harmful behavior because they are aware of them. Instead, they need encouragement to commit to action. People in the preparation stage need encouragement and support, as well as assistance in strategies to carry out their plans. It is a waste of time to discuss negative health effects of smoking with a person who has already decided to quit but who is backsliding. That individual would benefit more from specific suggestions on avoiding backsliding (e.g., nicotine replacement) and from increased support and encouragement. Those in the action stage are expending a significant amount of energy in behavioral change, and they need support and encouragement. People in the maintenance stage need strategies to prevent backsliding.

It is abundantly clear that facilitating behavioral change requires a lot more than passing on information, such as a giving someone a brief lecture or a pamphlet to read at home. If these alone were effective, nobody would smoke! The factors that keep people engaged in behaviors that are harmful to their health are complicated, as are the strategies to facilitate behavior change in others. The following strategies have been shown to be effective in patient education and counseling and are adapted from the *Guide to Clinical Preventive Services.*[3]

1. **Frame the teaching to match the patient's perceptions.** For example, a person who asserts she is unable to exercise may be asked to reframe her definition of exercise and commit to exercising five minutes a day.
2. **Fully inform patients of the purposes and expected effects of their behavioral change and when to expect to see these effects.** For example, advice to an elder may be that mus-

cle strength should increase over a year so that in six months he should be able to lift five pounds and in 12 months he should expect to lift ten pounds. Advice may also emphasize that patients may experience muscle soreness over the first few weeks.

3. **Suggest small changes rather than large ones.** Make recommendations that you are sure the patient can accomplish, and set small goals. For example, suggest walking only ten minutes twice a week at first. Once an individual has been successful in establishing a healthy habit, he or she is more likely to be able to continue or expand that activity.

4. **Be specific.** It is much more helpful to suggest walking around the block three days a week with your dog than, "You should get more exercise and drop a few pounds."

5. **It is sometimes easier to add new behaviors than to eliminate old behaviors.** For example eating more fruits and vegetables may be easier than reducing dietary fat. Adding exercise may be more easily accomplished than stopping smoking.

6. **Link new behaviors to old behaviors; help the patients find where the behavior change will fit into their usual routines.** For example, people who say they have no time to exercise may agree to walk to a friend's house twice a week instead of driving, or ask the friend to go for a walk instead of sitting and talking.

7. **Use the power of the profession.** Patients listen to what physicians and other health professionals tell them. Be direct about what you want the patient to do.

8. **Focus on the positives, not the negatives.** Reward works better than punishment, and the best rewards are those intrinsic to the activity. For example, it is better to say, "Exercising will give you more energy," than "If you exercise, you can have a candy bar" or "If you don't exercise, you can't go to the movies."

9. **Get an explicit commitment from the patient.** Asking clients to describe what they plan to do helps them focus on the specifics of their plan. This process may also reveal difficulties with the plan. For instance, "I will walk every day after dinner, but sometimes it is dark. Well, then maybe I will ask my husband to go with me." Saying something aloud to another person about one's plans helps in following through.

10. **Use a variety of strategies.** Combine written materials, verbal encouragement, and use of office staff or other professionals to help people change behavior.

11. **Monitor progress through follow-up contact.** A telephone call to assess whether changes are being made and to evaluate difficulties can be very effective.

Specific Health Promotion Interventions

Many health behaviors can be changed with health promotion activities. A visit with a doctor or other health professional is an ideal opportunity to encourage healthful behavior change. However, these activities are generally underutilized by elders and their health care providers. The following section will outline a variety of health behavioral interventions that can occur between elders and their medical providers. This section will outline community-based and federal health promotion efforts.

The following interventions have been shown to reduce the rate of illness and death and increase the quality of life. The chapters on nutrition, physical activity, chronic illness, acute illness, and accidents have already illustrated the benefits of modifying the following personal health behaviors. As mentioned earlier, it is never too late to stop the following harmful behaviors because even the very old can benefit.

Smoking Cessation

Smoking is the most important factor that contributes to premature death and disability in the United States. At least 20 percent of all deaths are linked to smoking cigarettes. Smoking has been implicated as a causal factor in many diseases, including lung cancer, head and neck cancer, bladder cancer, pancreatic cancer, cervical cancer, heart disease, stroke, peripheral vascular disease, chronic obstructive pulmonary disease, death from fires, and pneumonia. The deleterious health effects of secondary smoke on those who live with a smoker have also been repeatedly documented.

About one in four Americans smoke, most beginning in childhood or adolescence. Cigarettes contain nicotine, an addictive substance that induces people to continue to smoke. The more cigarettes smoked a day, the greater the nicotine addiction. Because of the addictive quality, smoking is a habit that can be quite difficult to change. Further, many people smoke for relaxation and stress release and depend on cigarettes psychologically. Most smokers who quit reported they tried multiple times prior to succeeding, and often periods of stress can induce backsliding.

Although it is ideal never to begin smoking, multiple studies have documented the positive effects of quitting smoking, even at an advanced age. Smokers who quit before age fifty reduce their risk of dying in the next fifteen years by half. The mortality rate is significantly reduced even for those who quit smoking after age seventy.[8] Five to ten years after a person quits smoking, cancer risks start to drop, and risk of stroke and heart attack fall even faster. Quitting smoking also reduces the progression and morbidity from lung diseases.

It is widely recommended that health professionals frequently discuss quitting smoking with their patients. Studies show that when physicians recommend to smokers that they quit, the recommendation alone is an inducement to quit. In addition, doctors should provide or refer smokers to individual or group cessation groups, distribute written materials, ask the patient to set a specific quit date, and follow-up to assure compliance. Sometimes nicotine gum or patches may be helpful. It is important that clinicians provide highly directive advice to quit smoking combined with information about the health effects of tobacco and advice about how to quit. Guidelines for health specialists to assist patients and clients to stop smoking have

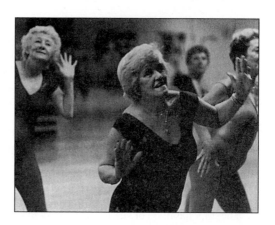

been developed by a group of experts and published by the Agency for Health Care Policy and Research.[9]

Physical Activity

A sedentary lifestyle is associated with multiple diseases, including heart disease, hypertension, obesity, osteoporosis, diabetes, and mental disorders (see chapter 4). Professional groups recommend a regular and moderate to vigorous level of physical activity for all age groups that is tailored to their capabilities. It is not clear whether physician advice is enough to compel people to exercise, but it should be offered. Physicians should determine the current activity level of their patients, ascertain individual barriers to increasing activity, and teach them the benefits of physical activity. Physicians should assist elders to design an exercise program appropriate for their needs and lifestyle (see chapter 4). Health care providers should emphasize both regular, moderate aerobic physical activity (e.g., walking, swimming) and regular muscle strengthening exercises.

Promotion of a Healthy Diet

Diet plays a role in the cause of many chronic illnesses, including cardiovascular disease, cancers, hypertension, obesity, adult-onset diabetes, osteoporosis, constipation, and anemia. Diets high in fats (particularly saturated fats) and low in fiber have been linked to poor health outcomes. The elderly often have special nutritional requirements due to disease, reduced caloric intake, medication use, or functional status. Multiple clinical trials have demonstrated that counseling and education can be effective at changing dietary habits. However, often these interventions were community-wide or conducted by dieticians, not physicians. Ideally, dietary counseling should include specific recommendations about dietary components. For example, adults should limit dietary fat intake to less than 30 percent of total calories, especially saturated fat (10 percent), maintain a balanced diet, eat at least five servings a day of fruits and vegetables and at least six servings of whole-grain products or legumes containing fiber. Dietary counseling should include a dietary history; address potential barriers to change in diet; offer specific guidance about food selection, preparation and meal planning; and recommend follow-up with a counselor skilled in this area (see chapter 5).

Prevention of Motor Vehicle Injuries

Motor vehicle fatalities are a significant cause of mortality among the elderly. Although the elderly have a relatively low rate of motor vehicle accidents, they drive many fewer miles. However, when they are involved in motor vehicle accidents, they are more likely to suffer serious illness or death than younger adults. The most important risk factors for motor vehicle injuries include driving under the influence of alcohol or drugs, and failure to properly use seat belts. Additionally, elders are at high risk of death from pedestrian injuries. There is little evidence regarding whether advice provided at medical visits is effective at reducing risk factors for motor vehicle injury. However, at minimum, clinicians are urged to recommend use of seat belts, motorcycle helmets, and air bags. All elders should be cautioned against drinking and driving and educated about which of their medications may impair their driving ability. Physicians are also obligated to report to the Department of Motor Vehicles individuals with certain diagnoses (e.g., seizures) or an inability to drive safely. Although not being able to drive can be a severe blow to an elder's self-esteem,

it is important for health care professionals to comply with these reporting requirements to protect other drivers.

Injury Prevention

Falls are a leading cause of unintentional injury and death in the elderly. Risk factors for falls are well-documented and include individual factors (e.g., sensory decrements, diminished strength, gait instability, age changes, medication use) and environmental characteristics (e.g., stairs, poor lighting, inadequate footwear). Multiple types of interventions have been attempted to reduce elders' risk of falls and fall-associated morbidity, including education, environmental modification, and strength, flexibility, or balance training. However, providing education about falls is not enough. In one study, elders were visited in their home by a public health nurse and were educated on safety, while a control group received information on influenza. At the two- to three-month follow-up there were no differences between the groups in the safety changes made in the home.[10]

The most effective programs seem to have a multipronged approach—assess risk factors, adjust medications, initiate exercise and education programs, and reduce the number of environmental hazards. However, even the effectiveness of these programs is mixed. One randomized controlled trial reported a reduced fall risk for community-dwelling elders over age seventy compared to a control group.[11] However, another randomized controlled study reported no difference in propensity or severity of falls between the intervention and control group.[12]

It is recommended that physicians perform fall risk assessments and counsel elders about ways to reduce falls. These measures include exercise (particularly balance training), safety behaviors, environmental hazard reduction, and medication review. More intensive intervention programs for elders show some promise and should be considered for high-risk elders: those over age seventy-five, those using more than four prescription medications, those using antihypertensive or sedative medications, and those with impaired cognition, balance, or gait.

Health Promotion in Community Settings

Although community-based health promotion programs have the potential to improve the health of elders, they have only recently been instituted and studied on a wide scale, but initial results are promising. These programs may target a particular health problem (e.g., accident prevention, smoking cessation, disease screening) or include many topics as part of a comprehensive wellness program. They may occur through health maintenance organizations or in community settings, such as senior centers, assisted living facilities, and nutrition sites. Health promotion efforts are increasingly being provided in workplace settings because corporations see the benefits of a healthy workforce in reducing absenteeism and health insurance costs and increasing satisfaction. However, because the proportion of elders employed in the workforce is relatively small, workforce health promotion efforts are less important to elders.

A disadvantage of some community health promotion programs is they are accomplished without knowledge of the participants' primary care providers. Thus, information obtained or exchanged in these settings (e.g., health fairs) may not be transmitted to the primary care physician for evaluation and follow-up. Some individuals may undergo unnecessary screening (e.g., monitoring one's cholesterol monthly at health fairs and grocery stores is not appropriate), while others will not have follow-up for abnormalities found in community screening. Ideally, these programs are multidisiplinary and incorporated with elders' primary medical providers.

PREVENTION AND HEALTH PROMOTION ON A NATIONAL SCALE

Healthy People is a federal government initiative to define a strategic plan for the nation to improve the health of its citizens. Out of years of collaboration from multiple groups, a document specifying specific goals and objectives was developed. It identifies the most significant preventable threats to health and focuses public and private sector efforts to address those threats. *Healthy People* offers a simple but powerful idea: provide the information and knowledge about how to improve health in a format that enables diverse groups to combine their efforts and work as a team. It can be envisioned as a road map to better health for all that can be used by many different people. *Healthy People* is based on the best scientific knowledge and is used for decision making and action at many levels. The goals can be implemented by states, counties, communities, professional organizations, groups whose concern is a particular health problem, or a particular population group.

The *Healthy People* concept was developed as the first set of national health targets published in 1979 in *Healthy People: The Surgeon General's Report on Health Promotion and Disease Prevention.* This report included five goals: to reduce mortality among four different age groups (infants, children, adolescents and young adults, and adults) and increase independence among older adults. Specific numbers were targeted for each of these areas to be achieved by 1990. Although goals were met for infants and children, they were not achieved for adolescents, and there were insufficient data to assess whether goals for elders were achieved.

The next initiative, *Healthy People 2000,* built upon the lessons of the first Surgeon General's report, is the product of unprecedented collaboration among government, voluntary and professional organizations, businesses, and individuals. *Healthy People 2000* was based on an expanded science base for developing health promotion and disease prevention objectives. Many of the year-2000 objectives specify improving the health of groups of people that bear a disproportionate burden of poor health.

The framework of *Healthy People 2000* consists of three broad goals:

• increase the span of healthy life for Americans,
• reduce health disparities among Americans, and
• achieve access to preventive services for all Americans.

Organized under the broad umbrella of health promotion, health protection, and preventive services, the more than 300 national objectives are organized into twenty-two priority areas. *Healthy People 2000* was built on comments from more than 10,000 individuals and organizations. Ongoing involvement is ensured through the Healthy People Consortium—an alliance of 350 national membership organizations and 300 state health, mental health, substance abuse, and environmental agencies.

Building upon scientific advances and experience, *Healthy People 2010* continues to evolve. The plan to be unveiled in January 2000 has two overarching goals for Americans through the year 2020: increasing the quality and years of healthy life and eliminating health disparities. These goals are to be achieved in four areas: (1) promoting healthy behaviors, (2) promoting healthy and safe communities, (3) improving systems for personal and public health, and (4) preventing and reducing diseases and disorders. *Healthy People 2010,* in cooperation with the Healthy People Consortium, has developed more than 500 specific objectives to be monitored during the years 2000 to 2010. The document will serve as a guide for policy and program development at the local, state, and national levels. For more information refer to the web site: http:\\web.health.gov/healthypeople.

PREVENTION: PROBLEMS AND PROSPECTS

Although most people would agree that prevention of illness and disability makes more sense than treating illnesses that have already damaged the body, care for end-stage diseases dominates the health care provided in the United States. Treating advanced chronic illnesses, such as chronic obstructive pulmonary disease (COPD), cardiac disease, stroke, and cancer, consumes the majority of the health care resources in the United States, and these diseases are preventable. Preventive services, on the other hand, comprise just 3 percent of health care expenditures in the United States.[13]

Because there is a high prevalence of disease in older persons, the potential to prevent or decrease severity of these diseases is great. However, prevention and health promotion programs are woefully underused. Medicare and insurance companies seldom reimburse for preventive services, physicians are less likely to offer them, and patients are less apt to make appointments or follow-through on preventive health recommendations. It is far easier for a physician to prescribe medication for high blood pressure than to discuss weight loss, the specifics of an exercise prescription, smoking cessation, and dietary changes. Also, it is much easier for a patient to take a pill every day than to initiate and sustain a physical fitness program or to lose weight healthfully.

Our health care system is oriented toward the management of acute and chronic issues, rather than towards the prevention of illness. The upfront costs of prevention may also seem high, and the benefits may seem intangible because the benefits occur years later. Although some preventive measures are cost savers, others are expensive because they prolong life expectancy—dead clients do not use many health care resources. A classic example is that smoking cessation may cost money because smokers die earlier.

Physicians get reimbursed for medical procedures, but often not for the counseling that is entailed in health promotion and prevention. Patient turnover makes it hard for the physician to track the preventive activities of their elder patients that they have received elsewhere (such as receiving an influenza vaccine or getting screened for diabetes at a a local health fair). People live in the moment and are crisis-oriented, so they may agree with the concept of prevention but neglect to make the appointment to follow-through.

Only half of the nation's citizens receive recommended preventive health care services. Studies repeatedly document that patients are not asked key questions during their check-ups about unhealthy lifestyles. Although three-fourths of older adults have routine checkups, only about half of all adults age sixty-five and older were asked about any one of four health behaviors (diet, physical activity, tobacco use, or alcohol use) during a checkup in the last three years.[14] Less than half of patients who smoke report that their doctor advised them to quit.[15, 16] Among women age sixty-five and older, less than three in five report receiving a Pap smear in the preceding three years, and only half had received a breast exam and mammogram in the last two years.[14] Only one-third of elders report receiving a tetanus immunization in the last ten years, and a little more than one-fourth report receiving a single pneumococal vaccination recommended for all elders over age sixty-five. About half of all elders reported receiving an influenza vaccination (flu shot) in the last year. Further, the use of preventive services is much lower for ethnic minority and poor elders.

Health promotion efforts and public education campaigns have made a significant difference in the lives of many Americans. Our television and print media discuss the latest advances in health, most people are more knowledgeable about dietary fat and physical fitness, states and communities have initiated mandatory seat belt laws and antismoking ordinances, and most people know something about prevention of HIV infection. These campaigns and the efforts of public health professionals, industries and government have resulted in positive health trends among Americans. Since 1964, the percentage of U.S. residents who smoke cigarettes has fallen from 40 percent to 25 percent. About one-third of the population consumes a low-fat diet, and one-fourth exercise regularly.[17] Between 1988 and 1993, the percentage of those living in cities with clean air increased from fifty to seventy-seven percent.[17] In this same period, the proportion of women over age fifty who had had a recent mammogram more than doubled.[17] As more Americans are adopting healthful behaviors, they are living longer and healthier lives as evidenced by decreases in death rates from heart disease (28 percent reduction), stroke (37 percent reduction), and injuries (32 percent reduction) and by an increased life expectancy.[18]

Summary

There is an increased focus on disease prevention and health promotion for adults of all ages. A large proportion of illnesses in this country are caused or aggravated by unhealthy lifestyles and personal health behaviors and are amenable to prevention. Increased efforts in this area have led to a reduction in cardiovascular disease, accidents, and other illnesses. Interventions to prevent disease from occurring in the first place, such as immunizations, constitute primary prevention. Early detection and treatment of illness to prevent mortality and morbidity constitutes secondary prevention and includes many screening tests. Multiple groups issue recommendations regarding screening tests, and even though there are some well-publicized disagreements, there is a core of tests recommended by most groups. Tertiary prevention involves treatments to reduce the impact of disease on the person's ability to function.

Health promotion activities, including counseling and education, assist people to make positive lifestyle changes and are provided on an individual or community-wide basis. Health care practitioners face barriers to encouraging and implementing health behavioral changes. Too few elders receive needed preventive health services. Health promotion methods should take into consideration the individual factors necessary to make positive lifestyle changes.

Activities

1. Develop a health education module (or outline) for a particular population of older people. Clearly specify the problem, measurable objectives, an outline of subject matter, teaching methods, and any educational materials you would use.

2. Survey a group of adults of various ages regarding their knowledge of and compliance with recommended screening guidelines.

3. Design a single-page advertisement for older individuals on a topic related to prevention or health promotion.

4. Collect screening recommendations from a variety of groups on a single topic (e.g., mammography, prostate cancer screening) and compare them. Can you determine why different organizations came to different conclusions with the same set of data? How might you explain these differences to a layperson? Which guidelines do you trust/would you follow?

5. Ask your friends and family members of various ages to recall their visits with a physician in the last year. Were they asked about personal health behaviors? What screening tests were they offered? Was health promotion counseling offered? How many of the elders had complied with the recommendations outlined in this chapter?

6. Ask friends and family members to define "risk factors" and to discuss the concept as it relates to their own health and the health of the general population. What misconceptions do you notice? Can you explain these concepts to others?

Bibliography

1. Steering Committee of the Physician's Health Study Research Group. 1989. Final report on the aspirin component of the ongoing Physician's Health Study. *New England Journal of Medicine* 321:129–35.

2. Manson, J.E., Stampfer, M.J., and Colditz, G.A., et al. 1991. A prospective study of aspirin use and primary prevention of cardiovascular disease in women. *Journal of the American Medical Association* 266:521–27.

3. U.S. Preventive Services Task Force. 1996. *Guide to clinical preventive services,* 2nd ed. Baltimore, MD: Williams and Wilkins.

4. Manolio, T.A., Pearson, T.A., and Wenger, N.K., et al. 1992. Cholesterol and heart disease in older persons and women: review of an NHLBI workshop. *Annals of Epidemiology* 21:161–76.

5. Woolf, S.H., Jonas, S., and Lawrence, R.S. 1996. *Health promotion and disease prevention in clinical practice*. Baltimore, MD: Williams and Wilkins.

6. Westberg, J., and Jason, H. 1996. Fostering healthy behavior: The process. In *Health promotion and disease prevention in clinical practice,* S.H. Woolf, S. Jonas, and R.S. Lawrence. Baltimore, Maryland: Williams and Wilkins, pp.145–62.

7. Prochaska, J.O., Velicer, W.F., and Rossi, J.S., et al. 1994. Stages of change and decisional balance for twelve problem behaviors. *Health Psychology* 13:39–46.

8. Department of Health and Human Services. 1990. *The health benefits of smoking cessation: A report of the Surgeon General.* Pub No. DHHS (CDC) 90-8416. Rockville, MD: Department of Health and Human Services.

9. Fiore, M.C., Bailey, W.C., and Cohen, S.J., et al. 1996. *Smoking cessation: Information for specialists. Clinical practice guidelines.* AHCPR Pub. No. 96-0694. Rockville, MD: U.S. Department of Health and Human Services, Agency for Health Care Policy and Research and Centers for Disease Control and Prevention.

10. Ploeg, J., Black, M.E., and Hutchinson, B.G., et al. 1994. Personal, home and community safety promotion with community-dwelling older persons: Response to a public health nurse intervention. *Canadian Journal of Public Health* 85:188–91.

11. Tinetti, M.E., Baker, D.I., and McAvay, G., et al. 1994. A multifactorial intervention to

reduce the risk of falling among elderly people living in the community. *New England Journal of Medicine* 331:821–7.

12. Vetter, N.J., Lewis, P.A., and Ford, D. 1992. Can health visitors prevent fractures in elderly people? *British Medical Journal* 304:888–90.

13. U.S. Centers for Disease Control and Prevention. 1992. Estimated national spending on prevention—United States, 1988. *Morbidity and Mortality Weekly Report* 41:529–31.

14. National Health Interview Survey. National Center for Health Statistics 1995.

15. Anda, R.F., Remington, P.L., Sieko, D.G., and Davis, R.M. 1987. Are physician's advising smokers to quit? The patient's perspective. *Journal of the American Medical Association* 257:1916–19.

16. Frank, E., Winkleby, M.A., and Altman, D.G., et al. 1991. Predictors of physician's smoking cessation advice. *Journal of the American Medical Association* 266:3139–44.

17. McGinnis, J.M., and Lee, P.R. 1995. Healthy People 2000 at mid-decade. *Journal of the American Medical Association* 273:1123–29.

18. Kochanek, K.D., and Hudson, B.L. 1995. Advance report of the final mortality statistics, 1992. *Monthly Vital Statistics Report* 43(6 suppl). Hyattsville, MD: National Center for Health Statistics.

12

Medical Care

You, the individual, can do more for your own health and well-being than any doctor, any hospital, any drug, any exotic medical device.

Joseph Califano

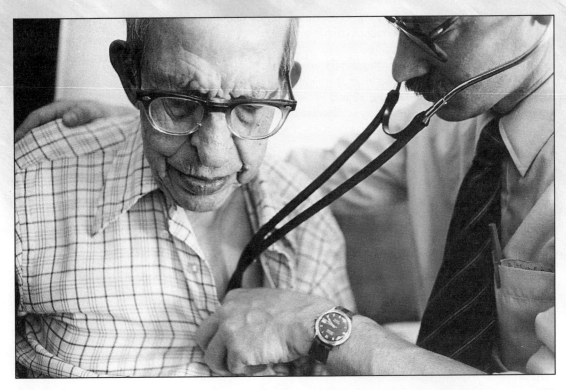

The United States has one of the largest, most technologically advanced health care systems in the world. A multitude of high-tech services and highly skilled providers are available throughout the United States. However, medical care in our country comes with a high cost: it is by far the most expensive of all developed countries. The payment mechanism for those under sixty-five is through private health insurance, often at least in part by employers, and sometimes by individuals themselves. The source of payment for those over sixty-five, the disabled, and poor of all ages is the federal and state government. Because of the stable source of government payment, elders are more likely to have better medical care coverage when compared to those under sixty-five whose coverage is more transitory as they move from one job to the next. However, the costs of government programs to pay for medical care are rising as the numbers of elders in the population increase.

This chapter will examine the use of medical care by older people, how such care is financed, problems that affect the quality of care, and ways in which the medical system is being modified to increase its effectiveness. Treatments commonly used that are outside the medical mainstream will also be discussed. The following chapter will focus on institutions and community services that comprise long-term care in our country. Mental health services, both acute and long-term, were discussed in chapter 7.

Elder Use of Medical Services

As might be expected from their higher rate of chronic illness, disability, and death than other age groups, elders use a disproportionate amount of medical care services. They visit physicians about twice as often as younger adults. Elders over age sixty-five average six physician visits annually.[1] About one-third of those age sixty-five and older are admitted to a hospital at least once a year, and the hospital admission rate for elders over eighty-five is almost twice as high as the sixty-five to seventy-four age group. Once admitted, they average longer stays, receive more medications, and undergo more medical procedures than their younger counterparts. The average length of hospital stay also increases with advancing age. In 1996, patients between the ages of forty-five and sixty-four stayed an average of 5.3 days, while those sixty-five and older stayed 6.5 days. That same year, the rate of medical procedures among hospitalized elders was more than triple that for people aged fifteen to forty-four, and more than double that of those aged forty-five to sixty-four.[2]

Multiple factors influence medical service use. In general, elders who visit physicians are sicker. However, many ill elders do not seek care, and many well elders are high users of services. Perceived health status, health beliefs, financial status, ethnicity, degree of isolation, and availability of medical care are only a few influences. Cost concerns, travel difficulties, belief that symptoms are due to age, or trouble making appointments are often cited as reasons to delay seeking care. Those who tend to worry about their health, or those who feel that their poor health keeps them from doing the things they want to do visit doctors more often.

Financing Medical Services

In 1997, annual health care spending surpassed $1 trillion (almost $4,000 per year per person), and the spending continues to rise. This figure includes monies spent on direct physician services, hospital bills, prescription drugs, medical supplies, and administrative costs. Health care expenses in the United States comprise 14 percent of the gross domestic product, higher than any other country in the world. Other countries have some form of national health care in which the government either provides and/or pays for health care. Our government, however, does not finance health care for all its citizens. In the United States, the government contributes toward the financing of medical care for elders, the poor, veterans, and the disabled, while other adults and children either buy private insurance, have employer-sponsored insurance, or go without. It is estimated that more than 43 million U.S. citizens are uninsured.

In the United States, several sources finance health care for elders: government-sponsored programs such as Medicare, Medicaid, and Veteran's health benefits, private insurance, and funds from the elders' own pockets. Medicare and out-of-pocket expenses are the largest payers of medical expenses, each contributing about 40 percent of the total expenditures. The remainder is paid by Medicaid, the Veteran's Administration, and private insurance policies to supplement Medicare. As health care becomes increasingly expensive, the amount financed out-of-pocket is rising. Approximately one-fifth of the average older person's income is spent on health care. The following section details the various financing mechanisms for health care of the elderly.

Medicare

Medicare, Title XVIII of the Social Security Act, was initiated in 1966 to provide selected medical benefits for those age sixty-five and older who qualify for Social Security, regardless of income. In 1972 and 1973, further legislation expanded the coverage to those age sixty-five and older who previously did not qualify for Social Security, as well as certain disabled people. When Medicare was first enacted, over half of all elders lacked health insurance, and many faced bankruptcy when they became seriously ill. Medicare offers protection from catastrophic losses due to high medical care costs. Currently about 95 percent of the nation's elder population, about 40 million elders, are enrolled, making Medicare the largest entitlement program in our country.

The majority of Medicare funds come from taxes levied on working adults. Upon reaching age sixty-five, elders are eligible to receive its benefits. Over $100 billion is paid into the Medicare fund annually, primarily through payroll deductions under Social Security and general income taxes. Elders also contribute to Medicare through the payment of premiums. Unfortunately, the cost of health care, the increasing numbers of elders, and their increased life expectancy are rising faster than workers' contributions. Because there are currently a relatively large number of workers (and a relatively small number of elderly beneficiaries), the fund is still solvent. However, experts predict that the Medicare fund will have a deficit in the future as the cohort of baby boomers retires. These predictions have sparked a great deal of interest in modifying the Medicare system, and a variety of solutions are being proposed.

Medicare insurance coverage is divided into two parts: Part A and Part B. Each part is funded differently and designed to cover different services. Part A reimburses the cost of hospital services and is financed by a hospital insurance payroll tax levied on employers, employees, and the self-employed and is available to all elders. Although Part A is directed primarily toward hospital care, it will reimburse home health care, hospice care, and limited stays in a nursing home following hospitalization.

In contrast, Part B reimburses the cost of medical services and is financed through the general revenues of the federal government and through the monthly premium payment of those who enroll. It is a medical insurance that reimburses 80 percent of reasonable charges for medically necessary physician and surgeon fees, medical supplies, physical and speech therapists, diagnostic tests, home health care, and outpatient hospital and lab services after meeting a yearly deductible. Part B is voluntary: individuals who want this coverage must pay a monthly premium. In 1999, this premium was $45.50 a month. That year, over 97 percent of those over age sixty-five elected Part B.

Neither Part A nor Part B covers all needed medical services or reimburses fully for any benefit. Although Medicare pays about 40 percent of elders' personal health care expenditures, the benefits vary according to the service.

Medicare is a complex program. Both Parts A and B have deductibles (a set price that a beneficiary must pay for each type of service each year before Medicare pays) and copayments (percentage of charge for each service paid by the patient). Unlike most private insurance plans, Medicare has no cap on what a person has to pay out-of-pocket. Although numbers change, in 1999, Part A required individuals to pay the first $768 of their hospital bill for the first sixty days, required a $192 per day copayment for days 61 to 90, and $384 per day for days 90 to 150. Coverage ceased if hospitalization was prolonged beyond 150 days. Part A covered skilled nursing home care for twenty days if the care followed a hospital stay and other conditions were met and up to 190 days of psychiatric hospitalization. In addition, Medicare Part A financed needed home health services and hospice services for the terminally ill without copayments or deductibles if certain guidelines were met. In 1999, Part B Medicare had a deductible of $100, which means that elders paid the first $100 of the year out of their own pocket. For mental health services, Part B had a 50 percent coinsurance premium. Likewise, Medicare Part B had a copayment of 20 percent, which means that if a doctor's visit cost $200, the elder would be responsible for a $40 payment.

Elders may finance copayments and deductibles through supplementary policies: they may purchase Medigap insurance, continue with an employer-sponsored insurance plan, or qualify for Medicaid funds. If an elder elects to join a managed care organization under Medicare, there are fewer deductibles and copayments, but they must give up free choice of health care providers.

Reimbursement to Hospitals and Physicians

Unlike nationalized health plans in other countries in which the doctors and hospitals are government-owned, Medicare provides public funds to private practitioners. That is, hospitals and doctors who see Medicare patients bill Medicare for those services. Because Medicare finances the health care of so many Americans, the government has bargaining power to set prices and standards that doctors and hospitals must follow to get paid. In an attempt to stem the rising costs of Medicare and to provide fairness and incentives to lower costs and improve services, changes have been made in the way Medicare reimburses physicians and hospitals. The following section describes some innovations developed by Medicare policy makers as an attempt to improve medical care and reduce its costs.

Diagnosis Related Groups   In the past, Medicare reimbursed hospitals based on its expenses after services were rendered, called "retrospective." This system, however, rewarded hospitals with higher costs and longer hospital stays and provided no incentives for efficiency of care. In an attempt to reduce costs, Congress amended the reimbursement process for hospital care (Part A). In 1983, Congress mandated a new system of payment before the service is rendered, a "prospective" payment system, that is based on diagnosis related groups (DRGs). When a Medicare patient is admitted, the hospital receives a fixed fee for treatment based on the average cost to treat that particular diagnosis in a particular geographic region. This fixed amount must cover all diagnostic tests, treatments, and hospital costs incurred for that patient. If the hospital can treat an elder for less, a profit is made on that patient; if a patient needs more care, the hospital loses money on that patient. The intent of the legislation is to reward hospitals for managing resources well and keeping costs down by decreasing hospital stays, diagnostic testing, medical supplies, and therapy. In fact, the implementation of DRGs has resulted in significantly shorter hospital stays, a decreased reliance on hospitals, and increased use of outpatient treatments. However, patients are often discharged in a more debilitated condition, so they may require increased home health care or temporary nursing home placement.

When physician services are billed for a Medicare patient, in most states, a physician must agree to "accept assignment," which means that the physician agrees to accept what Medicare determines as "reasonable" for that procedure as full payment. The reasonable charge is determined by experts, and the amount varies by geographic location. If the yearly deductible is met, Medicare pays 80 percent of the reasonable charge directly to the physician. The physician may then bill the patient for the remaining 20 percent copayment. In some states, a physician can choose not to accept assignment and may charge an additional cost over and above the 20 percent copayment. However, this additional charge must be 15 percent or less. For instance, Medicare agrees that $100 is a reasonable charge for a particular medical procedure. If the physician accepts assignment, Medicare pays the physician $80, and the patient pays the $20 copayment. If the physician does not accept assignment, the charge may be not more than $115 for the same medical procedure. Medicare will still only reimburse the physician $80, but the patient then must pay $35. In many cases, the patient must pay the physician the entire charge and wait for partial reimbursement from Medicare at a later date. The majority of the nation's physicians accept assignment because state and federal regulations have made balance billing less appealing, and in many states, illegal.

Resource-Based Relative Value Scales   In 1989, Congress made a significant change in the way Medicare reimburses physicians for their services. The change was implemented in order to save money for the Medicare program and make the reimbursement to different types of physicians more equitable. Previously, reimbursement was based on physicians' usual charges and the prevailing rate in a geographical area. Physicians in some areas of the country (for example, big cities) charged more for the same service than their counterparts in other areas, and their reimbursement from Medicare reflected these differences. Services of specialists or procedures were reimbursed at a much higher rate than patient evaluation/counseling services in which a physician likely spent more time with a patient rather than providing a procedure.

The method, called the *resource-based relative value scale,* was initiated in 1992 and fully implemented in 1996. The fee schedule for physician services is based on the relative value of the medical procedures and the resources needed to perform that procedure (e.g., malpractice insurance expenses, costs for specialty training). Currently, a base national fee has been developed for each of approximately 7,000 different medical charges. Geographical location was also taken into consideration, and the reimbursement now varies only 15 percent among regions.

The two major outcomes of the relative value scale are reduced Medicare reimbursements to sur-

geons and other specialists, and increased reimbursements to primary care physicians for their timeconsuming patient evaluation and management services. After implementation of the new payment scale, the average payment to a family doctor was about one-third more than it would have been under the old system. In addition, physicians in rural areas and those who serve a high proportion of poor patients receive increased Medicare reimbursements than before relative value scales were enacted. Physicians in urban and affluent areas receive less than they did in the past.

Medicare Health Maintenance Organizations (HMOs)   As Congress looks for ways to cut costs in the Medicare system, more attention is directed toward encouraging elders to enroll in managed care organizations. The health maintenance organization (HMO) is the most common type of managed care for elders. Instead of paying physicians a fee for each service rendered, individuals who enroll in an HMO pay a fixed monthly premium that covers all required medical services. In a staff model HMO, a group of physicians employed by the HMO serve patients in one location (e.g., Kaiser Permanente). More common are managed care plans that contract with physician groups and hospitals to provide care for their enrollees at reduced rates. These doctors and hospitals may be paid a fixed rate per month for each enrollee or a modified fee for service plan whereby the physicians receive reduced reimbursement for services provided. The financial health of an HMO depends on keeping costs within the total monthly premiums the organization receives. HMO physicians generally have a strong incentive to keep services to a minimum, so unnecessary or expensive diagnostic tests, drugs, surgery, or hospitalization are discouraged.

The 1982 Tax Act authorized Medicare to pay prepaid benefits to any HMO that enrolls Medicare patients. By 1997, almost 10 percent of those sixty-five and older in our country were enrolled in Medicare managed care organizations. Elders join HMOs because of their generous benefit packages and lower premiums. Development of new HMOs has become a big and profitable business.

Unfortunately, many of the small health mainte- nance organizations are "here today and gone tomorrow," while large for-profit health care con- glomerates owning a variety of health care services and products are providing care to elders in many states. Because of the low profit margin, many orga- nizations are not as interested in staying in rural areas, which is problematic for elders who previ- ously depended on them for their medical care. When the organizations close, the recipient needs to find another group or, if none is available, must reen- ter the traditional Medicare program.

There are many differences between tradi- tional Medicare and Medicare HMOs, but the most fundamental difference is in how these programs finance health care services. With traditional Medicare reimbursement, hospitals and physicians are reimbursed for services rendered. If an older person visits a physician often or is hospitalized frequently, the physician and hospital would receive more fees than they would for an elder who never visited the doctor or used a hospital. In con- trast, Medicare HMO plans cover all Medicare- covered services to enrolled beneficiaries. In turn, they receive a fixed payment for all services pro- vided, rather than payments based on individual services (called capitation). This means that the doctor or hospital gets paid according to the num- ber of elders enrolled, whether or not services are used. Exactly how much the doctor or hospital is paid is determined by approximating the costs for 95 percent of enrollees with similar demographic characteristics enrolled in traditional Medicare. Thus, the HMO providing Medicare will profit if it can reduce costs and services provided to its bene- ficiaries.

When Medicare recipients enroll in health maintenance organizations, they agree to a set of terms or conditions that include at least some of the following. In general, they sacrifice choice for increased benefits and decreased costs. For example, they are limited in their choice of doctors to those who participate in the HMO plan; if their private doctor is not reimbursed under the plan, they must switch doctors. Enrollees must generally seek care from a single primary care provider, rather than rely-

ing on various specialists. Many times, they need a written referral from their primary care doctor authorizing any visits or treatments by specialists. In addition, enrollees are generally restricted to one hospital system or geographic area (except in a true emergency). They may have to wait for health plan authorization before a particular medication, treat- ment, or specialized visits can be "covered." They may disagree with their physician or health plan about whether a given test, treatment, or specialist is needed, and resolving these disagreements can be a source of anxiety or result in delayed care. However, there are several benefits of joining a Medicare HMO. Elders enjoy added coverage such as pre- scription drugs, lower or no copayments or deductibles, and, ideally, more coordinated care.

Because the method of reimbursement differs between traditional Medicare reimbursement and Medicare HMOs, the incentives of hospitals and physicians under each plan differ. Each has its own set of problems. With traditional Medicare, physi- cians can easily order more tests, hospitalize patients, encourage repeat visits, and refer to spe- cialty care. This may result in unnecessary services and, consequently, unnecessary costs. Care may also be uncoordinated because elders seek care from various providers in various systems. However, with Medicare HMOs, there is an incen- tive to provide less care to increase profits. That means fewer tests, hospitalizations, surgeries, and referrals to specialists. This model could result in greater coordination of care and an expansion of preventive services. However, some fear it is more likely to result in denial of needed, but expensive, diagnostic and therapeutic interventions.

It is very difficult to accurately compare the true costs of traditional Medicare and Medicare HMOs. However, there is a general consensus that HMOs reduce patient expenditures. This is accom- plished by reducing hospitalization and referrals to physician specialists. Ideally, these organiza- tions have a greater emphasis on prevention and more highly coordinated care. Often there is a process of utilization review where those who need specialist care, surgery, or expensive diag- nostic tests must have their claims reviewed in advance to be sure the services are medically indicated. However, some assert that their costs appear deceptively low because HMOs tend to enroll healthier enrollees. Others complain that costs are reduced because services are reduced and that health care may suffer. Both state and federal governments are developing regulations to better monitor managed care organizations and assure quality of care.

Just as it is difficult to assess costs, it is also difficult to compare quality. Evaluating quality of care and patient satisfaction is a burgeoning area of research; however, there is still very little standardization. Insurance plans generate a type of "report card" where they list how satisfied their members are and how well they do in providing care. As might be imagined, the results they report may be those that are the easiest to measure, rather than the most important. For example, it is much easier to measure and report what percentage of members received a mammogram in the last year than it is to evaluate the quality of care received by patients with breast cancer.

In general, elders are relatively satisfied with the care they receive under Medicare health maintenance organizations, although a substantial number return to the traditional Medicare program. Unlike younger adults who are more limited in their ability to change their health insurance plan, elders can switch back and forth between Medicare and Medicare managed care, depending on which program better suits their needs. A disadvantage, however, is that elders may let their supplementary Medicare insurance lapse when their premiums are being financed by the managed care group, then find the coverage hard to find when they want to move back to the traditional Medicare plan.

Benefits and Limitations of Medicare

Medicare is unique among government entitlement programs in that it is not based on need, but rather is available to all those over age sixty-five and some disabled individuals. Medicare pays both hospital and physician costs of a group with a high level of disease and disability who would otherwise find it difficult to purchase private insurance. By its universal availability, Medicare equally spreads the costs of health care between the ill and the healthy. Medicare offers something that private insurance policies are increasingly eliminating—free choice of providers. An elder can see any physician who accepts Medicare as often as desired and does not have to get special permission to seek specialty care. Elders can choose to seek care from HMOs if it suits them, or return to traditional Medicare at any time if they are dissatisfied. However all this choice can be confusing, and the best choice often depends heavily on personal situation and preference. For example, if personal prescription drug costs are very high, an elder may elect to join a managed care plan that pays for prescription drugs. However, the available managed care organization may have restrictions on prescription drugs, or may not include the individual's long-time family physician. An excellent discussion of the bewildering array of choices and how to decide is found in the article, "Medicare: New Choices, New Worries" in *Consumer Reports.*[3]

Medicare provides many other benefits besides choice and low cost. Medicare has multiple mechanisms for assuring physician compliance, and it covers many preventive services. Because Medicare is such a large payer to hospitals and physicians, the program exerts particular clout in changing the health care environment (for example, initiating peer review to evaluate quality of care and medical practice). Medicare has consistently been one of the most popular social programs ever implemented.

Despite its benefits, Medicare has been criticized on a number of counts. A major criticism is that Medicare does not reimburse many medical needs. Although Medicare reimburses nursing homes or home health services after hospitalization, it does not cover home or institutional custodial care for long-term chronic conditions, a much more common situation among elders. In addition, Medicare does not reimburse for prescriptions used outside the hospital, dental care and dentures, routine physical examinations, vision or hearing exams and appliances, routine foot care, or orthopedic shoes.

Some criticize Medicare for being too complex with its copayments, deductibles, Parts A and

B, and benefit restrictions. However, regulations now require physicians and hospitals, not patients, to fill out paperwork for claims, which will significantly help frail elders. Others believe the program discriminates against minorities because they have a shortened life expectancy and are less likely to be alive at age sixty-five to receive its benefits. Still others criticize Medicare for providing the same benefits to all elders regardless of financial need, while many poor people who are not elderly are unable to afford health insurance.

Perhaps the biggest concern about the Medicare program is its tremendous cost. Medicare is projected to grow at a rate of about 8 percent annually with expenditures nearing $403 billion in 2005. These increases are driven primarily by the aging of the population and increased number of older people receiving Medicare benefits, but increasing technology and other factors are driving health care costs up as well. Health care costs have been rising more rapidly than the cost of living for at least the last twenty years. These costs will continue to rise as the elderly population swells with the aging of the baby boomers and as there are fewer workers to pay into the coffers of Medicare. In fact, rising health care costs mean that yesterday's workers (who are today's beneficiaries) did not pay into the system as much as they are taking out. Payroll taxes have been increased to partially remedy this problem. It has been predicted that in the future there will not be enough workers to support the health care costs of the nation's elders.

Several proposals have been made to increase Medicare solvency into the next century. One suggestion is to reduce costs by enrolling a greater percentage of the nation's elders in managed care systems. Although managed care reduces health care choices, it may result in reduced rates of specialist use, diagnostic tests, and hospitalization. Other suggestions include raising copayments and deductibles, increasing payroll taxes paid by working adults and employers, privatizing Medicare, reducing payments to hospitals or physicians, and providing means-testing for Medicare. Some suggest that Medicare should not be available to elders who are wealthier, and others suggest that copay-

ments and deductibles might work on a sliding scale, depending on income and assets. Some believe that the age of eligibility should be increased to sixty-seven or even older. However, changing the Medicare system is difficult and fraught with political difficulties, and few legislators are interested in risking their political careers by proposing changes to the system.

Medicaid

Medicaid, Title XIX of the Social Security Act, was enacted at the same time as Medicare to provide protection against the high costs of hospital, nursing home, and physician care for the poor, blind, and disabled of all ages. Although Medicaid was initially implemented to assist poor families, the majority of its funds are now used to supplement the expenses of long-term nursing home care, hospital care, and other medical and rehabilitation services not covered by Medicare for poor elders. Medicaid (called MediCal in California) is financed jointly by the state and federal government, but it is administered by each state. In 1997, Medicaid spent $54 billion in federal and state funds and served 35 million individuals. The majority of those expenditures were spent on nursing homes (42 percent) and hospitals (25 percent).

Eligibility for Medicaid is based on monthly income and assets. Because each state administers its own program, there is much variation among states regarding which groups of people can be covered, the financial criteria for eligibility, the amount, duration, and scope of coverage, and the rate of reimbursement for services. In addition to mandated coverage for many special younger populations, states are required to provide services for older persons who fit into the following two categories: those who receive Supplemental Security Income (SSI), and Medicare beneficiaries with incomes at or below 85 percent of the federal poverty level and resources at or below twice the standard allowed under the SSI Program. A few states provide Medicaid coverage for all below the poverty level, while others do not. Nationwide, only about 40 percent of those living below the poverty level receive Medicaid.

Although states vary in their range of services, the federal government mandates that each state provide the following as a minimum to older people who qualify: in- and outpatient hospital care, physician services, skilled nursing facility services, lab and X-ray diagnosis, home-care nursing services, screening mammograms, and some home health services. In addition, some states provide private nursing, dental care, physical therapy, drugs, dentures, glasses, and hearing aids. Most states use fixed-fee schedules to reimburse medical procedures. That is, those physicians who agree to participate must accept the state's Medicaid reimbursement as full payment and cannot bill the patient for any additional expenses.

Approximately 12 percent of elders on Medicare also receive Medicaid benefits. For these "dual-eligible" elders, Medicaid finances the yearly deductibles, copayments, and monthly premiums required of all Medicare recipients. Some individuals receive partial Medicaid benefits. Those who are Qualified Medicare Beneficiaries, characterized by incomes below the poverty levels and limited financial assets, can receive Medicaid assistance to pay the Medicare monthly premiums for physicians, copayments, and deductibles. Specified Low Income Medicare Beneficiaries have incomes between 100 to 120 percent of the federal poverty level and limited assets. For these elders, Medicaid assists in the payment of Medicare premiums, but not with copayments and deductibles.

Coordination of care for those with dual eligibility for Medicare and Medicaid is complicated because these individuals represent some of the sickest and poorest older Americans. They often have multiple chronic illnesses and disabilities and have difficulty in negotiating the health care system. Because this small population uses a disproportionate amount of health care resources, attention has been focused on improving health care delivery and reducing costs for that group. There is some overlap between services covered by Medicare and Medicaid, creating confusion about which program is responsible for certain costs. Managed care has been proposed as a solution, and most states now have managed care programs for their Medicaid recipients. However, there remains some conflict between the proportion of costs billed to Medicare versus Medicaid. In addition, there is widespread concern about assuring quality care for chronically ill, disabled beneficiaries.

Private Insurance (Medigap)

Although Medicaid "fills in the gaps" for low-income elders by paying premiums, copayments, and deductibles of Medicare, those with higher incomes generally purchase a private "Medigap" insurance policy to help with costs not covered by Medicare. Private policies usually reimburse hospitalization costs not paid by Medicare and pay the deductibles or copayments. Catastrophic policies are available to finance the high cost of serious injury or illness, while other policies provide coverage for nursing home care. However, the latter is very expensive. Elders without Medicaid are encouraged to purchase a single, complete Medigap policy that will pay many of the medical bills only partially covered by Medicare. Some elders continue their employer-sponsored health insurance plans that serve the same function.

In the past, many private insurance policies to supplement Medicare had a poor return on investment for those who purchased them. Because of strong advocacy efforts, the federal government passed legislation that requires private insurance companies to standardize and simplify their policies so elders can more easily compare benefits. All Medigap policies are now based on one of ten model packages, ranging from basic coverage of physicians' fees and extended hospitalization coverage, to more complete policies with extended prescription drug and home-care benefits. Each policy must offer core benefits, such as payment of the patient's 20 percent share of Medicare-approved physicians' fees and the patient contribution to the cost of a long hospital stay. The basic benefits package may cost from $40 to $200 per month, depending on the type and extent of coverage. Additionally, regulations require all policies be renewable, even if an elder becomes disabled, and provide elders with a set "loss ratio" of the policy (the percent of each premium dollar returned in the form of benefits).

To discourage unscrupulous salespersons and enable comparison shopping, policies sold by various insurers offering the same benefits must be labeled in the same way. These policies are now labeled A through J to allow the consumer to easily compare prices. The least expensive plans include basic benefits such as copayment for hospital days 61 to 150 and full coverage for additional days, the 20 percent of Medicare-allowed charges for doctor's visits, and the first three pints of blood. More expensive policies may include coverage for hospital deductibles, personal care at home, prescription drugs and some preventive services. These policies should ideally be purchased around the sixty-fifth birthday (one month before to five months after) because Medigap insurance companies cannot turn anyone down during that period. Further information is available in the "Guide to Health Insurance for People with Medicare" from the Health Care Financing Administration Medicare hotline: 800-638-6833.

Despite the legislation to control Medigap policies, there are still loopholes in laws regulating the sale of private insurance policies to elders, resulting in billions of dollars of unnecessary spending by elders on insurance policies they do not need. Some of these policies duplicate Medicare's benefits; others cover only certain illnesses. A good overview is found in "Filling the Gaps in Medicare" in *Consumer Reports.*[4]

Veteran's Health Care Benefits

The federal Department of Veteran's Affairs (VA), opperates the largest centrally directed hospital and medical service system in the United States. It is a tax-financed agency that delivers care directly through salaried physicians and goverment-owned facilities and relies on annual federal appropriations for its money.[5] It operates 173 hospitals, 401 clinics, 133 nursing homes, and 205 counseling centers. Over 95 percent of all veterans are men. There is at least one Veteran's Administration hospital in every state except Alaska and Hawaii.

The VA system was developed in response to the need to treat and rehabilitate veterans with service-related injuries and disabilities. Over the years, the system has helped poor veterans with medical needs unrelated to their military service. Currently, four overlapping groups of veterans are eligible to receive VA medical care: veterans with service-connected disabilities, recipients of VA pensions, veterans age sixty-five and older, and medically indigent veterans. Veterans with service-connected disabilities receive top priority; however, other veterans may be cared for when there are available resources. All veterans over age sixty-five are classified as disabled, making the VA a major health care resource for that group. The Veteran's Administration facilities also play an important role in medical education and research because they are staffed by medical school faculty and physicians in training. Schools of nursing, dentistry, rehabilitation medicine, and social work have also developed affiliations with the VA hospitals

The system has been undergoing rapid and substantive changes in the past decade. The role is changing from a hospital-based specialty-focused health care system to outpatient primary care, including case management and preventive services that are linked with local physicians. In order to be more efficient, the management of the Veteran's Administration was decentralized, and the existing medical sites are now grouped into twenty-two Veterans Integrated Service Networks (VISNs). Their charge is to create a continuum of care by integrating the VA resources with local general practitioner groups.

The major challenge currently facing the VA system is to accommodate the increased utilization of its medical services due to the aging of the veteran population. In the year 2000, more than three of every five older men in the United States, or almost nine million people, will be veterans.

Private Funds

Despite the huge outlay of federal dollars, elders still pay for a significant proportion of their medical bills out of their own pockets. Medicare was originally

What Is Your Opinion? Should Health Care Be Rationed?

Everyone would agree that our nation's health care costs are too high, and efforts need to continue to reduce them. But, how much money should be spent? How much is too much? Should everyone have access to every procedure, no matter what the cost? Lawmakers, health professionals, and health consumers seldom tackle the question. Generally, when individuals are well, their estimate of what is reasonable is quite different from the care they want when they are ill; most wish to have access to every available service. Health care decisions differ from many other economic decisions in that they may affect whether an individual lives or dies. Certainly there is a ceiling on the amount of money the state and federal government, employers, family members, and individuals can spend on medical care. Thus, a method of rational distribution of the available funds should be considered. Health care rationing may regulate who should have organ transplants or kidney hemodialysis, mandate use of generic or low-cost drugs, or restrict access to certain surgical procedures or diagnostic tests.

Decisions about medical treatments are made on a case-by-case basis, rather than whether they are cost-effective. For example, $1,000 spent on prenatal care would save money and provide more days of meaningful life for more people than the same money spent on an experimental chemotherapy for cancer that may extend life expectancy of one person by only days. However, when a patient is diagnosed with cancer, the experimental treatment is offered. Some theorists suggest that health care rationing decisions should be made as a society, not on a case-by-case basis. Even though families and physicians of sick individuals may want to do everything possible to keep the patient alive, the high costs are ultimately borne by the entire society, not only directly in tax dollars, but indirectly by depriving other citizens of medical care that may have greater long-term benefits.

Most commonly, rationing occurs on an individual level with health plans, physicians, or families not electing certain services for certain individuals. A difficulty with this approach, however, is that there is a tendency to fund more acute services to the exclusion of preventive services. As a society, it is difficult to ignore the plea of ill individuals and their families for a treatment that may cure them or extend their life and instead choose the less tangible benefit of preventive or basic health care services for a faceless group of people. When a patient will die without kidney hemodialysis, it is difficult to refuse that patient or to envision that the same money could be spent to vaccinate thousands of children or to expand prenatal care to underserved women.

Several years ago, Oregon undertook the arduous task of making rationing decisions more explicit in regard to the services covered by their Medicaid program. For example, Oregon has modified its Medicaid program to provide services to all persons below the poverty level by prioritizing health care services. A group of citizens, health professionals, and legislators worked together to devise a list of priorities for health care, ranking 709 medical conditions. How many of these 709 conditions will be treated depends on the amount allocated by the legislature each year. High-priority items, such as prenatal care, contraception, immunizations, general medical care, emergency psychiatric care, and acute care for chronic conditions are covered for all. Illnesses such as mononucleosis, the common cold, alcoholic cirrhosis of the liver, and organ transplants, among others, will not be treated unless all eligible citizens already had their basic health care needs met. There has been some controversy as individuals who are denied services have mounted campaigns to increase sympathy and raise private funds for care. Overall the program has been applauded as a sane effort at distributing a scarce resource as equitably as possible.

implemented decades ago because elders were paying about 15 percent of their income for health care, necessarily reducing money left for food, shelter, and other basic needs. Ironically, after all these years, elders now pay an average of 18 percent of their income for medical expenses; their out-of-pocket expenses for medical care are greater now with Medicare than before Medicare was implemented. However, given the increasing relative and absolute costs of health care services, Medicare does substantially reduce elders' out-of-pocket costs.

OUR HEALTH CARE SYSTEM: PROBLEMS AND PROSPECTS

The United States has the most technologically advanced medical care system in the world. Physicians have a myriad of diagnostic tests, drugs, surgical treatments, and modern equipment and facilities at their disposal, and research continues to expand knowledge and treatment of many diseases. Despite these advances, our medical care system has several deficiencies that reduce the quality of care offered to many elders. This section will highlight some of the characteristics of the medical system that reduce effective care for older people. New developments that will enhance traditional medical care will also be explored.

High Cost of Care

The United States spends more in total dollars, a greater percentage of its gross national product, and more money per person on health care than any other nation in the world. It seems there is no end in sight. Americans spent $250 billion for health care in 1980, and by 1997, the bill had increased to over $1 trillion. On the average, over $4,000 per person per year is spent on physicians, hospitals, and related medical services.

At its best, for those who can afford it, the quality of care is unsurpassed, but millions of Americans in this affluent nation do not have health insurance or have inadequate insurance. In 1998, the estimate was 43 million uninsured. Children, minorities, and those who work at low-paying jobs

are the most likely to be uninsured. Elders are protected somewhat because Medicare pays a proportion of their total medical care bill. However, because elders often have very high medical care costs, many still must pay a large proportion of their income for medical care. Additionally, health care costs for older people are rising faster than their incomes.

There are a number of complex reasons for the high cost of medical care in our country. The expense of hospitalization, physician services, prescription medications, and high-technology procedures and diagnostic tests are exorbitant. Furthermore, each year our country is facing increasing proportions of those who are high users of health services (e.g., the frail elders, those with AIDS, and premature infants), consequently placing an increasing burden on the health care system. Those age sixty-five and older are responsible for one-third of the nation's health expenditures even though they account for about 13 percent of the total population. Profits made from prescription drugs and health insurance and the high cost of fraud and waste by unscrupulous physicians and hospitals are commonly cited as areas in which medical costs might be reduced. Finally, our nation spends a higher proportion of health care dollars than any other country for administration. Hospital administration costs in the United States were approximately 25 percent of the total hospital bill in 1994, nearly twice that of Canada.[6]

Hospitalization expenses account for the largest single item in the national health bill, and this figure continues to rise, taking a 40 percent bite out of the total tab. In addition to the administrative costs, hospital costs are high because of the services it provides to the patient. Further, the hospital must maintain constant readiness to provide care. For example, even if the hospital beds are half-empty, extra staff must be on duty to respond to emergencies. There is a tremendous amount of duplication of hospital services in urban communities, which adds to hospital costs. For example, there may be multiple hospitals within a few miles of each other, each fully staffed, and each running at much less than capacity. Duplication also extends to diagnostic tests or specialty services offered. For example, it is not necessary for each hospital to have a MRI (magnetic resonance imaging) machine or a coronary care unit. However, in the United States, most hospitals have these things and are unwilling to "share" because the presence of the latest technology is important in drawing patients and providers into their facility.

In our country, health care spending differs from almost all other types of spending because both the provider (the physician) and the consumer (the patient) are insulated from the actual costs of the services. In other words, neither doctors nor patients are aware of the cost, nor are the costs even considered in their decision-making process. For almost every other industry, the consumer may "shop around" for the best prices, or even may elect not to purchase higher cost items. Not so with health care. There is an illusion in health care that "someone else is paying," which may prompt increased use of services. People commonly say that they do not have to pay for most of their health care because it is covered by insurance. However, consumers do pay, both directly by increased out-of-pocket expenses and insurance premiums, and indirectly through increased federal taxes. Most people do not realize that health care costs add to the costs of consumer goods, and their wages might be higher if their employers were not paying high premiums for employee health insurance.

Even those individuals who finance a significant proportion of their health care costs out-of-pocket are insulated from the real cost of the service. There is a great deal of shifting of costs charging less to some consumers (often those paying out-of-pocket) and charging more for insured patients when the company will pay the bill.

Medical Malpractice

The practice of medicine itself is criticized because it is not more standardized. Many laypersons assume that a known standard of care exists and that doctors always agree on diagnosis, prognosis, and optimal treatment. Unfortunately, none of these assumptions is true. Physicians constantly debate the safety, efficiency, and utility of various medical

practices in their offices, at conferences, and in medical journals. Physicians' decisions and treatment modalities are influenced by where they went to medical school, in what part of the country they trained, their personal experiences, and what journal they have read recently. For some conditions, there are established protocols outlining the most effective treatment plan, but many treatments have never been thoroughly studied in randomized, placebo-controlled trials. Thus, even when physicians practice medicine to the best of their ability, choosing one of several strategies, there is still a chance of a bad outcome. Thus, every bad outcome is not malpractice. For example, a certain percentage of people die during surgery, because, even if the surgery is performed perfectly, death is a possibility.

Malpractice generally involves negligence and incompetence: the failure to diagnose or treat an illness, failing to get informed consent before a procedure is done, making treatment errors that lead to a bad outcome, or failing to follow up with a patient. When physicians are negligent, providing substandard care in diagnosing or treating illnesses, this is medical malpractice. It is unclear exactly how much medical malpractice occurs in our country, but patients and physicians are in agreement: any medical malpractice is too much. One large study estimated that 80,000 persons die and up to 300,000 more are injured from medical negligence in hospitals alone, suggesting that medical malpractice is the third leading cause of preventable death in the United States (behind cigarettes and alcohol).[7]

It is apparent that medical practitioners are imperfect, and some patients are injured while under their care. However, the current malpractice system, which should compensate the victims and act as a deterrent for poor medical care, in fact, does neither very well. Most victims of medical malpractice never receive compensation and never end up in court. In fact, it is estimated that less than 2 percent of medical negligence results in malpractice claims.[8] Of those who do go to court, less than half are compensated for their injuries.[7] Because most malpractice suits are filed by lawyers on a "contingency" basis, they often receive a large proportion of the financial settlement. Further, there is no evidence that the current malpractice system deters malpractice.

Physicians purchase insurance policies to cover their malpractice claims; often, they are not at financial risk when a claim is filed or a settlement is won, and the majority continue to practice medicine. In fact, a small number of physicians are responsible for a large percentage of the country's malpractice claims. However, maintaining malpractice insurance is expensive: for physicians may pay thousands of dollars annually. Companies that sell medical malpractice insurance show some of the highest profits in the industry, and these costs are passed on to patients, employers, and the government. There is also a concern that fear of malpractice may lead physicians to practice "defensive medicine," ordering diagnostic tests and procedures that they would otherwise not recommend, to protect themselves against malpractice suits. A survey of physicians by the American Medical Association found that more than 80 percent of the respondents said they ordered more tests that they might otherwise believe are not needed as a defense against malpractice suits.[9]

Elders are the least likely to seek redress from the court system for malpractice because it is more difficult to show "loss" when individuals are not working, are not responsible for children, or are at the end of their "natural" life span.[10] For example, a young mother with small children who died because her treatable illness was misdiagnosed will gain far more jury sympathy and a larger judgment than an elderly widow who had a missed diagnosis of cancer.

One suggested alternative is a nofault system whereby all victims of adverse medical outcomes could apply to a general fund for compensation. This fund would compensate victims of medical negligence, as well as victims of "bad outcomes." The awards would likely be smaller, but quicker. Other countries, such as Sweden and New Zealand, have had success with this concept and have extended coverage to victims of other accidents. Two states, Virginia and Florida, provide such compensation to all parents with a child injured at birth, and a national program provides compensation to parents of children injured as a result of vaccinations. It has also been suggested that medical boards take their responsibility of "policing" their own more seriously by locating and disciplining negligent and incompetent physicians.

For-Profit Medical Care

Medical care in the United States is becoming a big business industry run by large corporations for profit. Increasingly, private and nonprofit hospitals are being bought up and subsumed into larger corporations or shut down altogether. Although the for-profit chains often tout their business acumen as important in reducing waste in the system, studies show that for-profit enterprises are costlier and less efficient than public or not-for-profit hospitals. They spend more on administration and less on direct patient care.[6] In addition, for-profit hospitals are less likely to have nonprofitable, but important services, such as neonatal intensive care units, AIDS treatment, and trauma care, and are less likely to provide charity care.

Not only are more hospitals operating for profits, but health maintenance organizations need to make a profit for their shareholders. Thus, the companies that sell insurance attempt to make a profit, as do the physicians and hospitals where care is received.

In addition to an increase in for-profit health care, there have been changes in the way that health care is financed that affects profitability. As described earlier, there has been a shift in how physicians are paid. Traditionally, they submitted bills for services provided, which insurance companies generally paid. "Fee-for-service" medicine was criticized because it was believed that physicians had no incentive to cut costs, and a high incentive to provide more care and services than were really needed. Enter "capitation," the financing mechanism of most managed care systems. Under capitation, a physician or group receives a set amount of money per patient per month to pay for all their medical expenses. If the patient never sets foot in the office, the practitioners get to keep the money they "saved." Conversely, if the patient is a high user of services, requiring costly hospitalization or visits to specialists, the group loses money.

Patient-Physician Relationship

Although most patients report satisfaction with their physician, multiple studies document inadequacies in the physician-patient relationship that may contribute to health care problems and poor compliance with treatment. The patient-physician relationsip is very important. Highly personal, emotionally charged information and decisions, often regarding life and death, are made. Within the past three decades, the relationship has changed from a paternalistic doctor treating an ignorant but trusting patient toward a patient-physician partnership. Consumers have become more assertive and knowledgeable, and physicians are more likely to share information and admit lack of knowledge. However, despite these changes, what used to be called "bedside manner," is still important. The quality and length of the doctor-patient relationship strongly influences a patient's decision to pursue a malpractice suit.[10]

One area of concern in the patient-physician relationship is the amount of time spent in the average office visit. Even though elders generally have more health problems than younger groups, and the diagnosis and treatment of chronic illness are more complex, physicians do not spend more time with elders when compared to younger patients. Elders need longer visits because they may have cognitive or sensory deficits that impair communication, multiple coexisting illnesses, or may need to discuss treatments they are receiving from other practitioners. One study reported that almost half of elders' health problems were unknown to their physicians. While cardiac, pulmonary, and major nervous system disorders were commonly diagnosed, incontinence, mobility problems, feet problems, depression, sensory decrements, alcoholism, and social needs were rarely noticed.[11]

The physician may not be aware of the extent of functional English illiteracy among their patients, which creates a significant barrier to receiving proper health care. It is estimated that over 90 million adults in our country are either totally or marginally illiterate, and the proportion increases among elders. In order to function as a partner in health care, the patient must be able to read appointment slips, labels on medications, consent documents, insurance forms, health education materials, and discharge instructions. One study of over 2,000 public hospital patients reported that inadequate or marginal health literacy among elders was over 80 percent, significantly higher than in younger patients.[12] Considering the average visit time is approximately fifteen minutes, it is easy to understand the communication problems that arise. Having health educators or other health professionals on staff to supplement the physician's communication would be an important step in increasing compliance among elders.

Furthermore, it is known that patient satisfaction with their physician increases with the amount

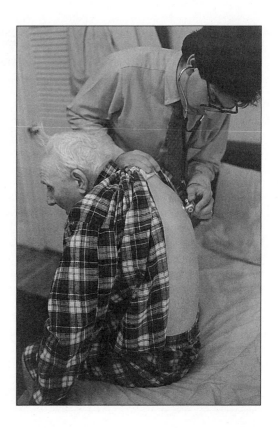

of information given to them. Even a few more minutes spent with patients may translate into increased understanding and compliance. Even if time is tight, the patient-physician relationship can be improved with more discussion of the psychosocial issues accompanying health problems.

Certain areas of patient-physician communication are notoriously poor. These include discussing advance directives and resuscitation, counseling on health behavior change, "breaking bad news," discussing areas such as sexuality, alcoholism, death, and depression, and assisting patients and families in withdrawing care at the end of life. Patients and physicians often leave office visits with different understandings of what has occurred. For example, what doctors believe to be their patients' more serious health problems are not recognized by the patient. A classic study found that even with nurses trained to advocate for patients to the physicians, most physicians did not

ascertain or follow patient's wishes regarding care at the end of life.[13]

There is concern that, with managed care, the physician-patient relationship will deteriorate. Patients often must choose a physician based on who is covered under their health plan, sometimes having to terminate a long-term association with another physician. Because physicians working under a managed care plan are monitored for productivity, they may feel pressure to see more patients, further reducing the time spent with elders. Some insurance policies have so-called gag clauses that prohibit physicians from making referrals or discussing treatments not covered under that particular policy. Physicians complain that they are employees, answering more to the insurance company's bottom line than to their patients.

Good communication skills of general practice physicians have been associated with reduced malpractice claims. One study conducted an audiotape analysis of several routine visits comparing the

---

Improving Patient-Physician Communication

- Before a visit with a doctor, write down your concerns and known medical problems. Be prepared to leave this list with the doctor. Prioritize your concerns, realizing you may only have time to address three to five of these issues.
- Talk to other members of the health care team, such as the pharmacist or nurse, to get questions answered.
- Bring to the doctor a list of all medications you are taking, even those you take only occasionally or those you buy over-the-counter. Include laxatives, eye drops, vitamins. Some physicians prefer you bring in all the bottles in a bag for the doctor to review.
- Wear/bring your glasses and hearing aids.
- Update your doctor on changes in your condition, visits to specialists or other physicians, and visits to the hospital or emergency room. Also update the physician on other important changes in your life, such as divorce, death, or change in job.

- Take notes or tape the conversation (with permission) to improve memory.
- Be honest with the doctor about your health and your reaction to the information given to you.
- Be prepared to initiate conversations on sensitive areas, such as sexuality, alcohol abuse, or death and dying concerns.
- Practice brevity in discussing your concerns. The first item you bring up should be the most important.
- Consider bringing someone with you to the visit.
- At the end of the visit, summarize what you heard the doctor say to you.
- Ask for clarification or further explanation if you do not understand.
- Ask the doctor to write down a list of all your current medical problems for your records. Including risk factors and treatments is also helpful.

Adapted from "Talking with your doctor: A guide for older people." National Institute on Aging National Institutes of Health, 1994, 30 pp. NIH Pub. 94-3452.

communication behaviors of physicians who had malpractice claims against them with those who did not. They reported that those who had no claims against them were more likely to educate patients about what would happen in the visit, laughed and used humor more, and tended to solicit their patients' opinions, encouraged them to talk, and checked their understanding. Further, their visits lasted three minutes longer than their counterparts who had claims against them. The authors suggested that physicians could be trained to be better communicators, helping both their patients and reducing their malpractice risk.[14]

Lack of Training in Geriatrics

Medical care in this country has been traditionally oriented toward drugs and procedures to cure or manage illness. Physicians are often inadequately trained to consider the myriad of environmental variables influencing the development and course of a chronic disease, such as marginal nutrition deficiencies, stress, psychosocial problems, or negative health behaviors. Physicians may look at their inability to cure elders or the death of older people in their care as personal failures in healing. Thus, it is important that physicians understand the special needs and problems of elders in order to serve them more effectively.

Shifting demographics continue to increase the need for physicians to have expertise in treating elders: by 2030, it is estimated that elders will comprise one-half their patient load. The majority of elders are cared for by generalists and specialists without special training in the care of older people. One national study indicated that only 3 percent of recent medical school graduates had taken an elective in geriatrics. Only three medical schools in the country have departments of geriatrics. According to the Association of American Medical College's curriculum directory, only fourteen of 126 medical schools require students to take a course in geriatrics, and eighty-five schools offer geriatrics as an elective. Experts debate whether geriatric specialists are needed or whether all primary care physicians should be trained in geriatrics. In any case, it is agreed that there are far too few physicians educated about the health needs of the elderly.

Inequities in Medical Treatment

Multiple studies have extensively documented the racial and ethnic disparities in health care. Researchers consistently find that blacks are less likely to use physicians and hospitals and to undergo diagnostic and surgical procedures than their white counterparts, even though they have more chronic illnesses, higher disability rates, and higher death rates. The discrepancy between blacks and whites has been reported for treatments of several health problems and is consistent among those receiving Medicare, private insurance, Medicaid, or Veteran's benefits. One study of Medicare beneficiaries demonstrated that whites were more likely than blacks to receive twenty-three medical services, including many preventive services. Whites had particular advantage in access to higher technology or newer services than did blacks.[15] Another study reported that black Medicare beneficiaries lacked the most basic components of clinical care, even though both groups had Medicare coverage.[16] Black elders have a very high rate of heart disease but are less likely to undergo a number of coronary procedures, including life-saving treatments of coronary artery bypass surgery and angioplasty. Studies vary, but generally there is a two- to threefold difference in the rate of coronary artery bypass operations between whites and blacks.[17, 18]

On the other hand, the rates for surgery for hysterectomy, prostatectomy, and leg amputations among black elders were significantly higher than for white elders.[19] Even though the incidence of prostate cancer and diabetes is somewhat higher for blacks than whites, the difference in those procedures is too great to be explained by disease rate alone.

As elders with varying income levels and of different races presumably belong to "equal-access" medical systems (Medicare, Veteran's benefits, Medicaid), financial access to care cannot account fully for these differences. Multiple reasons have been put forth to explain this disparity, including financial barriers, organizational barriers, physician and patient decision making, differences in patient treatment preferences, and differences in disease severity. However, racially discriminatory rationing by physicians and health care institutions, probably unconsciously, may play a role. One researcher wrote, "Lynching makes no contribution to the excess mortality among blacks in the United States today, [but] health inequality persists . . . we must begin to focus on the problem of racial inequality with the rigor and attention given to other public health concerns of similar magnitude."[20]

One expert suggests that every system of health care have an ongoing examination of racial disparities in the use of their services and in the physician's choices of diagnostic and treatment alternatives for racial and ethnic minorities. Also, an awareness of the dilemmas associated with race and health care should be part of every physician's training.[21] A study of seventy-eight medical schools revealed that only one-sixth of them offered a course on cultural sensitivity: in only one school was it a required course.[22]

Studies have also shown gender-based inequalities.[23] It is well-documented that women, despite their longer life expectancy, have greater rates of chronic illness and disability than men. These increased rates translate into higher use of physician services, prescription drugs, home-care services, and nursing homes. Despite the higher rate of chronic illness and disability among women, they are less likely to receive some procedures than men (e.g., coronary artery bypass grafting or angiography). Men, however, are more likely to be hospitalized than women. Women are less likely to have private insurance related to employment and are more likely to use Medicaid services.

Many studies document that physicians recommend different diagnostic and treatment strategies to older groups than they do with their younger patients, revealing an ageist perspective. In one study, seriously ill elder patients were reported to receive less costly and extensive hospital services than their younger counterparts, irrespective of the degree of illness, patient preference, or prospects of getting better.[24] Another study reported that hospi-

The Home Visit: One Physician's View
Rebecca Ferrini, M.D.

Mrs. Garcia was a 98-year-old Spanish-speaking woman who had been relatively healthy and active until about a month ago when she had a stroke. After the stroke, she had been unable to walk or even get out of bed, her appetite had lessened, and she spent more time asleep. About three weeks later, she suffered another stroke and completely lost the ability to speak. Her family physician agreed with the family's desire to keep her home and comfortable and referred her to hospice services. While with hospice, she received visits a few times a week from a nurse, and a social worker assisted the family in coping and provided referrals for low-cost burial. A home health aide assisted her granddaughter with bathing her and taught her to move and turn her in bed to prevent bedsores. However, one morning Mrs. Garcia became completely unable to swallow, and the granddaughter could no longer give her medications to her. The nurse noted Mrs. Garcia was restless and moaning.

Mrs. Garcia had expressed a wish never to go back to the hospital and was unable to get to my office, so a house call was arranged later that morning. I drove to her tiny apartment, which was in a very poor neighborhood with bars on the windows and doors. I was led into a dim house, overflowing with belongings, but scrupulously clean. Mrs. Garcia, a tiny lady of not more then 70 pounds, lay curled in a hospital bed in the living room, surrounded by medications, diapers, and religious artifacts, which her daughter felt gave her comfort. I was shown multiple medications and was able to tell her which were useful and which should be discarded: the granddaughter took careful notes. I gave Mrs. Garcia a small amount of morphine under her tongue, and she seemed to relax.

In a 15-minute visit, I learned more about Mrs. Garcia and her family than I knew about patients for whom I had cared for years. Mrs. Garcia died peacefully about two days later in her home—comfortable and surrounded by those she loved.

talized elder diabetics received less adequate care than younger diabetics.[25] Further, among women, physicians are less likely to advise older women to get mammograms, even though they are at highest risk for breast cancer. Elder women also receive less aggressive breast cancer treatment than young women and may not be offered the option of breast reconstruction.[26] In another study of women who had just been diagnosed with breast or colorectal cancer, older women were less likely to be offered a variety of treatments or be sent to radiology and oncology specialists.[27] No studies on treatment of

early stage breast cancer have included women over seventy, despite their high cancer risk.[28]

Overspecialization and Fragmentation

The United States has one of the highest rates of physician specialists in the world. With the expansion of medical technology and medical knowledge, many U.S. physicians have elected to specialize in one area of medicine to better keep abreast of new knowledge. Further, specialists make more money. Specialist care has many advantages for the patient

---

Physician Specialties

Allergy and immunology: Management of disorders involving the immune system, such as asthma, immune deficiency, autoimmune diseases, allergy.

Anesthesiology: Administration of anesthesia, management of chronic pain.

Cardiology: Nonsurgical management of diseases of the heart.

Dermatology: Surgical and nonsurgical treatment of the skin.

Endocrinology: Management of diseases and imbalances of hormones.

Family medicine: Delivery of basic health care to all members of the family with emphasis on prevention and psychosocial issues. Includes sports medicine and geriatrics subspecialties.

Gastroenterology: Nonsurgical care of the digestive tract.

Hematology: Diagnosis and treatment of blood diseases, including leukemia.

Internal medicine: Delivery of basic medical care as well as more sophisticated testing for most medical illnesses. Subspecialists include immunology, endocrinology, cardiology, geriatrics, hematology, infectious disease, oncology, pulmonology, nephrology, and rheumatology.

Nephrology: Management of kidney disease.

Neurology: Management of neurological problems, including headaches, spinal cord problems, brain tumors, and neuropathies.

Nuclear medicine: Diagnosis and treatment by using radioactive substances.

Oncology: Management of tumors or cancers.

Ophthalmology: Treatment of the eye.

Orthopedics: Treatment and rehabilitation of deformities or injuries of the skeletal system.

Otolaryngology: Ear, nose, and throat surgical specialty.

Pathology: Examines body organs, fluids, and tissues, and determines type of disease. Performs autopsies.

Physical medicine and rehabilitation: Evaluation and treatment of patients with disabilities to restore function and reduce pain.

Preventive medicine: Health promotion and disease prevention.

Psychiatry: Diagnosis and management of mental disorders.

Pulmonology: Diagnosis and treatment of lung diseases.

Radiology: Diagnosis with X-ray, ultrasound, and CT scan, and radiation therapy for cancer.

Rheumatology: Management of diseases of joints, muscles, bones, and tendons. Treatment of arthritis, back pain, and some autoimmune diseases.

Surgery: Includes general surgery (multiple body systems) and surgery that specializes in certain body areas. Surgery on female reproductive system is generally performed by a gynecologist.

Urology: Diagnosis and treatment of problems in the urinary tract of both sexes and the male reproductive system.

as well, especially for those with complex or severe illnesses. Elders generally manifest multiple, coexisting physical conditions that need attention from more than one specialist to diagnose and treat their different health problems. Whereas elders may have previously relied on their family doctor to provide comprehensive medical care, most older people now must seek care in a system full of "ologists." In the hospital setting, elders may receive simultaneous care by a number of specialists, each ordering tests and prescribing treatments. Unfortunately, when an elder sees a number of specialists, often no one is responsible for coordinating care.

Another barrier to comprehensive care for older people is a lack of connection between physicians and community resources, and among the community resources themselves. Services needed by older people are varied and are usually in different locations. Treatment, rehabilitation, prevention, and support services may not be coordinated. Furthermore, medical, health, and social services differ in eligibility requirements, administration, and financing mechanisms. The increase of for profit medical and health facilities and community based health agencies may further decrease cooperation because these compete with one another for clients. Finally, there is an insufficient range of health services in many communities.

Obtaining proper care for multiple health problems and coordinating medical services and treatment are formidable tasks at any age, but the problem is particularly evident among the old. Effective use of the current health care system requires mobility, strength, competitiveness, money, and a keen awareness of ways to gain access to splintered services—characteristics not possessed by many frail elders.

Medicare managed care has been proposed as a solution to the lack of coordination for those sixty-five and older. As discussed earlier in the chapter, under managed care, one primary care provider is responsible for the patient's medical care and must approve all specialist care. In theory, managed care promotes improved communication between the various doctors caring for the patient. There is yet no evidence that this is occurring.

Programs have been implemented to expand the managed care concept to include long-term care services to its elderly participants, called the social/health maintenance organization (SHMO). Currently, this federally funded demonstration project is being implemented at four sites around the country. The goal is to coordinate needed medical services with a broad range of health care services to delay or eliminate the need for hospitals and nursing homes. Although the idea is good, its effectiveness in coordination of acute and long-term care has not been realized. The programs are currently trying to overcome those deficiencies. If successful, the model will likely become popular among elders because of the emphasis on rehabilitation, continuity of care, and avoidance of unnecessary hospitalization or nursing home placement.

The interdisciplinary team approach is an excellent way to ensure comprehensive care, especially for older people. Each member contributes specialized knowledge and skills to develop a plan to meet the varying needs of the patient. The team approach is commonly employed in the hospital and in home care or hospice services, but is seldom seen in outpatient clinical settings. Even though comprehensive medical care under one roof is uncommon, medical and allied health and social service personnel can integrate care by providing appropriate linkages to other services.

Inaccessible Services

Use of the medical care system depends on an individual's decision to go to a physician and the ability to travel to the site of care. The paucity of outreach services is a major shortcoming in medical care for elders since many lack transportation or have health problems that interfere with their mobility. Many elders no longer drive so they rely on friends and family members to drive them. Some older people cannot use public transportation and cannot walk easily, and some lack the strength to sit through long waiting periods in the waiting room, or even to leave their homes. Adequate transportation services and outreach to elders who are unable to travel are needed. For the homebound,

Team Approach to Geriatric Care

Mrs. M. repeatedly visited the emergency room with episodes of shortness of breath brought on by exacerbations of her congestive heart failure. Each time she was admitted, she required days to stabilize her condition and often underwent many medical tests. Once she went to a nursing home for rehabilitation after a longer hospitalization that left her weaker. However, she insisted on going home to live alone.

An interdisciplinary team was appointed to assist Mrs. M. in managing her symptoms at home and avoiding unnecessary hospitalizations. A nurse visited Mrs. M. (with her neighbor Joan present to write things down) and provided instruction on how the heart worked and what each of her medications did. She helped her to learn about which foods were high in salt and should be minimized and taught her to weigh herself every day or so and check her ankles for edema. The nurse noticed that Mrs. M. was not taking an ACE inhibitor, which can improve function in heart failure and called her physician, who wrote out a new prescription. The nurse also found Mrs. M. had two bottles of the same medication, but Mrs. M. was taking them both because one was labeled with the generic name and one with the brand name. Mrs. M. was instructed to get all her medications from the same pharmacy; the pharmacist was notified and did a review of all her medications to look for interactions. The nurse returned every week or two and weighed Mrs. M., reviewed her medications to assure she was taking them properly, and communicated with her physician about her condition.

A social worker visited Mrs. M. in her home and helped her to complete a durable power of attorney for medical care naming her neighbor Joan as her decision maker and clearly specifying her wishes about her end-of-life decisions. The social worker also hooked up Mrs. M. with the local Meals on Wheels program and a beeper system that alerted the local hospital in the event of an emergency. Finally, the social worker facilitated conversations with Mrs. M.'s son, who lived out of the state and had little contact with his mother. Through her urging, Mrs. M. made a telephone call and updated her son on her medical problems, and her son arranged to bring out his new family to see her.

A home health aide helped teach Mrs. M. how to use the walker and bath aids and helped her to accomplish personal tasks, such as washing her hair once a week. A homemaker provided help with light cleaning and took her grocery shopping.

The team met on a monthly basis to share information about Mrs. M., both her medical status and her psychosocial state. After one of these meetings, the home health aide noted Mrs. M. was much more short of breath and seemed "puffy." She called the nurse, who made a visit, and found that Mrs. M. was developing an exacerbation of congestive heart failure after skipping her medications for a few days. She called the physician and was instructed to increase the dosage of her diuretic medication and to carefully monitor Mrs. M.'s weight. Over the next few days, the shortness of breath improved, and Mrs. M. resumed her normal medications and activities, avoiding a costly hospitalization.

outreach workers should be available to visit in the home to conduct physical assessments, develop a treatment plan, provide linkages to appropriate resources, and make regular follow-up visits. In some cases, Medicare and Medicaid provide reimbursement for these interdisciplinary home-care services.

House calls from physicians, common in the past, are now rare. Only 1 percent of Medicare patients receive house calls, and most of these are very sick or in their last year of life.[29] However, multiple studies document the positive effects house calls have on elders. House calls may be used to assess the safety of the living situation, educate caregivers, diagnose and treat illnesses, and improve functional status. Information gathered through a visit to a patient's home is invaluable in understanding the needs and resources of elders. One study reported that an average of two problems per patient were uncovered in home visits: 30 percent were

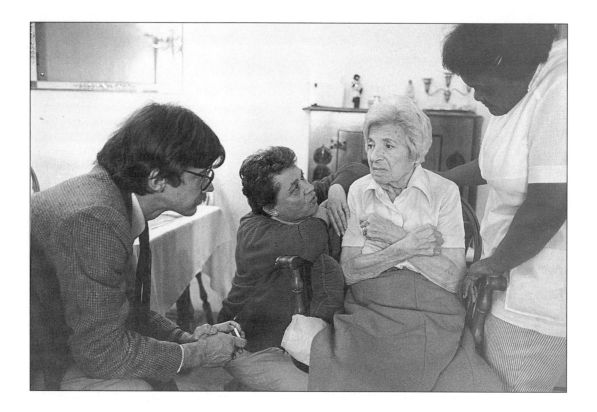

medically related, 38 percent were behavioral, and 36 percent involved serious safety hazards.[30] Another found that those receiving home visits (an average of ten visits in three years) required significantly less assistance with activities of daily living and fewer nursing home admissions than those receiving routine care.[31]

Unnecessary Diagnostic Tests

Historically, physicians relied predominantly on their trained observations to diagnose illnesses, and laboratory testing was unavailable or tedious. With the advent of many new technologies, tests are much easier to perform, and physicians rely more and more on the results of these tests to guide their treatment decisions. Some estimate that more than five billion medical tests are performed in the United States each year, an average of more than twenty tests per person. Tests are

ordered by physicians to detect a disease before it causes symptoms, establish a diagnosis, and monitor treatment. As discussed earlier, diagnostic tests are also being used for another purpose: defensive medicine.[9]

Diagnostic tests include a wide variety of procedures: laboratory examinations of blood, semen, urine, sweat, sputum, or tissues; radiographic tests such as X-rays, ultrasound, computer tomography (CT) scans, or magnetic resonance imaging (MRI); invasive medical tests where dye or tubes are inserted into the blood vessels of the body (angiography); or tests where flexible scopes are inserted into the stomach, colon, bronchi, uterus, or urethra.

Elders undergo more diagnostic tests than the rest of the population because they visit doctors and hospitals more often and they have a higher rate of chronic illness. Although many of these tests are helpful, multiple studies have documented that

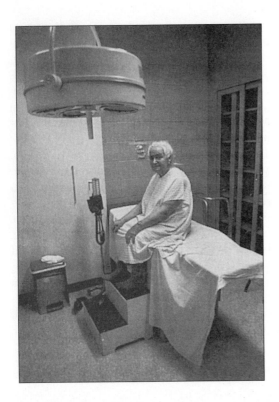

Further, test results are misinterpreted, prompting even more tests. In addition, because of the manner in which "normal" values are established, even normal healthy people may have abnormalities on lab tests, especially when a large number of such tests are drawn.

Diagnostic tests can be outright harmful for the patient, and older people are at the highest risk. Complications from diagnostic tests can result in a need for further hospitalization or therapy. For example, although rare, a colonoscopy might cause a perforation of the colon. Even the process of taking blood for diagnostic tests may result in adverse effects. One study showed that patients in intensive care had an average of two pints of blood drawn during their hospital stay and 17 percent had losses from blood draws significant enough to require a transfusion.[32] Diagnostic testing can cause needless anxiety, personal discomfort, and increased health care costs.

To reduce unnecessary testing, multiple federal, state, and organization regulations have been established. For example, hospitals or health insurance plans may require doctors to get approval for certain tests before they are permitted. Preapproval is commonly required for expensive or invasive tests. Regulations also make it more difficult for physicians to order panels of laboratory tests and require written rationale for each test requested. Governmental regulations strictly control quality of laboratories and restrict physicians from performing some diagnostic tests in their offices.

The elder consumer and family members can play a significant role in reducing unnecessary medical tests. The following questions should be asked before consenting to a medical test:

Why is the test needed?

Will the results make any difference in how I will be treated?

Are there enough symptoms to warrant a test?

Is the test dangerous?

What might the side effects be?

Is a test the most cost-effective way to gather information?

some laboratory tests are unnecessary, redundant, or ineffective. A difficulty in making this determination is that a test may be useful in one situation, but the same test may not be important in another. For instance, mammography every one to two years to detect breast cancer has been found useful in women of fifty to sixty-five years, but the same test has not been proven effective in women age twenty to thirty-nine, and there is controversy about its use for women in their forties. Other tests may be unnecessary if their results will not change treatment choices. For example, a chest X-ray is not needed if signs consistent with pneumonia were found on physical examination and the same treatment would be prescribed no matter what the X-ray shows.

Various studies have shown that physicians order tests that are not needed, that they fail to follow-up on some abnormal test results, and that they order "panels" or collections of tests when they really only want the results of a few specific ones.

Patients and their families should always ask for an interpretation of test results. In some cases, retesting or a second opinion is helpful. In addition, home-testing kits for some conditions are available.

Surgery: Too Much or Too Little

Surgery is one of the most invasive medical treatments, and there has been little research to document exactly when it is indicated and when it is not. This phenomenon first came to the attention of the public when studies were published documenting a geographic variation in surgical procedures. Analyses of these studies suggest that many surgical procedures are unnecessary, or that the criteria used to determine whether an individual needs surgery are not well-established. Procedures where there is a wide variation include back surgery, gallbladder surgery, prostatectomy, coronary artery bypass surgery, carotid endartectomy, and hysterectomy. Research is underway to help determine in which patients these procedures are useful.

On the other hand, there is evidence that some elders may not be receiving needed surgery, especially those who are very old. Many health care practitioners, patients, and their families may erroneously believe that surgery is not indicated in the very old or that the risks are too high. This misconception ignores the fact that surgery can be curative for many illnesses (e.g., cardiac conditions, hip fractures, cancer) and can improve functional status and quality of life in the remaining years. Although it is true that surgery in the elderly brings higher rates of death and complications, it is also true that older people progress remarkably well after major surgery, even into their nineties and older.

The qualifications and experience of surgeons performing the same surgical procedure may be highly variable. It is documented with some diseases that those surgeons who frequently perform a particular surgery have a better patient survival rate (practice makes perfect). Unfortunately, there are few data to assist the consumer in determining whether an operation is necessary and whether the surgeon is competent.

Because of cost considerations, many surgical procedures are now being performed on an outpatient basis that used to require hospitalization (e.g., cataracts, breast cancer). For older people, this switch in the location of care has resulted in increased out-of-pocket spending, increases in Medigap policy premiums, and increased use of home-based services for aftercare.

To avoid unnecessary surgery, or to be sure surgery is not needed, elders should be encouraged to get a second opinion when any type of surgery is recommended. In addition, elders and their families should question the physician about alternative treatments, why the procedure should be done, risks and benefits of surgery, and their outlook if surgery is not chosen. If surgery is necessary, elders should request information about how often the physician performs the surgery, the surgeon's success rate, and experience in performing that surgery on elders.

Iatrogenic Illnesses

A cardinal principle of geriatric medicine, especially when the course of a patient turns suddenly for the worse, is to ask first, 'What have I done to the patient?' rather than 'What has the environment done.'

William Hazzard

When diagnostic tests, medical treatments, or the hospital environment make people sick, the person is said to have an *iatrogenic* illness. Iatrogenic illnesses include a wide variety of conditions, such as adverse effects from the medical procedure itself as well as negligence of a health professional. They may also include adverse drug reactions, caused by the nature of the drug itself or medication errors of health professionals in prescribing or dispensing the medication. Although aging itself is not a risk factor for iatrogenic illness, the accompaniments of aging—multiple diseases, high drug use, age-associated decrements, and higher rates of hospitalization—create a higher risk for iatrogenic illnesses. The costs are more than monetary and may include lengthened hospital stay, physiological complications, depression, deterioration, and even death in some instances.

Iatrogenic illnesses are common in hospital settings because of the procedures that may accompany hospitalization and the presence of virulent microorganisms in the environment. Nosocomial infections (infections acquired in the hospital) are the most common iatrogenic illness and occur when bacteria or viruses are passed from one patient to the next through equipment or by health care workers. The most common sites of infection are the urinary and respiratory tract, blood, and wounds. Likewise, many hospital treatments carry adverse effects that can worsen a condition, such as the insertion of indwelling catheters.

Nursing homes are also sites of frequent nosocomial infections such as tuberculosis, urinary tract infections, bedsores, and respiratory infections. Residents are often in close contact with each other, are unable to care for themselves, and have chronic illnesses that increase susceptibility to illness. The lowest-functioning patients are at highest risk of infection.[33] Depending on the problem, the risk of nosocomial infections can be minimized; handwashing by staff, isolation of those infected, pneumonia and flu immunizations of staff and patients, patient surveillance, and screening for disease.

The Educated Health Consumer

Consumers need information to make educated choices about their health care and to select low-cost, effective health care products and services. The consumer health movement involves the education of individuals about their rights and responsibilities so they can maximize their health care. Increasingly, consumers are learning more about health matters and are becoming more assertive in directing their medical care. The myriad of health-related articles in newspapers, magazines, and self-help books attest to the increasing responsibility that individuals are taking for their own well-being. As a group, elders are somewhat less educated about health, disease, and their bodies and are more likely to accept a submissive role when talking to a physician. Further, not all elders are able to act on their own behalf, especially if weakened by illness.

Patient advocates assist elders in making important health care decisions and help them to negotiate the complex medical care system. Advocates are generally nurses or trained laypersons, but can be often elders themselves, or a family member or friend. Many accompany patients to their physicians to ensure the patient understands the information and that questions are adequately answered. Some advocates may find and coordinate needed health care services with the assistance of the physicians. Because advocates generally follow individuals throughout the course of their treatment, they are in a prime position to deal with the psychosocial issues surrounding the illness. In a hospital setting, advocates may provide key information to health care personnel. Patient advocates may also assist older people to deal with red tape of medical bills and reimbursement issues.

The single disadvantage of advocates is that their presence can interfere with the doctor-patient relationship. The health care team may address their questions to the advocate rather than the patient. Advocates need to be certain not to set up an antagonistic posture with physicians and to separate their own ideas of "what is in the best interests of the patient" from the patient's actual wishes. Because of cultural differences, elders may desire and expect a different relationship with their doctors than younger people (e.g., relying more on the doctor for decision making) and advocates need to respect their wishes. Family members in particular need to separate their own agenda from that of the patient. The federal government has formalized patient advocacy in nursing homes by mandating that ombudsman programs be implemented throughout the nation through local Area Agencies on Aging.

Alternative Healing Approaches

Modern conventional medicine (sometimes called Western, orthodox, or allopathic medicine) arose out of a mix of diverse traditions. In the mid-nineteenth century, a biologic basis of disease and its treatment was developed with the discovery of the role of bacteria and immune system–generated antibodies in response to infection. However, conventional medicine, and its approach to disease causation and cure, has always been accompanied by other types of healing philosophies and practices. These have been called alternative medicine (sometimes called unconventional, complementary, or integrative medicine).

A survey conducted in 1997 reported that about 40 percent of the adults in our country use at least one type of alternative medicine, and visits to alternative practitioners now exceed visits to traditional physicians. That study also estimated that $27 billion was spent out-of-pocket yearly for alternative therapies, similar to out-of-pocket expenditures for conventional medical care.[34] However, this does not mean that there is widespread dissatisfaction with conventional care because all but four percent use it as an adjunct to their regular medical care.[35]

A plethora of treatment strategies to treat illness, reduce pain and suffering, and restore health have been around for centuries. Obviously some are more successful than others. Although any treatment other than physician-directed is decried as unscientific by some, a number of alternative healing strategies are becoming more accepted among the public and the medical community. An analysis of these complementary medicine strategies is beyond the scope of this book. However, it is important to realize that not all are created equal—some have more potential for toxicity, and others have more documentation of effectiveness. For a thorough description and discussion, please refer to *Alternative Medicine: Expanding Medical Horizons* from which most of the information for this section is derived.[36]

Individuals choose alternative healing strategies for a variety of reasons. Some elders may be more likely to use alternative methods of healing because they do not have the same faith in medical science as younger groups. Others are fearful of doctors and hospitals and are more comfortable with their traditional cultural healing practices. Still others have been unsuccessful in obtaining relief from Western medical procedures. Many may see it

as a less expensive option. In some cases, refusal to also consult conventional medical practitioners may delay needed drugs or procedures.

Studies support the fact that positive expectations can improve health and immune system function. The time and attention spent with a practitioner of alternative medicine may be healthful. Often these practitioners focus on the whole body and encourage alteration of diet, increased exercise, and stress reduction. Alternative medicine practitioners spend more time with their patients, provide them with an understanding or meaning or their illness, and empower them to improve their health. Through a gentler focus on healing the self, many alternative healing strategies are far less toxic and invasive than conventional drugs or surgery. Even if they do no good, at least they do no harm. In addition, costs of alternative medical treatments are generally less than conventional medical treatments.

Increasingly, the lines are becoming blurred between conventional and alternative medicine. As research supports some alternative medicine practices, they are being integrated into conventional medicine. Ideally, medicine would become truly integrative, encompassing the best of all worlds with an emphasis on personalized care, empowering the patient to heal themselves, a focus on diet and exercise, and other behavioral changes and evidence-based interventions when needed.[37] A brief overview of the most common alternative treatments will be discussed below. Some are systems of medical practice, while others are more focused treatments for specific problems.

Osteopathy

Doctors of osteopathy (D.O. degree) use conventional therapies in combination with spinal manipulation to treat several health problems. Osteopaths are licensed on the same basis as medical doctors to practice medicine, perform surgery, and prescribe drugs. These doctors emphasize the relationship between body structure and function and tend to be general practitioners, rather than specialists. In the past few decades, osteopaths have received increasing responsibilities and privileges and many are indistinguishable from traditional physicians

What Is Your Opinion? Alternative Medicine Meets Science

There is no alternative medicine. There is only scientifically proven, evidence-based medicine supported by solid data or unproven medicine, for which scientific evidence is lacking. Whether a therapeutic practice is Eastern or Western, unconventional or mainstream, or involves mind-body techniques or molecular genetics is largely irrelevant except for historical purposes and cultural interest. We recognize that there are vastly different types of practitioners and proponents of the various forms of alternative medicine and conventional medicine, and that there are vast differences in the skills, capabilities, and beliefs of individuals within them and the nature of their actual practices. . . . Nonetheless, as believers in science and evidence, we must focus on fundamental issues—namely the patient, the target disease or condition, the proposed or practiced treatment, and the need for convincing data on safety and therapeutic efficacy.

Despite the increasing use of alternative medicine in the United States and throughout the world, most alternative therapies have not been evaluated using rigorously conducted scientific tests of efficacy based on accepted rules of evidence. The lack of properly designed and conducted randomized controlled trials is a major deficiency. . . . However, some advocates of alternative medicine argue that many alternative therapies cannot be subjected to the standard scientific method and instead must rely on anecdotes, beliefs, theories, testimonials, and opinions to support effectiveness and justify continued use.

Regardless of the origin or type of therapy, the theoretical underpinnings of its mechanism of action, or the practitioner who delivers it, the critical questions are the same. What is the therapy? What is the disease or condition for which it is being used? What is the purported benefit to the patient? What are the risks? How much does it cost? And, perhaps most important, does it work? For virtually all medical therapies and interventions, whether conventional or alternative, determination of effectiveness and recommendations for clinical application should be based on the strength of the scientific evidence

While acknowledging that many therapies used in conventional medical practice also have not been as rigorously evaluated as they should be, we agree that most alternative medicine has not been scientifically tested. However, for alternative medicine therapies that are used by millions of patients every day and that generate billions of dollars in health care expenditures each year, the lack of convincing and compelling evidence on efficacy safety and outcomes is unacceptable and deeply troubling.

Fontanarosa and Lundberg. 1998. Alternative medicine meets science. *Journal of the American Medical Association* 280:1618.
Copyright 1998 American Medical Association

(M.D.s). However, some have a tendency to focus more on health behavior change—diet and exercise—and rely less on drug therapy.

Chiropractic

Chiropractors are the third largest group of health professionals who have primary contact with patients (physicians are first, and dentists are second). Every state requires that they have a license to practice. Chiropractic differs from conventional medicine in that treatments do not include drugs or surgery, but depend on the body's ability to heal itself. Chiropractors facilitate that healing by correcting spinal misalignment through the use of spinal adjustments. Chiropractors believe that partially dislocated vertebrae cause pressure on the nerves, and these pressures are the cause of discomfort. It is fairly well-documented that chiropractic is effective in relieving acute low back pain and neck pain.

Physicians generally accept that chiropractic is effective in treating selected musculoskeletal problems. However, using chiropractic to treat other disorders raise some concern. In any case, the proportion of people going to chiropractors for health problems outside the musculoskeletal system are small, so it is not a major issue. Many Americans are very satisfied with the treatment they have received from doctors of chiropractic. Medicare covers chiropractic services for certain spinal problems. In almost all states, some chiropractic benefits are required to be included in all insurance plans.[38]

Chinese Medicine

Acupuncture is an ancient Chinese form of medicine that has been practiced for at least 2,500 years. The theory of acupuncture is based on the premise that there are patterns of energy flow through the body that are essential for good health. When these patterns are disrupted, illness occurs. It is believed that the flow of natural energy, Qi (pronounced "chee"), can be restored to normal by the insertion and manipulation of very thin needles into specific points in the body. Acupuncture is part of an entire system of diagnosing and treating illnesses. Diagnosis relies on taking a careful history, talking to the patient, and carefully examining the body, particularly the pulse and the tongue.

Much work has been devoted to try to understand how acupuncture works. Studies thus far indicate that acupuncture is effective because it reduces pain by triggering endorphin release (a natural chemical that acts like morphine). It also might trigger the release of hormones and other substances that act to fight inflammation and help wounds heal faster.

Multiple studies have been conducted on acupuncture that suggest benefit in many areas. However, it is difficult to design studies to document the effectiveness of acupuncture. A consensus statement from the National Institutes of Health concluded, after reviewing the literature on acupuncture, that research supports the use of acupuncture in alleviating nausea and vomiting after surgery or chemotherapy and relieving pain after dental surgery. Acupuncture was also believed to be useful as an adjunct treatment in the following: addiction, stroke rehabilitation, headache, tennis elbow, menstrual cramps, fibromyalgia, osteoarthritis, low back pain, carpal tunnel syndrome, and asthma.[39] The greatest risks are from unclean needles; all needles should be disposable. Practitioners should be certified.

Acupressure utilizes the same theories as acupuncture, except pressure is applied to the points where needles might be inserted. Acupuncture is often combined with other aspects of traditional Chinese medicine such as prescription for exercises, meditation, and herbal remedies, generally in the form of teas. One large well-conducted study found that irritable bowel syndrome symptoms responded better to Chinese herbal remedies than placebo treatments.[40]

Ayurveda

Ayurveda is a traditional system of medicine originating in India that has been around for more than 5,000 years. These practitioners believe that all illness is the result of imbalance or stress in the awareness or consciousness of the individual. Mental stress leads to unhealthy lifestyles, which is a stress upon the body. The focus of ayurvedic medicine is the prevention and treatment of illness through alterations in lifestyle, and natural remedies. Three basic physiological principles in the body (known as "doshas") may suffer imbalance, according to Ayurvedic tenets. These three doshas include vata, pitta, and kapha, and are evaluated primarily by feeling the pulse at the wrist. Treatments include specific exercises, sleeping patterns, diet, yoga postures, and herbal remedies are used. These practitioners also note a process of accumulation of toxins in the body that are treated by panchakarma. Panchakarma involves massage with oils impregnated with herbs, heat, and treatments designed to purge the bowels.

There are ten Ayurvedic clinics in North America, and some physicians incorporate these techniques in their daily practice. In India, Ayurvedic practitioners are trained in both Western and traditional Ayurvedic techniques. Studies of Ayurvedic techniques, including both herbal remedies and yoga, suggest the potential for success in prevention of cancer, reducing blood pressure, heart rate and stress hormones, improving symptoms of chronic diseases, and improving sense of well-being.

Homeopathy

Homeopathy has a long history in the United States, but was largely replaced by Western medicine in the twentieth century. Developed by Samuel Hahnemann in the nineteenth century, homeopathy attempts to trigger symptoms in the patient that stimulates the patient's immune system to fight a particular disease. Homeopaths subscribe to the principle of "like cures like" which means that they administer a very small amount of a substance that causes a reaction that mimics the patient's symptoms. For example, an itchy rash may be treated with poison ivy, or a flushing reaction may be treated with hot peppers. The homeopath also attempts to concoct a single dose that treats all the patient's symptoms simultaneously because they view symptoms as being related. Finally, the homeopath treats illness with very dilute medications.

Homeopaths believe that the more the substance to be administered is diluted and vigorously shaken, the more potent it is in treating illness. Thus, to prepare an extract, a practitioner starts out with one part of the remedy and ninety-nine parts of distilled water and makes serial dilutions. Some products are so dilute that not even one molecule of the original substance could be found in it; however, the homeopaths believe that the remedy maintains the energy, essence, or imprint of the agent. It has been suggested that homeopathic remedies act through electromagnetic energy. Studies have been conducted to determine the effectiveness of homeopathy, but most do not conform to the research standards of conventional medicine, so the results are not yet conclusive. However, there is an indication that homeopathy produces benefits for some illnesses, particularly for hay fever, allergic asthma, fibromyalgia, rheumatoid arthritis, migraine headaches, and diarrhea.

Physicians in other countries often integrate homeopathic remedies with Western medicine, and homeopathy is reimbursable in many European countries.

Native Healing Practices

Certain ethnic-cultural groups, including Native Americans and Latin Americans, often seek care from traditional medical practitioners. Native American practitioners emphasize certain practices, including herbal medicines, sweating, and purging (often accomplished in a sweat lodge), and shamanistic practices. Shamans are common in Native American and other traditional communities around the world. Shamans are recognized healers with specific spiritual powers who make a journey to the spiritual world to gain guidance to assist in the healing of others. Shamans may journey through a trance (similar to hypnosis or meditation), which they might achieve through ritual drumming, dancing, or consuming hallucinogenic plants. Shamans help people to understand the meaning of their illness, and they attempt to heal physical, psychic, and community wounds. Shamanistic activities have been likened to psychotherapy.

Latin American traditional medicine or "curanderismo" encompasses a method of classifying and diagnosing illness, physical activity, food, and drugs, as well as a series of folk illnesses. Illnesses or imbalances may be diagnosed or treated at home, or through traditional healers, called curanderos (men) or curanderas (women). Illnesses and other objects are classified as having characteristics akin to hot, cold, dry, or moist. Good health is achieved by maintaining a balance between these extremes. For example, a meal might include both hot (chili peppers) and cold (milk) food, or a person with a moist disease would require drying medicinals or activities. Folk illnesses include a set of recognized syndromes. Two of the most common are "mal de ojo" and "susto." Mal de ojo, also known as "evil eye," is a disease concept believed by people all over the world. Evil eye illnesses occur when one individual makes another sick by looking at them, generally not with the intent to harm. "Susto" or fright develops when a person has suffered a grave threat or shock to his or her system. Symptoms include daytime sleepiness and night-time insomnia, irritability, heart palpitations, anxiety, and sadness. Some aspects of traditional medicine are practiced by the majority of those of Mexican descent in the United States, and is especially common among the less educated or assimilated.

Natural Healing

There is increased attention directed to *naturopathy*, which encompasses herbal medicine, meditation, massage, physical exercise, healthy diet, fasting, vitamin therapy, and vegetarianism. The public's appetite for these therapies is evidenced by looking through any popular magazines and recently published books. Most individuals have adopted at least some of these changes (for example, eating less meat, taking vitamin supplements, or visiting a massage therapist. However, some programs offer more intensive approaches.

Use of herbal medications is becoming more popular, and herbs such echinacea, goldenseal, saw palmetto, and St. John's Wort are becoming household words. Herbs are used for many health problems, ranging from cold symptoms, to depression, to cancer treatment. Many herbs are the basis for many modern medications, and it is clear that herbs have many positive and negative effects on the body. The difficulty with herbal remedies is that there are no assurances of quality, purity, or concentration of herbs sold. Because the Food and Drug Administration does not regulate herbal remedies, there is no guarantee that any of these products even contain the ingredient listed on the label. Or, the formulation may be such that the body cannot absorb it. In some cases, the amount of "active ingredient" may be small or vary significantly from one pill to another, or from one brand to another.

A further discussion of herbal remedies can be found in chapter 10. The roles of vitamin supplementation in health and disease are discussed in chapter 5.

Mind-Body Approaches

The diverse approaches to healing addressed in this section have one thing in common: what one thinks or feels plays a crucial role in health and disease. Any discussion of mind-body responses includes a discussion of the placebo effect, one of the most widely observed and least understood phenomena in health and medicine. When patients are given a placebo (an inert substance with no physiological effects, most often a sugar pill) with a suggestion that it may have certain effects, they may (from 10 to 50 percent of the time) experience the effects they expect. Not only are the effects psychological, they are also physiological.

Although many discount the placebo effect, stating "it's all in your mind," this is inaccurate. In

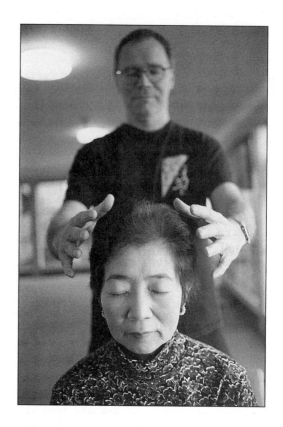

fact, the placebo effect suggests how powerful suggestion and expectation can be in changing health. What is also interesting is that placebos can also cause negative side effects when physiologically they are not supposed to. This further suggests the power of the placebo. The placebo effect is so great that researchers sometimes have trouble demonstrating that their treatment is better than a placebo.

This section will briefly address biofeedback, hypnotherapy, imagery, meditation, the power of prayer, and yoga. Many assert that the effects of these treatments are due to the placebo effect: individuals feel better because they expect to feel better. It is likely that at least some methods are more effective than the placebo effect alone. Evidence is mounting of the importance of the mind in stimulating immune function. However, placebos can be effective treatments and can change psychological reactions to illness as well as physiological processes.

Biofeedback Biofeedback is a treatment modality that uses instruments to measure and feed back information of a physiological change to patients so patients can learn to control their own physiology. Patients learn by trial and error how to adjust their heart rate, temperature, or blood pressure by watching monitors while adjusting their thinking or other mental processes. Generally a therapist assists the patient in learning appropriate techniques.

Biofeedback teaches individuals to control their bladder or bowels, reduce their stomach acid production, avert migraine headaches, control seizures, lower blood pressure, or improve sleep. Professionals in many areas of health care, including physical therapy, medicine, dentistry, and psychology practice biofeedback, and there are more than 10,000 practitioners in the United States. The American Medical Association has endorsed the use of biofeedback for muscle contraction headaches.

Hypnotherapy Hypnosis has been part of healing for centuries, and evidence of hypnosis is found in ancient Greek temples. There has been a recent resurgence of interest in this therapy among physicians, dentitsts, addiction counselors, and psychotherapists. Hypnotherapy uses suggestion to encourage deep relaxation. While in this relaxed state, the individual is susceptible to suggestions, such as to feel less pain, to heal one's own body, or to stop smoking. Hypnosis is a state of focused concentration in which people are relatively unaware of their surroundings. Unlike the stereotypes of hypnosis, encouraged by those who see it as a parlor game, all hypnosis is self-hypnosis. Those undergoing hypnosis will not follow suggestions against their own wishes: they must be willing to concentrate their thoughts and follow suggestions. In addition, those under hypnosis are not completely unaware of their surroundings and are able to respond to emergencies.

Studies show hypnosis is effective in many areas, including reducing pain during childbirth and in the dentist chair, treating emotional problems and headaches, and aiding in weight loss or other behavioral modification. Hypnotherapy is increasingly being used to reduce addiction to drugs, cigarettes, or alcohol. Hypnotherapy has been shown to stimulate immune function, reduce allergic or asthma attacks, even increase breast size and cure warts. Although studies of its success in treating these conditions are far from conclusive, it seems to have broad application and few side effects. One can receive hypnotherapy from a licensed hypnotherapist or from a physician or counselor who has received a variable amount of special training.

Imagery Imagery, similar to hypnosis, is a mental process of imagining or actively changing one's thoughts. For example, cancer patients may imagine their immune system is an efficient vacuum cleaner, ridding their body of the "dirt" of cancer cells. An elder woman may imagine herself in another situation (e.g., the top of a mountain with cool winds blowing over her) when she has pain. Imagery has been found to affect physiological processes throughout the body, including changes in function of the immune system, hormone levels, heart function, brain waves, and body temperature. Imagery has been found to be effective in controlling symptoms such as nausea, pain, and anxiety.

Meditation An ancient practice originating in the East, meditation is increasingly used by Westerners for relaxation and spiritual growth. While meditating, individuals relax the body and calm the mind by focusing on a single thought, sound, or process (e.g., breathing). The goal is to quiet the mind and stop the mind from racing. Meditation originally had a religious or spiritual purpose but is increasingly being used for presumed health benefits.

One of the most common types of meditation is transcendental meditation, introduced in the United States in the 1960s by Maharishi Mahesh Yogi. This technique is associated with reduced use of health services, reduced anxiety and chronic pain, decreased serum cholesterol, reduced substance abuse, increased intelligence, and other benefits. Through an examination of the positive effects of meditation, Benson identified "the relaxation response."[41] This response encompasses a constellation of psychological and physical symptoms that are altered by mind-body techniques (e.g., hypnosis, prayer, meditation). This relaxation response has been found to be helpful in many acute and chronic conditions and in stimulating immune function.

Prayer and a higher power may be accomplished by one individual on behalf of another. Prayer may involve touch and laying on of hands, or healing from a distance.

Anecdotal evidence about the power of prayer is as common as reports of its ineffectiveness. However, a few studies do suggest that prayer may have a variety of effects by altering physiological processes.[42] These studies do not directly look at prayer as a communication with a higher power, but more as a state of focused and general caring, compassion, or love toward another. Little is understood about the physiological mechanism by which prayer may promote healing.

Yoga Yoga is more than a set of exercises, it is an entire way of living in India that includes a special diet, exercises, and a daily routine. Practitioners of yoga have legendary abilities to modulate physiological functions that many believe are beyond the ability of humans to regulate. In the United States, yoga is practiced in a modified manner, generally as a series of exercises or poses, accompanied by breathing techniques or meditation designed for relaxation, health, and spiritual growth. Yoga has been reported to promote relaxation, increase resilience to stress, improve heart efficiency, lower blood pressure, improve physical fitness, and decrease dietary cholesterol and blood sugar. Yoga reduces diverse chronic illnesses, ranging from asthma to cancer to heart disease, hypertension, migraine headache, arthritis, and drug addiction.

Yoga can be accomplished alone or in a class setting. Videotapes are available to use at home, if desired. In general, a session begins with gentle postures to relax tension, then moves to more difficult positions while emphasizing a positive attitude, comfort, relaxation, and breathing. Yoga is particularly appealing to older people because it is a gentle form of exercise that improves flexibility and balance.

Increasingly, physicians are successfully integrating aspects of complementary therapy to more mainstream medicine. One attempt at integration, publicized by Dr. Dean Ornish in the Lifestyle Heart Trial, has shown promise in improving cardiac function and reducing risk of death.[43] In this intervention, individuals with heart disease participate in a program of comprehensive lifestyle changes such as eating a very low-fat vegetarian diet and participating in aerobic exercise, stress management, smoking cessation, and a psychological support group. A variety of similar programs are available, some associated with hospitals or universities in other parts of the country. Some of these programs also include psychological counseling, meditation, dietary supplements, or other interventions.

SUMMARY

Because of their higher rates of illness and death, elders utilize physician and hospital services more than any other age group. The majority of health care for those over sixty-five in the United States is financed through the federal health insurance policy, Medicare. Medicare is a very complex program with deductibles and copayments, and does not reimburse all services at a similar rate. Private Medigap insurance is available for elders to reduce their out-of-pocket costs not covered by the Medicare program. In addition, the nation's poorest elders may qualify for the federal/state program that supplements what Medicare does not reimburse, called Medicaid. The Veterans Administration provides health services to those elders who have been in the armed forces. Despite the multiple programs to finance elders' health care, they still pay a higher proportion of their health care expenses out of their own pockets than they did before Medicare was enacted.

The quality of our medical care, with its highly skilled medical practitioners, myriad of diagnostic tests, drugs, surgical treatments, modern equipment, and facilities are unparalleled in the world. Nevertheless, our health care system is not working for everyone. Many of its characteristics negatively impact health care delivery to elders. The high cost of medical care, its profit motive, quality of the patient-physician relationship, lack of training in geriatrics, inequities in medical treatment, overspecialization and fragmentation of services, unnecessary procedures and diagnostic tests, an ineffective malpractice system, and a high incidence of iatrogenic illness are significant barriers to effective health care. These problems are prompting multiple proposals for change. A number of trends have emerged that are changing the face of medical care in this country, such as increased attention to prevention and health promotion services, reliance on complementary medicine, and legislation promoting consumer rights.

ACTIVITIES

1. Review advertisements for health plans in your area or nationwide. Which plan is being highlighted, and what group of beneficiaries is being sought? What kind of strategy or claims are used by these companies? How might you select a plan?

2. Informally survey several physicians in your community by telephone to determine if they accept Medicaid. How many accept Medicare patients? How many accept Medicare assignment? Do those who accept Medicare or Medicaid have a limit on how many patients they will take?

3. Research the health care system of another developed country. What might be the advantages and drawbacks of such a system in our country? What special considerations does the system have for its elders? Is rationing occurring? Do you think this system would be more or less effective in meeting the needs of our country's elders than our current system?

4. As part of a class project, debate the pros and cons of the statement, "Medical care is the right of all individuals in our country, regardless of ability to pay."

5. Find out if your community offers the following health services to elders: free or reduced-rate medical care, mass screening programs, health promotion programs, medical outreach into elders' homes or neighborhood sites, transportation to medical care, and other medical services.

6. Many hospitals are reaching out to serve the special needs of elders. Find out what special services are offered to elders by the hospital(s) in your community.

7. Hold a class discussion in which students discuss their views of how the health care system might be improved without increasing the cost of health care.

8. Review some of the current proposals by federal and state governments that attempt to alter the medical care system. What problem is being addressed? Which constituents are actively influencing the debate and in which manner? Who is "right"? Write a letter to your representative outlining the reasons the proposal should or should not be passed.

9. Collect advertisements and articles on particular alternative healing techniques from both lay sources (e.g., magazines, health food stores) and medical literature. Visit a practitioner of an alternative technique and undergo a treatment, if interested. What claims are made? What do you experience? What might be the special risk and benefits of this treatment for the elderly? How might you evaluate the effectiveness of these therapies?

Bibliography

1. Woodwell, D.A. 1999. National Ambulatory Medical Care Survey: 1997 summary. *Advance Data from Vital and Health Statistics,* no. 305. Hyattsville, MD: National Center for Health Statistics.

2. Graves, E.J., and Owings, M.F. 1998. 1996 Summary: National Hospital Discharge Survey. *Advance Data from Vital and Health Statistics,* no. 301. Hyattsville, MD: National Center for Health Statistics.

3. "Medicare: New choices, new worries." 1998. *Consumer Reports* (September):27–33.

4. "Filling the gaps in Medicare." 1994. *Consumer Reports* (August):523–29.

5. Inglehart, J.K. 1996. Reform of the Veterans Affairs health care system. *New England Journal of Medicine* 335:1407–11.

6. Woolhandler, S., and Himmelstein, D.U. 1997. Costs of care and administration at for-profit and other hospitals in the United States. *New England Journal of Medicine* 336:769–74.

7. Harvard Medical Practice Study. 1990. *Patients, doctors, and lawyers: Medical injury, malpractice litigation, and patient compensation in New York.* Cambridge, MA: President and Fellows of Harvard College.

8. Localio, A.R., Lawthers, A.G., and Brennan, T.A., et al. 1991. Relation between malpractice claims and adverse effects due to negligence. *New England Journal of Medicine* 325:245–51.

9. McCormick, B. 1992. Most doctors say they practice defensive medicine. *American Medical News* (May 25):3, 58.

10. Penchansky, R., and Macnee, C. 1994. Initiation of medical malpractice suits: A conceptualization and test. *Medical Care* 32:813–31.

11. Stultz, B.M. 1984. Preventive health care for the elderly. *Western Journal of Medicine* 141:832–45.

12. Williams, M.V., Parker, R.M., and Baker, D.W., et al. 1995. Inadequate functional health literacy among patients at two public hospitals. *Journal of the American Medical Association* 274:1677–82.

13. The SUPPORT Principal Investigators. 1995. A controlled trial to improve care for seriously ill hospitalized patients. *Journal of the American Medical Association* 274:1591–98.

14. Levinson, W., Roter, D.L., and Mullooly, J.P., et al. 1997. Physician-patient communication. *Journal of the American Medical Association* 277:553–59.

15. Escarce, J.J., Epstein, K.R., Colby, D.C., and Schwartz, J.S. 1993. Racial differences in the elderly's use of medical procedures and diagnostic tests. *American Journal of Public Health* 83:948–54.

16. Kahn, K.L., Pearson, M.L., and Harrison, E.R., et al. 1994. Health care for black and poor hospitalized Medicare patients. *Journal of the American Medical Association* 271:1169–74.

17. Goldberg, K.D., Hatz, A.J., and Jacobsen, S.J., et al. 1992. Racial and community factors influencing coronary artery bypass graft surgery rates for all 1986 Medicare patients. *Journal of the American Medical Association* 267:1473–77.

18. Peterson, E.D., Wright, S.M., Daley, J., and Thibault, G.E. 1994. Racial variation in cardiac procedure use and survival following acute myocardial infarction in the Department of Veteran's Affairs. *Journal of the American Medical Association* 271:1175–80.

19. Gornick, M.E., Eggers, P.W., and Reilly, T.W., et al. 1996. Effects of race and income on mortality and use of services among Medicare beneficiaries. *New England Journal of Medicine* 335:791–99.

20. Cooper, R.S. 1993. Health and the social status of blacks in the United States. *Annals of Epidemiology* 3:137–44.

21. Geiger, H.J. 1996. Race and health care—An American dilemma. *New England Journal of Medicine* 335: 815–16.

22. Lum, C.K., and Korenman, S.G. 1994. Cultural sensitivity training in U.S. medical schools. *Academic Medicine* 69:239–41.

23. Miles, A., and Parker, K. 1997. Men, women and health insurance. *New England Journal of Medicine* 336:218–21.

24. Hamel, M.B., Phillips, R.S., and Teno, J.M., et al. 1996. Seriously ill hospitalized adults: Do we spend less on older patients? *Journal of the American Geriatrics Society* 44:1043–48.

25. Fletcher, A.K., and Dolben, J. 1996. A hospital survey of the care of elderly patients with diabetes mellitus. *Age and Ageing* 25:349–52.

26. Rosenberg, A. 1993. Breast cancer: Options for older patients. *Geriatrics* 48(Suppl 1):9–13.

27. Newcomb, P.A., and Carbone, P.P. 1993. Cancer treatment and age: Patient perspectives. *Journal of the National Cancer Institute* 85:1580–84.

28. Silliman, R.A., et al. 1993. Breast cancer in old age: What we know, don't know, and do. *Journal of the National Cancer Institute* 85:190–99.

29. Meyer, G.S., and Gibbons, R.V. 1997. House calls to the elderly—a vanishing practice among physicians. *New England Journal of Medicine* 337:1815–20.

30. Ramsdell, J.W., Swart, J.A., Jackson, J.E., and Renvall, M. 1989. The yield of a home visit in the assessment of geriatric patients. *Journal of the American Geriatrics Society* 37:17–24.

31. Stuck, A.E., Aronow, H.U., and Steiner, A., et al. 1995. A trial of annual in-home comprehensive

geriatric assessments for elderly people living in the community. *New England Journal of Medicine* 333:1184–89.

32. Smoller, B.R., and Kruskall, M.S. 1986. Phlebotomy for diagnostic laboratory tests in adults: Pattern of use and effect on transfusion requirements. *New England Journal of Medicine* 314(19):1233–35.

33. Alvarez, S., Shell, C.G., and Woolley, T.W., et al. 1988. Nosocomial infections in longterm facilities. *Journal of Gerontology* 43:M9–17.

34. Eisenberg, D.M., Davis, R.B., and Ettner, S.L., et al. 1998. Trends in alternative medicine use in the United States, 1990–1997. *Journal of the American Medical Association* 280:1569–75.

35. Astin, J. 1998. Why patients use alternative medicine: Results of a national study. *Journal of the American Medical Association* 279:1548–53.

36. Office of Alternative Medicine. 1994. *Alternative medicine: Expanding medical horizons.* Washington, D.C.: National Institutes of Health. NIH Publication No. 94-066.

37. Jonas, W.B. 1998. Alternative medicine—learning from the past, examining the present, advancing to the future (editorial). *Journal of the American Medical Association* 280:1616–17.

38. Shekelle, P.G. 1998. What role for chiropractic in health care? *New England Journal of Medicine* 399:1074–75.

39. NIH Consensus Development Panel on Acupuncture. 1998. Acupuncture. *Journal of the American Medical Association* 280:1518–24.

40. Bensoussan, A. 1998. Treatment of irritable bowel syndrome with Chinese herbal medicine: A randomized control trial. *Journal of the American Medical Association* 280:1585–89.

41. Benson, H. 1975. *The relaxation response.* New York: Morrow.

42. Braud, W.G. 1992. Human interconnectedness: Research indications. *ReVision* 14:140–8.

43. Ornish, D., Scherwitz, L.W., Billings, J.H., and Gould, K.L., et al. 1998. Intensive lifestyle changes for reversal of coronary heart disease. *Journal of the American Medical Association* 280:2001–7.

13

Long-Term Care

Everyone who is born holds dual citizenship, in the kingdom of the well and in the kingdom of the sick. Although we all prefer to use only the good passport, sooner or later each of us is obliged, at least for a spell, to identify ourselves as citizens of that other place.

Susan Sontag

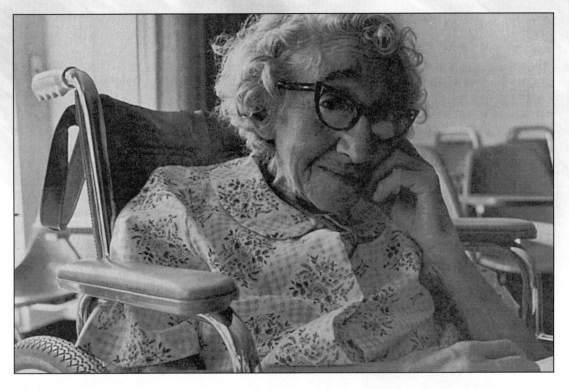

Long-term care includes a wide range of health, social, and personal care services designed to assist those who are chronically ill or are recovering from an acute illness to live as independently as possible by maximizing their level of physical and psychological functioning. Long-term care services may be formal or informal, and may occur within the home, in the community, or in an institutional setting. Those needing long-term care have many types of physical and mental disabilities that require different kinds of care. The care needed does not involve high technology, but personal assistance from others. They include services provided by family and friends, and staff from community agencies and institutions. Both informal and formal services assist millions of Americans who are physically and/or mentally disabled from birth defects, accidents, or chronic diseases that prohibit them from engaging in activities of daily living without assistance. Because more people are living to be old, long-term care services and facilities will need to be expanded to fill the increasing demand.

This chapter will explore the extent of elders' need for long-term care, whether they are at home, in sheltered living arrangements, or in institutional settings. An important consideration is how the health and supportive services they receive will be paid. This chapter will continue the discussion of the federal and state financing for long-term care. Several of the more common home-care services will be explored. Selected community-based services, including sheltered living arrangements, will also be reviewed. A number of important issues regarding institutional care will also be addressed. Because most of the care of frail elders in our country rests on the caregiver, their special needs and problems will be considered.

The Need for Long-term Care

It is difficult to determine who needs long-term care. Although individuals with heart disease and arthritis are more likely to be disabled and need care, the need cannot be determined by disease diagnosis alone. Not everyone needs the same level of care, and a person's need will inevitably change over time.

Measures that go beyond medical diagnosis of disabling disease have been developed to identify needs for long-term care. One measure is based on the ability to perform activities of daily living (ADL) that generally include the ability to function independently in the following ways: eating, bathing, dressing, getting to and using the bathroom, getting in or out of a bed or chair, and mobility. Inability to complete these tasks without assistance can be life-threatening. To live an independent life, it is also necessary to go outside the home, keep track of money or bills, prepare meals, do light housework, use the telephone, and take medicine. These are called instrumental activities of daily living (IADL). If there is no friend or relative to assist the frail person to perform these necessary activities, formal services are needed. Many factors must be considered in the decision of whether home and community-based services or institutionalization care would best meet those needs.

Approximately 13 million individuals of all ages in our country need long-term care. Although all age groups use long-term care services, those over age sixty-five are the prime recipients since they have more physical impairments than any other age group: they comprise more than half of all those using long-term care services.

Despite higher rates of disability and poor health among ethnic elders (particularly African-Americans), they use a smaller proportion of long-term care services, including nursing homes, community services, and home health care.[1] A number of hypotheses have explained the differences in use of services between whites and ethnic elders: discrimination of those who provide care, reduced access to high-quality care, economic insufficiency, cultural bias against outside help, and reliance on informal support networks.

Disability rates among the elderly have been declining over the last two decades. For example, more than a million fewer elderly people were disabled in 1994 compared to the number expected based on disability rates in 1982. This positive trend is likely a combination of four phenomena. First, higher educational level of the population makes it more likely that people are more receptive and compliant in changing negative health behaviors. Second, medical technologies are reducing the risk of developing a disabling chronic disease (e.g., reduction in the prevalence of circulatory disease and dementia). Third, over the years, Medicare has been improving the health care for elders, reducing the prevalence of some disabling chronic diseases. Finally, the decline in disability may be due to cohort differences in the type and degree of disability and mortality risk due to early life experiences.[2]

Despite the trend toward lower disability rates, the need for long-term care is on the increase in our country, primarily due to the rapid increase in the elder population. A large proportion of this is the baby boom generation, because they will enter the elderly years between 2010 and 2030. The population over age seventy-five is growing the fastest, and is projected to increase almost 50 percent in the next twenty years. This group has the greatest need for long-term services. Medical technology and advancements are keeping the very sick and very old alive longer; more long-term care services are needed because many will spend those extra years in a disabled state.

In addition, changes in living patterns are causing a shift from family-oriented care toward a greater need for formal services in our country. The number of older people living alone is increasing. In 1950, less than 15 percent of elders lived alone, but since then, that figure has more than doubled. Furthermore, the increased percentage of women in the labor force reduces the number of wives and daughters available at home to care for frail family members.

LONG-TERM CARE FINANCING

Federal and state funding have made institutional and community-based services more available to elders, the poor, and the chronically ill. In 1995, long-term care expenditures for the United States exceeded $100 billion: more than half this total was financed by the state and federal governments, and one-third was shouldered by individuals or

family members.[3] The major sources of funding for long-term care will be discussed in this section.

The Social Security Act of 1935 guaranteed a monthly income to eligible elders and the disabled. Almost all the nation's elders receive monthly *Social Security* payments throughout their old age paid for through taxes the federal government withdrew from their pay during their working years. Payments may begin as early as age sixty-two. Financed through equal contribution of employer and employee wages, it provides a low-cost, federally sponsored insurance to partially provide for participants and their surviving spouses in old age.

If Social Security benefits are less than that needed to survive, public assistance is available from the *Supplemental Security Income programs (SSI)*. The SSI program was established in 1974 to assist all aged, blind and permanently and totally disabled people who have inadequate income and assets. Program eligibility is not tied to participation in the work force. The program is financed by the federal government and managed by the state. The monthly payments to individuals and couples are set by the federal government and are the same in every state. Both Social Security and SSI programs provide elders with a guaranteed monthly income to allow them to choose to either remain in their own home or move into more sheltered settings.

In addition to Social Security, all older citizens in the United States receive guaranteed federally funded health care benefits through *Medicare,* regardless of income. Medicare was originally intended to support hospitalization and physician visits, so benefits are restricted for nursing home care and home care. Currently, Medicare will finance a nursing home stay for a limited amount of time for rehabilitation purposes for a particular illness or injury only if it directly follows at least a three-day hospitalization. Further, the physician must order that nursing care is required every day for the same condition that caused the hospitalization. Skilled nursing facility care coverage is limited to 100 days each benefit period and must follow a hospital stay of at least three days. For the first twenty days, all covered services are paid fully by Medicare. For the next eighty days, the elder must pay $96 coinsurance per day. After 100 days, the elder is responsible for all charges (1999 figures).

Home-care benefits under Medicare have increased almost tenfold in the last ten years. They now account for almost one-third of all Medicare expenditures. Both the number of beneficiaries and the number of visits by a home-care provider per person have more than doubled. There is significant concern that the lax controls over the use of the home health benefit are contributing to its rapid growth.[4]

In order to receive home health care under Medicare, elders must be homebound, under a physician's care, and must require part-time or intermittent skilled nursing care and/or physical or speech therapy services or rehabilitative therapies. Medicare does not pay for full-time nursing care, prescription drugs, or custodial care (homemaker or personal care services). Also, it does not cover services to assist with activities of daily living that permit individuals to remain in their own homes, such as bathing, dressing, and housekeeping. The services must be prescribed by a physician and be part of a treatment plan. Skilled nursing services are covered a maximum of eight hours daily and no more than twenty-eight hours weekly. In addition, Medicare provides hospice services to aid the dying and respite care to relieve those caring for a Medicare beneficiary.

Home health care under Medicare was originally intended to finance as transitional care to facilitate earlier hospital discharges. Currently only about 20 percent of home health care is used in this way. These services are now used primarily to provide long-term care: over half the users receive home health care for six months or more.[5]

The largest public funding source for long-term care is *Medicaid* (called MediCal in California), funded jointly by the federal and state government. Those who are eligible for SSI are automatically eligible for Medicaid. Other eligibility requirements are based on personal income and assets and vary by state. Medicaid provides medical and rehabilitation services to the disabled, blind, and poor of all ages. It also covers long-term care for those formerly middle-income older people who have exhausted their

financial resources for nursing home expenses. It is the payer of last resort, paying nursing home and home-health care bills not covered by Medicare and private insurance. For those poor enough to qualify, Medicaid pays for unlimited nursing home care without previous hospitalization.

Medicaid also finances a wide range of both medical and personal care services in the home and nursing home. The services must be authorized by a physician and be part of a treatment plan that is reviewed every sixty days. Currently, Medicaid is responsible for paying the bills of almost two-thirds of the nation's nursing home residents. This number is expected to continue to rise annually with the graying of the population.

In order to qualify for Medicaid funding, elders must prove they have few to no assets. For those elders who can't afford to pay for home or institutional care out-of-pocket, but are above the cutoff for Medicaid, they often "spend down" their remaining assets in order to qualify. However, they may retain $2,000, a car, a wedding ring, up to $5,000 in burial funds, some home furnishings, and a small life insurance policy. If married, the spouse may keep the house and some income and assets, with the amount varying by state.

A new legal industry has evolved to assist middle class and wealthy seniors to protect their assets for their children while allowing them to qualify for Medicaid. Elders may "give away" their assets to their relatives and protect themselves from some losses. Thus, the downside of Medicaid funding is that many people who could afford to pay for nursing home care with their own funds are relying on Medicaid, causing governmental expenditures for Medicaid to skyrocket. In an attempt to slow down asset-shifting, a federal law was passed that requires any transfer of assets (except to a disabled child or spouse) to occur at least three years before nursing home admission, and for trusts to occur at least five years previous to nursing home admission. In 1997, another law was passed that made asset-shifting a criminal offense, with up to a $10,000 fine, one year in jail, or both.

Although some states passed laws earlier, the federal Omnibus Budget Reconciliation Act of 1993 mandated that every state must try to recover the money the Medicaid program spent on long-term care by claiming assets left behind by deceased Medicaid recipients. However, states cannot make an estate claim if there is a surviving spouse or a child who is disabled, blind, or under 18. Recovery programs are now in effect in almost every state, and several have hired private contractors to collect at least a proportion of what Medicaid spent.

Medicaid reimburses nursing homes less than the true costs of care. Because of this, many nursing homes, especially those who cater to residents in the middle- and upper-income bracket or who have no trouble filling their beds, do not admit applicants who qualify for Medicaid or who have few assets. Some nursing homes will only allow a small proportion of their residents to be Medicaid-eligible. Those facilities that do accept Medicaid often place elders in multibed wards.

In 1965, the *Older Americans Act (OAA)* was passed with the goal of improving the lives of all people sixty and older by funding a broad range of health and social services and supporting education and research in gerontology. This legislation established the Administration on Aging, which drafts regulations and provides funds for health and social services for anyone age sixty and older. Each state has a Department of Aging that receives funds and direction from the Administration on Aging, then disperses those funds to the network of Area Agencies on Aging that reach every area of that state. Each Area Agency on Aging plans and coordinates services to benefit elders in its region, then contracts out the services needed in their area to other public or nonprofit providers. A large proportion of the funds is used for the following services: information and referral, in-home support, nutrition, transportation, and legal services. In addition, each Area Agency on Aging is mandated to offer ombudsman services to protect the rights of those in nursing homes and assisted-living facilities in its area. Although all elders were originally eligible for service with no regard to income, because of limited funding, many of the services are based on a sliding scale, dependent on income.

Title XX of the *Social Security Act,* implemented in 1975, significantly expanded the availability of home health care services to the poor and disabled of all ages. Under Title XX, the federal government matches the state's contribution to fund selected social services. Each state must determine income criteria, the populations to be served, and how the federal government funds will be allocated. Ten percent of Title XX funds is spent on in-home services, mainly for homemaker and home health services. Eligibility and available funds for the services vary from state to state.

The *Department of Veterans Affairs* provides institutional care for those who have served in the military, spending about $2.5 billion annually on long-term care. The VA administers 130 nursing homes and contracts with thousands of others to serve their veteran beneficiaries. The administration also pays for home health assistance to disabled veterans with service-connected disabilities. Several VA hospitals have established their own programs to deliver home-health care services.

Medicare supplemental insurance, commonly called Medigap insurance, is a voluntary, private insurance that gives elders a choice of policies with many benefit levels—the more coverage, the higher the premiums. Medigap insurance is designed to supplement Medicare coverage, generally paying for the noncovered costs of Medicare covered services, such as hospital deductibles and physician copayments. In the past, these insurance policies were not regulated, leading to confusion on which policy covers what, and many elders purchased coverage they didn't need. Subsequently, legislation was passed in almost all states to limit the number of Medigap policies that can be sold to no more than ten standard Medigap plans. It is now easy for consumers to comparison shop for Medigap insurance. Depending on the plan chosen, Medigap policies may pay for any or all of the following long-term care expenses: copayment for skilled nursing home care, a portion of outpatient prescription drug expenses, and some coverage for short-term in-home assistance.

A small proportion of nursing home expenses is paid by *private long-term care insurance.* Such insurance policies vary greatly. Each has its own eligibility requirements, restrictions, monthly premiums, and benefits. The cost depends on the extent of coverage. It often covers skilled nursing home care and home health care, not the lower level of custodial care that is most commonly needed. Although the federal government did attempt to add long-term care coverage to Medicare in the late 1980s, fierce opposition from the American Association of Retired Persons and other political action groups led to the defeat of this legislation, mainly because it was costly and had limited usefulness.

Even though it is possible to purchase insurance policies specifically to finance the costs of long-term care, very few people do because premiums may be thousands of dollars annually. Unfortunately, many elders are ineligible to purchase long-term care insurance because of policy restrictions: those with any signs of dementia, major illnesses, disabilities, and those who were recent residents of nursing homes may not qualify. Further, there are restrictions on type and length of long-term care covered. In addition, policies may have other types of restrictions that limit their usefulness. For example, some policies cover only certain diseases or cover only individuals with physical limitations in some activities, but not in others. Finally, many do not offer inflation protection, and premiums may increase without notice.

The rich can afford home care or nursing homes, and the poor who qualify can get their care provided by Medicaid. However, elders of middle incomes who hope to be able to leave an inheritance to their children or spouse may benefit from long-term care insurance. Buyers of these policies must be astute and should contact local experts before making a decision to purchase. See the special report on long-term care insurance for details on costs and benefits and ratings of different policies in *Consumer Reports,* "How Will You Pay for Your Old Age?"[6]

Out-of-pocket expenses paid by elders or their family for long-term care are substantial. In 1995, about one-third of all long-term care expenditures was paid by elders or their families. Not only do the expenses of long-term care deplete most elders' assets, but also they place a significant burden on their families, especially if the elder must be institutionalized.

HOME CARE

The primary consumers of home-based services are those recuperating from hospitalization, the chronically ill who need rehabilitation or help with daily living activities, the acutely ill who can be managed at home with help, and the dying. Most people want to deal with their chronic conditions and disabilities at home as long as possible. Staying at home gives a person control over when, how, and what type of personal care is received, unlike the care in a nursing home. Also, there is pressure to keep elders at home as long as possible to avoid, or at least delay, the higher cost of a nursing home. Much of the care in nursing homes can be effectively provided in the home because there are few disabilities or care needs that cannot be attended to in the home setting.

Formal care to enable a frail elder to remain as independent as possible at home includes a wide range of services. Skilled services include medical (physician services, nursing services) and rehabilitation services (physical, speech, and occupational therapy). Personal care services, provided by nursing assistants and homemaker aides, include bathing, toileting, dressing, and meal preparation. These services will be discussed in the following pages. Home care may be provided by one individual who lives in the elder's house, or by several individuals (generally under the auspices of one agency) who go into the home to perform various services.

Companies that offer home medical equipment (e.g., hospital beds, respiration devices, medical and surgical supplies, and home infusion therapy) are also expanding in response to an increased need for such services. Home infusion therapy allows an individual to receive intravenous medications (e.g., antibiotics, pain medications, tube feeding) at home instead of having to stay in the hospital.

The highest users of home-based care are likely to be white, disabled, and widowed women who are seventy-five and older who qualify for Medicaid coverage.[7] The most commonly used services are skilled nursing visits, and the most frequent diagnosis is heart disease. The decision to utilize home care is influenced by the elder's needs and desires, the elder's financial situation, and the availability of the service in the community. However, only about one-third of frail elders needing these services use them. And, for those elders with severe limitations, more than half use no formal services. Unfortunately, funding of in-home services by health insurance is often minimal and is restricted to skilled nursing services rather than the personal care and housekeeping services needed by most frail elders. Further, home

---

What Will You Do With Mother?

Your mother no longer can live on her own. Now comes the difficult decision about what to do. Should you bring her to live with you? Find someone to live with her? Explore expensive options for outside care, such as nursing homes or supportive housing? It seems each of these solutions has major drawbacks—the loss of privacy, the cost. The hardest part, though, will be telling mom.

At one time or another, most of us are likely to find ourselves in a situation much like this. You might be a child wrestling with these decisions about long-term care for your parent. Or a spouse or relative of someone needing ongoing care, someone who isn't necessarily older. Younger adults and children with chronic illness need long-term care too. You also might be worried about what you will do, especially if there are no family members or friends to rely on to help you. Long-term care is not just an issue that concerns older persons—it affects us all.[8]

---

care is expensive, and, if 24-hour care is required, the costs are similar to institutionalization ($2,000 to $4,000 monthly).

The number of agencies providing home services to frail elders has increased tremendously in the last decade for a number of reasons. Revisions in Medicare financing encourage shorter hospital stays and expanded funding for home health services. The increase in federal and state funding sources, combined with a rise in the number of elders wanting and needing home care, and the skyrocketing costs of institutionalization have created a tremendous demand for home-care products and services. Many for-profit organizations have become involved in the home-care market because it can be very lucrative. It is now the fastest growing segment of the health care system.

Benefits and Limitations of Home Care

The availability of home-care services may postpone, or even eliminate, the need for a nursing home. Most elders and their families are more comfortable with home care than the more impersonal care received in an institution. When the elder is able to remain at home, the network of family and friends remains intact. Furthermore, the individual and family can select particular services that meet their needs without financing unnecessary care. However, many frail elders choose institutional care because they do not want to be a burden to their family, their family members are not capable of caring for them, or they have no family.

If round-the-clock care is not needed, home care can be less expensive than institutionalization. And live-in care can be less expensive than care provided by those working in shifts. Costs for 24-hour care in one's home are generally close to the expenses of a nursing home. Even if costs are similar, home care provides one-on-one contact with a caregiver, compared to institutionalization where one caregiver's time is spread out among multiple patients.

For the elder poor who qualify, Medicaid finances home health and homemaker services, although not full twenty-four-hour medical care. And, those who do not qualify as poor must bear the costs of home care from their own assets, especially if the care required is nonmedical. Thus, whether or not an elder is eligible for governmental financial support is often a significant factor in deciding between home care and institutionalization.

Home care does have its limitations. Home care does not have quality and training standards; thus, the quality of home care is less carefully monitored than that received in a nursing home, which must comply with multiple federal and state regulations. This is especially true in cases where a caregiver is hired privately and not through an agency. Formal safeguards for consumers of in-home care vary widely among programs and types of providers. Although most states license or regulate some or all home-care organizations, few have licensure requirements for workers in the home-care industry. While all states must maintain a registry for nursing

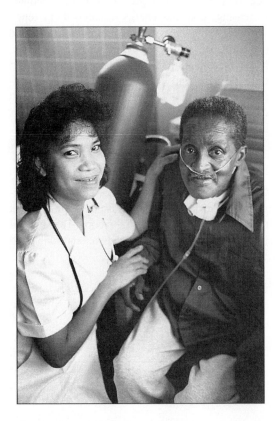

home aides according to federal law, only about a quarter of the states have their home-care workers registered, or they have developed a separate registry. Also, about a quarter of the states require criminal background checks on some types of home-care workers, and are primarily limited to criminal records within their own state.[9] In response to this concern, some states have initiated licensing requirements and criminal background checks for home-care workers before they will be hired by an agency.

In theory, home-based care is comprehensive and accessible, but in practice, the services may fall short of these goals. Despite the rapid growth in home-health care, most small communities have only a few types of services. When services exist, they are often underdeveloped and fragmented, focusing on a specific health need or professional specialization instead of fully meeting the need of the client. And, when many different services are utilized, none has full responsibility. This fragmentation makes it difficult for elders, especially those with multiple disabilities and language difficulties, to coordinate their home-care services to meet their needs. Even when all needed services are available, elders may be unaware of them and may not know whether they might qualify for reduced or free services. There is disturbing evidence that elders in managed care plans do not receive as many home-care services as those who are not enrolled, suggesting that the insurer's efforts at cost-cutting may deprive some elders of beneficial and needed services.[10]

Family Providers of Home Care

Families, not formal services, provide the majority of home care to frail elders. It is estimated that over 90 percent of those needing long-term care in a community setting are getting at least some informal care, and two-thirds depend completely on family and friends for their long-term care services. The most important consideration in determining whether a frail elder can remain at home is whether there is a close family member or friend willing and able to perform the physically and emotionally taxing role of the caretaker. For example, half of those frail elders with no family are in institutions, while only 7 percent are in institutions if they have a family caregiver.

Caregiver effectiveness depends on a number of factors: the frail elder's degree of disability and dependence, the caregiver's own health and mobility, and the availability of emotional support. The caregiver's other roles and responsibilities in the family and community and the degree to which the caregiver can obtain relief can also affect the ability to serve a frail elder.

In nearly one of four households, there is at least one adult caring for someone fifty and older. The average caregiver is a working woman in her mid-forties who is also caring for children under 18. Three-fourths of caregivers are women, and the majority are relatives of the care recipient. The prevalence of caregiving is higher among Asian and black households than among Hispanic and white households. The average duration of caregiving is 4.5 years. About one in five caregivers lives in the same house as the care recipient. In most cases, the recipient has a long-term illness, and an estimated 20 percent have Alzheimer's disease.[11]

Caregiving encompasses a wide variety of behaviors and commitments to a frail relative, from visiting or running errands a couple of hours a week to living with the relative and being responsible for round-the-clock care. Such care commonly includes the following: medically related care, personal care, household maintenance, transportation, and shopping. Family members might choose to care for elder relatives at home because of a bond with the loved one, an obligation to help a family member in need, financial reasons, or an aversion to institutionalization.

Demands of caring for a frail elder can be physically, financially, and emotionally draining. Often caregiving is hard physical work, particularly if one must move the patient or if the patient is violent. Disruption of sleep during the night is common. Caregivers often need to quit their jobs or reduce their hours to provide care to a family member, often at great financial expense. They must deal with the sadness of watching their loved one deteriorate physically. Also, watching a loved one deteriorate mentally, sometimes to the point of not recognizing the caregiver, can be very depressing. Furthermore, juggling the demands of a disabled parent with their spouse and children, career responsibilities, and their own health needs can be overwhelming. Caregivers who are old themselves may have to deal with their own disabilities, failing health, and declining energy.

Parental or spousal care is less predictable than child care and becomes increasingly difficult with time as the elder becomes more and more dependent rather than more independent, as with children. Caregiving can impact family relationships, creating or exacerbating conflicts among relatives regarding who does what care and how much. Another common consequence of caregiving is the accompanying confinement within the home and restriction of outside activities. In many cases, caregivers become as housebound as the family member they serve. Caregiving activities demand increasing time and energy, often without relief. Isolation from friends, other family members, and even alienation from the frail elder may occur. Many have feelings of guilt because they sometimes wish the frail elder would die. Some individuals experience a "loss of self" with prolonged caregiving as their world becomes confined to caring for their disabled relative.[12]

Formal Support for Caregivers

Given the multiple stresses placed upon those caring for an invalid at home, it is not surprising that many families find it difficult to cope. The stress of caregiving can create or worsen emotional and physical health problems. Because of this, it is important that caregivers obtain help, either formally or informally. The services outlined below are available in many areas to provide support to caregivers.

Education programs can increase caregivers' feelings of competence and skill development in dealing with the medical needs of their frail relative. Such education might include information about the patient's illness or disability, how to deal

Life of a Caregiver

"At first, although he couldn't remember what day it was or what he had for breakfast, his memory of long-ago events was still sharp. So we'd talk a lot about our wonderful years together and the great times we'd shared.

But soon, those memories left him too. Now they're fading for me as well. Because the person who sits across from me staring blankly into space is *not* the same person from those memories. He no longer even knows who I am.

The dreams we had for our "golden years"? *Forgotten.* The money we saved to make those dreams come true? *Gone.* Used up for medical expenses and supplies. Even though our little house is paid for, I can barely pay the taxes on it. Our friends are enjoying retirement, always making travel plans. *I have to make plans just to take a walk!*

The worst part is, I look at my husband and sometimes find myself hating him. Then I hate myself for feeling that way. But I can't help it. At least when someone dies, the grief eventually ends—you accept the loss, pick up the pieces of your life, and go on. With Alzheimer's, *the grief doesn't end because death doesn't come even though you find yourself praying it will!*"

(Letter to the Alzheimer's Family Relief Program, 15825 Shady Grove Road, Suite 140, Rockville, MD 20850.)

with crises as they arise, use of special equipment, transport techniques, rehabilitation strategies, and how to administer medications. They also need to learn about available community services and their eligibility standards.

Support groups provide emotional and practical support to caregivers, providing them with an opportunity to share experiences, develop coping strategies, enhance knowledge about disease and treatment, and gain access to community resources. Support programs also can assist caregivers in making the difficult decision of continuing home care or placing their ailing relative in a nursing home. Support groups encourage members to air feelings of resentment, anger, or hopelessness. Some groups become political advocates to bring about legislative change and development of respite care programs in the community. A professional facilitator may or may not be present. Some group membership is specific to the illness of the frail elder (e.g., Alzheimer's disease). One study reported that providing support to spouses of those with Alzheimer's disease delayed nursing home placement by about a year.[13]

Respite care is a service that offers temporary, infrequent care or supervision of frail and disabled adults to provide relief for caregivers from the stress of constant care. For example, a frail elder may be temporarily placed in a specialized wing of a hospital or a nursing home, especially for longer periods. More often, a worker comes into the home to oversee the frail elder for a couple of hours, giving the caregiver time for a short trip, shopping, or a visit with friends. Adult day-care facilities and homemaker and home health aides may also provide respite care. Respite care can prevent institutionalization by temporarily relieving the intolerable level of stress experienced by the caregiver. Medicaid and Medicare both provide some funding for limited respite services, but restrictions apply.

Elder Abuse

As older persons become more frail and dependent upon others, they become more susceptible to abuse by their caretakers. Elder abuse encompasses a wide range of behaviors, including physical or sexual abuse, psychological abuse, financial exploitation, and neglect. An elder might experience more than one form of abuse. Variable definitions of what constitutes abuse and neglect result in conflicting data on its prevalence. Since many cases never come to the attention of authorities, many believe that for every case reported, there are fourteen more unreported.[14] It is estimated that one million Americans sixty and older are abused in their own homes each year.[15] The abused might not report the problem because of shame, fear of retaliation, or loyalty to the abuser. They may also fear that they will have to be moved to an institution. Further, when confronted, they may even deny they have been abused or internalize the blame and believe they caused or deserved the abuse.

Victims have one characteristic in common: they are vulnerable. They are physically or cognitively impaired, socially isolated, and dependent on a caregiver, who is often the abuser. In two-thirds of the cases, the abuser is a relative who lives with the elder. Usually the abuser is the spouse, adult child, or grandchild of the victim. In 1996, the most frequent abusers were adult children, accounting for more than a third of the abuse

cases.[15] Experts once believed that the stress of caring for a disabled elder was the major contributor to elder abuse. However, recent studies show that abuse occurs because of personality problems of the caregiver. For instance, adult children who are financially dependent on their elder relative are much more likely to abuse that relative. Relatives with mental illness or substance abuse problems, a history of violent or antisocial behavior are also higher risk for being an abuser. The abusers are often part of a cycle of violence; they may have been abused children, child abusers, or wife abusers. More than half suffer from alcoholism, drug abuse, or psychological problems.[16]

Elder abuse may also occur in institutional settings, but few data are available, and no national studies have documented its presence.[16] One random-sample survey of nursing home staff in one state reported that more than one-third of respondents had witnessed at least one episode of physical abuse in the last year, the most frequent abuse being

Elder Abuse Case Study

Helen Mitchell is a 78-year-old woman who still loves to garden. One day when watering rosebushes in her backyard, she slipped on the wet patio and broke her hip.

While Mrs. Mitchell recuperated from the injury, she turned to her only son, Richard Montgomery, 42. Recently divorced and a heavy drinker, Richard is a laid-off construction worker. Without an income and a place to live, Richard offered to move in with his mother and care for her during her recovery. He took over some household duties, including writing checks to pay bills and making deposits or withdrawals.

As complications in Mrs. Mitchell's recovery arose, she started to presign the checks for Richard to pay the bills. What she didn't know was that Richard had begun to steal money by writing checks to himself or using them to pay his own mounting bills. After looking over one bank statement, the

elderly woman noticed suspiciously large ATM withdrawals made after her accident, so she confronted Richard.

He reacted with anger and accused her of not being grateful for the cooking, cleaning, and twenty-four-hour care that he provided her while she was bedridden. Richard threatened to "pack up and leave you all alone in the house." He started to isolate her, turning visitors away and intercepting her mail. He continued to threaten and intimidate his mother whenever financial questions were brought up. The relationship deteriorated, and Mrs. Mitchell became depressed, giving up hope, and feeling she had no way out of the situation.

Lifeline. . . preventing elder abuse. Crime prevention Center, California Attorney General's Office and California Department of Aging, 1992, p. 1.

excessive restraining of a patient. Pushing, grabbing, shoving, or pulling a patient was the second most common type of physical abuse. In addition, about 80 percent of respondents had witnessed psychological abuse by other staff: yelling, insulting, swearing, excessive isolation, threatening, and denying privileges. Interestingly 10 percent of respondents reported they themselves had engaged in physical abuse, while many more (40 percent) recalled emotionally abusing a patient.[17] Although this study used self-report, it provides preliminary evidence that abuse of elderly residents is significant in long-term care facilities and warrants concern.

Often physicians and other health providers overlook telltale signs of abuse and don't even consider the possibility. Further, many of the signs of abuse could be mistaken for aging or other common chronic conditions, such as surface bruises, malnutrition, and recurrent fractures.[18] In the past, most physicians have been unresponsive in dealing with the issue of elder abuse in their practice. In order to help physicians identify and treat the problem, the American Medical Association developed guidelines for physicians to enable them to diagnose and treat elder abuse and neglect.[19]

In 1976, the Older Americans Act established nursing home ombudsman programs to respond to the abuse and neglect of residents of long-term care facilities. Local Area Agencies on Aging are responsible to train volunteers to regularly visit all nursing homes and assisted-living facilities in their area, and to visit with residents to determine whether their rights have been violated.

All states have enacted elder abuse laws to require health care providers to report any type of suspected elder abuse, generally to Adult Protective Services within the county Department of Social Services. For abuse in long-term care settings, the local ombudsman should be contacted. Usually there should be a "reasonable belief" that a vulnerable adult has been or is likely to be abused, neglected or exploited. If the health care workers fail to make a report, they could be found guilty of a misdemeanor, and in some states, be reported to their licensing agency for disciplinary action.[20] States differ in the process of reporting elder abuse. Usually the abuse must be reported within twenty-four hours of an incident, and the agency is obligated to quickly investigate the case.

Types of In-Home Services

In-home services encompass a wide range of care options to meet the needs of the frail individual, such as medical services, personal care and housekeeping services, home-delivered meals, emergency response services, and personal reassurance programs. However, the funding methods differ, and their availability varies. A wider range of services is more likely to be available in metropolitan areas. This section discusses the most common types of services offered in the home.

Homemaker and Home Health Services
Homemaker and home health services are the most common and most important services to postpone or prevent institutionalization. *Homemaker aides* perform a full range of homemaking activities, including light housekeeping, laundry, shopping, and meal preparation. Since elders often are limited in performing daily activities, these individuals can be instrumental in helping an elder remain at home. *Home health aides* provide personal care, such as assisting with bathing, grooming, toileting, or therapy. In many cases, one worker performs both housekeeping and personal care activities. The need for both homemaker and home health aides currently far exceeds the supply. In many cases, the frail elder relies on family members for this type of assistance.

Funding for homemaker and home health aides differs. Home health services may be reimbursed by Medicare, but homemaker services are not. Furthermore, Medicare has very stringent criteria for eligibility and number of allowable home health visits. For those poor enough to qualify, homemaker and home health aide services are funded through local departments of social services (funded by Title XX). Sometimes, a family member will be paid for caregiving services through Title XX monies. For those who do not qualify for the above programs, some agencies funded by the Older American's Act offer services and charge a variable fee based on income and assets.

Skilled Nursing Services

Nurses commonly visit sick individuals in their homes to evaluate their condition and determine the type of nursing care required to fulfill the prescribed medical treatment plan. They provide direct patient care, monitor treatment, and refer the client to other social and medical supports as needed. Nurses provide health education and instruct the patient and family on basic home-care techniques, such as changing sterile dressings, catheter care, and insulin injections.

Nursing services are commonly provided by registered nurses or licensed vocational nurses from visiting nurse associations, public health departments, or home health agencies. Nurses working under the auspices of health departments provide free services, mainly to poor inner-city elders. Other agencies adjust fees based on the client's income or may be reimbursed by Medicare or Medicaid. The provision of skilled nursing care service is a requirement for all home health agencies certified by Medicare.

Physician Services

Although physicians commonly made home visits decades ago, physicians now prefer to see the patient in an office setting. Some doctors complain that they do not earn enough money by visiting patients; others feel uncomfortable being separated from the medical and diagnostic testing equipment in the office.

Although still rare, a few cities have agencies that employ physicians to make house calls when frail older people cannot leave their homes. These physicians assess the patient, then develop a treatment or rehabilitation plan. In general, the family or home health agency staff implements the plan and periodically informs the physician about the patient's health status. Agency physicians may be involved in short-term home care after hospitalization as well as maintenance care for those with chronic illnesses.

Physical, Speech, and Occupational Therapists

Rehabilitation therapists help patients who have suffered a debilitating illness or injury to improve their ability to care for themselves. A physical therapist is needed to improve patients use of limbs or muscles. A speech therapist helps patients whose speech has been affected to relearn and maintain this skill. An occupational therapist helps patients with their ability to perform routine functions. Activities and devices are also introduced to maintain or restore skills needed to function independently (such as walkers). Elders who suffer a stroke or bone fracture are the most likely to need these rehabilitation services.

To qualify for Medicare, individuals may receive physical, speech, or occupational therapy at home if prescribed by a physician. After assessing the client, the therapist develops a treatment schedule and may routinely visit the home, or the client may go to the agency until therapy is no longer needed. A therapist may also instruct the patient and family on rehabilitation activities that can be accomplished between visits. Some studies find that rehabilitation at home provides quicker results and increased patient satisfaction than visits to a rehabilitation site.

Emergency Response System Services

Elders living alone may use an emergency response system to decrease their isolation and reduce the fear that they won't be able to summon help in medical crisis. These services vary in the way they monitor a frail elder; monitoring services may be personal or electronic.

Some communities offer a program in which a volunteer, often an elder, will make a phone call at a prearranged time every day to a homebound elder to check on physical status. If the caller receives no answer after several calls within an hour, a friend, neighbor, police officer, or nurse is dispatched to the home to check if the elder has had an accident or needs help.

Although they cost more, electronic emergency response systems are more reliable because the elder is able to get emergency help at any time of the day or night. The frail older person wears a portable help button, or a help button is located in an easily accessible place. When the button is pushed, a device attached to a standard telephone automatically dials a central office, where a trained professional can dispatch help. The person then calls the elder to determine the problem. If there is no answer, the staff person contacts a relative or neighbor who has previously agreed to be called to check on the person, or dispatches an ambulance to the home. In many assisted-living facilities, call buttons are commonly placed in the bathroom and bedroom. Electronic technology using pagers and cell phones allows other types of monitoring as well.

Telephone and Visiting Programs

Perhaps the most effective programs to reduce isolation of frail elders who live alone are those that provide volunteers to make home visits. For instance, friendly visitor programs send volunteers, who are usually old themselves, to the homes of isolated or homebound elders once or twice a week. The visitors are trained to recognize health problems and environmental dangers, and serve as an information and referral source for local services. Some communities have friendly visitor services that, in addition to visiting, help the elder with errands, writing letters, or other helpful activities. Some programs contact elders by phone instead of visiting their homes. In some communities, mail carriers are trained to check up on homebound elders on their routes.

Home-Delivered Meals

Meals delivered to the home are an important support for those elders who cannot prepare their own meals. Home-delivered meal programs, usually called Meals on Wheels, provide homebound elders

---

No Meals for Many Homebound Elders

Randall Mueck's job at San Francisco's meal clearinghouse is to decide who will get food and who will wait. In mid-January, 411 of the city's homebound elderly were on Mueck's waiting list, 100 more than a few months earlier. All qualify for a hot, home-delivered meal under the federal Old Americans Act, but there isn't enough money to feed everyone.

Seniors who move up the fastest are those in the custody of adult protective services, the dying and the very old. Twenty-five percent of the people asking for food are over 90. "I try to think of all 411 and fit someone in accordingly," Mueck explains. "Age is going to bump somebody way up."

That means Audrey Baker, 79, must wait. When she asked for help last September, Mueck assigned her 750 points out of the 900 or so she needed to qualify for a meal. In January, her score had reached 877. (Each day on the list adds a point.) Baker, a thin woman, is blind, falls a lot, and is on the mend from a broken back. She also has hypertension and diabetes.

"I've outlived everybody else in my family," Baker says. "I don't have any friends." Her only help is an aide who comes for two hours on Fridays. Like many seniors, Baker is vague about what she eats. "It's whatever I can afford," she says. What will she eat this week? "I'll eat all right, but I don't know exactly what." Tonight it's an apple and some nuts.

Food isn't far from her mind, though. On the table beside the armchair in her tiny living room is a copy of the food magazine *Cooking Light,* in braille. "She's clearly struggling," says Frank Mitchell, a social worker with San Francisco's Meals on Wheels program. "How do you say, 'I know you're hungry. We'll serve you in three months.'?"

For many, there are no meal lists to get on. In Big Springs, a speck on the Nebraska prairie, 134 of the town's 495 residents are eligible for a meal. But there's no money to start a food program. Vic Walker, director of the Aging Office of Western Nebraska, doesn't even have enough money to feed those living outside the city limits of Scottsbluff, the largest town in the area. One man living on a ranch three miles over the line "needed a meal so desperately," recalls Irma Walter, Walker's case manager. "He was so debilitated, but there was no access to food."

Excerpted from "Hunger in America" by Trudy Lieberman. *The Nation,* March 30, 1996, pp. 11–12, 14–16.

one hot meal a day, five days a week. The programs will also prepare meals for those with special dietary restrictions. Sometimes the service also provides an additional meal to be refrigerated for the evening. The services are usually provided by voluntary organizations, and costs vary widely. Often, the program is funded through city government, the United Way, or senior organizations. The demand far exceeds the service capability in many communities, and often there is a long waiting list.

For those needing tube feeding, private agencies provide this service in the home. This program is reimbursed by Medicare and costs significantly less than hospitalization.

Hospice Care

Hospice care was developed as a more humane alternative to dying in a hospital. In order to qualify, the individual must have a physician's prognosis that they have six months or less to live. A team of medical and social service personnel and trained volunteers provide physical and psychological care to the dying person and family. Hospice services may be provided in hospitals and skilled nursing facilities, but are most commonly provided in the home. For elders with terminal illnesses, hospice services offer the advantage of skilled nursing, social work, home health aide, and homemaker services at home. Medicare reimburses these services without the stringent requirements imposed on home health services. Hospice services will be discussed in more detail in the following chapter.

Types of Community-Based Services

The following paragraphs describe several types of services available in the community that support elders' desire to live in their own homes with assistance. Also described are the variety of sheltered living arrangements that permit those who can no longer live without assistance, but do not yet need the level of medical care provided in nursing homes, to function in the community.

Congregate Meal Services

For those who are ambulatory, congregate meal programs serve a hot lunch and an opportunity to socialize at selected community sites. Transportation to and from the site is included. Additionally, the sites are often used for education, outreach, health screening, and social activities. Funding for this service is primarily by the federal monies from the Administration on Aging to the local Area Agencies on Aging, which then contracts with local providers. Although this service is free to everyone, donations are encouraged. This service was discussed more fully in chapter 5.

Adult Day-Care Centers and Adult Day Health Centers

Day-care centers provide supervised social, recreational, and health-related activities in a group setting to elders who are too frail to be left alone during the day. Several have special programming for those with Alzheimer's disease. Meals and transportation to and from the site are usually included. Adult day health centers, in addition to services mentioned above, offer nursing and rehabilitation services. Sometimes adult day health centers or day hospitals are located in a wing of a nursing home or hospital. Both adult day-care centers and adult day health centers are especially valuable for working families who care for a dependent adult. For many families, if a day-care center were not available, the frail relative would have to be placed in a nursing home. Even for family members who do not work, the program provides a welcome respite to the caregiver.

Adult day health care is reimbursable through Medicaid, but for those who do not qualify, many centers adjust cost according to ability to pay. However, many communities do not yet have adult day centers, and those who do often have long waiting lists. There are more than 3,000 centers in the nation, but it is estimated that more than three times that number is needed.[21]

The term "day-care center" is unfortunate because many believe that it is similar to a day-care center for children. The following comments provide us with a different perspective:

> We object to the comparison to child care because it is inaccurate. We are not a place where people are left in safety as children are left, until someone is ready to "pick them up" again. Our services have an

objective, and those who are consumers are not children. They are adults who may be limited for shorter or longer periods of time in their capacities for total self-care—but they are participants in their own care programs with everything that the term implies.[22]

Multipurpose Senior Centers

Multipurpose senior centers were designed to be the community focal point for elders—a place to come together to receive services and participate in activities that increase their involvement in the community and support their independence. Two basic types of programming are available: recreation/education and service. The recreation/education component is generally seen as the most central component of the senior center. Ideally, the program reflects the needs of the elders in the area and should be developed in cooperation with elders who participate in the center. The types of activities can be as varied as the interests of the center participants and as resources permit.

The service component is also important to the success of the center. The types of services offered are dependent upon the facility, the local community resources, and the defined needs of elders in the area and of the center participants. The services might be provided directly by center staff, or outside agencies might come to the center on a rotating basis. The services with the highest number of participants are congregate meals, information and referral, and sedentary recreational activities. The success of the senior center can be measured by the variety of services and activities provided and the degree of volunteer participation. Depending on the survey, between 10 and 20 percent of the older population utilizes senior centers. The challenge is to make the senior centers appealing to all older people, not just one subgroup of elders.[23]

Transportation Services

In our society, the ability to drive is a sign of independence, providing ready access to visit friends, go to the doctor, attend social functions, and shop for life's necessities. However, some older people choose not to drive: vision deficits or health problems, increasing insecurity in driving, or the high cost of maintaining an automobile are significant reasons. In order to freely move within the commu-

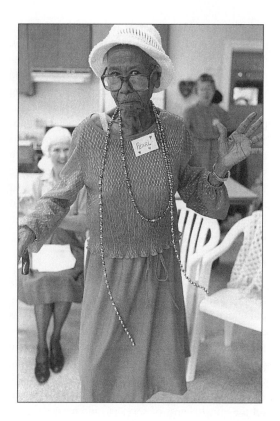

nity, those who do not drive must rely on their family or friends, utilize public transportation, or walk to their destination. Cities are more likely to have good public transportation than small communities. Even when public transportation is available, it may no longer be suitable for an elder who is frail or wheelchair-bound. The population groups most needing transportation services are frail elders eighty-five and over and those in rural areas.

The goal of elder transportation services is threefold: to enable formerly isolated elders to reach needed agencies and programs, to enable elders to obtain the medical and mental health care they require, and to enable the elderly to make the necessary shopping trips to avoid doing without important goods or becoming dependent on any local store and its possibly inflated prices. After communities get these three important goals solved, then expanding transportation services to enable elders to attend social and cultural events should be next on the agenda.[23]

Transportation services are sometimes part of other community-based services. Many nutrition programs and adult day-care programs have transportation services (usually a wheelchair-accessible van) built into their programs. Many assisted-living facilities also provide service for residents for physicians, shopping, and selected social events. Some communities have implemented a senior taxi service that responds to calls, taking elders to wherever they need to go for a low fee: others have a wheelchair-accessible minivan service that responds to elders' calls. Many times the cost of such service is subsidized by federal funds through the local Area Agency on Aging.

Case-Management Services

The delivery of long-term services to older people has become complicated, mainly due to the varying qualification standards and payment mechanisms among the services offered. Case managers, sometimes called care coordinators, assist the client and family to design the optimal package to meet an elder's special medical and social needs: arrange for and coordinate the appropriate services, monitor the effectiveness of services, and reassess them as needed. Ideally, the frail person makes the decisions regarding the type and amount of services to be utilized. However, as the person becomes more debilitated, the family and/or the case manager might need to make health care decisions. For complex levels of care, a multidisciplinary team may be needed, with the case manager as the team leader.

Hospitals and some local Area Agencies on Aging offer case-management services, as do private companies. The fees range from $40 to $120 an hour. These programs enable elders who would otherwise be institutionalized to remain in the community. Case-management services are proving to be especially helpful for children of frail elders who live some distance away. These services enable the relative to work with a case manager by phone to ensure the elder is receiving appropriate care. Although these services are not inexpensive, the case manager is more skilled in accessing local health and social services than a frail elder or an out-of-town relative.

Not only can a good case manager coordinate many services to enable the older person to remain in the home, she or he can also facilitate the move to an appropriate sheltered setting when needed. Even if the individual is placed in an assisted-living facility or a nursing home, periodic visits by a case manager to communicate with the elder and the health care providers can facilitate continued appropriate care.

Comprehensive Community-Based Care

Comprehensive community care facilities provide more than the case-management services listed above. They offer an extensive evaluation by a multidisciplinary team, then develop a treatment plan, arrange for needed health and social support services, and periodically evaluate the client to determine changing needs. The comprehensive care facility may employ its own medical and social support staff, but more often the program arranges needed care through other providers in the community.

These services are most often found in large population centers. Two well-publicized programs of this type are the Minneapolis Age and Opportunity Center and On-Lok Senior Services in San Francisco, both nonprofit organizations. Services may be offered on location or in close cooperation with other agencies. Services include home-delivered meals, chaplain contacts, dietary counseling and referral, legal and employment services, telephone reassurance programs, emergency food supply, volunteer visitors, pharmacy, individual and group counseling, health screening, and homemaker and home-health care services. The centers are financed through both public grants and private contributions.

Another type of comprehensive community-based care is the social health maintenance organization (SHMO), a managed-care approach originally financed through Medicare to improve the continuity of care and patient outcomes for those living in the community. The service offers a range of benefits through one umbrella organization. This idea was modeled after the health maintenance organization concept of acute and chronic illness care, but with the added benefit of social and long-term care services. Four demonstration projects were funded with Medicare monies in the mid-1980s and are still functioning.

Although the SHMO concept is in theory a good one, several studies to determine their effectiveness report that they are not meeting their intended goals. One study found problems with access to services, continuity of care, and satisfaction with physicians. Further, there was no difference in mortality rates between those SHMO members and those enrolled in the traditional fee for service. Although two organizations were providing satisfactory medical care, they fell short in the concept of integrating acute, social, and long-term services. For instance, the SHMO appointment system did not allow flexibility for longer or emergency visits with elder participants. Further, they employed few trained geriatric practitioners. Also, although SHMOs offered long-term care services, there was no coordinated system of care between the acute and chronic medical services. SHMO physicians seldom interacted with case managers and community-based long-term care providers. Many physicians were not even aware of the SHMO benefits and eligibility for long-term care services. Finally, the physicians were not involved in the development of a comprehensive geriatric assessment and management plan for frail participants.[24]

Evaluations of the SHMOs have spurred several recommendations to improve their effectiveness. Continuing evaluation and adjustments will improve the program so that the potential benefits of these types of coordinated care projects can be realized.

Community-Based Sheltered Living

This section will briefly describe the sheltered housing alternatives based in the community for those who cannot live independently but do not need the medical care offered in nursing homes. Common terms for sheltered living vary, and often the types are used interchangeably: adult congregate living facilities, residential care facilities, domicilliary homes, personal care homes, boarding houses, board and care homes, and the newest term, assisted living. The terms used for the types of sheltered facilities discussed in this section may not fit with what the resident actually receives because these living environments are poorly regulated.

Boarding houses provide room and board to frail and disabled adults who are fairly independent, but need help in some personal care and daily living activities. Some homes might also offer other services, such as transportation, laundry, and housekeeping, but medical care and supervision are not available. In general, boarding houses serve the poor. These homes are the primary repository for the chronically mentally ill and house many other groups of people who need sheltered living, such as those with developmental disabilities. The rent varies, and might cost as little as $350 per month. Many residents rely on public funding (SSI) to pay for room and board. If that is not sufficient, most states will supplement the SSI income to make up some of the difference between monthly board-and-care fee and residents' income, allotting the resident a small allowance for personal needs.

These homes ideally provide for social needs in a safe, secure living arrangement. However, in practice, they often fall far short. Problems with board-and-care homes have been well documented and include physical and sexual abuse of residents, inadequate staffing, overreliance on psychotropic medications, neglect, malnutrition, overcrowding, inappropriate placement, or misappropriation of funds. States differ widely in licensing requirements: in some states only those facilities with three or more residents must be licensed. About half the board-and-care homes in the United States are not licensed.

Adult foster care is geared to an adult population who is unable to live independently. Adult foster care is a type of sheltered living arrangement in which a substitute family provides care and protection for one to four older people in a homelike setting. Usually, the programs are administered by local social service departments and have strict income limitations. The family is paid a monthly fee for caring for one or more older persons in their home. A limitation of this program is that it is difficult to recruit foster families and the demand is higher than the available homes. This type of care has been found to be especially effective for mentally ill elders discharged from mental institutions.[23] Oregon has implemented a very successful foster care program that has allowed Medicaid patients to move from nursing homes to adult foster care homes.[25]

Assisted living is a relatively new type of supportive housing with an emphasis on meeting the needs of elders who want to maintain independence and privacy, but no longer want to maintain a home or prepare their own meals. As mentioned earlier, this term is also used to encompass boarding houses and continuing-care facilities. Although several assisted-living facilities offer little more than room and board, others have many services and offer a continuum of care. Generally, elders have private living areas, with some shared facilities, such as dining rooms, exercise and craft rooms, and sitting rooms. Meals are generally provided in a communal dining room, although in times of illness may be delivered to the resident's room. Call buttons and grab bars are usually installed to increase elder's safety. An attendant is on duty around-the-clock daily to check on residents, remind them about medications, and respond to emergencies. Often staff is available to assist with personal care and housekeeping services. Social activities and transportation services also may be provided.

The costs and quality of assisted-living facilities vary greatly. The monthly fee may range from $600 to $4,000. Ownership of the facility may be church-sponsored or government-subsidized, but most often are private for-profit endeavors. State governments often regulate these facilities, sometimes under similar regulations as board-and-care facilities. However, the rapid growth in this industry, uneven standards, and varying contracts make oversight somewhat patchy.[26]

Although several federal agencies have jurisdiction over consumer protection and quality of care in assisted-living facilities, states have the primary responsibility for developing standards and monitoring the care. Some states regulate facilities under board-and-care standards, others developed new standards specific to assisted living, and still others are in the process of developing standards. There is a concern that the rapid growth in assisted-living facilities will make it difficult for the state to effectively monitor the standards they do set. Because of this, contracts are very important to the consumers because they will help them to determine whether the facility meets their needs.[27]

Because of the confusion of what these facilities provide and the spotty regulation, it is important that many questions be asked of the owner before any decisions are made. When staff from *Consumer Reports* reviewed the quality of a sample of these facilities, they concluded that, no matter what it was called, "the operators promised to provide at least a place to sleep and food to eat. Beyond that, services and assistance offered vary enormously from facility to facility. Some claim to be able to give the same level of care one might expect at a nursing home. Others offer what they call a "continuum of care, allowing a resident to move from a setting with light supervision to one affording heavier care. Still others offered little in the way of any services outside of room, board, and an occasional ride to a shopping mall."[26]

Continuing-care retirement communities offer a range of living accommodations from independent-living facilities to skilled nursing home care in one location. In these communities, the resident can move from one level to another, as needed. The services provided usually include living space, one or two meals a day, 24-hour emergency call service, laundry and housekeeping service, recreational facilities, transportation, and a variety of health and social services. Elders usually begin their stay in apartments or cottages, and move to assisted care, and skilled nursing care when necessary. The sicker one becomes, the more medical supervision is available. The advantage of continuing care is that relationships formed in the community may be easily maintained, and the stresses of relocation are reduced because moving from one level of care to another is easily accomplished. This type of care eliminates the problem of finding an appropriate level of care in the community with short notice. It also eliminates the problem of financing the high cost of skilled nursing care and gives elders a sense of security.

Generally, elders buy into the community with an initial fee that may range from $30,000 to $300,000 or more with a contractual agreement that the facility will finance care at whatever level is needed for life. In addition, elders pay monthly fees from $800 to $3000, depending on the amenities. However, if the resident decides to leave the multilevel care home, he or she may lose the initial fee. Some of these facilities have gone bankrupt, losing the life savings of elders who lived there. Membership in one of these communities is a major investment decision and should not be undertaken without a great deal of thought and review of the solvency of the organization.

No matter what type of sheltered living is under consideration, the questions below can be asked of the owner or manager to help decide which

Questions to Ask in Choosing a Sheltered Living Facility

- **Where will the resident live?** In almost all assisted-living arrangements, residents simply reside in a unit or room; they have no ownership rights. Nevertheless, contracts should provide for flexibility when it comes to furnishings, modifications to the unit, who can come to live or visit, and whether the same unit will be available after a temporary absence, such as a hospital stay.
- **With or without meals?** Most contracts specify what meals will be provided. However, some facilities don't provide special diets. Some states require homes to post menus, but the rules are not always followed.
- **How do you get about?** Whether a resident can freely leave the facility to shop, dine out, attend religious services, or visit a doctor is key to quality of life and independence. Contracts should specify who will provide what kinds of transportation and where.
- **What help is available?** Contracts should describe staffing. How many people are on duty on the premises? Are they trained to give medical care? Have they attended classes or merely read manuals? What happens in an emergency?
- **What services are provided?** Facilities should specify exactly what services—housekeeping, laundry, nursing care, activities, meals—they'll provide, how often, and whether they can stop providing them.
- **What about privacy?** Residents need their privacy, but at the same time need some assurance that they're safe.
- **What's the cost?** What are the costs of living in the facility? What about entry deposits, cleaning charges, vacating fees, processing fees, and fees that increase as more intensive care is needed? Contracts should address fee increases.

- **Can you see your own doctor?** Can the resident choose the doctor, or is it determined by the owner?
- **Who's in charge of medicine?** Contracts should say who is responsible for administering, coordinating, and scheduling medications. Is it the facility, the resident or family member, or a visiting nurse?
- **Suppose health fails?** Few contracts specify what happens when a resident's physical or mental status declines. What happens if a resident's eyesight goes, or if he or she can no longer walk to the dining room? Ideally, contracts should specify that an individual program will be devised to accommodate those needs.
- **Who decides about transfers?** Knowing who makes the decisions regarding transfers (e.g., to different levels of care or to other units in same care level, or to a nursing home), the factors they're based on, and whether a resident has any say in the matter are crucial. Ideally the facility should provide for a committee composed of staff and other residents. Also, residents should be allowed to have a say when such transfers are recommended in nonemergency situations.
- **Can they kick you out?** Contracts should allow for a minimum of thirty- days notice if the facility wants to end the agreement, something the facility should have the right to do if a resident fails to pay or harms others. Contracts should also provide for a probationary period to see if a resident is suited to assisted living. If not, the facility should offer a prorated refund of fees.

Adapted from "Can your loved ones avoid a nursing home?" *Consumer Reports,* October, 1995, pp. 657–659.

living facility in the community is best for a client, a family member, or yourself. The answers to the questions should be formalized in the contract. The contract is very important because it should clarify what is and what is not offered by the facility and the rights and responsibilities of the resident.

LONG-TERM CARE INSTITUTIONS

Long-term institutional care can be divided into three categories: *sheltered care* is designed for those who need room and board and assistance with personal care, but medical care is not needed. They will not be included in this section because they were discussed earlier. *Mental institutions* are also long-term care institutions and were dis-

cussed in chapter 7. *Nursing homes* are designed for those who need 24-hour care and supervision by a health professional. Nursing homes meet the needs of those who are chronically ill or who are recovering from an accident or acute illness and need extended medical care but not hospitalization. These homes have traditionally been divided into "skilled" facilities, which offer around-the-clock nursing care by RNs or LVNs (also called LPNs), and "intermediate"-level care homes, which offer less medical care. New nursing home regulations abolish this distinction in the naming of the homes. However, nursing homes still offer either skilled or intermediate-level care or both. This section will primarily focus on nursing homes.

History of Long-Term Care Institutions

Early long-term care institutions in our country were almshouses built to house the poor, sick, and old who had no relatives to provide for them. Almshouse residents were expected to work for low wages to partially defray the cost of their care, and the remainder of their expenses were the responsibility of the towns in which they were located.

In the early 1900s, privately endowed foundations and philanthropists began to fund boarding homes for elders that replaced many of the almshouses. At first, these boarding facilities offered only custodial care, but as the residents became older and sicker, the homes began to provide nursing care. The passage of the Social Security Act of 1935 resulted in a tremendous increase in the number of nursing and board-and-care homes since more elders were able to afford them. In the 1950s, the government authorized grants and loans for the construction of long-term care institutions. This legislation was prompted by the shortage of hospital beds because patients with chronic illnesses were taking up beds needed for acute care.

In response to an increased concern over rising health care costs for the old and poor, two pieces of

important legislation were added to the Social Security Act that significantly increased the expansion of nursing homes. Medicare and Medicaid helped elders finance nursing home care and spurred the development of profit-making nursing homes previously managed by religious and philanthropic organizations. These federal programs set national standards for staffing, physical facility, and services provided by the institutions that they reimbursed. In the 1970s, federal legislation awarded monthly Supplemental Security Income to the aged, blind, and disabled who were poor enough to qualify, giving them more purchasing power in sheltered living environments.

Within the last thirty years, the number of nursing homes and sheltered living facilities have increased tremendously to respond to the increase in the frail elder population, the deinstitutionalization of the mentally ill from mental institutions to nursing homes, and the expansion of Medicaid reimbursement for institutional care.

Adapted from Gelfand, D.E. 1999. *The aging network: Programs and services.* New York: Springer.

NURSING HOMES

Nursing homes in the United States have a bad reputation. They conjure up visions of frail, dying, drugged, hopeless individuals, sitting in front of an out-of-focus TV or shuffling aimlessly down dimly lit halls smelling of urine, all waiting for death. To most, nursing homes are seen as the last resort—a place to die. The deplorable quality of care in nursing homes is commonly reported in the media, generally with accompanying examples of neglect or abuse of patients. Because of its reputation, most families are hesitant to place a loved one in an institution. Even when the nursing home is of good quality, institutionalization may be accompanied by trauma for both the elder and family. Despite their tarnished image, nursing homes are an important component of long-term care since they are the only alternative when care at home or other living arrangements are not suitable or available.

There is tremendous variability in the physical structure, the quality of care, the price, and the atmosphere of nursing homes. Some homes provide excellent, personalized care in a homelike setting, while others provide impersonal, uneven, or even substandard care. They may house only a few residents or be extremely large; elders may have private rooms or share with others; homes may vary in their composition of ages or illnesses.

In the past few years, the total number of nursing homes in our country has declined while the number of total beds has increased. As of 1996, the number of beds per home was 106, thirty more per facility than twenty-five years ago. Thus, there is a trend towards larger-capacity nursing homes. A little more than half the nation's nursing homes are part of national chains. There are also differences in their ownership type. In 1996, nearly two-thirds of all nursing homes operated for profit, as opposed to nonprofit voluntary or government-sponsored homes.[28] Some experts assert that administrators cannot maximize profits without sacrificing quality. Evidence is accumulating that for-profit nursing homes are of lower quality than nonprofit homes. Those not operating for-profit have better staffing and better outcomes among high-risk residents.[29]

A relatively new concept in service delivery to care for demented patients has been implemented within the nursing home setting. It is hypothesized that, since demented residents have special needs, separating them from other nursing home residents might enable staff to care for them more effectively. Special-care units (SCUs) are becoming more prevalent in nursing homes. The unit is usually locked to prevent access to the outside without supervision. Staff is usually trained to care for cognitively impaired residents and to provide specialized programs and services. The units usually cost more and provide more services than the rest of the facility.

Although there are no national regulations on such units, many states have implemented standards or regulations in an attempt to improve the quality of care and to protect the consumer. Regulations often include the following: physical design, staffing ratios, staff training, admission criteria, assessment and care planning, and therapeutic services.

Studies on the effectiveness of special-care units in reducing physical decline of those with dementia have shown no positive effect. One large-scale study of nursing home residents with Alzheimer's disease compared their speed of physical decline in both traditional nursing home care and care in the SCUs. They found no difference in speed of physical decline when residents from each group were compared.[30] Patient and family satisfaction with the care received in the special unit was not measured.

Nursing Home Population

In 1995, about 1.4 million elders lived in almost 16,700 nursing homes across the country.[31] Ten percent of nursing home residents were under age sixty-five.[28] The risk of institutionalization increases steadily with advancing age. While only 1 percent of those aged sixty-five to seventy-four are in nursing homes, 15 percent of those aged eighty-five and older are institutionalized. Approximately 4 percent of the nation's elder population is in nursing homes at any one point in time, but the probability an elder will spend time there is much higher. It has been estimated that two out of five people sixty-five and older in the United States will spend some time in a skilled nursing facility.[32] Because the proportion of old, especially the oldest-old, will continue to rise, the number of nursing home residents in the year 2025 is expected to reach over three million, more than double the current rate. Although elders remain at a higher risk of institutionalization, growth in the home-care industry, combined with lower-than-expected rates of disability, has caused the growth in nursing home placement to be slower than anticipated.

In 1995, elderly residents in nursing homes were predominantly women (75 percent), white (89 percent), and widowed (66 percent). The average age of admission into a nursing home was eighty-two. Most elders are admitted to nursing homes because of poor physical health (78 percent), but some are institutionalized for mental illness (7 percent), mental retardation (4 percent), or social, economic, or other reasons (11 percent). Those admitted into a nursing home generally have multiple chronic illnesses and cannot perform many of the tasks of daily living. One study of nursing home residents found that 96 percent needed assistance in bathing, 87 percent in dressing, 58 percent in using the toilet, 45 percent in transferring from bed to chair, 40 percent in eating, and 55 percent were incontinent (bowel and/or bladder).[31] Studies vary, but up to half the residents in nursing homes are reported to have some form of dementia.

Nursing home admission is strongly related to whether a frail elder is married or not: those who are married have almost half the risk as those who are not married. And, having at least one daughter or sibling reduces the chance of nursing home admission by one-fourth.[33]

Frail elders stay in nursing homes for varying periods of time. A little more than half (54 percent) stay less than a year, primarily those admitted for rehabilitation or recovery after a hip fracture or those who enter the nursing home very ill and die within a few weeks or months. In contrast, close to 25 percent of all residents stay more than two years, 12 percent stay between five and ten years, and 4 percent stay for more than ten years.[34] The mean length of stay is twenty-eight months.[31] This figure is six months less than what it was ten years ago, possibly because of the increased availability of home-care services that postpones the need for institutionalization.

Ethnic groups are underrepresented in nursing home populations, even though they are reported to have a higher level of disability. Researchers offer many hypotheses for this disparity. One explanation is that African American populations are congregated in the South where few elders of any ethnicity are institutionalized. Another reason is that ethnic groups may have greater kinship networks that minimize the need for institutionalization. They may also have a strong cultural bias against institutionalization or not be able to afford nursing home placement. Furthermore, African Americans, Hispanic Americans, and Native American elders have a shorter life expectancy, and fewer survive to need a nursing home. A lower risk of hip fracture among non-white elders, a predominant risk for institutionalization, may also explain some of the differences. Finally, racial discrimination is a likely barrier that keeps many from receiving such care. In one survey of several nursing homes in Texas, it was reported that the Mexican American residents were significantly more disabled by acute and chronic illness than the white residents.[35] It may be that this population waits until they are sicker than their white counterparts before they enter a nursing home, possibly for one or more of the reasons mentioned above.

The Nursing Home Reform Act

In response to serious concerns regarding the quality of care in nursing homes, Congress established the Nursing Home Reform Act, part of the Omnibus Budget Reconciliation Act of 1987, to increase the quality of care in nursing homes and to address the common complaints regarding such homes. The regulations in this act attempt to improve physical and mental assessment of patients, increase the effort that goes into planning of care, expand residents' rights (particularly regarding physical restraints and psychoactive medications), and encourage an inter-disciplinary team approach to care. Physicians were given a more important role in the day-to-day care at nursing homes under those federal regulations. They must participate in continuing assessment and plan-ning of care and must visit the resident at least once a month.

According to the federal mandate, a resident admitted to a nursing home must undergo a thor-ough assessment by a multidisciplinary team that develops measurable objectives and timetables to meet his or her medical, nursing, and psychosocial needs. Staff is expected to aggressively prevent deterioration of the resident's medical and func-tional condition and justify any invasive procedure, such as a catheter or feeding tube. In addition, the use of psychoactive medications and physical restraints are only allowable under certain condi-tions and must be frequently assessed and closely monitored.

Regular medical visits are required—every thirty days for the first three months of care, then every ninety days for Medicaid and every sixty days for Medicare residents. A physician, or a nurse practitioner or physician's assistant under the physician's direction, must review each resi-dent's treatment plan and medications at every visit. In addition, patients' rights are expanded, and nursing homes are required to survey resi-dents to determine how to increase their quality of life.

The Health Care Financing Commission trains reviewers to oversee nursing homes and assure compliance. The act also tightens up its inspection procedures to ensure compliance with the regula-tions. Previously, state inspectors made prean-nounced visits to each nursing home once a year. The new law mandates that they make unan-nounced visits on a nine- to fifteen-month survey cycle. Previously, inspection procedures were com-posed of looking at menus, activity schedules,

staffing records, and nursing notes—so-called paper compliance. Currently, the inspectors must interview a sample of residents and observe their daily routine, meet with the home's residence council, the ombudsman, and a sample of family members.

If a nursing home has performance deficien-cies, the inspector completes a report. The nursing home must respond in writing, stating its plan to correct the problem and when it will be corrected. These reports are available to the public at the local Social Security office, the state health depart-ment, and the nursing home itself. Unfortunately, many facilities repeatedly violate regulations, including regulations critical to good patient care. Often, regulations are not strictly enforced until a family member files a complaint. When a nursing home is cited for lack of conformance to regula-tions, its license is generally not even temporarily revoked because the need for nursing home beds is so great in most communities. The political influ-ence of the nursing home industry combined with erratic enforcement, few/low fines, and only extremely rare shutdowns of poor quality homes combine to make nursing home placement a "let the buyer beware" endeavor.[36]

Nursing Home Costs

Nursing home care is expensive, costing the nation $80 billion in 1995, and the price tag con-tinues to increase. Nursing home care is causing a substantial drain on both federal and state budgets and personal finances. In 1995, the annual cost of residing in a nursing home averaged more than $46,000, with costs as high as $90,000 in some geographic areas. Over half the residents in nurs-ing homes use Medicaid as their primary source of payment.[31] Despite the substantial contribution of public funds, on the average, elders still pay almost one-third of the nation's total nursing home bills out of their own or their families' pockets. In fact, the cost of institutionalization is the highest single medical expenditure paid for by elders.

Nursing home costs impoverish most residents within two years after entry. After personal assets are depleted, they will likely qualify for Medicaid funding to continue their care. A federal law now prevents spousal impoverishment. The healthy spouse is permitted to maintain some resources and income while depleting the frail spouse's share to become eligible for Medicaid to pay the nursing home bills. These figures change annually and vary by state. In 1997, on the average, the healthy spouse was able to keep less than $1,500 a month in income, half the couple's assets with a ceiling of $75,000, the primary home, a car, and personal goods.

Nursing homes typically try to minimize the number of patients they serve on Medicaid because they are reimbursed less than those qualifying for Medicare or those paying out of their own pockets. Also, the rates quoted to the family may be confusing. Typically, one rate might be quoted as a daily rate, but the resident may be charged for all extras at high rates—including diapers, pressure ulcer care, laundry, incontinence care, speech or occupational therapy, even turning and positioning—to compensate for the low reimbursement for the daily rate.

Nursing homes may be overused in this country because the government does not fund sheltered living facilities offering only personal care. One survey found that between 15 and 70 percent of nursing home residents could be cared for in less-intensive settings, depending on the criteria they used. Even though the cost savings would be great if individuals were transferred to a lower level of care, the researchers stated that policies to encourage such use would be difficult to design.[37]

Benefits and Limitations of Nursing Home Care

Nursing home care has significant advantages. The resident has access to twenty-four-hour medical supervision, and most of the services needed are in the home itself. The staff is able to collect information on the resident's behavior, enhancing the opportunity to make effective treatment decisions. Coordination of care is facilitated because many services are located under one roof. Furthermore, the group-living environment provides elders with opportunities for social interaction. Nursing homes are carefully monitored by multiple governmental regulations, which are designed to reduce use of unnecessary medications. Finally, nursing homes provide a safe, secure environment to frail elders when nobody else is available to adequately care for them.

Nursing homes are an important component in the continuum of long-term care, but they have their limitations, and, even though the full implementation of the Nursing Home Reform Act goes a long way to improve these homes, many problems are still unresolved.

A major complaint about nursing homes is *the difficulty in recruiting, training, and retaining qualified, sensitive staff.* Nurses and nurses aides are not attracted to nursing home work because it may be depressing and does not pay well. Registered nurses who do work in nursing homes generally perform administrative duties rather than direct patient care, leaving poorly trained and poorly paid nursing assistants to provide one-to-one patient contact. The work of nursing assistants is especially hard and frustrating when given responsibility for more patients than can be handled effectively. Because they are overworked, nursing assistants are often more concerned with finishing the necessary "bed and body work" than spending time to encourage independence in their patients and offering emotional support. Because of the hard work and low pay, many nursing assistant positions are vacant at any one time, compromising the quality of care.

Governmental regulations attempt to address staffing issues by mandating a minimum staff-resident ratio. Nurse's aides are required to undergo seventy-five hours of training and to be registered by the state. Further, nursing homes must have a registered nurse on duty twenty-four hours a day. However, the lack of nurses available to work in skilled nursing facilities makes compliance difficult. Very few nursing homes have suffi-

Problems and Joys of Working in a Nursing Home
Interview of Priscilla Frails, Nursing Assistant

My job can be very stressful, frustrating at times, I find it especially so when we are understaffed. When there are three nurses in the wing, three nursing assistants, it's really beautiful. Because you have even extra time to spend with them. A lot of times they just want to express themselves and how they feel inside. When I go in to make their bed or just go in to say hello to them, they want you to sit down, to talk for a few minutes. So when we are fully staffed, you are able to do extra things for them. But when you're understaffed, the work load is tremendous. It's just tremendous. When I go home, I feel good in my heart, but my body physically is just exhausted. . . .

A lot of times you learn about their families and many trials and tribulations that they went through, and how God blessed them and gave them the courage to continue to press forward. I say to myself, "Oh, God did this for you. I know He could do the same for me if I had to go through a similar experience." And then they tell you about their country and how they lived and what they went through, and how they themselves were enriched, how they were strengthened through all the trials they went through. . . .

I give baths. I do TPRs—which is temp, respiration, and pulse. I take blood pressures, I do weights, I have to serve two meals. Footcare, handcare. Make sure that their nails are cleaned and trimmed. I like to soak their feet because it's so refreshing—they love it. Yes. And while I'm soaking their feet, then we have a chance to chat, you know? So that's very enjoyable. We can't do it every day. Sometimes they give us an extra girl, but when we don't get the extra girl on, I just do the major things.

Even though we're understaffed a lot of times, and it can be very stressful and frustrating, I still love my work. I wouldn't give it up for anything in the world. . . .

The majority of my residents are very grateful and they're very thankful, very appreciative. Only a few, I would say, aren't. Every now and then, perhaps someone will come, like the supervisors will say, "You did a great job" or whatever. But you're not always appreciated. You're not.

It can be really difficult at times. Because you're dealing with so many people. Not just your residents, not just your coworkers, but their families, social service, even dietary, people from activities. It's very involved.

One time I went in to my resident to greet her and she told me that had had an encounter with this nursing assistant on the 11:00 P.M.–7:00 A.M. shift. And she told me that she had had an accident and she called the nursing assistant—rang the buzzer—the resident was incontinent of feces. You know what the nursing assistant told her to do? Told her to clean it up herself! When she told me that, I was so upset. Immediately I went and informed the nurse, and the nurse informed the supervisor. She isn't here today. We don't need those kinds of people here. We really don't. We need more dedicated people. . . .

There are a lot of people in this profession, but only a few dedicated ones, only a few dedicated ones that really love their work. You really have to love people. You do. You have to love people to do this kind of work. Because it's not easy. Everybody knows it's not easy.

From R.R. Shield. 1988. *Uneasy endings,* Ithaca: Cornell Press, pp. 223–224.

cient staff to meet the federally mandated staff-resident ratio.

There is a lot of concern about the *overuse of certain medications* (particularly antipsychotics and sedatives) prescribed to nursing home residents. In the 1980s, these medications were likely overused; depending on the home, from one-fourth to one-half the residents received antipsychotic medications. These medications were often used for long periods of time with inadequate monitoring, exposing elders to unacceptable side effects and drug interactions.[38] Concern about overuse prompted regulations regarding medication regulation in the 1987 Nursing Home Reform Act. The amendment stipulates very careful monitoring of those medications that affect mental function, such as antidepressants, benzodiazepines, pain medications, sedatives, and antipsychotics. The new regulations specify certain indications, length of treatments, and drugs that can be used, as well as alternative nondrug therapies that must be considered. Written consent is mandated to use these medications. Frequent review and frequent attempts to discontinue the medication are also required. Studies of medication use after the Nursing Home Reform Act went into effect report a significant reduction.[39] Nevertheless, these regulations have been criticized. Even though these medications have been reduced, studies need to be conducted to distinguish the discontinuation of appropriate and inappropriate prescriptions by observing the outcomes upon the residents. There is also some concern that nursing home administrators might be so fearful of violating the regulations that they may unnecessarily limit the use of these helpful drugs, consequently undertreating elders who have pain, agitation, and depression.

The use and misuse of *physical restraints* on nursing home residents has been getting much attention in the medical literature. The most commonly used restraints are safety vests with ties on the sides to keep patients strapped to a bed or chair, lap trays to hold elders in a chair, and wheelchair belts to keep elders from sliding out. Mittens and wrist and ankle restraints are also used. Nursing homes are required to get patients up each day; some patients are quite weak and unable to support themselves well, so restraints are used to hold them in the wheelchair. Restraints may also be used on elders who tend to fall out of bed or who do not call for help before attempting a trip to the bathroom. Additionally, restraints are used on elders who tend to wander. Elders who are most likely to be restrained are those with physical or cognitive impairments who are taking antipsychotic medications, have a history of falls, or have problems with mobility.[40]

Before the implementation of the Nursing Home Reform Act, restraint use was very prevalent: an estimated 41 percent of nursing home residents were restrained in 1988.[41] Evidence suggests that restraints cause more harm than good. Those who are involuntarily restrained are likely to become more agitated and even combative when trying to free themselves from the restraint. Further, there is no evidence that elders who are restrained have a diminished risk of injury. In fact, restraining increases injuries.[42] In addition, those who are regularly restrained become less mobile and may suffer loss of bone or muscle mass, pressure sores, and pain. They suffer psychologically as well: being restrained can be a frightening and humiliating experience. Improper application or monitoring of the restraints increases the risk of injury or death by causing fractures and strangulations.[43]

Because of the increasing concern over overuse of restraints without any clear benefits, the Nursing Home Reform Act includes guidelines to restrict the use of physical restraints, forcing nursing homes to look at alternatives. The Act (regulation 483.13a) states that "residents have the right to be free from . . . any physical or chemical restraint imposed for purposes of discipline or convenience and not required to treat the resident's medical symptoms." These regulations have significantly reduced restraint use. About 22 percent of residents in skilled nursing facilities were restrained in the first half of 1996, but there is wide variation among homes and geographic areas.[44]

Several alternatives to restraints have been suggested: modify the physical environment, provide mobility programs to reduce the need to wander, work with staff to reduce resistance, highlight at-risk residents and modify care practices for them, use alarms to alert the staff when a resident is getting out of bed, and place those at high-risk closest to the nurses station. However, studies need to be conducted to determine the effectiveness of these restraint-reduction practices.[45] One study was able to reduce the percentage of restrained residents by implementing a step approach to releasing residents from restraints, starting with those who need the restraints the least. Further, this approach was reported to decrease staff resistance to restraint reduction.[46]

Because of their significant physiological and psychological effects, physical restraints should be used only as a last resort. Even then, the least restrictive choice should be used, with staff regularly observing and assessing the resident's condition to document whether continued restraint is needed.

Another problem with many nursing homes is that they may *exacerbate residents' existing sensory deficits.* Unvarying appearance of rooms and corridors can cause orientation problems. Glare, caused by enameled walls, waxed floors, and fluo-

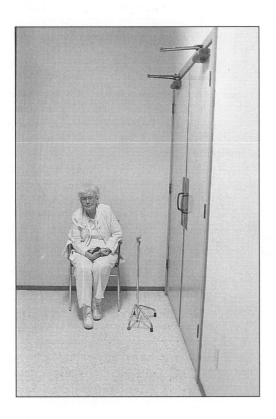

rescent lights, reduces vision. Background noise, such as piped-in music and institutional clatter, can make hearing even more difficult for the hearing-impaired. Also, the monotony of the days may reduce the type and amount of sensory input. Further, an estimated one-fourth of nursing home residents have uncorrected vision and hearing problems,[31] exacerbating an already serious problem of sensory deprivation.

Although *too much care* sounds like an oxymoron in an institution caring for the very frail, it can undermine the residents' ability and confidence to care for themselves, causing further disability. For instance, aides may insist on feeding elders or using wheelchairs to transport them because it is quicker and easier than allowing patients to do it themselves. Also, putting in a catheter instead of assisting a frail elder to the bathroom every hour or two, although it saves time for staff, encourages dependence and feelings of inadequacy in the patient. Often frail elders may receive excessive care because staff is concerned about meeting the regulations. For example, an elderly man with end-stage Alzheimer's disease who is no longer eating adequately and whose family elects not to insert a feeding tube, may be encouraged to leave the nursing home because the staff may fear that they will be accused of "starving" a patient or elder abuse.

Institutional life, no matter what its type or quality, creates an *impersonal and depersonalizing environment.* The prominent sociologist, Erving Goffman, asserted in his book, *Asylums,* that many types of total institutions (e.g., prisons, mental institutions, nursing homes, army barracks, monasteries) contribute to the "mortification of self," or profound loss of individuality of those residing there.[47] A total institution has the following characteristics:

1. All aspects of resident life (sleep, work, and play) are conducted in the same place under the same authority.
2. Daily activities are carried out in the immediate company of many others, all of whom are treated alike and required to do the same thing.

3. The day's activities are tightly scheduled; the sequence of events is imposed by those in authority.
4. Activities are carried out for the sake of the institution, not for those residing there.

A number of factors contribute to the self-mortification of nursing home residents. Upon entering an institution, some self-identity is lost because most new residents bring little clothing or few personal items with them. Institutionalization detaches individuals from their previous lifestyle, friends, and society at large. Institutionalized elders are often unable to enter or leave a facility at will, visiting hours may be restricted, phones may be inaccessible, and residents may lack access to newspapers or radios.

MY WORLD NOW.
Life in a Nursing Home, From the Inside.

This is my world now. It's all I have left. You see, I'm old. And, I'm not as healthy as I used to be. I'm not necessarily happy with it but I accept it. Occasionally, a member of my family will stop in to see me. He or she will bring me some flowers or a little present, maybe a set of slippers—I've got 8 pair. We'll visit for awhile and then they will return to the outside world and I'll be alone again.

Oh, there are other people here in the nursing home. Residents, we're called. The majority are about my age. I'm 84. Many are in wheelchairs. The lucky ones are passing through—a broken hip, a diseased heart, something has brought them here for rehabilitation. When they're well they'll be going home.

Most of us are aware of our plight—some are not. Varying stages of Alzheimer's have robbed several of their mental capacities. We listen to endlessly repeated stories and questions. We meet them anew daily, hourly or more often. We smile and nod gracefully each time we hear a retelling. They seldom listen to my stories, so I've stopped trying.

The help here is basically pretty good, although there's a large turnover. Just when I get comfortable with someone he or she moves on to another job. I understand that. This is not the best job to have.

I don't much like some of the physical things that happen to us. I don't care much for a diaper. I seem to have lost the control acquired so diligently as a child. The difference is that I'm aware and embarrassed but I can't do anything about it. I've had 3 children and I know it isn't pleasant to clean another's diaper. My husband used to wear a gas mask when he changed the kids. I wish I had one now.

Why do you think the staff insists on talking baby talk when speaking to me? I understand English. I have a degree in music and am a certified teacher. Now I hear a lot of words that end in "y." Is this how my kids felt? My hearing aid works fine. There is little need for anyone to position their face directly in front of mine and raise their voice with those "y" words. Sometimes it takes longer for a meaning to sink in; sometimes my mind wanders when I am bored. But there's no need to shout.

I tried once or twice to make my feelings known. I even shouted once. That gained me a reputation of being "crotchety." Imagine me, crotchety. My children never heard me raise my voice. I surprised myself. After I've asked for help more than a dozen times and received nothing more than a dozen condescending smiles and a "Yes, deary, I'm working on it," something begins to break. That time I wanted to be taken to a bathroom.

I'd love to go out for a meal, to travel again. I'd love to go to my own church, sing with my own choir. I'd love to visit my friends. Most of them are gone now or else they are in different "homes" of their children's choosing. I'd love to play a good game of bridge but no one here seems to concentrate very well.

My children put me here for my own good. They said they would be able to visit me frequently. But they have their own lives to lead. That sounds normal. I don't want to be a burden. They know that. But I would like to see them more. One of them is here in town. He visits as much as he can.

Something else I've learned to accept is loss of privacy. Quite often I'll close my door when my roommate— imagine having a roommate at my age—is in the TV room. I do appreciate some time to myself and believe that I have earned at least that courtesy. As I sit thinking or writing, one of the aides invariably opens the door unannounced and walks in as if I'm not there. Sometimes she even opens my drawers and begins rummaging around. Am I invisible? Have I lost my right to respect and dignity? What would happen if the roles were reversed? I am still a human being. I would like to be treated as one.

The meals are not what I would choose for myself. We get variety but we don't get a choice. I am one of the fortunate ones who can still handle utensils. I remember eating off such cheap utensils in the Great Depression. I worked hard so I would not have to ever use them again. But here I am.

Did you ever sit in a wheelchair over an extended period of time? It's not comfortable. The seat squeezes you into the middle and applies constant pressure on your hips. The armrests are too narrow and my arms slip off. I am luckier than some. Others are strapped into their chairs and abandoned in front of the TV. Captive prisoners of daytime television; soap operas, talk shows and commercials.

One of the residents died today. He was a loner who, at one time, started a business and developed a multimillion-dollar company. His children moved him here when he could no longer control his bowels. He didn't talk to most of us. He often snapped at the aides as though they were his employees. But he just gave up, willed his own demise. The staff has made up his room and another man has moved in.

A typical day. Awakened by the woman in the next bed wheezing—a former chain smoker with asthma. Call an aide to wash me and place me in my wheelchair to wait for breakfast. Only 67 minutes until breakfast. I'll wait. Breakfast in the dining area. Most of the residents are in wheelchairs. Others use canes or walkers. Some sit and wonder what they are waiting for. First meal of the day. Only 3 hours and 26 minutes until lunch. Maybe I'll sit around and wait for it. What is today? One day blends into the next until day and date mean nothing.

Let's watch a little TV. Oprah and Phil and Geraldo and who cares if some transvestite is having trouble picking a color-coordinated wardrobe from his husband's girlfriend's mother's collection. Lunch. Can't wait. Dried something with puréed peas and coconut pudding. No wonder I'm losing weight.

Back to my semiprivate room for a little semiprivacy or a nap. I do need my beauty rest, company may come today. What is today, again? The afternoon drags into early evening. This used to be my favorite time of the day. Things would wind down. I would kick off my shoes. Put my feet up on the coffee table. Pop open a bottle of Chablis and enjoy the fruits of my day's labor with my husband. He's gone. So is my health. *This* is my world.

The author, Anna Mae Halgrim Seaver, lived in Wauwatosa, Wis. Her son found these notes in her room after her death. From *Newsweek*, June 27, 1994. All rights reserved. Reprinted by permission.

Privacy is rare in institutions. Facts about the patient are listed on medical charts for anyone to peruse. Personal acts, such as dressing, bathing, toileting, and catheter care, become public. Elders can seldom find a place or time to be alone because doors are usually left open, and staff enter and leave at will. Privacy during visits with relatives or friends is difficult. Institutions remove an elder's freedom of personal choice. Social activities, mealtimes, waking and retiring, toileting, even naps are arranged without the resident's input. Individuals seldom have sufficient living space, and privacy may be further compromised by a lack of barriers between the beds. Because of their proximity, elders must associate with each other, even with those who are irrational and confused.

Nursing Home Advocacy

In an attempt to improve care of those residing in nursing homes, federal and state legislation mandate that residents of nursing facilities who are reimbursed by Medicare and Medicaid have certain rights protected by law. These rights were updated in the Nursing Home Reform Act in 1987. Some states and individual nursing homes have expanded these rights even further. Each state has guidelines regarding the steps an individual can take to report to the proper state authorities if a patient's rights have been violated. For a detailed, updated version of these rights, request a copy from a local nursing home, or write AARP Fulfillment, 601 E St., NW, Washington, D.C. 20049.

RESIDENTS' RIGHTS

Persons who live in a skilled nursing home or board and care home keep the rights they have had all their lives, plus they gain special rights under federal and state law. Some of the basic rights for residents are outlined below. If a person is unable to exercise these rights, family members or legal representatives can act on their behalf to protect and promote these basic rights.

FAIRNESS

Residents Have the Right To:
- Be treated with courtesy, respect, dignity and compassion
- Be free from discrimination because of age, race, religion, physical or mental disability, gender, sexual orientation, financial status, nationality or family status
- Information about all services and their costs, policies and procedures, and written notice of any changes in a language that is understandable
- A written description of legal rights and responsibilities
- A safe and clean place to live.

SELF-DETERMINATION

Residents Have the Right To:
- Refuse treatment
- Voice grievances to the facility staff, public officials, the ombudsman or any other person, without fear of reprisal or retaliation
- File complaints and have them promptly addressed and resolved
- Understand and participate in their plan for care and treatment
- Choose their doctor, pharmacist and other health care providers
- Be given all information about their medical condition and health
- Have information about Medicare/Medicaid eligibility and benefits
- Make their wishes known about medical treatment, and have advance directives, such as living wills and durable powers of attorney for health care
- Express preferences with respect to room, roommates, food and activities
- Keep and use personal belongings, without loss or damage
- Manage and control personal finances, or be given a written record of all transactions made on their behalf
- Organize and participate in a resident council and to recommend changes and improvements in the facility's policies and services. (Note: Family has a right to organize and participate in family groups.)

FREEDOM

Residents Have the Right To:
- Be free from physical and chemical restraints
- Be free from physical, emotional and verbal abuse and neglect
- Be free from financial abuse
- Freely participate in religious, social, community and other activities
- Leave the facility freely and return without unreasonable restriction
- Be free from unjustified room transfers or discharge (eviction) from the facility
- Appeal any transfer or discharge (eviction) decision.

PRIVACY

Residents Have the Right To:
- Private and confidential medical care and records
- Privacy in their room and during bathing, medical treatment, and personal care
- Personal privacy, including private visits, telephone calls and unopened mail
- Communicate privately and freely with any person.

Adapted from materials prepared by the New Mexico Office of the State Long Term Care Ombudsman and Long Term Care Ombudsman Program, Janet Levy Center, Chico, CA.

The federal ombudsman program was legislated to assure that all residential facilities and nursing homes ensure patients' rights and provide good patient care. In addition, ombudsman programs in each state have the authority to respond to complaints on behalf of their residents. Each Area Agency on Aging in the country is mandated to have an ombudsman program. Ombudsmen, assigned to particular nursing homes, are trained to respond to specific complaints, document significant problems, work as an advocate for improving quality of care, and help build a constructive working relationship among staff, administration, patient, and the family. Ombudsmen must report cases of abuse to the state office if discussions with the nursing home administrators do not resolve the problem. One analysis of abuse reporting for the long-term care institutions in Oregon found that the presence of ombudsmen was related to increased abuse reporting and complaint substantiations, more facility deficiencies, and higher sanction activity.[48]

The ombudsman programs use trained volunteers who are often elders themselves. To contact a local ombudsman, or become one yourself, contact your local Area Agency on Aging. In addition to dealing with complaints, the ombudsman can provide general information regarding how to select a nursing home or residential care facility, whether any enforcement actions have been taken against facilities in your area, and whether the inspection reported any deficiencies.

All nursing homes are mandated to have residents' councils that enable residents to discuss problems encountered with the administration or staff. Unfortunately, these councils may only be used to make small decisions (e.g., what movies to see) instead of dealing with the larger issues of good patient care and patient rights. Some institutions have grievance boards within the homes to enable patients, family, staff, and administrators to air their differences and arrive at workable compromises without outside intervention.

One way to stimulate patients, decrease maltreatment, and increase the quality of care is to make sure nursing homes have frequent and many visitors. Members of the community may act individually or as an organized group to improve nursing home care in their locale. Some individuals, especially the relatives of residents, can make unannounced visits to nursing homes to ensure conformity to the Residents' Bill of Rights and report any suspected abuse, neglect, or mistreatment. Case managers can be hired to check up on elders, review medical records, and arrange other services as needed. A recent phenomenon is to use legal action to sue nursing homes for poor-quality care. Many sizable damage awards, including punitive damages, have been granted.

Families of Nursing Home Residents

One of the pervasive myths is that elders are "dumped" in nursing homes by their uncaring kin. However, this is not true in the vast majority of cases. For every frail person in a nursing home, there are four people outside who are being taken care of by the family. Elders often must be placed in homes because they are very disabled and need a high level of care. Some elders are institutionalized because they have no family to care for them, and many times, those who do have family have medical needs greater than family members can provide. Further, many children of nursing home residents are old themselves and cannot perform the physically taxing work of caring for a parent.

Spouses and children commonly need emotional support to cope with feelings of guilt and personal failure in placing their loved one in a nursing home, especially if the decision was made without the elder's consent. The nursing home staff are in a good position to ease the adjustment for families. They can implement self-help groups to offer families of the institutionalized an avenue to address feelings about placement. They can educate families on ways to assist their loved one with common problems, such as resident adjustment. They can also educate families about institutional routines and prepare an elder for adjustment

Nursing Home Checklist

Call in advance for an appointment. Ask the Director of Nursing or Administrator to provide you with a tour or interview. However, schedule revisits unannounced (and if this is not permitted, choose another home). Schedule your visit to coincide with a meal. Talk directly with residents and their family members, as well as nursing and staff members, to inquire about their satisfaction.

Daily Living

What is the level of disability, age, and activity level of the other residents?

Are residents dressed for the season?

Does the staff know residents by name?

Does the staff appear rushed and busy?

Are observed staff interactions with residents gentle and respectful, or hurried and patronizing?

Does the staff respond quickly to resident's call for assistance?

Does the food appear attractive?

Do the menus vary depending on resident's preferences?

Observe residents being fed—is this hurried or respectful?

Are residents clean and well-groomed?

How does the facility select roommates? Can you switch?

Does the nursing home have a family council?

What activities are offered, and who participates?

What are visiting hours?

How are accommodations made for various religious preferences?

Level of Care

How involved are the resident and family in developing a plan of care?

How does the facility avoid the use of physical restraints?

Does the nursing home have an arrangement with a nearby hospital?

Does the nursing home have contracts with community groups?

Will your regular physician follow the resident in the nursing home? If not, what are the qualifications and reputation of the assigned physician?

How does the staff respect patient autonomy? Are residents free to refuse treatments?

What kinds of "therapies" or consultants are available (e.g., dental services, podiatry, optometry, physical therapy), and what are their costs?

Physical Environment

Is it located near enough for family and friends to visit?

Are there accessible outdoor areas?

Is the facility clean and in good repair?

Are there any visible hazards (e.g., wet spots on the floor)?

Does it smell?

Is it noisy?

Are there private areas for residents?

How are bedrooms furnished? Do residents display their personal belongings?

Are certifications and licenses on display?

How does the facility prevent residents from wandering?

Are there partitions or curtains to allow roommates privacy?

Is there fresh drinking water near each bed and a chair for each resident?

Financial Considerations

How much does it cost?

What amenities are included in the base costs, and which are extra?

What do Medicaid rooms look like?

How many residents share a room?

Look at Reputation

Ask discharge planners and social workers their opinion of the nursing home.

Ask for a list of references; call them.

Read the state inspection report on the facility. Do not expect it to be perfect, but instead discuss some of the problems with the staff, and see how they respond.

Call the local ombudsman or the local licensing office of the Department of Health Services for more information about a facility.

to the nursing home. Nursing home staff also might implement newsletters, lectures, or discussions on topics of interest to families to keep them involved in the care. Periodic meetings between staff and family members can also serve to update the treatment plan, clarify institutional policies, and resolve complaints. At times, professional counseling or an ombudsman may be brought in to resolve problems between the nursing home staff and the resident or family.

Planning Long-Term Care

All elders, regardless of their current health and ability, should consider their eventual long-term care needs. Elders who do not currently need such services may plan for their future by surveying programs and institutions in the community and discussing their preferences with family and friends, should such a need arise. In addition, they must consider how long-term care might be financed. For example, they may determine whether they wish to purchase insurance, pay out-of-pocket, or whether they may qualify for Medicaid. Reverse mortgages are another possibility for those who have little savings, but own their own home. In this case, the bank agrees to pay the owner a specified amount each month in return for the bank recovering the property upon the owner's death.

Ideally, planning for long-term care is accomplished before the need arises. Too often the recognition that long-term care is needed occurs when an elder is hospitalized from an accident, an acute illness, or crisis in a chronic illness and is too weak to be sent home without additional help. Many times the need is not recognized until the home situation fails (e.g., an elder who falls and is not discovered for some time). When this occurs, hospital nurses and physicians assess the elder's current level of function and potential to be rehabilitated, then recommend increased level of care or surveillance. Social workers, case managers, or hospital discharge planners are responsible to discuss long-term care options and financial issues with elders and their families. They can also make

appropriate referrals and arrange for home-care services or institutional placement. Many times, these plans must be made over the course of only hours or days because hospitals are under pressure to discharge patients rapidly.

When individuals need 24-hour care or can no longer live independently, families must make the difficult decision between home and nursing home care. When given a choice, most individuals prefer to remain in their own homes as long as possible. Often, family members make promises to an older relative that they will never "put them in a nursing home." However, home is not always the best choice. Frail spouses and working children often cannot provide the care needed and cannot afford to pay for further help. If an individual needs more care than the family or community can provide, institutionalization may be the only option. Further, elders may dislike their current living situation and prefer to move to a safe, sheltered environment. Some elders would rather move into an institution than move in with grown children. Finally, caring for frail elders who have severe and debilitating illnesses, such as severe dementia, is often best accomplished in an institutional setting where patients are less isolated and can consistently receive the extent of personal and medical care they require.

When choosing a nursing home, families are often given a list of nearby facilities and instructed to visit. Each Area Agency on Aging has a list of nursing homes in its region and record of violations. Generally, the time frame under which families must select a home is short. A number of inventories have been developed to assist them in evaluating nursing homes. In addition, *Consumer Reports* has reviewed and rated many major nursing home chains.[36] Although different individuals may place different weights regarding the relative value of nursing home characteristics, the importance of the physical environment should not be the overriding consideration because daily care provided by staff is more important. No matter how carefully a placement is selected, nothing can substitute for frequent visiting and monitoring of the care.

Summary

Long-term care includes a wide variety of health and social services and living arrangements for frail elders in the home, the community, and nursing homes. The need for long-term care services and facilities in this country is increasing drastically as the population ages. Federal and state funds finance much of long-term care expenditures, but a significant proportion must be paid out-of-pocket by the elder or family.

In-home services and community-based services include a wide variety of services and living arrangements provided in the home or community to frail elders to delay or avert institutionalization. Despite the variety of services available, family members still provide the lion's share of homecare services to their loved ones, often at great emotional cost. Support programs and respite care services are available in some communities to reduce their stress.

Nursing homes are very expensive for the federal and state government, and half the residents must use their own funds to pay for care. The risk of nursing home placement increases with advanced age, and the vast majority of residents are widowed white women. There are many advantages and disadvantages to institutionalization. However, to the public, the disadvantages are more evident. Nursing home advocates have pressed for legislation to protect residents' rights and increase their quality of care.

Before a rational decision can be made on whether to institutionalize a frail elder, a thorough assessment should be made by medical professionals. The factors to consider are the level of function, financial resources, availability of a caretaker, accessibility of formal services, and personal preferences of the client and family.

Activities

1. If you were preparing to enter a nursing home, what five personal items would you consider most important for your comfort and well-being? Contact a local nursing home and question them about types of personal belongings permitted in the facility.

2. Tour a local nursing home as if you were planning to place a loved one there. Inquire about the following: daily costs, admission requirements, personal items permitted, how roommates are matched, available interaction between resident and the community, activities offered within the home, and nutrition services. Observe the activity of the residents. Are services available for residents' families? Use the checklist provided to gather added information. For a group project, compile your work, developing a directory of nursing homes for the public. Alternatively, have two groups go to the same facility and assess it separately. What differences were reported?

3. Compile a list of home-care services for elders in your community. Check with the local Area Agency on Aging. What services are not available that are discussed in this chapter?

4. Would you prefer home or institutional care? Why? What health problems would convince you that your own institutionalization was necessary?

5. Using material from this chapter and other information about health needs of elders, design a topic outline for nurse's aide training in a nursing home. How might it differ from training home health aides?

6. If you were given unlimited funds to build a nursing home, what would it be like? Include physical environment, staffing, food service, rehabilitation, social and educational activities, admission procedures, residents' rights, services for families, system of how residents would participate in decision making, and interaction with the community. Remember that most residents have moderate to severe disabilities.

7. You have just been hired as a nursing home administrator. List five policies or procedures you would want to implement to enhance the residents' quality of care. What arguments would you use to convince the board of directors of the cost-effectiveness or benefit to patients?

8. Do you or your parents or grandparents have long-term care insurance? Why or why not? Contact a broker who sells this type of policy and inquire about its purchase. Compare rates and benefits among various policies.

9. Interview a case manager or discharge planner from a local hospital regarding his or her opinions about local community home-care programs and nursing homes. How much time do families typically have to arrange placement? What options does he or she recommend? How is the determination between institutional and home care made? What happens if elders refuse to follow recommendations for institutionalization or long-term care?

10. Attend a support group meeting for caregivers. Who is there? What issues are addressed? Who is facilitating the group?

Bibliography

1. Mui, A.C., and Burnette, D. 1994. Long-term care service use by frail elders: Is ethnicity a factor? *The Gerontologist* 34:190–98.

2. Manton, K.G., Corder, L., and Stallard, E. 1997. Chronic disability trends in the U.S. elderly populations: 1982–1995. *Proceedings of the National Academy of Science: USA* 94:2593–98.

3. National Academy on Aging. 1997. *Facts on long-term care.* Washington, D.C.

4. U.S. General Accounting Office, 1996. *Medicare: Home health utilization expands while program controls deteriorate.* Washington, D.C.: General Accounting Office GAO/HEHS 96-16.

5. Welch, H.G., Wennberg, D.E., and Welch, W.P. 1996. The use of Medicare home health care services. *New England Journal of Medicine* 335:324–29.

6. "How will you pay for your old age?" 1997. *Consumer Reports* (October):35–50.

7. Dey, A.N. 1996. Characteristics of elderly home health care users: Data from the 1994 National Home and Hospice Care Survey. *Advance data from vital and health statistics.* Publ. no. 279. Hyattsville, Maryland: National Center for Health Statistics.

8. "Ensuring a responsive long-term care system: New challenges for a new century." 1997. *Perspectives in Health and Aging* 12(November):1. American Association of Retired Persons.

9. U.S. General Accounting Office. 1996. *Long-term care: Some states apply criminal background checks to home care workers.* Washington, D.C.:General Accounting Office GAO/PEMD 96-5.

10. Schlenker, R.E., Shaughnessy, P.W., and Hittle, D.F. 1995. Patient-level cost of home health care under capitated and fee-for-service payment. *Inquiry* 32:252–70.

11. The National Alliance for Caregiving and the American Association of Retired Persons. 1997. Family caregiving in the U.S.: Findings from a national survey. Bethesda, MD: National Alliance for Caregiving.

12. Skaff, M.M., and Pearlin, L.I. 1992. Caregiving: Role engulfment and the loss of self. *The Gerontologist* 32:656–64.

13. Mittelman, M.S., Ferris, S.H., and Schulman, E., et al. 1996. A family intervention to delay nursing home placement of patients with Alzheimer's disease. *Journal of the American Medical Association* 276:1725.

14. American Medical Association. 1992. *Diagnostic and treatment guidelines on elder abuse and neglect.* Chicago: American Medical Association.

15. Tatara, T. 1997. *Summaries of the statistical data on elder abuse in domestic settings for FY 95 and FY 96.* Washington, D.C.: National Center on Elder Abuse.

16. Lachs, M.S., and Pillemer, K. 1995. Abuse and neglect of elderly persons. *New England Journal of Medicine* 332:437–43.

17. Pillemer, K., and Moore, D.W. 1989. Abuse of patients in nursing homes: Findings from a survey of staff. *Gerontologist* 29(3):314–20.

18. Wolfe, S. 1998. Look for signs of abuse. *RN* (August):48–49.

19. American Medical Association. 1992. *Diagnostic and treatment guidelines on elder abuse and neglect.* Chicago: American Medical Association.

20. Steigel, L.A. 1995. *Recommended guidelines for state courts handling cases involving elder abuse.* Washington, D.C.: American Bar Association.

21. Adult day care centers vital, many more needed. 1993. *Journal of the American Medical Association* 269:2341–42.

22. Trager, B. 1976. *Adult day facilities for treatment, health care and related services.* Washington, D.C.: U.S. Government Printing Office.

23. Gelfand, D.E. 1999. *The aging network: Programs and services.* New York: Springer.

24. Harrington, C., Lynch, M., and Newcomer, R.J. 1993. Medical services in social health maintenance organizations. *The Gerontologist* 33:790–800.

25. Kane, R.A., Kane, R.L., and Illston, L.H., et al. 1991. Adult foster care for the elderly in Oregon: A mainstream alternative to nursing homes? *American Journal of Public Health* 81:113–20.

26. "Can your loved ones avoid a nursing home?" 1995. *Consumer Reports* (October):656–62.

27. U.S. General Accounting Office. 1997. *Long-term care: Consumer protection and quality-of-care issues in assisted living.* Washington D.C.: Department of Health and Human Services GAO/HEHS 97-93, May 15.

28. Strahan, G.W. 1997 An overview of nursing homes and their currrent residents: Data from the 1995 national nursing home survey. *Advance data from vital and health statistics.* Publ. no. 280. Hyattsville, MD: National Center for Health Statistics.

29. Aaronson, W.E., Zinn, J.S., and Rosco, M.D. 1994. Do for-profit and not-for-profit nursing homes behave differently? *The Gerontologist* 34:775–86.

30. Phillips, C.D., Sloane, P.D., and Hawes, C., et al. 1997. Efffects of residence in Alzheimer disease special care units on functional outcomes. *Journal of the American Medical Association* 278:1340–44.

31. Dey, A.N. 1997. Characteristics of elderly nursing home residents: Data from the 1995 National Nursing Home Survey. *Advance data from vital and health statistics.* Publ. no. 289. Hyattsville, MD: National Center for Health Statistics.

32. Kemper, P., and Murtaugh, C.M. 1991. Lifetime use of nursing home care. *New England Journal of Medicine* 324:595–600.

33. Freedman, V.A. 1996. Family structure and the risk of nursing home admission. *Journal of Gerontology* 51B:S61–69.

34. Murtaugh, C.M., Kemper, P., Spillman, B.C., and Carlson, B.L. 1997. The amount, distribution and timing of lifetime nursing home use. *Medical Care* 35:204–18.

35. Mulrow, C.D., Chiodo, L.K., and Gerety, M.B., et al. 1996. Function and medical comorbidity in South Texas nursing home residents: Variations by ethnic group. *Journal of the American Geriatrics Society* 44:279–84.

36. "Nursing homes when a loved one needs care." 1995. *Consumer Reports* (August):518–27.

37. Spector, W.D., Rechovsky, J.D., and Cohen, J.W. 1996. Appropriate placement of nursing home residents in lower levels of care. *Milbank Quarterly* 74:139–60.

38. Harrington, C., Tompkins, C., Curtis, M., and Grant, L.. 1992. Psychotropic drug use in long-term care facilities: A review of the literature. *The Gerontologist* 32:822–33.

39. Shorr, R.I., Fought, R.L., and Ray, W.A. 1994. Changes in antipsychotic drug use in nursing homes during implementation of the RA-87 regulations. *Journal of the American Medical Association* 271:358–62.

40. Castle, N.G., Fogel, B., and Mor, V. 1997. Risk factors for physical restraint use in nursing homes: Pre- and post-implementation of the Nursing Home Reform Act. *The Gerontologist* 37:737–47.

41. Strumpf, N.E., and Tomes, N. 1993. Restraining the troublesome patient: A historical perspective on a contemporary debate. *Nursing History Review* 1:3–24.

42. Tinetti, M.E., Wen-Liang, L., and Ginter, S.F. 1992. Mechanical restraint use and fall-related injuries among residents of skilled nursing facilities. *Annals of Internal Medicine* 116:369–74.

43. Miles, S.H., and Irvine, P. 1992. Deaths caused by physical restraints. *Gerontologist* 32:762–66.

44. Medicare/Medicaid Automated Certification Survey. 1991–1996. Arlington, VA:Health Care Financing Administration.

45. Castle, N.G., and Mor, V. 1998. Physical restraints in nursing homes: A review of the literature since the Nursing Home Reform Act of 1987. *Medical Care Research and Review* 55:139–71.

46. Ejaz, F.K., Folmar, S.J., and Kaufmann, M., et al. 1994. Restraint reduction: Can it be achieved? *The Gerontologist* 34:694–99.

47. Goffman, E. 1961. *Asylums.* New York: Doubleday.

48. Nelson, H.W., Huber, R., and Walter, K.L. 1995. The relationship between volunteer long-term care ombudsmen and regulatory nursing home actions. *The Gerontologist* 35:509–14.

14

DYING, DEATH, AND GRIEF

Don't be afraid your life will end: be afraid that it will never begin.

Grace Hansen

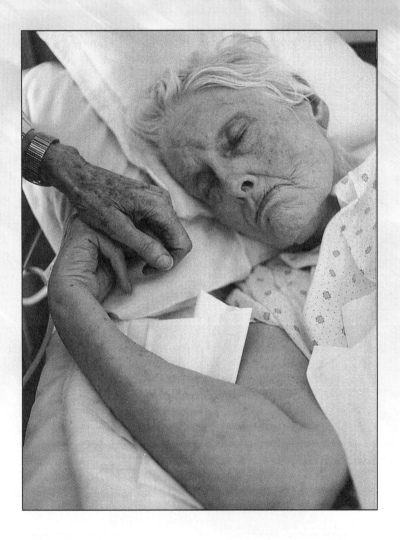

A text on health and aging is not complete without a discussion of dying, death, and grief since death occurs more frequently among elders than other age groups. Although this seems elementary, it has not always been true. In 1900, those aged sixty-five and older comprised only 17 percent of all deaths; now more than three-fourths of those who die are sixty-five and older. Reductions in infectious disease; infant mortality, and deaths from childbirth have contributed to this changing pattern. Not only are deaths more common among older people, but also they experience the deaths of family and friends more often than younger groups.

Professionals working directly with elders, especially those in the health and social services, will inevitably confront death, whether they work with people who die while in their service, or deal with others' grief. To be effective, professionals will also have to face their own attitudes toward death and dying. This chapter will address issues commonly faced by the dying, the bereaved, and those who work with them.

DEATH DEFINED

The moment of death used to be easy to determine; a person was pronounced dead when the heart stopped beating. However, the availability of new technology now blurs the distinction between life and death. Sophisticated medical technology can now keep the body functioning whether or not the individual is capable of thinking, eating, or breathing. Machines can ventilate the lungs, feed a patient through a tube or a vein, and remove waste products from the bloodstream through dialysis.

The federal Uniform Determination of Death Act in 1981 mandated that each state define death as the loss of all brain function. The brain cells involved in higher thought and voluntary action are the most sensitive when trauma, heart attack, or stroke robs the brain of oxygen. Some believe these cells are irreversibly damaged after less than six minutes without oxygen. If an individual is revived after the brain has been deprived of oxygen for more than a few minutes, the lower brain, less sensitive to oxygen deprivation, can be revived, and

heart beat and respiration will continue. However, these individuals show no evidence of higher brain functions as measured by an electroencephalogram (EEG), and are considered "brain dead." In practice, an EEG is rarely done to determine death: absence of spontaneous heartbeat and breathing and the loss of pupil response to light are used as indicators.

Death is more difficult to define in the relatively rare *vegetative state*. Affected individuals who have suffered extensive brain damage may pass into a chronic state of unconsciousness and have no self-awareness. They may spontaneously open their eyes, make unintelligible sounds, or make facial movements; however, they cannot speak coherently, comprehend speech, or make any voluntary movement. When the condition lasts for more than a few weeks, it is called a *persistent vegetative state*. These patients retain the functions necessary to sustain life; however, recovery is very rare and is usually only partial.[1]

WHO SHOULD DECIDE?

The advances of technology have created many complicated ethical dilemmas. Most will agree that maintaining life at any cost is not necessarily better than death. However, there is a controversy surrounding the role of individual choice in dying and who should decide; the patient, the family members, the physician, or the law? Although most people support the right of conscious, mentally stable adults to refuse medical treatment, even if it means death, who decides when very frail individuals are not able to decide for themselves? Should life be artificially prolonged if there is only a minute chance of recovery? If not, then who should decide when a life is no longer of worth and death should be allowed? Although it is generally accepted that life-sustaining measures, such as feeding tubes or ventilators, may be refused, once they are in place, who should decide whether they are to be removed? If a person suffers a heart attack, who should determine whether or not to resuscitate? Should family members be permitted to request that everything be done to keep the patient alive, even if the chance of recovery is minimal, the treatment causes pain for the patient, and the cost of the treatment is exorbitant? When does the cost of care become a part of the decision?

> Most of us would like a quiet, dignified death. Anyone who works in a hospital knows that this reasonable wish is almost never fulfilled and most of us now die in hospitals. The last rites of respirators, dialysis machines, nasogastric tubes and gastrostomy tubes along with cardiopulmonary resuscitation and the nth round of chemotherapy are wonderful when prolonging useful life but have changed death into a mechanized spectacle in which no sane person would like to be the main actor.[2]

Whether or not measures are implemented to maintain life depends upon the patient's age, income, preferences of the patient and family, type and severity of illnesss, and prognosis. For example, an elderly person with widespread cancer who finally succumbs to pneumonia will generally not be resuscitated vigorously, tube fed, or put on a ventilator. On the other hand, a young college student involved in a motor vehicle accident would most likely be aggressively treated. Even in the face of extremely poor prognosis, some patients or their families are adamant that "everything be done," including treatments that may be medically futile. In other cases, people with a good chance of partial recovery may refuse life-extending treatment, perhaps motivated by fear of prolonged suffering.

Ethical issues surrounding care at the end of life become more complex when the cost of treatment is considered. Although patients themselves are somewhat insulated from the actual costs, it is true that money allocated to health care is limited.

What Is Your Opinion? Setting Limits on Care to Frail Elders

Bioethicist Daniel Callahan believes that the health problems of disabled elders should not be treated the same as younger adults. He believes that there is a time that the fight against death should stop. If the nation had infinite financial resources, treating elders equal to younger people would be acceptable. However, since Medicare puts no controls on payments for excessive life-prolonging technology, old people are favored. In order to counteract the drain of money to the 65 and older group, he developed the following principles, called the life-cycle approach to medical care. Others call it age-based rationing of care, setting limits on the medical care provided to frail elders.

1. After a person has lived out a natural life span (late seventies), medical care should no longer be oriented to resisting death.
2. Provision of medical care for those who have lived out a normal life span will be limited to the relief of suffering.
3. Although medical technologies are available to extend the lives of elderly who have lived out a

natural life span, it should not be presumed that they should be used for that purpose.[4]

Even though many doctors may follow this approach, there is a concern that once treatment is denied because of advanced age, it is a "slippery slope" to denying other groups, such as gender, race, ethnicity, or extent of disability.[5] Other ethicists argue that health care considerations should be based on the potential for treatment success, not on age.[6]

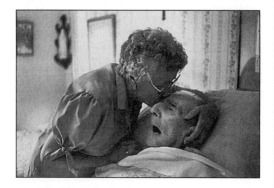

The aging of the population, combined with newer more expensive technology to prolong life, has markedly increased the costs associated with care for the dying, especially those in their last weeks or days of life. Medical care near the end of life consumes 10 to 12 percent of the total health care budget and 27 percent of the Medicare budget.[3] When health care resources (provided by the government or insurance companies) support a dying patient, fewer resources are available to other patients, many of whom have a better prognosis. Although it is difficult to place more value on one person's life than another, in the face of limited health care dollars, these decisions need to be faced. However, the dilemma takes on a different focus when the dying individual is you or your loved one.

Euthanasia

A topic that continues to engage heated public debate is euthanasia. *Euthanasia* is the painless putting to death of a person suffering from an incurable condition. *Passive euthanasia* is withholding treatment that would otherwise prolong life, allowing death to occur naturally. If a person with severe lung disease is not put on a ventilator or given antibiotics to prolong life, this is passive euthanasia. In contrast, *active euthanasia* occurs when someone takes an active step to deliberately end another's life, such as giving an overdose of medication. The differences between active and passive euthanasia are not always clear-cut. For instance, "pulling the plug" on a ventilator is sometimes considered passive because it allows the death to progress naturally, but it is active in that it is an intentional, conscious act to end life.

Advance Directives

Advance directives are legal documents that enable individuals to convey their desires about life-prolonging medical treatment when they are no longer able to make their wishes known. *Living wills* discuss specific medical treatments to be withheld or withdrawn in certain situations, and proxy, or *durable power of attorney for health care*

specifies an individual to assist in medical decision making for a person who is no longer physically or mentally competent. Living wills are usually generic and focus on choices of specific interventions, such as cardiopulmonary resuscitation (CPR), artificial feeding, or use of a ventilator machine. A durable power of attorney for health care is more flexible because the individual appoints a trusted person who ideally makes decisions based on the individual's wishes and in the individual's best interest.

Each state has its own specific requirements regarding advance directives. In general, these documents must be signed and witnessed when a person is mentally capable. A witness should not be a blood relative or beneficiary of property. Completed copies of the documents should be given to physicians and family members and should be taken to the hospital or nursing home to be included in medical records. Because older people are at higher risk of becoming ill or dying, they are encouraged to prepare advance directives and sign legally binding documents regarding medical treatments while still mentally competent. The federal Patient Self-Determination Act of 1991 requires all patients admitted to health care institutions to be informed about their right to participate in medical decisions about their care, to be aware of advance directives, and to document their wishes for life-sustaining treatments in certain situations. However, a study in 1993 reported that only 13 percent of nursing home residents had completed a living will or durable power of attorney, indicating that decisions on end-of-life care will fall to the family or a court-appointed guardian.[7]

Advance directives are theorized to provide proof of the patient's wishes when the patient is no longer able to make decisions and have been upheld in court. However, studies show they are not widely used in decision making for care of the dying. Why are advance directives not more widely used? First, few patients complete them. It is estimated that fewer than one in five Americans have made a living will,[8] and only one-third of frail elders in nursing homes had any advance directives.[9] Individuals only rarely discuss their wishes with their physician, and copies of advance directives (from home or nursing home) too often do not make it to the hospital to influence decision making there. Further, despite advance directives, if a family calls 911 in an effort to improve the comfort of a terminally ill relative, paramedics are required by law to provide CPR if the heart has stopped beating. (Some states will recognize "do-not-resuscitate" orders outside the hospital if they are signed by a doctor.)

There are other reasons why advance directives are underused. Healthy people may not complete a living will because their death seems so far off. Some people may not want to think or talk about their death, have cultural proscriptions about such preparations, or know nothing about living wills. Another difficulty with these documents is that healthy people may not be able to predict what they might wish if they were disabled. For instance, an individual may believe that if she was to become dependent on a ventilator that she would not wish to live. However, if this situation actually happened, she may change her mind. Individuals with multiple disabilities often have a high quality of life if they have appropriate supports and care.

Another difficulty with a living will is the inability to predict the situations that might come up and to write a directive detailed enough to handle all contingencies. There are hundreds of possible scenarios, and it is impossible to micromanage one's own dying before one becomes ill. For instance, a person may refuse chemotherapy for one type of cancer because of its poor success rate, but would undergo this treatment for another type of cancer. A person may not desire artificial feeding in one situation, but be willing in other circumstances.

The average citizen knows precious little about the realm of therapeutic possibilities that differ substantively from one diagnosis to another. Without knowing the benefits and risks of each type of life-extending procedure for one's personal situation, how can anyone make a good choice regarding cardiopulmonary resuscitation, artificial feeding, intravenous fluids, intensive care, chemotherapy, or surgery? To clarify the patient's intent, a medical directive form was designed to be used in conjunction with a living will that includes several scenarios and allows patients to select the treatments they would desire in each case.

Finally, it is often difficult for the patient and family to admit, or the physician to determine, that the patient is dying and that it is time for the provisions of the living will to be enacted. Studies show that physicians often only write do-not-resuscitate orders when patients are very near death. Because there is almost always more treatment possible and patients with terminal illnesses may live a long time, it is often difficult to decide when certain therapies are "heroic" or "ill-advised" and should be avoided or terminated. Doctors may not communicate to the patient their own opinions about his or her poor prognosis leaving the patient to believe that treatments may be helpful. Ideally, treatment alternatives should be communicated to the patient with specifics about the risks and benefits. Unfortunately, many of the treatments have not been rigorously tested.

Even if a living will is signed and given to the physician, there is no guarantee that the patient's wishes will be honored. In one pilot study, the treatment given to about one-fourth of the patients in one nursing home conflicted with the patient's advance directives. Most of the living wills were never transferred from nursing homes to hospitals when patients were moved. Even when they were transferred, there was little correlation with the course of treatment.[10] However, because so few patients understand advance directives, it is questionable whether advance directives truly represent the patient's wishes."[11] Although these documents may not influence the nuts and bolts of medical treatment, they may be an important step in initiating conversations with family and friends regarding desires and preferences. This communication between patients, families, and physicians has been shown to increase rates of satisfaction with care, as well as reducing hospital costs for end-of-life care.[12] However, even with improved communication between patient and physician and execution of advance directives, many physicians remain unaware of their patient's wishes and provide overly aggressive care at the end of life.[13]

Some of the problems with living wills are minimized by the durable power of attorney document,

What Is Your Opinion? Life and Death Choices Using the Medical Directive

In choosing the Medical Directive, you can give specific directions in advance about medical procedures to be used—or not used—in six situations where you would be unable to make decisions or speak for yourself. The complete Medical Directive form contains six grids identical to the one below. Above each grid is one of the six descriptions below, each applying to a different medical situation. By checking the appropriate box in the grid, a person makes his or her wishes clearly known.

Situation A. If I am in a coma or a persistent vegetative state and, in the opinion of my physician and two consultants, have no known hope of regaining awareness and higher mental functions no matter what is done, then my wishes—if medically reasonable—for this and any additional illness would be:

Situation B. If I am in a coma and, in the opinion of my physician and two consultants, have a small but uncertain chance of regaining higher mental functions, a somewhat greater chance of surviving with permanent brain damage and a much greater chance of not recovering at all, then my wishes would be:

Situation C. If I have brain damage or some brain disease that in the opinion of my physician and two consultants cannot be reversed and that makes me unable to recognize people, to speak meaningfully to them, or to live independently, *and I also have a terminal illness,* then my wishes would be:

Situation D. If I have brain damage or some brain disease that in the opinion of my physician and two consultants cannot be reversed and that makes me unable to recognize people, to speak meaningfully to them, or to live independently, *but I have no terminal illness,* then my wishes would be:

Situation E. If, in the opinion of my physician and two consultants, I have an incurable illness that involves mental disability or physical suffering and ultimately causes death, and in addition I have an illness that is immediately life-threatening but reversible, and I am temporarily unable to make decisions, then my wishes—if medically reasonable—would be:

Situation F. If I am in my current state of health (describe briefly) and then have an illness that, in the opinion of my physician and two consultants, is life-threatening but reversable, and I am temporarily unable to make decisions, then my wishes—if medically reasonable—would be:

	I want	I want treatment tried. If no clear improvement, stop.	I am undecided	I do not want
CARDIOPULMONARY RESUSCITATION (chest compressions, drugs, electric shocks, and artificial breathing aimed at reviving a person who is on the point of dying) **OR MAJOR SURGERY** (for example, removing the gallbladder or part of the colon)		*Not applicable*		
MECHANICAL BREATHING (respiration by machine, through a tube in the throat) **OR DIALYSIS** (cleaning the blood by machine or by fluid passed through the belly)				
BLOOD TRANSFUSIONS OR BLOOD PRODUCTS		*Not applicable*		
ARTIFICIAL NUTRITION AND HYDRATION (given through a tube in a vein or in the stomach)				
SIMPLE DIAGNOSTIC TESTS (for example, blood tests or X rays) **OR ANTIBIOTICS** (drugs to fight infection)		*Not applicable*		
PAIN MEDICATIONS (even if they dull consciousness and indirecly shorten my life)		*Not applicable*		

Emanuel, L. L. and Emanuel, E.V. 1989. The Medical Directive. *Journal of the American Medical Association* 261:3288–3293. Copyright 1989, American Medical Association.

where the patient appoints another individual (called a surrogate)—spouse, friend, child, or parent—to make medical decisions when he or she can no longer do so. However, there is some evidence that the surrogates may not be correctly interpreting the patient's wishes.[14] Without an advance directive, decisions about care are generally made quietly between family members and the health care team. In rare cases when family and the health care team disagree, then decisions are made by the court.

Each state is responsible for developing its own advance directive laws and unique procedures to enable a dying person's wishes to be carried out. State-specific advance directives are available from Choice in Dying, Inc., 1035 30th St. NW, Washington, DC 20007 (1-800-989-9455) or www.choices.org. Choice in Dying is a nonprofit organization that deals with end-of-life issues and provides public and professional education, advance directives, and counseling about the preparation and use of these documents.

Assisted Suicide

Although not euthanasia, a similar concept is *assisted suicide,* where a physician or other person knowledgeable in certain ways to assure death, helps a seriously ill individual to commit suicide by providing a lethal dose of an agent. The most publicized advocate of assisted suicide is Dr. Jack Kavorkian, a retired Michigan pathologist. Despite multiple arrests, imprisonment, loss of his medical license, and political censure, he facilitated the suicides of 130 terminally ill patients. Over the years, he had been tried for murder four times, resulting in three acquittals and one mistrial. Subsequently, in April 1999, he was convicted of second-degree murder after administering a lethal injection to Thomas Youk, a 52-year-old man with Lou Gehrig's disease, at Youk's request. Prosecutors charged him after he appeared on "60 Minutes" with a videotape of the act because he wanted to force the issue of assisted suicide into the limelight. In addition to the murder charge, he was also convicted for the possession of a controlled substance. He was sentenced to ten to twenty-five years in prison. The decision is currently under appeal.

What Is Your Opinion?

Jessica Cooper, the judge who sentenced Dr. Kavorkian to ten to twenty-five years for the videotaped death of Thomas Youk shown on "60 Minutes," said the following words to him at his sentencing:

> "This trial is not about the political or moral correctness of euthanasia. It was about you, sir. It was about lawlessness. It was about disrespect for a society that exists because of the strength of the legal system. No one, sir, is above the law. No one. You had the audacity to go on national television, show the world what you did and dare the legal system to stop you. Well, sir, consider yourself stopped." (Associated Press, April 14, 1999)

Assisted suicide is a very controversial issue. Depending on the survey, from one-half to two-thirds of the American public think physicians should be allowed by law to help terminally ill patients end their lives painlessly, although most people are also cognizant of the need for safeguards to protect the vulnerable. Proponents of assisted suicide argue that preventing prolonged suffering from incurable or terminal illnesses is necessary. Opponents argue assisted suicide is the first step on a "slippery slope" of devaluing human life and suggest that the pain and depression that kindle a desire to end one's life can often be effectively alleviated. Many believe that patients might choose euthanasia for the wrong reason, such as saving their family the burden of paying for nursing home care.

Although the majority of physicians oppose active euthanasia, most support a terminally ill patient's right to die, and some would practice euthanasia if it were legal. Results vary, but surveys reveal that about half the physicians in the United States support assisted suicide, with about one-third willing to participate in hastening the death of a patient. One survey of almost 2,000 physicians found that more than one in six of the respondents had received requests for physician-assisted suicide and euthanasia. About 6 percent had helped a patient commit suicide, either by pills or a lethal injection. Many more physicians reported they would practice it if it became legal.[15]

A combination of individual fears about dying in pain or "on machines" and personal experience with the "undignified death" of loved ones have initiated a new movement. Led by Derek Humphrey, author of *The Final Exit,* a how-to book on ending one's life painlessly, this group seeks to introduce state legislation and voter initiatives to legalize assisted suicide and some types of euthanasia. Its proponents argue that the right to take one's own life is as important as the right to life, that death with dignity is preferable to prolonged life with a terminal illness, and that the quality of life, not its duration, is the most important.

Through high court decisions, legislation, and voter initiatives, states are clarifying the limits of active and passive euthanasia and assisted suicide. In many states, voter initiatives have been put on the ballot, sometimes to permit physician-assisted suicide, other times to prohibit it. The states of Washington and New York passed statutes that prohibited physician-assisted suicide. The "right to die" groups in those states challenged the initiatives, asserting that there is a constitutional right to physician-assisted suicide. The cases went through the higher courts, and finally, in 1997, the Supreme Court unanimously ruled that physician-assisted suicide was not a constitutional right, allowing state laws permitting or outlawing assisted suicide to stand.

During their deliberations on physician-assisted suicide, the Supreme Court justices were very sensitized to the need of the terminally ill to be free of

Guidelines for Physician-Assisted Suicide

Multiple guidelines have been put forth to implement physician-assisted suicide if and when legislation permits it. These guidelines were developed by seven Michigan physicians and Dr. Kevorkian with the goal of putting the process of dying under the control of the patient, not prosecutors or politicians.

1. The request for help in committing suicide must be made in writing by the patients. The request must be signed (and notarized) by the patient, any physician involved in the request, and two competent adults who have no financial interest in the patient's life or death.

2. The request must be reviewed by a professional with experience in the area who will refer the patient to a specialist in the patient's illness, a pain-management specialist if that is relevant, and a psychiatrist.

3. Those doctors must verify that the patient is mentally competent to make the decision, and that the illness is incurable (some experts specify terminal), that the patient's pain cannot be controlled, or that the side effects of the pain medication are intolerable. The reports from these consultations will be reviewed by either the obitiatrist (the individual responsible for performing the act) or by another physician requested by the patient.

4. Within three weeks, the patient must decide the time and place for the assisted suicide in a signed informed consent that is also signed by the requesting physician and two competent adults.

5. The assisted suicide must be performed 24 to 72 hours after the informed consent's signing.

6. The patient can call off the assisted suicide at any time.

7. The obitiatrist will perform the assisted suicide for no fee; other physicians involved in the case may be present, but will not participate in the final act.

© Associated Press

pain and suffering while dying. They requested experts in the field, such as hospice groups and the American Medical Association, to make a statement about controlling pain during the dying process. The group assured the justices that pain can be controlled for most patients without heavy sedation, but for a few, sedation to a sleeplike state may be necessary in the last days or weeks of life to prevent the patient from experiencing severe pain.[16,17]

A part of the Supreme Court ruling that was not as well-publicized, but may be very important, is that individuals have the right to adequate palliative care (care to alleviate pain and other suffering). Further, the Supreme Court prohibited any state law or regulation from obstructing the provision of adequate care to alleviate pain and other physical symptoms of people facing death. So, although physicians may not intentionally hasten death, the ruling does permit them to use a drug to hasten death if the drug is intended for other purposes, such as pain relief. Thus, they asserted that terminal sedation intended to relieve symptoms is not assisted suicide, even though terminal sedation hastens death. This ruling will invalidate several states' regulations that unduly restrict the prescribing of opiates for pain relief and will also eliminate the disciplining of physicians who prescribe high doses of opioids to their patients by regulatory boards of some states.

Terminal sedation can often be used as a form of euthanasia and, some experts believe that terminal sedation is ethically more problematic than assisted suicide because it is can be a type of euthanasia without the safeguards, making it more vulnerable to abuse. For instance, physicians can prescribe terminal sedation without the patient's consent. One expert asserted that patients who undergo terminal sedation are required to accept a form of death that may be less desirable for them.[18]

Suicide

Choosing to kill oneself is the ultimate human decision. What are the circumstances in which it is justified? And when is it condemned? The act of suicide may range from an irrational act committed by a mentally unstable individual to a premedi-

tated, rational decision to end a life of physical or mental anguish. Suicide is a serious problem for all ages, but elders commit disproportionately more suicides than other age groups, and the rates have been rising since 1980. The suicide rate for each grouping older than sixty-five is higher than that for any other ten-year age grouping, including the youth population. Those elders seventy-five and older have a suicide rate nearly double the national average. In 1996, elders in the United States accounted for 13 percent of the population but almost 20 percent of the suicides.[19]

In our country, gender plays a large role in suicide rates, with men accounting for over 80 percent of suicides among those over age sixty-five. Race is also important: whites kill themselves at higher rates than non-whites. Elderly white men have the highest suicide risk of any other group.[19] Despite these high numbers, suicide rates are underestimated among older people because many suicides are reported as other causes of death (for example, drug overdoses, refusal of life-sustaining drugs, intentional starvation, and accidents).

Important risk factors for suicide at any age are depression, alcoholism, and poor physical health, especially if accompanied by chronic pain and disability. Those who are divorced or widowed are at higher risk that those who are married. Crises, such as the diagnosis of serious illness or the death of a spouse, may increase risk of suicide. The circumstances that lead an older person to suicide are unlikely to be one single factor, but many factors interacting with one another. The breakdown or failure of coping methods, social supports, and other resources occur when several conditions exist simultaneously, finally overwhelming or exhausting the person's ability to cope.

Elders who attempt suicide are more likely to succeed than are younger adults. Younger persons often act impulsively, but older people are more likely to plan their suicide attempts and to use highly lethal methods. Approximately three-fourths of the suicides among elders are accomplished with a gun. Elders may be more determined to kill themselves and less likely to attempt suicide for attention or to hurt another person.

Most elders provide behavioral and verbal clues to suicide prior to the act. Previous suicide attempts, preoccupation with suicidal thought, agitation, or expression of hopelessness are important indicators. An older person who is planning suicide may purchase a firearm, stockpile pills, make funeral arrangements, or give away valued possessions. Verbal clues may be direct (e.g., "I'm going to kill myself") or indirect (e.g., "I'm tired of life, what's the point of going on?") Family, friends, and professionals should be alert to prolonged depression or hints about suicide and should openly discuss the topic. When an elder suddenly seems happier after a period of depression, this can serve as a sign that he or she has made a plan and is at *higher* risk of suicide. Contrary to popular belief, talking about suicide will not increase suicidal intentions. Many suicides could be prevented if high-risk elders were identified and referred to appropriate help.

Most elders visit a physician within a month of the suicide event with vague somatic complaints that mask their anguish and helplessness. Whether due to lack of time, interest, or skill, few physicians are trained to recognize symptoms of depression or assess risk of suicide in their patients. Many doctors are still fearful of discussing death and suicide, mistakenly believing that these discussions will make individuals more likely to take their own life.

Unfortunately, few suicide prevention programs in our country are designed for elders. McIntosh discusses several approaches to suicide prevention for elders.[20] Primary prevention programs include information, education, and training programs about suicide and aging for people who are in contact with elders from a variety of settings, particularly health professionals and those working in senior programs. Secondary prevention (crisis intervention and therapy) includes seeking out those most at risk and providing them with services to reduce their depression and risk of suicide. Strategies for reducing suicide among older persons include peer-counseling programs, outreach efforts targeting high-risk persons, improvement of mental health services to treat depression, and pro-

Warning Signs of Suicide

- Depressed or irritable mood
- Withdrawal from usual pleasurable activities
- Overwhelming sense of helplessness, hopelessness, unworthiness, or guilt
- Difficulty in thinking or concentrating
- Self-neglect, including failure to take life-sustaining medications
- Neglecting home, finances, pets
- Weight change, loss of appetite, change in sleeping patterns
- Low energy or unexplained fatigue
- Physical complaints out of proportion to physical findings
- Sudden interest or disinterest in religion
- Giving away prized possessions
- Unusual behavior—buying a gun, stockpiling pills, changing a will
- Signs of frequent drinking
- Verbal statements suggesting desire to die
- Has a suicide plan
- Tried to commit suicide before

grams to increase awareness of risk factors among those with frequent contact with elders. One particular intervention in Italy was very successful in significantly reducing deaths by initiating a two-pronged telephone service. One was a monitoring service in which the user could send an alarm signal to activate a network of assistance and help. The second was a visiting service in which trained staff members visited each client twice a week to monitor the client's condition and offer emotional support.[21]

Some people take the controversial viewpoint that elderly suicides are more often "rational" suicides: individuals choose to take their own lives rather than live out their final days ill, in pain, disabled, or being a burden to their family. Suicides have a great impact on the survivors, who often feel guilty for not having noticed the victim's trauma or for not intervening soon enough. Many survivors feel responsible for the victim's action. Furthermore, because suicide is not a socially acceptable means of dying, survivors of a suicide may receive less social support from friends. For these reasons, those close to suicide victims may need counseling and support to allay their feelings of guilt, depression, and self-blame.

A useful source of information that includes support groups for survivors, clinical training and suicide prevention centers is the American Association of Suicidology, 4201 Connecticut Ave., NW, Suite 130, Washington, D.C. 20008.

ATTITUDES TOWARD DYING AND DEATH

A number of studies indicate that attitudes toward dying and death change throughout the life cycle. Because death is universal (we all will die) and frightening (we can never understand it), it is reasonable that death anxiety and fear are a part of everyone's life. However, many researchers believe that children think less about their own death than adults because they may believe death is impermanent or something that happens to "old" people. With advancing age, however, death looms somewhat closer and is more difficult to deny. Middle-aged individuals commonly reevaluate their life by assessing their accomplishments and envisioning future goals—what has been accomplished and what remains to be done. Time no longer stretches out endlessly as it did in adolescence and young adulthood.

Studies consistently report that fear of death diminishes with advancing age. This may be due to a number of factors. Richard Kalish, a leading thanatologist, asserts that death becomes more familiar with advancing age because older persons generally have more experience with the death of others than do younger groups.[22] In addition, the death of parents makes death more of a reality since parents generally die before their children. Furthermore, the urgency of staying alive diminishes when individuals no longer have dependent children. Finally, death is expected in the later

years, so older persons are more likely to be prepared and resigned to it.

Because death occurs more commonly among elders, it is not unusual that elders fear death less and think about death more than younger age groups. Some elders may talk about funeral arrangements or disposition of belongings; others may reminisce and take stock of their lives. Many elders cope with their impending death by preparation. Elders are more likely than younger people to have drafted a will, made funeral arrangements, paid for a cemetery plot, and arranged for someone to handle their affairs.[23] Older people who are institutionalized or those who are chronically ill, depressed, or disabled, may welcome death as a release from continued disability and pain. Many have already started to withdraw from family and friends, have lost much of their autonomy, and have been separated from the pleasures in life that made it meaningful.

Although older people are less likely to fear their own death than younger persons, they are more likely to fear the process of dying. Common fears include fear of prolonged illness or disability, being a burden on others, separation or rejection from loved ones, being dependent, and being in pain. Elders often fear dying alone, dying without dignity, and being forgotten after they die.[24]

OPTIONS ON WHERE TO DIE

Historically, the family has had the major responsibility of caring for dying relatives, and almost all the dying were cared for in the home. Over the years, institutions (hospitals and nursing homes) have taken more responsibility for the dying.

The transfer of responsibility from the family to the institution has altered the care of the dying. Families are motivated to care for their dying largely because of emotional ties, whereas institutions are motivated by economic gain. Because hospitals focus on control of physical problems, care is less personal and seldom meets the emotional or social needs of the patient. The advent of advanced medical technology and drugs have extended the length of life, but they also have prolonged the dying interval, isolating the terminally ill and placing added

What Is Your Opinion? How Do You Want to Die?

Harold M. hadn't felt well for the past three days and had actually been on his way to the doctor when he experienced sudden chest pressure. He decided to drive directly to the hospital emergency room. He was found dead in the driver's seat from a heart attack and fatal arrythmia in the parking lot of the hospital. His wife of thirty-seven years was shocked to learn of his death—he had been so healthy (except for a little high blood pressure and cholesterol) and had not yet retired. They had plans to travel the country in an RV upon his retirement later that year. She regretted they had not had a chance to say goodbye and knew little about the family finances. Their children, arriving for the funeral, thought it may have been better to die quickly, with a minimum of pain and suffering and worry about death. Their dad had been so independent and proud, they reasoned, he wouldn't have tolerated the indignities of a slow death.

Margaret S. had lost some weight over the past six months and had a nagging stomach ache, and her over-the-counter antacids were not working anymore. When her stomach cancer was diagnosed, it had already spread to most of her liver, and the doctors said there was little they could do. She underwent chemotherapy, but felt ill, and the tumor's growth was not slowed, so she elected to stop treatment. As she became weaker, her children were able to visit her and say goodbye, and she resolved a long-standing dispute with her eldest daughter. Her husband became overwhelmed with caregiving and hired a live-in helper (despite his concerns about spending their savings). He had promised never to put her in a nursing home. She had some pain, and this was treated with morphine. She spent the last two weeks of her life in a coma and died in her sleep with her husband in the bed next to her.

What are some of the advantages and disadvantages of a sudden death?

A more prolonged dying? Which would you prefer for yourself or your loved ones?

What have been your personal experiences with death and dying?

What are your biggest fears about dying? Your greatest hopes?

Do you think people have any control over the kind of death they have?

If you have six months to live, what would you want to accomplish in that time? What if you were very weak and unable to travel?

What issues do you think people must resolve before they die?

strain upon the family. In some cases, there are positive aspects to dying in a hospital or nursing home. The patient may receive better medication for pain or other symptoms, and the family may be freed from overwhelming responsibilities for body care, being able to focus on the patient's emotional needs. With the advent of cost-cutting measures in hospitals and the trend toward home recovery, the trend towards dying in hospitals may be reversed.

A number of factors influence where death occurs: the health condition of the person, amount of care required, and the availability of a willing caretaker and in-home services. People who live alone are more likely to go to an institution or hospital to die than those who live with family. Married men are more likely to die at home than married women since wives are more likely to be alive to care for dying spouses than vice versa. Personal preference also plays a role. Most elders prefer the familiar surroundings and personalized care at home, but some do not want to burden their families and prefer hospitalization.

Hospitals are the most common place of death, but some experts believe that they may not be the most appropriate place. Physicians generally subscribe to the view that death is pathological, not natural, so they value cure more than easing of symptoms. Their training is geared

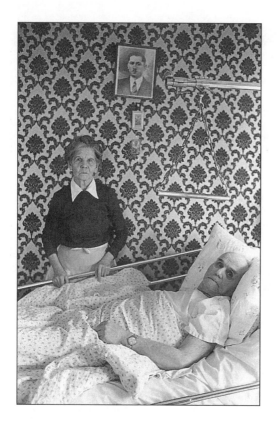

toward saving lives and controlling death rather than alleviating symptoms and meeting the psychosocial needs of the dying. Many doctors are fearful of using the high doses of opioid medications required to alleviate pain or are uneducated about the use of medications for symptom relief. Doctors and nurses must meet the acute medical needs of patients and have less time to provide a restful, supportive, and comfortable patient- and family-centered environment. Furthermore, the bureaucratic nature of hospital policies and procedures (for example, frequent blood draws, having to ask for pain medication) can deplete the scarce energy resources of the dying and depersonalize the patient.

In-home services can provide an alternative for the dying patient. Services may include everything from homemaking services to twenty-four-hour nursing care (see chapter 13). Elders who are disabled and slowly dying and who are unable to be

cared for at home by family or hired help generally reside in *skilled nursing facilities.* Although some individuals die in these facilities, others are transferred to a hospital for their final days or hours. Although many individuals in nursing facilities are dying, staff is often not trained to deal with the multiple medical, social, and psychological needs of the dying. Further, seldom is there education and support for staff to learn to work with dying patients.

Hospice care enables people to remain at home in the final phase of a terminal illness while offering support to the family. Hospice refers to a concept of supportive palliative care (making the patient as comfortable as possible). This includes efforts to relieve pain (with strong medication, if needed), reduce distressing symptoms, maintain alertness, provide a dignified death for the patient, and support and comfort the family. Hospice programs use multidisciplinary teams composed of clergy, physicians, nurses, social workers, and trained volunteers who offer medical services, personal care, and emotional and spiritual support for the dying, as well as respite care and grief counseling for bereaved family members. No curative, life-prolonging treatment is provided. About two-thirds of those using hospice care are over sixty-five. Over 80 percent of hospice patients have cancer, although some have other diagnoses, such as end-stage cardiac or pulmonary disease and AIDS.[25] Often hospice patients die at home, although they may be admitted to inpatient facilities for their final days for symptom relief.

Medicare finances hospice benefits for those who are already covered by Medicare. To be eligible, both the patient's physician and the hospice director must certify that the patient is terminally ill and has six months or less to live. The patient must sign a statement to choose hospice care rather than the standard medical benefits. When a patient receives hospice services, Medicare pays the entire cost of physician services, nursing care, medical appliances and supplies, drugs for pain and symptom relief, social services and counseling, and physical therapy. It also pays for up to five days per stay for care in a nursing home or hospital to provide time off for the person caring for the individual at home (respite care). There are about

1,800 hospice programs in the country, serving about 60,000 terminally ill patients.[25] Information on hospice services and referral to the nearest hospice can be obtained by calling the National Hospice Organization at 1-800-658-8898.

Many more seriously ill individuals could benefit from hospice; however, an acceptance of hospice care is an acceptance that death is inevitable, and many individuals continue to search for new treatments, even when death is near. Many endure pain and suffering in a hospital or nursing home, and seek hospice care when they have only a few weeks to live, reducing the benefits of pain-reducing medications and social services. Earlier referral to a hospice program may improve their quality of their remaining days by providing pain-relieving medicine and support services.[26]

Even with help from a hospice and other home services, managing the impending death of a terminally ill relative at home may be too anxiety-provoking for some families.[27] Further, having relatives care for physical needs may be humiliating and distressing for both the ill person and the family member. Finally, some patients may feel guilty that they are a burden on their loved ones, not only emotionally but financially. Thus, it is important to remember that home may not be the best place to die for everyone.

Grandpa Pat
by Wendy Gabrielle Evans, medical student, University of California, San Diego School of Medicine

Until Grandpa Pat died in the summer of 1995, I hadn't had much close experience with death and dying. He was diagnosed with prostate cancer about ten years before he died. The radiation treatment he underwent soon after his diagnosis did little to slow the course of his disease, and during the spring of my junior year in college, we learned that the cancer had metastasized to his bones and Grandpa Pat started to plan for his death. All his life, he had been a difficult man to get along with, reluctant to show his feelings and too proud to apologize to anyone or say he was wrong. While his stubbornness brought him great success as a leader in the longshoreman's union in San Francisco and later as a lobbyist in Washington, it left significant battle scars on his relationships. Coming closer to his end mellowed him, though, and he made many reconciliations. He had been estranged from his son Dan since Dan's teens, and my mother and I feared that Grandpa Pat would die without talking to his son. But Dan and Grandpa Pat proved us wrong. During that last year, Dan took care of my grandfather. He was there every day fixing his medication schedule, getting his food, taking him to the doctor.

My relationship with Grandpa Pat was different from his relationship with other members of our family in that it was not wrought with as many conflicts and hard feelings. He was infinitely proud of me, thought I was the smartest, most beautiful girl in the world. His pride in me was so unconditional and he talked about it so often that being around him always made me feel special. As his condition declined, we talked more and more on the telephone. He developed a real interest in his disease; I guess he wanted to figure out why he was dying. I tried to explain cancer to him in simple terms, translating from what I was learning in college biology, and went to the medical library and copied articles about prostate cancer for him. He said his doctors never explained his cancer to him in common terms, and it seemed to mean a lot to him to understand his illness.

The week my grandpa died was in late August. I was in Berkeley on vacation when my mom called to tell me that Grandpa Pat had been admitted to the hospital because he was acting strangely and seemed paranoid to Dan. We thought he was having trouble with the dosing of his hormone treatments and narcotics, but it turned out that tumors were encroaching on the drainage from his kidneys, so it wouldn't be long. His nitrogenous wastes would build up in his blood stream, he would slip into a peaceful coma, and die. Though my family told me that I didn't need

Grandpa Pat (*continued*)

to stay, I wanted to because I felt my presence would mean a lot to my grandfather. Staying with my family during that last week was one of the most wonderful experiences in my life. Working together to take care of Grandpa Pat, I felt closer to my family than I ever have before and that closeness stayed with us after he died.

I had always assumed that dying of cancer was not painful because drugs relieved the pain. I'm glad I was able to watch someone close to me suffer through his last week so that I will know what it is like for my patients. The narcotics, it is true, relieved the pain, but mentally made him feel awful. He became confused and agitated, so he was given another drug which made him groggy and sedated. We finally moved him home, where we cared for him—with much help from hospice, for the second half of the week. The hardest thing for us was determining when he needed more pain medication, especially when he could not communicate well through the drugs and uremia. Even when he could articulate how he was feeling, he didn't want to take the drugs because they took him away from us, but then his pain would become terrible and he would have to take more, but then he would become more groggy. It was an unending cycle.

For all of that, though, I have to say—and I know this sounds strange—that the last week of my grandfather's life was a fun and joyful time. Once he was home, my mom and I and my uncles took shifts staying with him. Once, when my mom and I tried to change his sheets, he resisted and resisted and kept whining "Wait, Wait" and we waited and finally he said okay he was ready and as soon as we started to lift him he started wailing "Wait, Wait" again. It turned out that he was embarrassed for us to see him naked, so when we closed our eyes and rolled it was okay. He laughed the whole time, though, becoming a comedian, and I think he loved having everyone there to pay attention to him and baby him.

Finally, I had to fly back to school and my mother back to work. Grandpa Pat could no longer speak, and could barely squeeze a hand. I think many people would wonder whether he knew at all what was going on around him. Before we left from our second to last day in San Francisco, I went to his room and sat with him and held his hand and explained that my mom and I were leaving the next day and that we were sorry we couldn't stay with him. I also told him that he should not be afraid, that he didn't need to hang on any longer and that he could just let go and leave us. He died three hours later.

Though we did mourn for my grandpa after his death, much of our grieving took place that week as we slowly said good-bye while watching him fade from a robust, overbearing man to a skinny, paralyzed vestige of what he once was. I also think that his week with us was what allowed him to die peacefully and happily. He was cremated, and we had a memorial for him a month later. There was more laughter than crying at the memorial. People told their stories about him and reminisced and we all heard some very funny stories. Afterwards, we scattered his ashes in the Pacific Ocean off San Francisco, so that he would always be near the city which symbolized his life and his work to him. The whole family gathered around my mother as she opened the bag that contained what was left of Grandpa Pat. The ashes were a beautiful purple color and glinted when the sun shone on them as they fell to the water, swirled around, and were gone.

THE DYING TRAJECTORY

When a person is diagnosed as terminally ill, his or her social status changes radically. Even though an individual was previously an important, contributing member of the community, the person now is forced to withdraw as it becomes obvious that time is running out. Former friends may ignore the sick individual because they are not comfortable in being around the dying. Alternatively, family members may travel great distances, become more open about their feelings toward each other, or renew estranged relationships. As weakness progresses, the social sphere of the sick person becomes very small. Even conversation may become difficult and the sick person may no longer desire to interact with more than a handful of friends and family members. Many former activities and broader interests disappear as the sick person becomes more focused on the tasks of dying and activities directly related to day-to-day comfort and survival. Although many people face their own death fully awake or die suddenly while sleeping, often the process of dying involves days, weeks, or months, characterized by a withdrawal from communication, diminished appetite, increased sleepiness, disorientation, and a dulling of consciousness.

It is commonly thought that the end of life is fraught with existential concerns, anguish, or spiritual rebirth. In actuality, the concerns of the dying more often revolve around symptoms, fear of pain and loss of control, indignity, and being a burden to their families. It may be that the fear of pain is well-founded. Although estimates vary widely, between one-third and three-quarters of cancer

patients report uncontrolled pain near the end of life. Among those with other illnesses, about one-third have pain at the end of life. In contrast, only a small proportion of patients (2 percent) under hospice care, which emphasizes symptom palliation, have inadequate pain control when dying. Guidelines on management of pain and other symptoms (shortness of breath, nausea, agitation) at the end of life are available for general physicians when physicians trained in palliative medicine are not available.[16]

It is commonly observed that those who are very old eventually undergo a decline in abilities, become increasingly apathetic, and lose the desire to eat and drink. This behavior ends in death, even in the absence of terminal disease. Even though this loss in the will to live is probably the most natural way to die, the accompanying symptoms are often medicalized by physicians, with subsequent efforts to reverse the decline.[28] Death has become

A Case of the Dwindles

H. Y. is a 94-year-old widow who was hospitalized three times in three months for dehydration, urinary tract infection, and stool impaction. Despite treatment for her illnesses and a trial of an antidepressant, she continued to lose weight and functional ability until she was bed-bound. She denied having sleep disturbances or problems with appetite, although she ate little. She had previously been married to a man with high rank in the military and still maintained a close-knit group of other widowed socialites. She missed her husband very much, but thought her life was "all right." Medically there was nothing found that could be treated to explain her decline. She developed a decubitus ulcer (bedsore) from lying in bed. She remained cheery, even when talking about death, but maintained she was "tired of living" and "ready whenever the good Lord wants to take me." She was very polite with caregivers and friends who attempted to motivate her to become more active, and vowed to "get on the ball after her birth-

day." She died peacefully of unknown causes after a brief decline only days before her ninty-fifth birthday.

Medical practitioners are noting a new phenomenon known as "the dwindles," or alternatively as "geriatric failure to thrive." These individuals manifest a gradual decline in physical and/or cognitive function, accompanied by weight loss, reduced appetite and social withdrawal that occurs without immediate explanation.[29] It seems that failure to thrive is a downhill spiral whereby poor nutrition affects cognitive function, which in turn leads to worsening nutrition, which increases susceptibility to disease and will to live as well as the ability to respond to stresses of life and illness. Failure to thrive carries a high rate of morbidity (e.g., poorer recovery from surgery, bedsores, repeated hospitalizations) and mortality and is sometimes considered a form of suicide. Some professionals have suggested that among the very old (individuals in their nineties and 100s), the "dwindles" may be what is meant by dying of "old age."

the enemy of medicine—a reminder of its limitations in diagnosis and treatment.[30] Mendes believes that the medicalization of dying trivializes the final event of our lives, distorting it from a natural event of great social and cultural significance into the end point of untreatable or inadequately treated disease or injury.[31] The case study on page 391 exemplifies this natural process. The attending physician called it a case of "the dwindles."

Based on her extensive work with the dying, Elizabeth Kübler-Ross, a Swiss-born psychiatrist, described five distinct stages through which many terminally ill patients pass, each a defense mechanism to cope with their impending death.[32] Kübler-Ross observed that the stages were not absolutes because the time spent in each stage and the sequence varied among individuals, and many stages overlapped. Superimposed on all the stages was hope, which remains possible in all five stages. The five stages are as follows:

Denial: When first learning that he or she is terminally ill, the patient registers shock and disbelief. The individual rejects the diagnosis, thinking that the lab reports must be mistaken or that the physician made a wrong diagnosis. This stage is generally short unless the family continues to deny the illness.

Anger: The diagnosed terminally ill patient will bemoan, "Why me?" The patient may become resentful that others are healthy while he or she must die. The individual may express anger at family members, health professionals, himself or herself, or the anger may be unfocused. Irritability and complaining are common.

Bargaining: During this stage, death becomes a reality, but the individual attempts to postpone the time of death by bargaining. Most deals are struck with God, even if one has never talked with God before, and most are secret. During this period, the dying individual may seek out alternative treatments, such as faith healers, unusual drugs, or vitamin supplements, to postpone death.

Depression: When it becomes obvious that a bargain cannot be struck, depression occurs. Death

is recognized as inevitable, and the feelings of loss become overwhelming. Whereas before the individual may have been talkative, crying, agitated, or seeking sympathy, during this stage the individual often withdraws from visitors and mourns silently. Mourning for loss of capability and lost relationships allows an individual to prepare for death and to attempt to make sense of life and death.

Acceptance: Individuals at this stage are often devoid of emotion and disengaged from the outside world. Many limit contact to one or two people who are very close. The dying are often tired and weak, and days are spent sleeping, resting, and reminiscing.

Kübler-Ross' work was revolutionary in that it sensitized the public and the medical profession to the needs of the dying. However, her research has been criticized on a number of counts. For one, there are no clear, observable behavior patterns for each stage; differentiation among stages relied on her subjective interpretation of the patient's emotions or motivations. Critics question her findings because they believe her subjects' emotions were probably highly vulnerable to suggestion and manipulation and may have been influenced by medications, since this variable was not controlled in her study. Another problem with the Kübler-Ross model is that, even though she did not envision these stages as a "correct" way to die, many health professionals erroneously interpret the stages as a prescription all must follow for a "good death." In some instances, this expectation leads to labeling patients and attempting to move them to different stages rather than helping them deal with their feelings and accepting their individuality. Many doctors and laypeople feel the dying need to get to the acceptance stage of their death. Finally, her findings were not confirmed by other studies.

Other research has revealed that there are many emotions associated with the dying process than those she described. Many experts agree with psychologist Edwin Schneidman's description of the dying process: "Rather than the five definite stages . . . . my experience has led me to posit a hive of affect, in which there is a constant coming and going. The emotional stages seem to include a constant interplay between disbelief and hope and, against these as background, a waxing and waning of anguish, terror, acquiescence and surrender, rage and envy, disinterest and ennui, pretense, taunting and daring and even yearning for death—all these in the context of bewilderment and pain."[34]

The general consensus is that the way one copes with the dying process is very individual. One expert's analysis of Kübler-Ross' work suggests that the most valuable lessons for families and professionals are (1) to assist the dying in resolving unfinished needs, (2) actively listen to those who are dying, and (3) help them identify their own needs. Further, we need to learn from those who are dying in order to come to know ourselves better.[34]

Kalish speaks for many when he expresses his views on his own dying process: "For some people and under some circumstances, acceptance of death is certainly the way to an appropriate death. For others, it is not. Perhaps anger, even fury, is the most appropriate way to die: what a mockery death is; how destructive it is; how absurd it is— there is nothing good about death, at least about *my* death and I have no intention of being peaceful or submissive or accepting!"[22] He echoes the words of Dylan Thomas' famous poem:

> Do not go gentle into that good night,
> Old age should burn and rave at close of day;
> Rage, rage against the dying of the light.

Rights of the Dying

Dying people are very vulnerable. The process of dying takes a lot of physical and psychic energy. Sedatives, painkillers, and some treatments can further reduce energy and cause disorientation and diminishing capabilities. As strength decreases, dying individuals are progressively less able to carry out daily activities. Because those who are dying are generally in a weakened state, family members and professionals are responsible to ensure that their rights are not violated. Following are some of these rights.

Right to Open Communication about Death

The majority of Americans believe individuals have the right to know about their impending death and would want to be told if they were dying. Because individuals commonly deny in the early stages that they are dying, it is generally most sensitive to inform them first that their condition is serious and allow them to ask more questions as they are ready to hear it. Knowledge of impending death allows dying persons to complete certain tasks before dying and to close their life in accordance with personal wishes. Additionally, full awareness of impending death allows an individual to make responsible decisions, such as where to die and what treatments to allow. However, individuals from some cultures do not believe that dying relatives should be informed of the severity of their illness.

Right to a Painless Death, to the Extent Possible

A common fear among elders is that their death will be painful. However, severe pain among the dying is not common, and most patients can become pain-free with proper medication. Physicians generally believe that painkillers, including strong opioids, should be given freely to the dying who are in severe pain. Other discomforting symptoms should be treated as well.

Right to the Presence of Concerned Others

Elders are more likely to die in lonely, isolated conditions than younger people. In fact, one of elders' greatest fears is abandonment at the time of death. A high proportion of elders may spend their dying interval without a concerned person to help make medical decisions or advocate adequate medical treatment. It is imperative that those who are dying alone be assigned a nurse or volunteer.

Right to as Much Control over Environment as Possible

Because the dying so often experience loss of control over their environment and declining health, it is imperative that health professionals and family allow the dying person as much control as possible. Allowing patients some choice over meals, frequency of nursing interruptions, visiting hours, roommates, and medical treatments can greatly enhance their feelings of autonomy.

Right to Have All Treatments Fully Explained and to Refuse Treatment

The dying, like other patients, have the right to have all medical treatments fully explained, including a description of the prognosis, methods of treatment, and potential risks, benefits, and side effects. For instance, chemotherapy, a common cancer treatment, has a variable success rate and is accompanied by many uncomfortable side effects, including hair loss and nausea. Because of this, many patients refuse the therapy, opting for a more comfortable, although perhaps shorter, life. As discussed earlier, patients have the right to refuse all heroic, artificial efforts to sustain life. On the other hand, it should not be assumed that all elders are ready to die and would refuse life-sustaining measures. Elders should have the right to all the technologically advanced equipment and treatments available to younger groups to prolong life and should be allowed to seek out alternative treatments, even those not condoned by the medical profession.

Tasks of the Dying

Individuals who know they are dying are often compelled to complete a number of tasks before they die. The importance of each task and the time spent on each varies with the degree of disability, the nature of the illness, the time left to live, the personality of the individual, and the environment, but will generally center around the following themes.[22,35]

Completing Unfinished Business

Individuals vary in the types of activities they wish to complete before death. The unfinished business may include reuniting with a distant family member, completing a photo album, or sharing intimate feelings with their family. It is important to let the dying person decide what tasks to accomplish and the ways the family and the health worker can help.

Dealing with Medical Care Needs

The dying need to understand their diagnosis and prognosis, learn of alternative treatments and pain-control methods, and decide on life-sustaining treatments. Furthermore, they need to tell others what measures should be taken if their condition worsens to a point where they are no longer in control. They may complete a living will or direct a family member to make medical decisions. The dying individual also needs to be involved in the decision whether to die in a hospital, in a nursing home, or at home.

Allocating Time and Energy Resources

We all have thought of what we would do if we knew we had five or six months to live. The usual answers—such as traveling or accomplishing a creative feat—generally include tasks that require more mental and physical energy than most dying persons possess. How much time and energy a dying individual can allocate depends on the nature of the illness and its progression. As the disease progresses, individuals generally become weaker and must be selective about which tasks can be accomplished before death and which must be left behind. Additionally, dying persons must choose who to spend time with during their last days.

Arranging for Death

Another important task for the dying is to arrange what will happen after death. The dying person may need to make a will and distribute valued possessions to loved ones before death. Many make decisions on cremation, burial, or donation of body organs. Some plan the details of their funeral. Others arrange for people to take care of finances and insurance policies as well as their pets.

Life Review

The dying often spend time reminiscing about their life and its meaning. Some contemplate on what it means to die and their belief in an afterlife. Many individuals turn to religion or God during this time to give them hope or justification for their suffering.

Caring for the Dying

Whether the seriously ill older person is dying at home or in an institution, the family is generally intensely involved. When the task becomes overwhelming or the sick person needs specialized care, institutionalization usually occurs.

The Family

Caring for a terminally ill patient brings about profound changes in family roles and interactions. A parent, once the caregiver for his or her children, now must depend on them for physical care, decision making, and emotional support. A husband may have to learn homemaking skills to care for an ailing wife. Caretakers must cope with feelings of loss and grief while dealing with the physical, emotional, and financial needs of a dying loved one. Family members may become overwhelmed with responsibility, and their feelings commonly

result in resentment and consequent guilt. For instance, the care of a very sick older person may require tremendous personal commitment, physical strength, and financial resources. At times, the caregiver may guiltily wish for the sick person to die. Although emotionally draining, caring for the dying can help the grieving process later on.

Open communication with the terminally ill about their illness and treatment, day-to-day concerns, death fears or anxieties, and life reminiscences can reduce isolation and bolster feelings of control. If the patient must be institutionalized, the caretaker may also serve as an advocate to ensure adequate care, as well as encourage patient compliance with necessary medical treatments.

Health Professionals

Many who work in the health and social services fields will have to deal with death and dying. However, many professionals are inadequately

Helping the Patient Who Is Approaching Death

The hospice staff realizes that this period of time is one of the most difficult times for the family to live through sometimes because "fear of the unknown" is greater than fear of the known. Our desire is to be as honest and straight-forward as possible in helping you through this period, so we offer you this information to help you prepare and anticipate symptoms that are indicative of approaching death. Your physician and the hospice nurse are available to help you clarify your concerns about this information. We want to describe each possible symptom to you in order to decrease your fear if one should appear suddenly. This will give you some guidelines about what you can do about the symptoms. The symptoms described are indicative of how the body prepares itself for the final stage of life; any one of the symptoms may be present, all may be present, or none may be present.

1. *Withdrawal:* Withdrawal is normal for the dying patient as they become less concerned about

their surroundings. Separation begins first from the world (no more interest in newspaper or television), then from people (no more neighbors visiting), and finally from the children, grandchildren, and perhaps even those persons most loved. With this withdrawal comes less of a need to communicate with others.

2. *Food:* Your loved one will have a decreased need for food and drink as the body is preparing to die. This is one of the hardest concepts for a family to accept. There is a gradual decrease in eating habits. Nothing tastes good. Cravings come and go. Liquids are preferred to solids. Please remember that it is okay for your loved one not to eat, if that is his/her choice.

3. *Sleep:* The hospice patient will gradually spend more and more time sleeping. It may be difficult for them to keep their eyes open. And then it may become difficult for you to arouse the patient. This is a result of a change in the

(continued on next page)

Helping the Patient Who Is Approaching Death (*continued*)

body's metabolism. Plan to spend more time with the patient during those times when he/she is most alert.

4. *Disorientation:* Your loved one may become increasingly confused about time, place, and the identity of people around him or her. Gently remind the patient what day it is, what time it is, and who is in the room talking to them, to allow for a peaceful transition. Provide your loved one with a comfortable, quiet environment and filtered light.

5. *Restlessness:* You may notice your loved one becoming restless and pulling at the bed linens. These symptoms are also a result of a decrease in the oxygen circulation to the brain and a change in the body's metabolism. Talk calmly and assuredly with the patient so as not to startle or frighten him or her.

6. *Decreased senses:* Clarity of hearing and vision may decrease. You may want to keep soft lights on in the room when vision decreases. *Never* assume that the patient cannot hear you, as hearing is the last of the five senses to be lost. Nothing should be said that would distress the patient should the conversation be overheard.

7. *Incontinence:* Incontinence (loss of control) of urine and bowel movements is often not a problem until death is very near. Your hospice nurse or home health aide can help direct you to where to obtain pads to place under the patient for more comfort and cleanliness, or the doctor may order a catheter. The amount of urine will decrease, and the urine becomes darker as death becomes near.

8. *Physical change:* There are changes that occur that show the physical body is losing its ability to maintain itself.

   a. The *blood pressure* often lowers and can cause dizziness.

   b. There are changes in the *pulse,* either increasing from a normal of 80 to upwards of 150, or decreasing anywhere down to zero.

   c. The *body temperature* can fluctuate between fever and cold.

   d. There is increased *perspiration* often with clamminess.

   e. The *skin color* changes: flushed with the fever, bluish with the cold. A pale yellowish pallor (not to be confused with jaundice) often accompanies approaching death.

   f. *Breathing changes* also occur. Respirations may increase or decrease. Breathing may become irregular with ten to thirty seconds of no breathing (apnea). This symptom is very common and indicative of a decrease in circulation and build-up in body waste products.

   g. *Congestion* can also occur, and a rattly sound may be heard in the lungs and upper throat. This occurs because the patient is too weak to swallow (saliva) secretions and/or cough them up. The congestion can be affected by positioning, may be very loud, and sometimes just comes and goes. Your doctor might order medication to dry these secretions. Elevating the head of the bed and swabbing the mouth with oral swabs gives comfort.

   h. The *arms and legs* of the body may become cool to the touch. The hands and feet become purplish. The knees, ankles, and elbows are blotchy. These symptoms are a result of decreased circulation. Cover your loved one with a light blanket.

   i. Generally a person becomes *non-responsive* (unable to respond to their environment) some time prior to death.

Courtesy of San Diego Hospice, CA.

prepared to deal with the physical or psychological needs of the dying or their own response to it, making their work frustrating and depressing. Furthermore, many people do not care to work with the dying, but do so because of a lack of career alternatives.

Health and social services professionals, like the rest of the population, do not like to be confronted with death. Physicians who see their role as restoring an individual to health and productivity may have intense feelings of failure and emotional conflict as they watch a patient deteriorate and die. On the other hand, if emotional involvement is withheld from the dying, the professional may be less effective.

People who work closely with dying patients need to have deep compassion for the terminally ill and their families, while preserving a distance from the death that keeps them from falling into depression every time a patient dies. Harper has conceptualized a one- to two-year process that new professionals undergo as they learn to be progressively more comfortable in working with dying patients.[36]

- *Intellectualization.* During their initial confrontation with death, people beginning to work with dying people are very intellectual regarding their tasks. There may be an abnormal desire for medical knowledge, and the patient and disease are discussed in a detached manner. This is generally a period of brisk activity. Tangible services to the dying and their family are provided, but no emotional involvement is displayed, and conversations with the dying are impersonal. The professional is uncomfortable, but concerned. However she or he is unable to discuss death or dying with the patient.
- *Emotional survival.* The move from intellectualization to emotional survival occurs when the professional realizes that death and suffering are unavoidable. As professionals confront the death of their patients, they are forced to deal with the reality of their own death and mourn and grieve for it. They may also pity the patient as they feel guilt and frustration at the contrast between their own health and another's illness.

They may try to fight back against death or illness, or question death. At times the professional is too emotional to face the patient.
- *Depression.* This is the most crucial stage, often referred to as the "grow or go" stage. Professionals may either quit their jobs or learn to accept the reality of death. They begin to question their ability to help the dying and their families. They commonly express feelings of anger, hurt, depression, or grieving. If the depression or frustration is too great, the professional may begin to avoid interactions with the dying and may resign.
- *Emotional arrival.* In this stage of mitigation and accommodation, the professional experiences a sense of freedom from such debilitating emotions as identification with the patient's symptoms, preoccupation with his or her own death, guilt feelings about personal health, and incapacitating depression. Sensitivity to the needs of the dying is sharpened, enabling a more appropriate emotional response.
- *Deep compassion.* During this stage of self-realization, professionals relate compassionately and sensitively to the dying while fully accepting their impending death. They learn to channel feelings of compassion into constructive and appropriate activities that assist the dying individual and the family. In this final stage, professionals have a full awareness and acceptance of their own death and so are able to help patients deal with their death compassionately. After reaching this stage, which takes one to two years, the caregiver has matured both professionally and personally.

For professionals to learn how to effectively care for the dying, they need information on the psychological needs of the dying and the bereaved. Historically, medical schools have offered little death education, although with medical education reforms, this is changing. Skills needed to work with the dying can be learned. Those students who attend classes on death and dying are better able to deal with the terminally ill and their families than those who had not. Health professionals need to

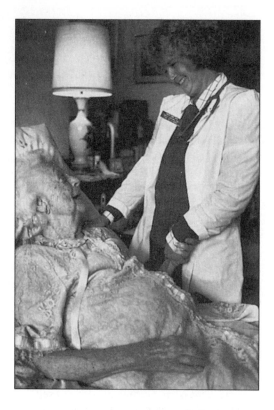

develop skills to assist the dying patient, the grieving family, and their own dealing with death.

Caring for the dying takes greater personal and time investment than working with any other patient population. However, this investment is seldom recognized. Often those who are serving dying patients (the nurses' aides in hospitals or nursing homes) are the lowest-paid paraprofessionals. Nurses' aides are commonly overburdened with more sick people than can be effectively served, increasing their physical and emotional load.

No matter what the level of professional training, *burnout* (emotional and physical exhaustion) is common among those who work with the dying. Burnout is characterized by job dissatisfaction, cynicism, withdrawal from the dying and their families, and, in some cases, termination of employment. If professionals do not deal with the stress of working with the dying, they will not only reduce their effectiveness with the dying and their families, they will also damage the quality of their personal life. Those

professionals who work alone with the terminally ill, such as home health aides and visiting nurses, need special support.

Hospital or nursing home administrators can support those who work with dying patients by providing in-service training on the psychological, physiological, and social needs of the dying and how to communicate with the dying and their families. Institutions may also offer both formal and informal support to staff, allowing them to vent their frustrations and concerns. Supervisors can also help employees to work through the complex emotions associated with caring for the dying. Supervisors may serve as role models for new professionals who are learning to give good care without burning out. However, supervisors need to be aware that not all employees are qualified to work with the terminally ill, and some staff may need to be transferred. Furthermore, supervisors need to recognize that even the most competent staff needs a periodic timeout from working with the dying.

BEREAVEMENT

Bereavement is a natural, even necessary, response to the death of a loved one and is generally manifested as an acute sense of despair. The process of grieving is very complex, involving a whole host of physiological, psychological, and social reactions. The grief response is highly individual and dependent on the personality of the aggrieved, whether death was expected or unexpected, and the intensity of the previous relationship. Additionally, the number of past losses experienced, the number of other love relationships, and the available social supports of the grief-stricken influence the extent of mourning. Grieving may invoke multiple, contradictory emotions: despair, anger, detachment, sadness, denial, guilt, and depression.

The Grieving Process

Many experts have attempted to classify stages of grieving in much the same way stages of dying are categorized. There is an extraordinarily wide range of healthy responses to death of a loved one; emotions such as relief, sadness, anger, disbelief, even happiness may all be normal appropriate responses. Stephenson described three stages of grief: reaction, disorganization and reorganization, and reorientation and recovery.[37] Although these stages may proceed in order, often the process of grieving is begun before a loved one dies (for instance, when a diagnosis of terminal illness is made, or when signs of dying are noted). Furthermore, these stages may sometimes be interrupted—grief is put aside for a while, then is endured again when reminded.

As in the dying process, it should not be assumed that everyone who is grieving should go through the grieving process in an orderly, stereotypical way. In fact, there is no prescription of proper grieving, and research is just beginning to uncover the wide variation in normal mourning patterns.

Survived by His Wife
By Margaret Flanagan

Eyes swollen she lay in their bed—
head covered, legs drawn up,
cold though her forehead was damp—
who had warmed herself on his warm flesh.

Now his absence was a constant companion:
his hairbrushes, his keys,
his clothes still smelling of him
in his closet, covered, like museum artifacts.

She shuddered, remembering the shoes he
 wore
were still beneath the bed
exactly as he left them,
as if covered by a glass case.

All of the things he had handled,
used, inhabited, and finally left
were covered or lying about
like the frames of stolen paintings left behind.

From *When I am an Old Woman I Shall Wear Purple. An Anthology of Short Stories and Poetry.* 1987. Manhattan Beach CA: Papier-Mache Press.

The state of recovery or resolution following loss, thought to be the goal of grieving, is also being reconsidered. It seems that grief, feelings of meaninglessness, painful memories and anxiety persist for years after the loss in many people.

Some degree of physiological disturbance is common among the bereaved, including a hollow feeling in the stomach, tightness in the chest and throat, breathlessness, muscle weakness, and lack of energy. Furthermore, after a loved one dies, the survivor is more likely to become ill or die than others their age who have not survived a recent loss. Experts think that grief may impair immune system function. Survivors, especially widowers, commonly experience insomnia, changes in appetite and weight, increased consumption of alcohol and other drugs, and increased physician visits and hospital admissions. Widowers suffer more than widows after the death of a spouse with higher rates of illness, alcoholism, depression, suicide, and death.[38]

Assisting the Bereaved

Methods to assist the bereaved in coping with the death of a loved one are highly variable and depend on the situation and personality of both the helper and bereaved. It is not uncommon for those approaching a newly bereaved person to be unsure how to act. Even though visits to the bereaved may be uncomfortable, friends should not avoid the bereaved or avoid discussion of the loss because of not knowing what to say. Visits and sympathy during the grieving process can be tremendously helpful in reducing social isolation and helping the bereaved express their grief. However, well-intentioned comments from friends and family may exacerbate the grief. Such comments as "don't question God's will," "your wife is at peace," and "I know how you feel," can be distressing to the bereaved. In contrast, nonjudgmental statements of support, such as "I'm here anytime if you need to talk" are more helpful.

Some physicians prescribe drugs to help individuals deal with grief, but others believe this practice may not be in the best interest of the mourner.

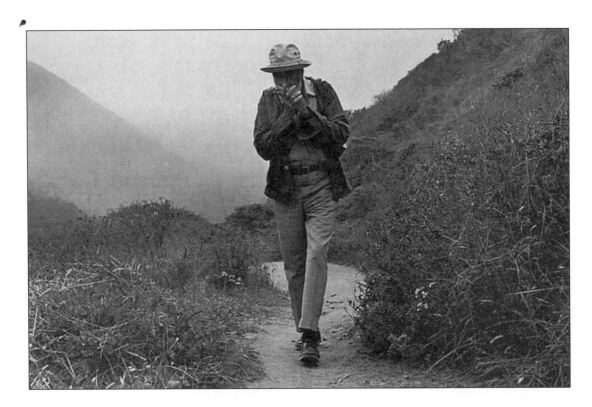

Sometimes the prescription of mild sedatives may relieve anxiety and insomnia closely following the death of a loved one. However, sedatives may have negative effects. The bereaved may be drugged during the funeral and miss this experience to grieve at a time when social support is available.

A number of resources are available for the bereaved, but vary significantly among communities. Although seldom used by older people, psychotherapy can help the bereaved release emotions, reminisce, and orient them to the future. Group therapy may be especially appropriate for widows and widowers, enabling them to deal with their grief and problems of living alone while facilitating social interaction. Perhaps the most inexpensive, accessible programs for the bereaved that offer both social and psychological support are widowhood programs. Some utilize volunteers, themselves widowed, who contact a recently bereaved person (from obituaries or funeral home referral) to provide psychological support. Other programs utilize social gatherings or discussion groups of widows or widowers led by a professional or trained layperson. Many hospice programs offer bereavement programs.

SUMMARY

It is important to learn about dying, death, and grief when studying aging and health because death occurs more frequently among those age sixty-five and older than any other age group. Furthermore, elders are more likely than younger persons to have to confront the deaths of friends and loved ones.

Modern technology allows the prolongation of life, but many ethical questions about euthanasia and the right to die accompany it. Suicide is a serious, growing, and often overlooked, problem among elders. More elders, especially white, single males, take their own lives than any other age group.

The dying can choose to die in a hospital, at home, or in a nursing facility. The dying have certain rights, such as the right to full knowledge of their condition and treatment, and the presence of supportive others. Furthermore, dying individuals have certain tasks to complete, such as finishing projects, planning funeral arrangements, and deciding on medical treatment.

Caring for the dying is physically and emotionally draining, and family and professional caretakers must cope with their own feelings while meeting the needs of the dying. Professional caretakers pass through certain stages in learning to work with the dying. Grief reactions are inevitable following the death of a loved one. Support groups and professional assistance are often available for those who need help in the grieving process.

ACTIVITIES

1. What type of advance directive would you be willing to sign now? Who would you appoint as the proxy to make decisions on your behalf? Would you be more likely to sign a living will to refuse treatment or to ask for heroic efforts? Give reasons for your choice. Discuss this issue with your family and friends. Find out statutes in your state related to living wills and the right of families and the dying to refuse treatment.

2. Make a will stipulating what should be done with your personal possessions in the event that you die and how your funeral should proceed. Discuss this with your family and close friends.

3. Question your parents and friends to determine who has made a will. Do you find it true that elders are more likely than younger persons to have plans for their death?

4. If you were given six months to live and knew your health would be failing considerably toward the end, what tasks would you wish to complete? What significant others would you like near you? Would you prefer to die in a hospital or at home? Why?

5. What services or programs in your community help bereaved elders (churches, senior organizations, funeral homes, or hospitals)? How are they publicized? What is the cost?

6. Design an administrative policy for a hospital or nursing home on care for the dying. Outline goals, policies, and procedures to meet the social, psychological, and medical needs of the dying and their families.

7. Visit a local nursing home or hospital and question staff on their policies regarding the dying. Is there a special section for the terminally ill? Are the patients told they are dying? Are there professionals or volunteers available who are trained to work specifically with the dying? How do other residents react to the death of an elder? What is their policy on advance directives?

8. Design a suicide-prevention program specifically targeted to the elderly. How would your program meet the needs of this high-risk group? How would you target elders at particular risk, and what mechanisms might serve to reduce their suicide rate? How might such a program be evaluated?

9. Are there any circumstances in which suicide would be a solution for you? Discuss these with the rest of the class.

10. Class debate or discussion: Assisted suicide should be legalized.

BIBLIOGRAPHY

1. The Multi-Society Task Force on PVS. 1994. Medical aspects of the persistent vegetative state. *New England Journal of Medicine* 330:1499–508.

2. Kjellstrand, C.M. 1992. Who should decide about your death? *Journal of the American Medical Association* 267:103–4.

3. Lubitz, J.D., and Riley, G.F. 1993. Trends in Medicare payments in the last year of life. *New England Journal of Medicine* 328:1092–96.

4. Callahan, D. 1994. Aging and the goals of medicine. *Hastings Center Report* 24:339–41.

5. Belsky, J. 1997. *The adult experience.* St. Paul, MN: West Publishing Co.

6. Jecker, N., and Schneiderman, L.J. 1994. Is dying young worse than dying old? *The Gerontologist* 34:66–72.

7. Teno, J.M., Branco, K.J., and Mor, V., et al. 1997. Changes in advance care planning in nursing homes before and after the Patient Self-Determination Act: Report of a 10-state survey. *Journal of the American Geriatrics Society* 45:939–44.

8. Greco, P.J., Schulman, K.A., Larizzo-Mourey, R., and Hausen-Flaschen, J. 1991. The Patient Self-Determination Act. *Annals of Internal Medicine* 115:639–43.

9. Terry, M., and Zweig, S. 1994. Prevalence of advance directives and do-not-resuscitate orders in community nursing facilities. *Archives of Family Medicine* 3:141–45.

10. Danis, M., Southerland, L., and Garrett, J., et al. 1991. A prospective study of advance directives for life-sustaining care. *New England Journal of Medicine* 324:882–88.

11. Jacobson, J.A., White, B.E., Battin, M.P., and Francis, L.P., et al. 1994. Patients' understanding and use of advance directives. *Western Journal of Medicine* 160:232–36.

12. Chambers, C.V., Diamond, J.J., Perkel, R.L., and Lasch, L.A. 1994. Relationship of advance directives to hospital charges in a Medicare population. *Archives of Internal Medicine* 154:541–47.

13. The SUPPORT Principal Investigators. 1995. A controlled trial to improve care for seriously ill hospitalized patients. *Journal of the American Medical Association* 274:1591–98.

14. Sulmasy, D.P., Terry, P.B., and Weisman, C.S., et al. 1998. The accuracy of substituted judgments in patients with terminal diagnoses. *Annals of Internal Medicine* 128:621–29.

15. Meier, D.E., Emmons, C.A., and Wallenstein, S., et al. 1998. A national survey of physician-assisted suicide and euthanasia in the United States. *New England Journal of Medicine* 338:1193–201.

16. Council on Scientific Affairs. 1996. Good care of the dying patient. *Journal of the American Medical Association* 275:474–78.

17. Burt, R.A. 1997. The Supreme Court speaks: Not assisted suicide but a constitutional right to palliative care. *New England Journal of Medicine* 337:1234–36.

18. Orentilicher, D. 1997. The Supreme Court and physician assisted suicide: rejecting assisted suicide but embracing euthanasia. *New England Journal of Medicine* 337:1236–1239.

19. Peters, K.D., Kochanek, K.D., and Murphy, S.L. 1998. Deaths: Final data for 1996. *National vital statistics reports,* vol. 47, no. 9. Hyattsville, MD: National Center for Health Statistics.

20. McIntosh, J.L. 1995. Suicide prevention in the elderly (age 65–99). *Suicide and Life Threatening Behavior* 25:180–92.

21. DeLeo, D., Carollo, G., Dello Buono, M. 1995. Lower suicide rates associated with a tele-help/tele-check service for the elderly at home. *American Journal of Psychiatry* 152:632–34.

22. Kalish, R.A. 1985. *Death, grief and caring relationships.* Monterey, CA: Brooks/Cole.

23. Kalish, R.A., and Reynolds, D.K. 1981. *Death and ethnicity: A psychocultural study.* Farmingdale, NY: Baywood.

24. Rando, T. 1984. *Grief, dying and death: clinical interventions for caregivers.* Champaign, IL Research Press.

25. Haupt, B.J. 1998. Characteristics of hospice care users: Data from the 1996 National Home and Hospice Care Survey. *Advance Data from Vital and Health Statistics.* Publ no. 299. Hyattsville, MD: National Center for Health Statistics.

26. Christakis, N.A., and Escarce, J.J. 1996. Survival of Medicare patients after enrollment in hospice programs. *New England Journal of Medicine* 335:172–78.

27. Arras, J.D., and Dubler, N.N. 1994. Bringing the hospital home: Ethical and social implications of high tech home care. *Hastings Center Report* 24:S19–S28.

28. McCue, J.D. 1995. The naturalness of dying. *Journal of the American Medical Association* 273:1039–43.

29. Braun, J.V., Wykle, M.H., and Cowling, W.R. 1988. Failure to thrive in older persons: A concept derived. *The Gerontologist* 26:809–12.

30. Callahan, D. 1993. *The troubled dream of life: Living with mortality.* New York: Simon and Schuster.

31. Mendes, O.E. 1993. Death in America: A clinician's perspective. *Critical Care Clinics* 8:613–26.

32. Kübler-Ross, E. 1969. *On death and dying.* New York: Macmillan.

33. Schneidman, E. 1973. *Deaths of man.* New York: Quadrangle/New York Times, p. 7.

34. Corr, C.A. 1993. Coping with dying: Lessons that we should and should not learn from the work of Kübler-Ross. *Death Studies* 17:170–76.

35. Butler, R.N., and Lewis, M.J. 1982. *Aging and mental health.* St. Louis, MO: CV Mosby.

36. Harper, B.C. 1977. *Death: The coping mechanism of the health professional.* Greenville, SC: Southeastern University Press.

37. Stephenson, J.S. 1985. *Death, grief, and mourning.* New York: The Free Press.

38. Martikainen, P., and Valkonen, T. 1996. Mortality after the death of a spouse: Rates and causes of death in a large Finnish cohort. *American Journal of Public Health* 86:1087–93.

INDEX

M

N